Springer
Tokyo
Berlin
Heidelberg
New York
Barcelona
Hong Kong
London
Milan
Paris
Singapore

Organizing Committee for the International Symposium on Spina Bifida

S. Matsumoto, H. Sato (Eds.)

Spina Bifida

With 156 Figures

Springer

Satoshi Matsumoto, M.D.
Chairman, The Japan Spina Bifida & Hydrocephalus Research Foundation
7-1-21 Tomogaoka, Suma-ku, Kobe 654-0142, Japan

Hiromi Sato, M.D
Department of Neurosurgery, Shizuoka Children's Hospital
860 Urushiyama, Shizuoka 420-0953, Japan

ISBN 4-431-70260-1 Springer-Verlag Tokyo Berlin Heidelberg New York

Printed on acid-free paper

Printed in Japan

Typesetting: Best-set Typesetter Ltd., Hong Kong
Printing and Binding: Hirakawa Kogyo, Japan
SPIN: 10730835

Preface

Spina bifida and the associated malformation of the central nervous system are initially managed by neurosurgeons. The disturbance of locomotion, deformity of the skeletal system, neurogenic bladder and bowel, and other malfunctions of patients with spina bifida have to be treated and managed by specialists such as orthopedists, urologists, pediatric neurologists, and physical therapists.

Generally, manifestation of these disorders is not limited to a definite age distribution, but the therapeutical importance of these malfunctions may vary by age group from infancy to adulthood. For these reasons, the spina bifida symposia were organized in three parts according to the age of patients.

The first symposium, under the leadership of the president, Dr. D. McLone, was held in Chicago in 1996 and focused on patients up to the age of five years. The third symposium, held in Verona in 1999 and led by C. DiRocco, focused on patients in adolescence and adulthood.

Our symposium, the second in the series, met in 1997 in Kobe and focused on patients from elementary school age to adolescence. The speakers included not only clinical specialists but also medical staff from all therapeutical fields. The contents of the symposium included current trends in the care, management, and treatment of spina bifida, as well as social welfare with the aim of improving the quality of life of these children. Therapeutical controversies related to spina bifida were thoroughly discussed from several points of view.

I express my sincere gratitude to the contributors for their participation and cooperation. I sincerely hope this volume will contibute to better management of patients with spina bifida and related disorders.

Satoshi Matsumoto, M.D.

Contents

Neurosurgery

Syringomyelia

Plenary Sessions

Parallel Sessions

Lipoma, Tethered Spinal Cord

Plenary Sessions

Parallel Sessions

Hydrocephalus

Plenary Sessions

Parallel Sessions

Ideal Management

Experimental Studies

Orthopedics

Gait Disturbance

Plenary Sessions

Spine Pathology

Foot Pathology

Urology

Neurogenic Bladder

Plenary Sessions

Parallel Sessions

Pediatric Neurology

Nursing

Spina Bifida: An International Perspective

Ethics, Social Welfare, and Psychosocial Adjustment

Neurosurgery

Syringomyelia
Lipoma, Tethered Spinal Cord
Hindbrain Anomalies
Hydrocephalus
Ideal Management
Experimental Studies

Pathophysiology and Surgical Treatment of Syringomyelia Associated with Spinal Dysraphism

Hiroshi Abe and Izumi Koyanagi

Summary. Since 1982, 43 patients with spinal dysraphism have been examined with magnetic resonance imaging or computed tomography myelography. Fifteen patients (35%, occult spinal dysraphism 8, meningomyelocele 7) were shown to have syringomyelia. In the present study, clinical and image features of syringomyelia in these 15 patients are described. Syringomyelia in this condition can be divided into two types according to the dysraphic state. The syrinx in patients with occult spinal dysraphism occurred immediately rostral to the lumbosacral lipoma and was localized to the lower thoracic to lumbar levels. In the meningomyelocele patients, the syrinx extended from the cervical to the thoracic levels. For syringomyelia with occult spinal dysraphism, four patients underwent syringo-subarachnoid shunting (S–S shunt), or syringostomy, during an untethering operation. In cases of meningomyelocele, a S–S shunt was placed in two patients. Collapse of the syrinx was achieved in all six patients.

It was concluded that, a symptomatic large syrinx in the case of spinal dysraphism should be surgically treated. A S–S shunt is effective in both types of syringomyelia.

Key words. Spinal dysraphism, Syringomyelia, Spina bifida, Meningomyelocele, Tethered cord

Introduction

Syringomyelia is known to be associated with spinal dysraphism. However, the pathogenesis, clinical characteristics, and optimal surgical treatment of syringomyelia with spinal dysraphism have not been determined. In this study, we analyzed the clinical course and diagnostic images of syringomyelia in some patients with spinal dysraphism. The purpose of this study was to clarify the clinical significance of syringomyelia associated with spinal dysraphism, and to determine the optimal surgical treatment.

Patients and Methods

Thirty-four cases of occult spinal dysraphism (lumbosacral lipoma 32, tight filum terminale 2) and 9 cases of spina bifida aperta (meningomyelocele) were examined by means of computed tomography (CT) myelography or magnetic resonance imaging (MRI) in our clinic

Department of Neurosurgery, Hokkaido University School of Medicine, North 15, West 7 Kita-Ku, Sapporo, Hokkaido 060-8638, Japan

from 1982 to 1995. These image examinations revealed syringomyelia in 8 (24%) of 34 occult spinal dysraphism patients and 7 (78%) of 9 meningomyelocele patients. Thus, out of 43 patients with spinal dysraphism, a total of 15 (35%) were revealed to have syringomyelia. In this study, a clinical and image analysis of these 15 patients was performed. There were 4 male and 11 female patients. The syrinx was recorded as "large" when its transverse diameter exceeded 70% of that of the spinal cord.

Each of the 8 patients with occult spinal dysraphism had a lumbosacral lipoma to which the elongated spinal cord was continued. These patients underwent untethering of the spinal cord with partial removal of the lipoma at 1 month to 9 years of age. The diagnosis of syringomyelia was made from preoperative images.

All 7 meningomyelocele patients had undergone repair of a meningomyelocele defect with muscle and skin flaps within 24h after birth. Ventriculo-peritoneal (VP) shunting was performed 3–42 days (mean 15 days) after birth because of hydrocephalus in all cases. Syringomyelia was diagnosed with MRI performed at 1 month to 9 years of age. Two of the meningomyelocele patients had suffered meningitis following VP shunting, which was treated with i.v. antibiotics, and 4 patients had undergone revision of their VP shunt before the diagnosis of syringomyelia.

Illustrative Cases

Case 1: Occult Spinal Dysraphism

This 4-year-old boy had presented with a cutaneous dimple in the sacral region. He was referred to our clinic with occult spinal dysraphism below the L4 level. Neurological examination on admission showed no abnormality. MRI revealed spinal cord tethering with lipoma at the level of L4–5. A large syrinx was identified at the T12–L3 levels (Fig. 1a). Partial removal of the lipoma and untethering of the spinal cord were performed. At the same time, a S–S shunt was placed at the L2 level. The postoperative MRI showed collapse of the syrinx (Fig. 1b). The patient has been free of neurological and urological signs and symptoms for 8 years since surgery.

Case 2: Occult Spinal Dysraphism

This 7-month-old girl had presented with a cutaneous angioma and subcutaneous lipoma in the sacral region since birth. She developed motor weakness of the lower extremities at 3 months old. Neurological examinations on admission revealed paresis of the feet and decreased tendon reflex of the patella and ankle bilaterally. Voiding cysturethrography performed in the Urology Department showed marked deformity of the bladder. MRI demonstrated a lipoma below the L2 level, with the spinal cord continued thus far. A small syrinx was identified at T12–L1 (Fig. 2a). At surgery, partial removal of the lipoma and untethering of the spinal cord were performed. No attempt was made to explore the associated syrinx. MRI 1 week after surgery revealed a decrease in the size of the syrinx (Fig. 2b). No neurological changes have been observed 1 year after surgery.

Case 3: Spina Bifida Occulta

This 9-year-old girl had undergone repair of a meningomyelocele defect in the lumbar region and VP shunting for hydrocephalus soon after birth. At 7 years old, she suffered a respiratory arrest owing to VP shunt malfunction and was resuscitated, after which the VP shunt was

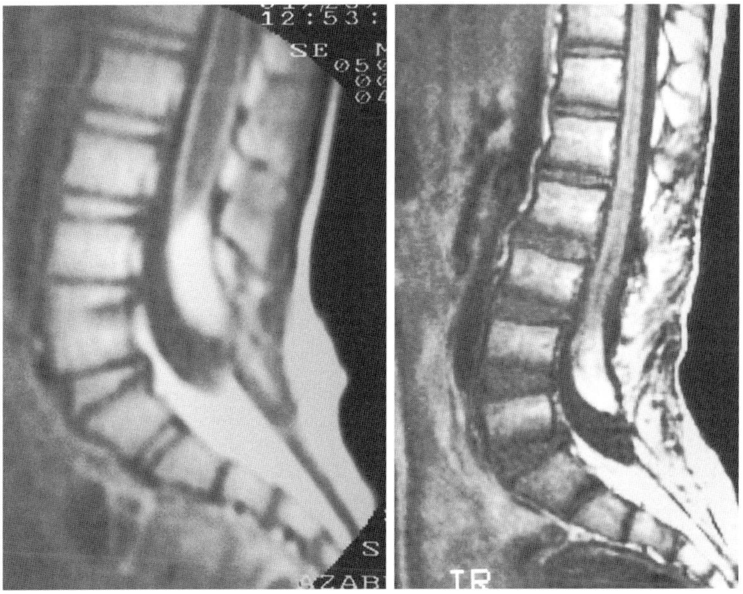

FIG. 1. **a** Preoperative MRI of case 1. The sagittal T1-weighted image of the lumbosacral spine shows the tethered spinal cord with lipoma at L4–5. A large syrinx is noted immediately rostral to the lipoma. **b** Postoperative MRI of case 1 taken 6 years after untethering of the spinal cord and an S–S shunt. The sagittal T1-weighted image shows the collapsed syrinx

revised. At 9 years old, she was admitted to our clinic because of grand mal seizure. On examination, she was found to have nystagmus, mild motor weakness of the upper limbs, and severe paraparesis. Intermittent catheterization was done for urination because she had a neurogenic bladder. Radiological examinations showed scoliosis and spina fibida below T11. MRI revealed Chiari malformation and a large syrinx from the C5 to the conus level (Fig. 3a). The level of the tonsillar tip was C3. VP shunting was effective. Because the patient had a large syrinx and had motor weakness of the upper limbs, a S–S shunt was placed via T7–9 laminotomy. The motor weakness of the upper limbs improved after S–S shunting. Postoperative MRI showed a decrease in the size of the syrinx (Fig. 3b). The follow-up period after placement of the S–S shunt was 8 years. Except for improved muscle power in the upper limbs, there have been no neuorological changes.

Results

Image Findings

Plain roentgenograms and a CT scan revealed that spina bifida was present in the sacral spine in 7 patients and in the lumbosacral spine in 6 patients. Two patients with meningomyelocele were found to have spina bifida below the thoracic level.

The extent of the syrinx is illustrated by MRI for each case in Fig. 4. In the case of occult spinal dysraphism, the syrinx was located immediately (7 cases) or 1 vertebral segment (1 case) rostral to the level of the lumbosacral lipoma and extended rostrally for 1–6 vertebral

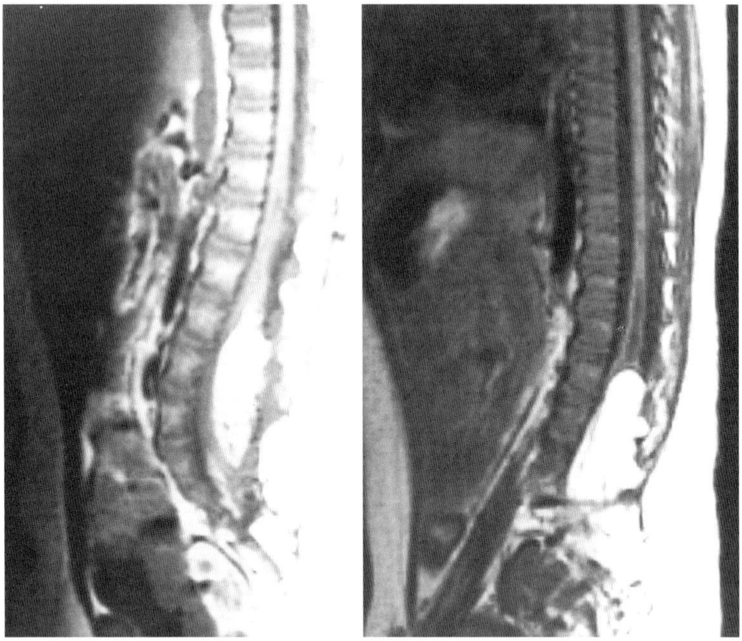

FIG. 2. **a** Preoperative MRI of case 2. The sagittal T1-weighted image of the thoraco-lumbar spine shows the tethered spinal cord with lumbosacral lipoma below the L2 level. A small syrinx is seen immediately rostral to the lipoma. **b** Postoperative MRI of case 2 taken 1 week after partial removal of the lipoma and untethering of the spinal cord. The sagittal T1-weighted image of the lumbosacral spine shows the decreased size of the syrinx

segments. No patients had the syrinx extending up to the cervical or upper thoracic levels (Fig. 4a). The syrinx was located in the center of the spinal cord and was small in 7 of 8 occult spinal dysraphism patients. One patient had a large syrinx extending from T12 to L3 (case 1). In none of these patients was hydrocephalus or Chiari malformation associated with the occult spinal dysraphism.

In the patients with meningomyelocele, hydrocephalus had been present and treated with a VP shunt soon after birth in all cases. No patients showed enlarged cerebral ventricles when syringomyelia was diagnosed. MRI examinations revealed Chiari malformation type II in all patients. The level of the tonsillar tip was C1 in 1 case, C3 in 5 cases, and C4 in 1 case. Syringomyelia was more extensive in the meningomyelocele patients than in the occult spinal dysraphism patients. The syrinx extended from the lower cervical to the lumbar level in 4 cases, and from the lower cervical to the thoracic level in 3 cases (Fig. 4b). In 3 (43%) of the 7 meningomyelocele patients the syrinx was large.

Neurological Status

Of 8 occult spinal dysraphism patients, 3 (38%) showed motor weakness of the lower extremities with decreased Achilles tendor reflex, and Babinski's sign was positive ipsilaterally in 1 of these 3 patients. Urinary incontinence was noted in only 2 patients, but urological examinations in the Urology Department of our hospital revealed a neurogenic bladder in 6 (75%) of 8 occult spinal dysraphism patients. There were no upper limb or cranial nerve signs or symptoms in the patients with occult spinal dysraphism.

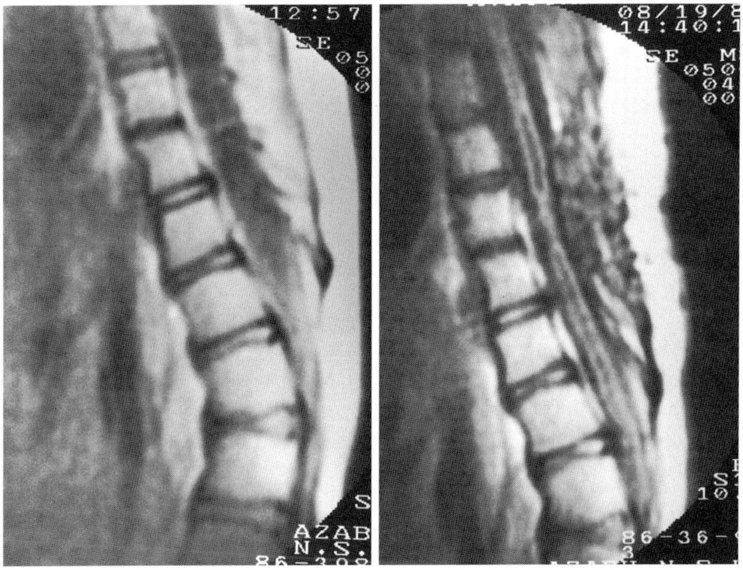

FIG. 3. **a** Preoperative MRI of case 3. Sagittal T1-weighted image of the lower thoracic spine shows an extensive and large syrinx in the spinal cord. **b** Postoperative MRI of the lower thoracic spine 6 months after an S–S shunt at T8. The sagittal T1-weighted image of the lower thoracic spine shows the collapsed syrinx

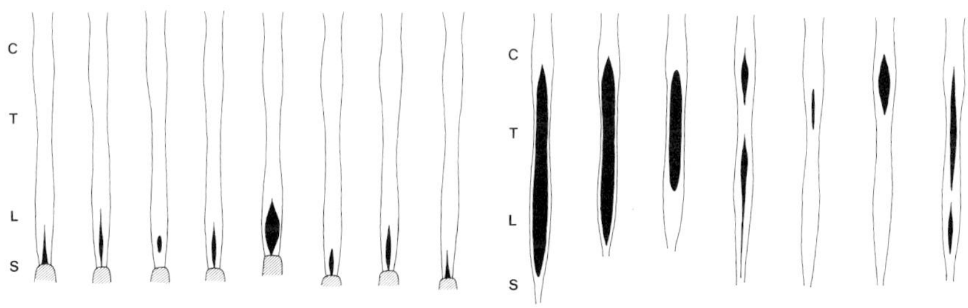

FIG. 4. The extent of the syrinx in each case of **a** occult spinal dysraphism, and **b** meningomyelocele. *C*, cervical; *T*, thoracic; *L*, lumbar; *S*, sacral

All 7 meningomyelocele patients had paraparesis since birth. One patient (case 3) showed mild motor weakness of the upper limbs. Nystagmus was noted in 3 cases. Decreased anal tonus and loss of urinary sphincter function were present in all 7 patients.

Surgical Treatment

The patients with occult spinal dysraphism underwent partial resection of the lipoma and untethering of the spinal cord. In 4 of the 8 patients, a midline syringostomy was performed at the dorsal spine and immediately rostral to the lipoma during untethering surgery. A S–S shunt was placed in 2 of those 4 patient. In the other 4 patients, no surgical procedures were attempted on the syrinx. The meningomyelocele patients had all undergone dural and skin plasty and VP shunting soon after birth. Repair of the dysraphic spinal cord had not been performed. Two meningomyelocele patients aged 3 and 9 years, who each showed a large syrinx on MRI, were treated with a S–S shunt at the thoracic level.

Follow-up Results

Follow-up periods after untethering of the spinal cord in 8 occult spinal dysraphism patients ranged from 1 to 8 years (mean 4.1 years). There were no serious complications or neurological deterioration in the early postoperative period in any of these patients. The syrinxes of 4 occult spinal dysraphism patients who underwent S–S shunting or syringostomy were markedly decreased in size after surgery. In 3 patients, postoperative follow-up MRI revealed a decrease in the size of the syrinx 1 week to 3 years after the untethering operation alone. In 7 patients there has been no neurological deterioration in the follow-up period, but 1 patient developed motor weakness of the left leg 1 year after surgery.

The follow-up periods of the 7 meningomyelocele patients ranged from 1 to 7 years (mean 3.4 years) after the diagnosis of syringomyelia. In 2 patients who underwent S–S shunting the syrinx was markedly decreased in size after surgery. The size of the syrinx in the other 6 patients did not change during follow-up. Neurologically, 1 of 2 patients who underwent S–S shunting showed improved muscle power of the upper limbs after surgery. No neurological changes were observed in the other 6 patients.

Discussion

Syringomyelia and the Dysraphic State

The incidence of syringomyelia in the case of occult spinal dysraphism has been reported to be 3–45% [1, 3, 7, 8, 11, 12, 16, 22, 25]. Higher incidences (38–53%) have been reported in the case of diastematomyelia [7, 12, 15] than in the case of lipomeningomyelocele (3–25%) [7, 11, 12, 25]. In the case of meningomyelocele, the incidence of syringomyelia has been reported to be 27–33% [1, 27], which is slightly higher than that in lipomeningomyelocele cases. In our series, syringomyelia was observed in 8 (24%) of 34 occult spinal dysraphism patients, which is comparable to the previously reported incidence. The meningomyelocele patients in our series showed a much higher incidence (7 of 9 cases, 78%) than previously reported. The reason for our higher incidence of syringomyelia in the meningomyelocele patients is not known. The meningomyelocele patients in our series had undergone repair of the dural and skin defects, but closure of the dysraphic spinal cord had not been performed. The method of repair of the dysraphic state might have played some part in syrinx formation in our series. In addition, in the present series the patients underwent MRI examination of the whole of the spinal cord to detect the syrinx. Because the syrinx was frequently located at the cervicothoracic junction in our cases of meningomyelocele, image examinations in early studies may have missed small syrinxes at levels remote from the level of the dysraphism.

In our series, syringomyelia associated with spinal dysraphism can be divided into two types by clinical states and MRI findings: occult spinal dysraphism and meningomyelocele. These two types of syringomyelia showed different MRI features. The former was observed immediately rostral to the lumbosacral lipoma to which the spinal cord was tethered. No other abnormality, such as hydrocephalus or Chiari malformation, was seen in these patients.

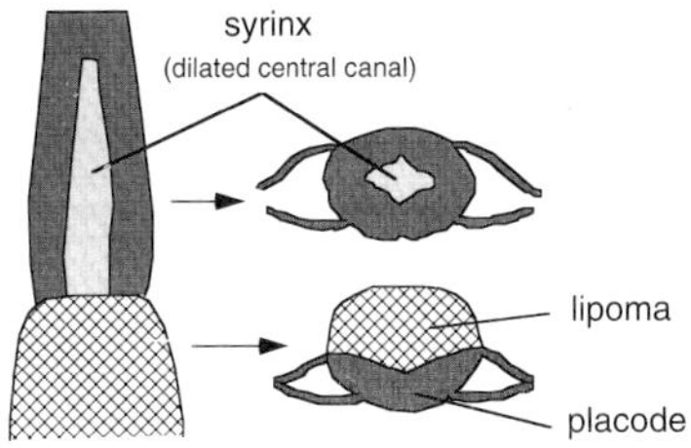

FIG. 5.

In most of the occult spinal dysraphism patients (7 out of 8 cases), the syrinx was small and located centrally in the spinal cord. These findings were consistent with the MRI features of terminal syringohydromyelia, which was defined by Ishander et al. [12] as a cystic dilatation of the lower third of the spinal cord and is frequently associated with occult spinal dysraphism. In the meningomyelocele patients the syrinx was more extensive and was located from the cervical to the thoracic level. All the meningomyelocele patients had associated Chiari malformation type II and hydrocephalus, although no intracranial ventricular dilation was present when syringomyelia was diagnosed.

There has been no clear explanation for the origin of syringomyelia and mechanisms of syrinx formation in patients with spinal dysraphism. It is likely that the small syrinx observed in our occult spinal dysraphism patients is an enlarged central canal, because the syrinx is located centrally in the spinal cord and immediately rostral to the lipoma (Fig. 5). The concept described by Naidich et al. [19], whereby the lumbosacral lipoma attaches intimately to the dorsal surface of the placode in a case of lipomeningomyelocele, seems to support the theory of central canal dilatation in our series. The large syrinxes in our occult spinal dysraphism patients may originate from the enlarged central canal, although the mechanisms explaining large syrinx formation are unknown. Recently, Cho et al. and Hida [5, 9] reported that a subarachnoid block secondary to adhesive arachnoiditis played an important role in syrinx formation in experimental posttraumatic syringomyelia. In that study, a combination of kaolin injection into the spinal subarachnoid space and a weight-drop injury of the spinal cord produced an extensive syrinx in a rabbit spinal cord. In an experimental study by Milhorat et al. [17], blockage of the central canal with an intramedullary microinjection of kaolin resulted in noncommunicating syringomyelia in the rat spinal cord. These experimental data seem to suggest that the large syrinx in the case of occult spinal dysraphism is caused by a blockage of flow in the enlarged central canal or around the spinal cord. However, we did not find evidence of a prior inflammatory process or arachnoiditis around the spinal cord of our cases at surgery. Chapman and Frim [4] reported 3 cases of symptomatic syringomyelia that occurred following an untethering operation for previously treated lipomeningomyelocele. They also reported that there was no significant arachnoiditis or infection that might have caused the syringomyelia.

In meningomyelocele patients, hydrocephalus and Chiari malformation are considered to have an important role in the pathogenesis of syrinx formation. It is well known that Chiari malformation type I is commonly associated with syringomyelia. Mechanisms proposed to explain syrinx formation in this lesion have included transmission of arterial pulsation of the cerebrospinal fluid into the central canal [6], drawing of the cerebrospinal fluid flow from the IV ventricle in the central canal owing to the pressure dissociation of the intracranial and intraspinal compartments [26], or penetration of the cerebrospinal fluid along the perivascular channel owing to subarachnoid obstruction [2]. Recently, Milhorat et al. [18] reported that obstruction of the upper end of the central canal or its continuity with the subarachnoid space at the foramen magnum produced a noncommunicating syringomyelia. Although the exact mechanism of syrinx formation in Chiari malformation has not been elucidated, a blockage of the subarachnoid space or the upper end of the central canal is likely to have some role in syrinx formation in meningomyelocele patients. The syringomyelia in these patients could be "isolated central canal dilatation" after shunting of intracranial ventricles [19].

Symptomatic Syringomyelia and Surgical Treatment

Although syringomyelia is sometimes seen in spinal dysraphism patients, symptomatic syringomyelia is considered to be rare. According to Azimullah et al. [1], segmental neurological signs attributable to the syrinx were recognized in 2 out of 10 meningomyelocele patients with syringomyelia. Chapman and Frim [4] reported 3 patients with symptomatic syringomyelia and lipomeningomyelocele who showed progressive deterioration of sensory and motor function in the legs after retethering of the spinal cord. This number was described as corresponding to approximately 10% of all patients who underwent surgery for retethering of lipomeningomyelocele in their hospital. In our series, only 1 (7%) of 15 patients with syringomyelia had shown motor weakness of the upper limbs as a result of the syrinx extending along the cervical cord. Because spinal dysraphism patients have shown neurological deficits attributable to the dysraphic state or spinal cord tethering, it is often difficult to identify neurological signs and symptoms originating from the associated syringomyelia. Scoliosis will be an important sign suggestive of syringomyelia in the case of spinal dysraphism [12, 14], although it is not specific for syringomyelia.

Neither indications for surgery nor a standard surgical method for treatment of syringomyelia in the presence of spinal dysraphism has been established. In our series, in 3 cases of occult spinal dysraphism the size of the syrinx decreased after an untethering operation alone. Why the untethering procedure resulted in collapse of the syrinx is unknown. A change in the cerebrospinal fluid circulation around the spinal cord and associated lipoma or surgical effects similar to those of terminal ventriculostomy might be responsible for such effects. Although we performed syringostomy during untethering operations in our early series of occult spinal dysraphism (2 of 8 lumbosacral lipoma cases) and achieved collapse of the syrinx, there is no need to attempt such direct surgical procedures aimed at the associated syrinx if the syrinx is small and asymptomatic.

Foramen magnum decompression with suboccipital craniectomy, upper cervical laminectomy and dural plasty is a commonly accepted surgical procedure for syringomyelia associated with Chiari malformation type I. Although its effects on syringomyelia in meningomyelocele patients (Chiari malformation type II) have not been determined, foramen magnum decompression may be the surgical treatment of choice in these patients. S–S shunting will also be the surgical treatment of choice for syringomyelia in meningomyelocele patients [23]. In our series, the large syrinx in meningomyelocele patients was successfully treated by S–S shunting. Recent clinical studies [10, 13, 21, 24] revealed that S–S shunting was effective in the case of syringomyelia with Chiari malformation type I. In our opinion, if a meningomyelocele patient has a large syrinx and shows signs and symptoms mainly caused by the syrinx, such as progressive motor weakness or pain in the upper limbs, S–S shunting will be the primary method of surgical treatment. If untreated hydrocephalus is present, placement of a VP shunt should be attempted, because the pathogenesis of syringomyelia in meningomyelocele patients might be closely related to the associated hydrocephalus [20].

Acknowledgment. This study was supported by a Research Grant (5B-3) for Nervous and Mental Disorders from the Ministry of Health and Welfare, Japan.

References

1. Azimullha PC, Smit LME, Rietveld-Knol E, Valk J (1991) Malformations of the spinal cord in 53 patients with spina bifida studied by magnetic imaging. Child's Nerv Syst 7:63–66
2. Ball MJ, Dayan AD (1972) Pathologenesis of syringomyelia. Lancet II:799–801
3. Brophy JD, Sutton LN, Aimmerman RA, Bury E, Schut L (1989) Magnetic resonance imaging of lipomyelomeningocele and tethered cord. Neurosurgery 25:336–340
4. Chapman PH, Frim DM (1995) Symptomatic syringomyelia following surgery to treat retethering of lipomyelomeningoceles. J Neurosurg 82:752–755
5. Cho KH, Iwasaki Y, Imamura H, Hida K, Abe H (1994) Experimental model of posttraumatic syringomyelia: the role of adhesive arachnoiditis in syrinx formation. J Neurosurg 80:133–139
6. Gardner WJ (1965) Hydrodynamic mechanism of syringomyelia: its relationship to myelocele. J Neurosurg Psychiatry 28:247–259
7. Gupta RK, Sharma A, Jena A, Tyagi G, Prakash B, Khushu S (1990) Magnetic resonance evaluation of spinal dysraphism in children. Child's Nerv Syst 6:161–165
8. Herman JM, McLone DG, Storrs BB, Dauser RC (1993) Analysis of 153 patients with myelomeningocele or spinal lipoma reported upon for a tethered cord. Pediatr Neurosurg 19:243–249
9. Hida K, Iwasaki Y, Imamura H, Abe H (1994) Posttraumatic syringomyelia: its characteristic magnetic resonance imaging findings and surgical management. Neurosurgery 35:886–891
10. Hida K, Iwasaki Y, Koyanagi I, Sawamura Y, Abe H (1995) Surgical indication results of foramen magnum decompression versus syringosubarachnoid shunt shunting for syringomyelia associated with Chiari I malformation. Neurosurgery 37:673–679
11. Hoffman HJ, Taecholarn C, Hendrick EB, Humphreys RP (1985) Management of lipomyelomeningoceles. Experience at the Hospital for Sick Children, Toronto. J Neurosurg 62:1–8
12. Iskandar BJ, Oakes WJ, McLaughlin C, Osumi AK, Tien RD (1994) Terminal syringohydromyelia and occult spinal dysraphism. J Neurosurg 81:513–519
13. Isu T, Iwasaki Y, Akino M, Abe H (1990) Syringo-subarachnoid shunt for syringomyelia associated with Chiari malformation (type I). Acta Neurochir (Wien) 107:152–160
14. Isu T, Chono Y, Iwasaki Y, Koyanagi I, Akino M, Abe H, Abumi K, Kaneda K (1992) Scoliosis associated with syringomyelia presenting in children. Child's Nerv Syst 8:97–100
15. Jaspan T, Worthington BS, Holland IM (1989) A comparative study of magnetic resonance imaging and computed tomography-assisted myelography in spinal dysraphism. Br J Radiol 61:445–453
16. Koyanagi I, Iwasaki Y, Hida K, Abe H, Isu Y, Akino M (1997) Surgical treatment of syringomyelia associated with spinal dysraphism. Child's Nerv Syst 13:194–200
17. Milhorat TH, Nobandegani F, Miller JI, Rao C (1993) Noncommunicating syringomyelia following occlusion of central canal in rats. Experimental model and histological findings. J Neurosurg 78:274–279
18. Milhorat TH, Miller JI, Johnson WD, Adler DE, Heger IM (1993) Anatomical basis of syringomyelia occurring with hindbrain lesions. Neurosurgery 32:748–754
19. Naidich TP, McLone DG, Multluer S (1983) A new understanding of dorsal dysraphism with lipoma (lipomyeloschisis): radiological evaluation and surgical correction. AJNR Am J Neuroradiol 4:103–116

20. Oi S, Kudo H, Yamada H, Kim S, Hamano S, Urui S, Matsumoto S (1991) Hydrodynamic hydrocephalus. Correlation of hydromyelia with various stages of hydrocephalus in post-shunt isolated compartments. J Neurosurg 74:371–379
21. Padovani R, Cavallo M, Gaist G (1989) Surgical treatment of syringomyelia: favourable results with syringosubarachnoid shunting. Surg Neurol 32:173–180
22. Scatliff JH, Kendall BE, Kingsley DPE, Britton J, Grant DN, Hayward RD (1989) Closed spinal dysraphism: analysis of clinical, radiological, and surgical findings in 104 consecutive patients. AJR Am J Roentgenol 152:1049–1052
23. Schlesinger AE, Naidich TP, Quencer RM (1986) Concurrent hydromyelia and diastematomyelia. AJNR Am J Roentgenol 7:473–477
24. Sgouros S, Williams B (1995) A critical appraisal of drainage in syringomyelia. J Neurosurg 82:1–10
25. Taviere V, Brunelle F, Baraton J, Temam M, Pierre-Kahan A, Lallemand D (1989) MRI study of lumbosacral lipoma in children. Pediatr Radiol 19:316–320
26. Williams B (1980) On the pathogenesis of syringomyelia: a review. J R Soc Med 73:798–806
27. Williamson MR, Glasier CM, Chadduck WM, Angtuaco EJC, Binet EF (1989) MRI in the evaluation of spina bifida patients in the remote period after meningomyelocele repair. Pediatr Radiol 19:442–443

Abstract

Chiari Malformation and Syringomyelia

Maurice Choux

Chiari I and Chiari II malformation may be associated with syringomyelia. The mechanisms proposed for the progression of syringomyelia with Chiari I are controversial. We know now that many Chiari I malformations are acquired, and are secondary to intracranial expanding masses. Preoperative dynamic MRI and quantitative cine-mode MRI are useful to analyse CSP dynamics. In symptomatic patients with progressive neurological symptoms, surgery is recommended, including a small suboccipital craniectomy, cervical laminectomy at C1, and more rarely at C2, and dural grafting using fascia lata or Gortex or lyophilized dura mater. In a few cases we have used obex plugging. We are not in favor of syrinx shunting.

What we do in Chiari I malformation may be done in Chiari II malformation in patients with myelomeningocele, with secondary symptoms such as diminution of motor function, progressive spasticity, upper arm weakness, or worsening of the spinal deformation. In these cases, CT and MRI could detect localized or extensive syringomyelia. The first step in management is to control the shunt function, and eventually to revise a nonfunctioning shunt. Decompression of the cerebellar tonsils is mandatory in other cases, using the same technique as in Chiari I malformation. We do not recommend a direct approach of the medullary cyst or a syrinx shunting.

Department of Pediatric Neurosurgery, Hopital des Enfants, La Timone, Marseille, France

Moderator's Comments on Sessions—Syringomyelia

Masashi Fukui

In this session, two experts presented papers on syringomyelia. Professor Abe, a well-known neurosurgeon in Japan, presented his experiences on the syringomyelia associated with spinal dysraphism. He has treated 43 cases of spinal dysraphism, among which 15 (35%) were found to have syringomyelia. According to his classification, the syringomyelia associated with spinal dysraphism can be divided into two types. The syrinx in patients with occult dysraphism occurred immediately rostral to the lumbosacral lipoma and was localized to the lower thoracic lumbar levels (7 cases). The syrinx associated with myelomeningocele extended from the cervical to the thoracic levels (8 cases). Four cases of the former type were treated by syringo-subarachnoid shunt (S–S shunt) or syringostomy during the untethering of lipoma. Collapse of the syrinx occurred in all surgical cases. In addition, the syrinx associated with lumbosacral lipoma was found to decrease in size by the untethering procedure alone. This phenomenon was also reported by the speakers in the lumbosacral lipoma session. In cases of a large syrinx associated with myelomeningocele, a S–S shunt was inserted with good results. Prof. Abe stressed the importance of surgical treatment for symptomatic syrinx associated with spinal dysraphism.

Professor Choux, the most active pediatric neurosurgeon in France, reported syringomyelia associated with Chiari types I and II malformations. Chiari malformations may accompany myelomeningocele, and the symptomatic syrinx in those cases were treated by surgical strategies as for Chiari malformations. The first step was to manage the hydrocephalus, if present, and decompression surgery of the cerebellar tonsils was given for a Chiari malformation. Prof. Choux did not recommend a direct approach to the medullary cyst or a syrinx shunting.

The syringomyelia associated with spinal dysraphism has not been well documented in the literature. Prof. Abe and Prof. Choux outlined these pathologies and treatments. Although their treatment policies are not always consistent, their reports are much appreciated as a guideline for the situation to date.

Department of Neurosurgery, Neurological Institute, Faculty of Medicine, Kyushu University, 60 Maidashi, Fukuoka 812-8582, Japan

Syringomyelia with MMC: Management with Reference to its Progression

Hiromi Sato and Noriko Sato

Summary. The authors evaluated the clinical spectrum and management of pediatric syringomyelia with myelomeningocele (MMC), focusing on its progression. Of 74 MMC patients, syrinxes of various sizes were detected in 24 (32%). Twelve (16%) of these were large and progressed, 6% disappeared, and the others remained small. Syringomyelia were divided into the tight foramen magnum (TFM)-related type, and the cord tethering (CTH)-related type. Of the large syrinxes, TFM-related syrinxes were diagnosed in neonates, while the CTH-related syrinxes were detected in patients older than 3 years. The likely deteriorating factors were the transobex CSF influx, the developmental craniocerebellar disproportion, the prenatally isolated central canal, and the spinal cord retethering. Osseous foramen magnum decompression (osseous FMD) or spinal cord untethering stabilized the syrinx. The collapse of a large syrinx was begun by osseous FMD in one patient, and by syrinx diversion in others. Procedures against the deteriorating factors prevent the progression. For an enlarged syrinx, direct shunting is promising for the maximal restoration of neurological function.

Key words. Syringomyelia, Hydromyelia, Myelomeningocele, Progression, Management

Introduction

Recent information is revising previous concepts about pediatric syringomyelia. However, the diverse etiology and dynamic changes which are reported features of pediatric syringomyelia still leave the pathogenesis unclear, and controversy remains about suitable management [2, 3, 11, 12], especially for those with myelomeningocele (MMC) [1]. The current therapeutic attitude demands less invasive modalities of treatment. In this regard, the authors evaluated the clinical spectrum of pediatric syringomyelia with MMC, focusing on its progression. An attempt is made to define a progressive syrinx and factors which might lead to deterioration.

Patients and Methods

Syringomyelia was used as the general term, including hydromyelia and MMC, for open spinal dysraphism. A syrinx was defined as large when it extends over four vertebrae, with a maximum syrinx/cord diameter ratio over 70%. According to the symptoms, the distribution,

---

Department of Neurosurgery, Shizuoka Children's Hospital, 860 Urushiyama, Shizuoka 420, Japan

and the direction of progression as shown on magnetic resonance imaging (MRI), syringomyelia was divided into two types: the tight foramen magnum (TFM)-related type, i.e., symptomatic Chiari malformation or caudally expanded syrinx from the cervicothoracic cord, and the cord tethering (CTH)-related type, i.e., symptomatic tethered spinal cord or rostrally expanded syrinx initially dominant in the thoracolumbar cord. Based on follow-up MRIs, large syrinxes were divided into the holocord, the progressive, the stable, and the collapsed syrinx. Progressive syrinxes were subdivided into two groups: those with or without a dilated 4th ventricle.

Since 1983, 42 pediatric syringomyelia patients have been enrolled in a prospective management trial. A recent series of 23 newborns with MMC were assessed on preoperative MRI. All patients were followed up on MRI, with neurological assessment at 3–24-month intervals. After extensive observation, large or progressive syrinxes were entered in a treatment protocol (see Fig. 4).

According to their symptoms and suggested causes, syrinx-oriented procedures were undertaken on an individual base. Direct approaches, e.g., syringosubarachnoid (SS) shunt or syringostomy, were followed by indirect procedures, e.g., laterally extended osseous foramen magnum decompression (osseous FMD) or spinal cord untethering, after confirming a functioning ventriculoperitoneal (VP) shunt.

Results

Clinical Spectrum

Of 119 spinal dysraphism patients, 33 (28%) were associated with syrinxes of various sizes. All syrinxes formed a centrally located single cavity, as shown on MRI. The incidence of syringomyelia in MMC was 32% (24/74). Eleven (42%) of these were large at diagnosis or progressed within 3–24 months. A half (52%) remained small, and 6% were seen to have disappeared on follow-up MRI (range 3–177 months). Of 11 large or extended syrinxes, 6 were TFM-related syrinxes diagnosed in a neonatal MRI survey of 23 MMC cases. In neonatal syringomyelia, females are common (83%), and the tonsillar shift was severe (C-4/5) in 83%. All were associated with myeloschisis, advanced hydrocephalus, and symptomatic Chiari malformation refractory to conservative treatment. Postrepaired and VP-shunted progression was noticed in 5 (83%). CTH-related syrinx was detected in 6 patients older than 3 years. All presented with symptomatic tethered cord after nonrepaired skin-flap closure. The mean age at diagnosis was 6.3 years (Fig. 1).

Factors Related to Progression

The likely deteriorating factors are transobex CSF-influx in 3 patients, developmental craniocerebellar disproportion in 1, prenatally isolated central canal in 2, and postrepaired spinal cord retethering in 6. A MRI survey showed the following features, which support the pathophysiological implications of these factors on the progression of syrinx with MMC.

Extension With the Dilatation of the 4th Ventricle

Case. A neonatal syringomyelia patient with sacral myeloschisis and Type I split cord at Th-9. The syrinx extended from C-4 and bifurcated along the split cord, forming a double syrinx. The syrinx extended after repairing and shunting, which was correlated with the progressive dilatation of the 4th ventricle (Fig. 2). The elongated 4th ventricle contained the deformed

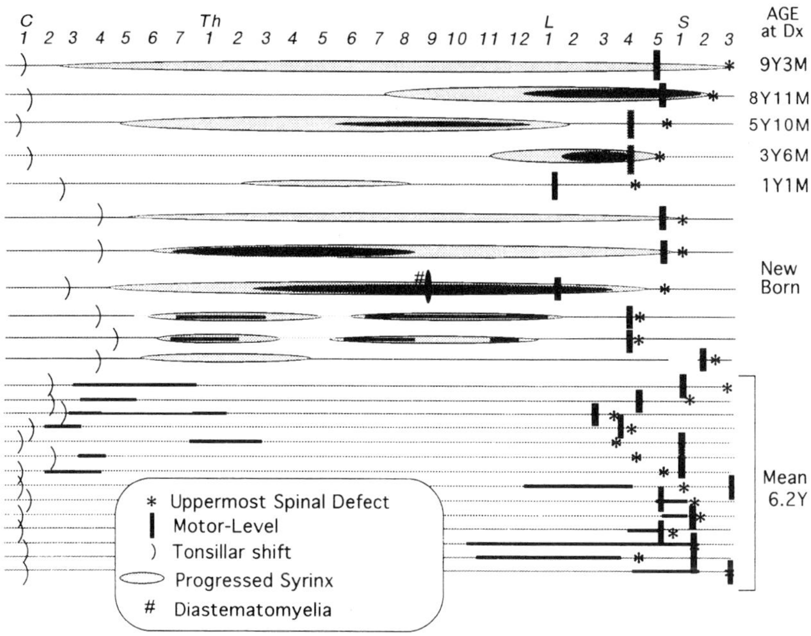

FIG. 1. Clinical spectrum of syringomyelia with MMC

lower vermis roofed by the posterior medullary velum. Contrast material introduced into the 4th ventricle directly filled the syrinx, which demonstrated transobex CSF influx. The fourth VP shunting with FMD reduced the syrinx.

Extension Without the Dilatation of the 4th Ventricle

Case. Syrinx gradually extended within 4 months after birth, while the 4th ventricle remained a slit. The hanging of the occipital lobes over the cerebellar vermis became marked even after VP shunting, and overlapping with the growth of the vermis, the tightness of the posterior fossa or the developmental craniocerebellar disproportion advanced further.

Neonatal Holocord Syrinx

Case. A holocord syrinx was visualized in a neonatal lumbosacral myeloschisis. The paramedian occipital lobes hung over the severely deformed cerebellar vermis, which was confined in the narrowed posterior fossa. The 4th ventricle extended up to the C5-level, together with the shifted tonsil.

Reduction After Repairing, VP Shunting, and Osseous FMD

Case. A neonatal syrinx which extended between the spinal cord levels C6-9 and Th5-11 as a centrally located cavity remained stable on MR images immediately after repairing and VP shunting. Additional osseous FMD against intractable sleep apnea at 2 months of age effectively ameliorated the brain stem compression symptoms. A satisfactory collapse was achieved 2 months after the procedure.

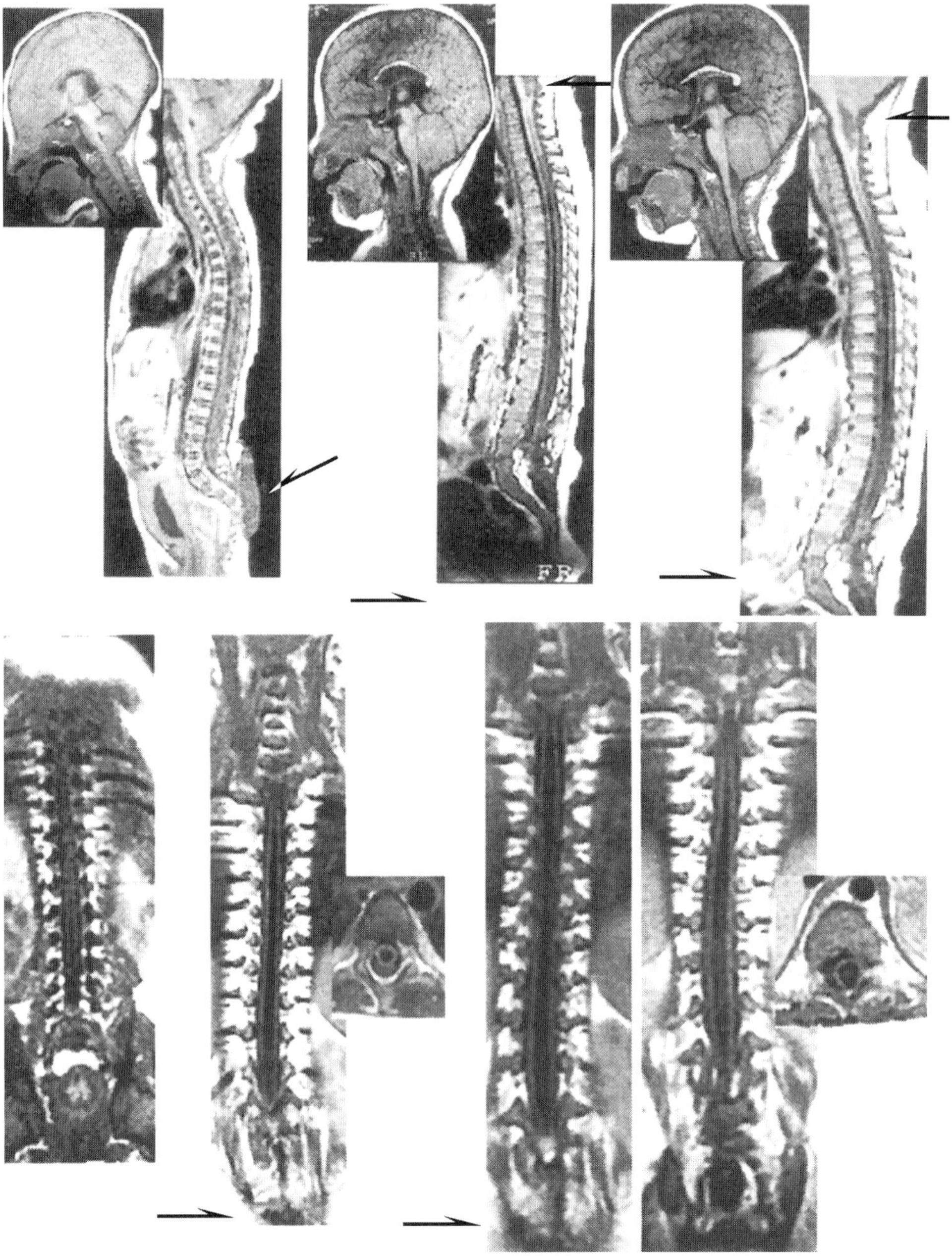

a

b

FIG. 2. Sequential alterations in a progressive neonatal syringomyelia with myeloschisis (*oblique arrow*) complicated by the isolated 4th ventricle (*arrows*). Magnetic resonance images in **a** sagittal and **b** coronal view. From left to right in both series, sequential images at birth, 9 months, and 12 months after repair and VP shunting

Cord-Tethering-Related Syrinx

Case. A 5-year-old boy with myeloschisis repaired and VP-shunted at birth developed a syrinx which extended from Th3 through L1. One year later, the syrinx progressed rostrally up to C2. Lumbago with diminished patellar tendon reflex (PTR) and progressive scoliosis were detected. On MRI, a flow void was confirmed at the foramen Magendie. SS shunting collapsed the syrinx within 2 weeks and improved foot joint weakness, with the reappearance of PTRs. After 10 years he remains stable without recurrence of the syrinx.

Surgical Results

All the tight foramen magnum-related large syrinxes with MMC were identified in the newborn period. Osseous FMD against syrinx relieved Chiari type II symptoms and stabilized the syrinx. However, except for one patient, additional syrinx diversion was inevitable to attain collapse. In cord-tethering-related syrinxes, small syrinxes disappeared or remained slit after untethering. However, for large syrinxes, the collapse of the syrinx was achieved only after additional SS shunting. Shunt revision was necessary for one patient 2 years after shunting.

Discussion

Clinical Spectrum

The most common signs and symptoms of syringomyelia were brain stem dysfunction refractory to conservative treatment in neonates and infants, and spinal cord tethering in school-aged patients. However, exact delineation of the features of syringomyelia was difficult owing to the overlapping symptomatology of MMC. For early detection, syringomyelia should be recognized as a potent condition which rapidly aggravates the clinical features of MMC.

Syringomyelia is most accurately diagnosed by MRI. Surveillance MRIs are essential to clarify the clinical spectrum of syringomyelia with MMC [9]. In our survey, the overall incidence of pediatric syringomyelia with MMC was 28%, and neonatal syringomyelia was diagnosed in 26% of cases. Large syrinx was detected in 50% of cases. In neurologically deteriorated patients with MMC diagnosed by MRI between 6 months and 10.5 years of age, the incidence of syringomyelia was reported as 48.5% [6], which is comparable with our findings for large syrinxes.

Pediatric syringomyelia with MMC diagnosed by MRI consists of (A) large neonatal syrinxes which are closely related to Chiari type II malformation or tight foramen magnum, (B) large syrinxes in toddlers or school-aged children which are related to spinal cord retethering, and (C) small or slit-like syrinxes. Small or slit-like syrinxes remain stable under the successful control of hydrocephalus with or without osseous FMD against symptomatic Chiari malformation. The primary repair of MMC might also reduce or stabilize the syrinx.

Progressive Syringomyelia and the Patent Spinal Central Canal in the Closing Process

Patency of the spinal central canal is classically claimed up to 2 years of age, and in 82% of patients during childhood [8]. Thus, pediatric syringomyelia progresses in the spinal cord with an open central canal in the closing process, which might form the morphological background of the more dynamic changes in pediatric syringomyelia. To prevent this progression, efforts should be made to evaluate the diverse factors which might lead to progression on an individual basis.

Possible Factors Which Might Lead to Progression

Sequential MRIs disclosed the likely mechanism of progression which relates to disturbed CSF bulk flow, tightened foramen magnum [5], and spinal cord retethering (Fig. 3). (1) A neonatal holocord syrinx might be formed by the isolated fetal spinal central canal if the fetal spinal central canal is a cavity equipped with a sink action, and CSF bulk flow exists in the canal [7]. (2) A progressive syrinx with a dilating 4th ventricle is formed by transobex CSF influx [4] from the isolated fourth ventricle. (3) A progressive syrinx with a nondilating 4th ventricle might be related to the developmental craniocerebellar disproportion which advances the periforamen magnum CSF flow dynamics, especially in the dorsal area; the tight foramen magnum. (4) Spinal cord retethering might impair the microcirculation of the tethered spinal cord and progress the preexisting syrinx [10]. (5) Reduction after repair, VP shunting, and osseous FMD supports the deteriorating role of the cord tethering and the tightened foramen magnum in the progression. Once enlarged, a syrinx might be influenced by hydrodynamically deteriorating factors such as the slosh and squeeze mechanism [13].

Proposed Management

The surgical goal is to achieve cord reconstitution with maximal functional restoration. Procedures should be aimed at ameliorating the deteriorating factors which might lead to the acquired formation and progression of the syrinx, as well as removing the mass effect. Pediatric syringomyelia has a long life expectancy. Moreover, it is a disease of the developing spinal cord. Thus, management requires less invasive procedures. Because pediatric syringomyelia progresses without delineable signs and symptoms, watchful observation by MRI is essential. A direct syrinx diversion should be planned for an enlarged or progressive syrinx even after treating the deteriorating factors (Fig. 4).

Efficacy of SS Shunt and Criticism Against Shunting

The SS shunt tube with a slit valve was designed to avoid CSF influx from the spinal subarachnoid space. To prevent this migration, the shunt tube was equipped with tiny wings for

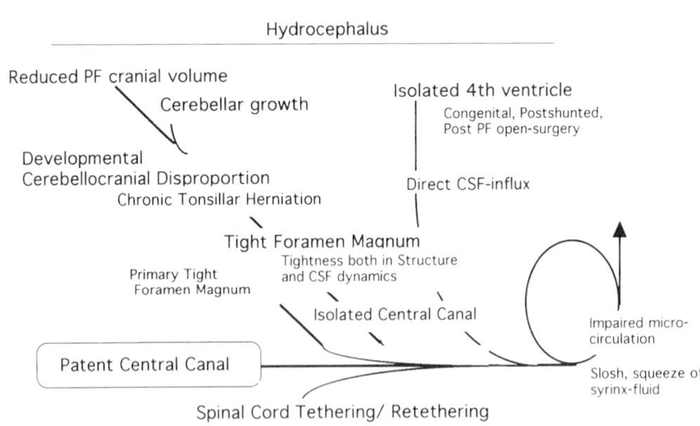

FIG. 3. Deteriorating factors in pediatric syringomyelia

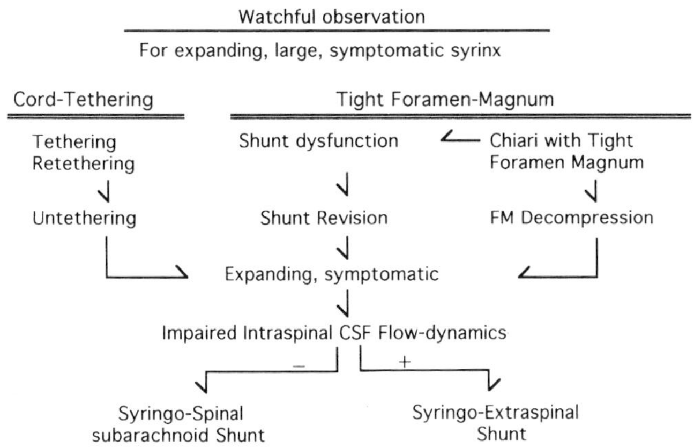

FIG. 4. Proposed guidelines for the management of pediatric syringomyelia

fixation. Meticulous closure of the arachnoid space and a bloodless operation is essential to prevent shunt dysfunction and spinal cord retethering. Some reports argue against the efficacy of SS shunting [11]. In our series, none showed intraspinal CSF retention, and the ventral spinal CSF space was opened even in cases with severely tethered cord. We believe that the drained syringeal fluid enters the bulk flow of the spinal CSF. Once a syrinx is collapsed, the fluctuation of the syrinx or the squeezing effect on the syrinx reduces, and reexpansion might be prevented.

Conclusions

The incidence of pediatric syringomyelia with MMC was 32%, and that of neonatal syringomyelia was 26%. Large syrinxes which indicate syrinx-oriented management were detected in 50% of cases. Surgical interventions against the suggested deteriorating factors are effective for a small syrinx to stabilize. For an enlarged syrinx with MMC, diversion of the syrinx is the procedure of choice to attain collapse in a short time, and promises to achieve maximal restoration of the neurological function.

Acknowledgment. This study was supported by a Research Grant (5B-3, 8B-5) for Nervous and Mental Disorders from the Ministry of Health and Welfare, 1994–1998.

References

1. Baztzdorf U (ed) (1991) Syringomyelia. Current concepts in diagnosis and treatment. Current neurosurgical practice [Wilson CB (ed)]. Williams & Wilkins, Baltimore, pp 1–3
2. Bertrand G (1990) Hydrosyringomyelia due to congenital and acquired lesions—common mechanisms, search for a logical treatment. Spinal Surg 4:3–9
3. Carmel PW (1991) Congenital syringomyelia. In: Batzdorf U (ed) Syringomyelia. Current concepts in diagnosis and treatment. Williams & Wilkins, Baltimore, pp 140–150
4. Gardner WJ (1965) Hydrodynamic mechanism of syringomyelia: its relationship to myelomeningocele. J Neurol Neurosurg Psychiatr 28:247–259

5. Kogness KG, Nyland H (1978) Early infantile hydrocephalus assessed by the posterior fossa ratio method. Acta Neurochir 45:115–121
6. La Marca, Herman M, Grant JA, McLone DG (1997) Prevention and management of hydromyelia in children with Chiari Type-II malformation. Pediatr Neurosurg 26:57–67
7. Milhorat TH, Johnson RW, Johnson WD (1991) Evidence of CSF flow in rostral direction through central canal of spinal cord in rats. In: Matsumoto S, Tamaki N (eds) Hydrocephalus. Pathogenesis and treatment. Springer-Verlag, Tokyo, pp 207–217
8. Milhorat TH, Kotzen RM, Anzil AP (1994) Stenosis of central canal of spinal cord in man: incidence and pathological findings in 232 autopsy cases. J Neurosurg 80:716–722
9. Oakes WJ (1997) Editorial comment. Pediatr Neurosurg 26:66–67
10. Sato H, Sato N (1994) Implication of tethering in expanding syringomyelia (abstract). Child's Nerv Syst 10:407
11. Sgouros S, Williams B (1995) A critical appraisal of drainage in syringomyelia. J Neurosurg 82:1–10
12 Williams B (1980) On the pathogenesis of syringomyelia—a review. J R Soc Med 73:798–806
13. Williams B (1993) Pathogenesis of syringomyelia. Acta Neurochir (Wien) 123:159–165

Treatment of Hydro/Syringomyelia Associated with Spina Bifida

MASSIMO CALDARELLI, CONCEZIO DI ROCCO, and FRANK LA MARCA

Summary. Patients affected by spina bifida show a higher incidence of hydro/syringomyelia compared with the general population. However, this incidence varies considerably depending on the modalities of patient recruitment; in fact, neuroradiological identification of a spinal cord cavitation is a much more frequent event than its detection on a clinical base. This observation obviously raises the question of whether the simple recognition of the abnormality is sufficient to indicate the need for surgical treatment. On these grounds, we have analyzed the actual incidence of hydro/syringomyelia in our population of myelodysplastic children, who were followed at the Spina Bifida Clinic of the Catholic University Medical School, Rome. One hundred and forty-two patients with complete magnetic resonance studies and sufficient follow-up were considered eligible for this analysis. Thirty-two patients (22.5%) presented various degrees of spinal cord cavitation on magnetic resonance images, although only 14 of them (9.8%) presented with clinical signs referable to the spinal lesion. Clinical manifestations included deterioration in motor and sphincter functions, scoliosis, and, less frequently, pain and sensory loss. The mean age at hydromyelia diagnosis for all patients affected was 3.9 years and, in particular, 4 years for those patients who presented with symptoms. All patients with symptoms due to the hydromyelia underwent surgical treatment. Two main forms of treatment were adopted, namely direct drainage of the spinal cavity in 6 cases, and surgical procedures aimed at correcting the filling mechanism of the malformation in the remaining 8 patients (5 posterior fossa decompressions, 2 CSF shunt revisions, and 1 spinal cord untethering procedure with terminal syringostomy). All patients improved postoperatively, except one who remained clinically stable at follow-up. The authors conclude that the incidence of hydromyelia is actually higher than that reported until now in the literature, although not all lesions are symptomatic. The radiological picture may be helpful in planning a more careful follow-up program for patients theoretically at risk from neurological deterioration. Surgical treatment, when indicated, permits the achievement of good results in the majority of cases, and should be carried out as soon as possible before further deterioration occurs.

Key words. Hydromyelia, Spina bifida, Chiari II malformation, Children, Treatment

---

Section of Pediatric Neurosurgery, Department of Neurosurgery, Catholic University Medical School, 8 Largo Agostino Gemelli, Rome 00168, Italy

Introduction

Patients affected by spina bifida can present with cavitating lesions of the spinal cord, either segmental or extended to its entire length, which take their origin from CSF accumulation escaping from the central canal, through a disruption of the ependymal lining. Such cavitating lesions are more and more frequently discovered in myelodysplastic children owing to the wider utilization of magnetic resonance imaging (MRI) as part of their follow-up [3, 7, 9, 12–14, 16, 23]. In fact neuroradiological investigation is not limited to cases presenting with neurological deterioration possibly related to a spinal cord disease, but is increasingly becoming a routine part of the postoperative follow-up of children operated on for myelomeningocele (MMC) as well as for other forms of spina bifida. For this reason the incidence of hydro/syringomyelia seems to be increasing in myelodysplastic children, although the neuroradiological demonstration of a spinal cord cavitation does not necessarily correspond to a clinical syndrome. Also in our experience [2, 8], the incidence of symptomatic hydro/syringomyelia is much lower than its recognition on a mere neuroradiological basis.

This discrepancy raises the question of whether all forms of spinal cord cavitation should require surgical treatment or only the symptomatic ones. Even here, however, the demonstration of signs and symptoms of neurological deterioration is not unequivocal. Indeed, clinical manifestations of hydro/syringomyelia in children include, either alone or in various combinations, motor weakness, spasticity, sensory loss, pain, gait disturbances, scoliosis, and bowel or bladder changes [1, 5, 12]. These symptoms and signs are not specific to this condition, but are similar to those related to tethered spinal cord, which is a consistent finding in myelodysplastic children. Conversely, the classical syndrome of hydro/syringomyelia is quite rare in these patients, especially in the younger ones. Once treatment is advised, the next question to be addressed is the modality of any surgical procedure.

On these grounds, we reviewed the MMC patients attending our Spina Bifida Clinic with the aim of analyzing the actual incidence of hydro/syringomyelia in neuroimaging investigations, the incidence and characteristics of the symptomatic forms, the indications for treatment, the modalities of surgical management, and the results of treatment.

Materials and Methods

Two hundred and thirty-two children, ranging in age between 1 and 15 years, are regularly checked at the Spina Bifida Clinic at the Catholic University Medical School in Rome. Most of them have been operated on in the Pediatric Neurosurgery Section since 1980, although about 1/8 of them have been referred to us from peripheral centres after receiving the initial MMC repair. Since MRI has become available in this hospital, all of them have undergone at least one MRI study either as part of their follow-up or because of the appearance of some neurological alteration, possibly referable to spinal cord (or cerebral) deterioration. One hundred and forty-two cases with complete MRI studies and sufficient follow-up were considered eligible for this study. For all the patients who had had more than one MRI study, the latest negative MRI, or the earliest positive MRI for hydromyelia, was taken into consideration for the analysis.

The criteria for classifying hydro/syringomyelia were the extent of spinal cord cavitation and the ratio between the transverse diameter of the hydromyelic cavity and that of the entire spinal cord, calculated at the level of maximal expansion of the lesion. Following these criteria, we subdivided the hydro/syringomyelia into a "holocord" and a segmental type, and among the latter we distinguished cervical, cervico-dorsal, dorsal, dorso-lumbar, and lumbar forms. As to the width of the spinal cavitation, we identified three degrees of increasing severity [2]: Grade I covered the forms where the diameter of the hydromyelic cavity was between one-quarter and one-third of the total spinal cord diameter; Grade II covered those with hydromyelia diameter between one-third and one-half of the total spinal cord diameter; Grade III covered those with a diameter greater than one-half of the total spinal cord diameter and associated with signs of tension such as severe reduction of the spinal subarachnoid space or thinning of the spinal cord parenchyma, with or without spinal cord atrophy.

Hydrocephalus was present in all these patients, although in two cases ventricular dilatation was so mild as not to require surgical treatment. Likewise, Chiari type II malformations and low-anchored spinal cords with or without an associated symptomatology were identified in all instances. The low-anchored spinal cords were classified into four grades of tethering [1]. Neurological, orthopedic, and urologic status were evaluated routinely every 6 months until the age of 3 years and every 12 months thereafter, and/or immediately at onset of referred clinical deterioration.

The follow-up period from the time the hydromyelia was diagnosed by MRI ranged from 1 year to 8 years (mean 4.2 years). All patients with hydromyelia who later underwent surgical treatment had at least one MRI study carried out within the first postoperative year. Those who underwent conservative treatment for hydromyelia, following a "wait-and-see" policy, also had at least one MRI study carried out within 3 years of the initial hydromyelia diagnosis.

Results

Of the 142 patients selected on the basis of the completeness of their neuroradiological investigations and a sufficient follow-up duration, 32 presented more or less extended spinal cord cavitations. The mean age at diagnosis was 3.9 years. The site of the previously repaired MMC was dorso-lumbar in 5 cases, lumbar in 10 cases, and lumbo-sacral in 17 cases. Seven patients presented a holocord hydromyelia, while the remaining 25 patients presented a segmental hydromyelia, of which 6 were at the cervico-dorsal level, 8 were dorsal, 8 were dorso-lumbar, and 3 were lumbar.

The classical neuroradiological manifestations of Chiari type II malformation were present in all subjects, although only 2 of them became symptomatic and required surgical treatment. A ventricular dilatation, generally of mild degree, was present in all patients. In 2 children, such mild hydrocephalus did not require treatment, whereas the remaining 30 children had been treated in infancy with ventriculo-peritoneal shunting. All these 32 patients had a low-lying or tethered spinal cord, which was judged as Grade I in 8 cases, Grade II in 16 cases, Grade III in 5 cases, and Grade IV in 3 cases.

Regarding the symptomatology, 9 of these 32 patients were asymptomatic at diagnosis for hydromyelia (or showed stable clinical pictures) (group A). In these cases, the syrinx was casually diagnosed on routine MRI control and a "wait-and-see" policy was followed. The remaining 23 cases with hydro/syringomyelia were symptomatic. However, in 9 children the clinical manifestations referred to conditions other than hydromyelia (group B), and in the remaining 14 patients they were attributed to spinal cord cavitation (group C).

Patients with Hydro/Syringomyelia and Without Clinical Signs (Group A)

Nine children who were completely asymptomatic (or clinically stable) were casually diagnosed to have hydromyelia in routine MRI studies. The spinal cavity was holocord in one patient and segmental in 8, of which 1 was cervico-dorsal, 2 were dorsal, 3 were dorso-lumbar,

TABLE 1. Extension of hydro/syringomyelia

Extension of hydro/syringomyelia	Group A	Group B	Group C	Total
Holocord	1	0	6	7
Segmental	8	9	8	25
cervico-dorsal	1	2	3	6
dorsal	2	3	3	8
dorso-lumbar	3	3	2	8
lumbar	2	1	–	3

Group A, patients with hydro/syringomyelia and without clinical manifestations; Group B, patients with hydro/syringomyelia and symptomatic for related conditions; Group C, patients with symptomatic hydro/syringomyelia.

TABLE 2. Degree of dilatation of hydro/syringomyelia

Degree of dilatation	Group A	Group B	Group C	Total
Grade I	4	7	–	11
Grade II	5	2	5	12
Grade III	–	–	9	9

Group A, patients with hydro/syringomyelia and without clinical manifestations; Group B, patients with hydro/syringomyelia and symptomatic for related conditions; Group C, patients with symptomatic hydro/syringomyelia.

and 2 were lumbar (Table 1). Dilation of the hydromyelic cavity was of mild degree in 4 cases and moderate degree in 5 cases (Table 2).

Seven patients had an associated hydrocephalus that was adequately shunted, while the remaining 2 did not present a need for hydrocephalus treatment. Ventricular size was considered to be small in 1 case and normal in 8 cases.

The patients' ages at the time the hydromyelia diagnosis was reached on MRI ranged from 2 months to 6 years (mean 2.8 years). The period of observation from the time of hydromyelia diagnosis ranged from 6 months to 9 years (mean 4.9 years). During this time, radiological and clinical status remained stable in all patients.

Patients with Hydro/Syringomyelia and Symptomatic for Related Conditions (Group B)

Nine children presented a symptomatology that was not considered to be due to the hydromyelia, but rather to a tethered cord (7 cases) or to a symptomatic Chiari type II malformation (2 cases) for which specific surgical treatment was carried out.

In the 7 patients who were considered to be symptomatic for spinal cord tethering, a Grade III or IV tethered cord was present. The hydro/syringomyelic cavity was located in the dorsal region in 3 cases, in the dorso-lumbar region in 3 cases, and in the lumbar region in 1 case (Table 1). The dilatation of the hydromyelic cavity was mild (Grade I) in 5 cases and moderate (Grade II) in 2 cases (Table 2). The symptoms in these children consisted of worsening muscle weakness in the lower extremities in 5 cases, worsening bladder function in 5 cases, spasticity in the lower extremities in 2 cases, scoliosis in 2 cases, and low back pain irradiating to the lower extremities in 1 case. The 2 patients with symptomatic Chiari II malformation had Grade II tethered cords and cervico-dorsal hydromyelia of mild degree in both cases. Clinical manifestations included stridor, swallowing difficulty, and neck rigidity.

All the patients had an associated hydrocephalus that was adequately shunted. Ventricular size was considered to be normal or near normal in all cases.

The patients' ages at the time the hydromyelia diagnosis was reached on MRI ranged from 8 months to 9 years (mean 3.9 years). The period of observation from the time of hydromyelia diagnosis (and/or treatment of the related pathological conditions) ranged from 1 to 10 years (mean 5 years). During this time, radiological and clinical status remained stable for all patients.

Patients with Symptomatic Hydro/Syringomyelia (Group C)

The last 14 patients presented with clinical manifestations which were attributed to the spinal cavitation. The hydromyelia in this group of patients was of the holocord type in 6 cases and segmental in 8 cases, of which 3 were cervico-dorsal, 3 were dorsal, and 2 were dorso-lumbar (Table 1). The spinal cord cavitation was moderate (degree II) in 5 cases and severe (degree III) in 9 cases (Table 2). All patients in this group presented an associated hydrocephalus. Ventricular dilation was mild to moderate but stable in 11 of the cases. One child presented an isolated lateral ventricle not drained by the original shunt system. The remaining 2 children were presenting a shunt malfunction, which was established by the increased size of the ventricular system as compared with earlier CT and/or MRI studies.

In this group, the following symptoms were observed: worsening motor deficits in 10 cases, progressive scoliosis in 8 cases, pain in 5 cases, pyramidal signs in 4 cases, worsening sensory deficit in 3 cases (upper extremity involvement or rising lower sensory level), neck stiffness in 3 cases, and worsening bladder function in 3 cases (Table 3). The age of these patients ranged from 18 months to 11 years (mean 4 years) at the time of diagnosis.

In the surgical treatment of hydro/syringomyelia, two main procedures were carried out: direct and indirect. Direct treatment, which was adopted in 6 cases, had the goal of draining the hydromyelic cavity by means of a hydro-peritoneal shunt in 5 cases and by means of a hydro-subarachnoid shunt in one case. Indirect treatment, which was used in the other 8 cases, was aimed at eliminating the filling mechanism of the hydromyelia (5 posterior fossa decompressions, 2 CSF shunt revisions, and 1 spinal cord untethering aimed at creating a "terminal ventriculostomy").

TABLE 3. Clinical manifestations and results of treatment in 14 cases of symptomatic hydro/syringomyelia

Clinical manifestations	Preoperative	Recovery	Postoperative improvement	Stable
Worsening motor deficit	10	6	2	2
Progressive scoliosis	8	–	3	5
Pain	5	5	–	–
Pyramidal signs	4	4	–	–
Sensory loss	3	–	3	–
Worsening bladder function	3	–	3	–
Neck stiffness	3	2	1	–

Five of the 6 children undergoing direct drainage of the hydromyelic cavity showed a marked improvement in their clinical condition (which was complete in 4 cases). At control MRI, these patients presented a marked or complete collapse of the spinal cavity (2 and 4 cases, respectively).

Five children underwent posterior fossa decompression: in two cases a simple laminectomy with widening of the foramen magnum was carried out; in 3 cases the dura mater was also opened and a larger subdural space was created by duroplasty. In one of the latter cases, the hydromyelic cavity was also opened by myelotomy and shunted into the subarachnoid space. Out of these 5 children, 4 improved clinically and one remained stable. In all five cases the hydromyelic cavity was seen to have decreased in size in postoperative MRI studies: in two cases slightly, and in three moderately.

Of the remaining 3 children who underwent CSF shunt revision (2 cases) and spinal cord untethering and terminal syringostomy (1 case), all clinically improved and MRI studies showed a reduction of the hydromyelic cavity.

The symptoms that responded best to surgery can be seen in Table 3. All 5 patients with pain and all 4 with pyramidal signs had a resolution of the symptoms. Eight out of the 10 cases with worsening motor deficits improved postoperatively, of which 6 returned completely to their initial clinical status. The remaining 2 children with progressive motor deficits stabilized after surgery. All 3 cases of neck stiffness improved, of which 2 had complete resolution. All 3 cases with worsening sensory deficit and all 3 with worsening bladder function improved, although none of them resolved the symptoms completely. Three cases of scoliosis improved partially, while the remaining 5 remained stable postoperatively.

The postoperative follow-up period ranged from 1 year to 8 years (mean 3.1 years).

Discussion

Although many theories have been propounded over recent years to explain the pathogenesis of hydro/syringomyelia, the most credited are those suggested by Gardner [4] and Williams [22]. According to Gardner's hydrodynamic theory [4], the central canal of the spinal cord is forced open and progressively distended by CSF pulsations transmitted to the central canal because of the reduced CSF outflow from the 4th ventricle. The "water-hammer" effect of the arterial pulsation generates an initial dilatation of the central canal, and secondarily rupture of its ependymal layer and the creation of a paracentral cavity inside the cord parenchyma which is contiguous with the canal itself. Williams [22] introduced some modifications to Gardner's theory and emphasized the effect of increased venous pressure as the driving force of spinal cord cavitation. In his theory, he postulates that the presence of hindbrain herniation into the cervical canal prevents CSF pressure increases (brought about by venous pressure increases, such as those occurring during coughing or Valsalva's maneuver) being dissipated caudally in the perimedullary subarachnoid spaces. The simultaneous increase in CSF pressure at the level of the cisterna magna and the corresponding drop in the spinal subarachnoid pressure favor the accumulation of CSF within the hydromyelic cavity. These two hydrodynamic theories, rather than being mutually exclusive, can help to interpret the genesis and progression of hydro/syringomyelia as a combination of the effects of arterial and venous pressures [23], particularly in myelodysplastic patients who often present an alteration of the outlet foramina of the 4th ventricle as well as more or less severe hindbrain herniation for the associated Chiari type II malformation.

The overall radiological incidence of hydromyelia in MMC patients, to our knowledge, has been reported in the literature to be 19% [15]. One report considered only patients who underwent MRI studies for deteriorating clinical status, and showed a 48.5% incidence in that particular group of patients [8]. In our series of 142 patients, the radiological incidence was observed to be 22.5%.

Hydromyelia does not seem to be present at birth or in early infancy, but appears later on. In fact, hydromyelia was not detected in a spina bifida population screened in infancy with cranial and spinal ultrasound [21]. We did not carry out MRI screening at birth, and the average age at hydromyelia diagnosis in our series was 5.1 years; however, that of asymptomatic children was 2.8 years. Such an observation could suggest that hydromyelia may start at an early age, although usually after the first year of life, and remain asymptomatic for a variable amount of time. The average age at which the hydromyelia became symptomatic in our series was 4 years.

As follow-up continues, we would expect the overall incidence of hydromyelia to increase, and therefore the average age at onset of symptoms to become greater, as reported in other studies [6, 12]. Spontaneous resolution of hydromyelia has been reported [17]. In our experience, however, a gradual and insidious onset of symptomatology seems to be more probable, especially in patients in whom it is associated with a subtle shunt malfunction. For this reason, an even closer follow-up is recommended for these children, preferably consisting of neurological checks to be performed every 6 months in patients who are clinically stable, and immediate spinal and cerebral MRI for patients showing any deterioration in their clinical conditions. The routine follow-up study should also include an evaluation of the ventricular system. Although ventricular size was not correlated with the presence of hydro/syringomyelia in our patients, the presence of a functioning shunt system seemed greatly to influence the clinical and radiological status of the patients. Subtle shunt malfunctioning can, in fact, result in a hydromyelia, regardless of the actual ventricular size. In suspected cases, an assessment of the functioning of the CSF shunt device should be carried out and any shunt malfunction corrected first, as the hydromyelia may improve with this alone [5].

In our study, the extension and degree of dilation of the hydromyelia appeared to be correlated with the presence of symptomatology. In fact, in the symptomatic group of children, there were 9 cases (100.0%) with severe hydromyelia dilation, while none were present in the asymptomatic group. There were also 6 cases out of 7 (85.7%) with holocord hydromyelia in the symptomatic group, while only 1 was present in the asymptomatic group. On the other hand, after MRI examination, some authors rule out any significant relationship between symptoms attributed to spinal cord damage and the size of the hydromyelia [20]. From the radiological evidence in our study, the association between a tethered spinal cord and a hydromyelic cavity appeared to be significant. It has been hypothesized that the filling mechanism, especially for distal segmental hydromyelia, is likely to be related to the tethering of the spinal cord itself [5]. From our data, neither the level of the spinal defect nor the degree of cerebellar tonsil herniation seemed to have an influence on the incidence of hydro/syringomyelia. However, the prevalence of hydromyelia has been found to be higher in patients with tonsillar herniation measuring 9–14 mm than in patients with lower or more severe degrees of herniation [10].

As regards the clinical picture, it is interesting to note that classic hydromyelia syndrome appeared to be very rare. Worsening motor deficits (present in 71.4%) and progressive scoliosis (present in 57.1%) were the most common symptoms to occur in our series, but sensory loss was less apparent than has been reported in other series [5, 11].

The overall incidence of symptomatic hydromyelia in our MMC series appeared to be 9.9%. This value is very similar to that of 9.4% reported in a study in which routine MRI screening was not applied, and only patients presenting neurological deterioration were radiologically examined [8].

Obviously, candidates for surgery are those who present clinical deterioration. Therefore, for the assessment of MMC patients, as in symptomatic tethered cord and Chiari II malformation, a clinical diagnosis of hydromyelia appears to be more important than a radiological one. However, although MRI screening of all MMC patients does not appear to be necessary, it permits the determination of a radiological baseline picture in case clinical deterioration of the patient were to occur. Early MRI evidence of a hydromyelia may also be helpful in planning a more careful and frequent control program for patients theoretically at risk of neurological deterioration due to the presence of hydromyelia.

The results of treatment showed that 93% of patients improved after surgery. The type of procedure carried out did not seem to affect the chances of a favorable outcome. However, in our series, precise criteria were followed in choosing the type of surgery. In fact, posterior fossa decompression was carried out in patients in whom packing of the foramen magnum was found by MRI, and/or who presented with neck rigidity. Ventriculo-peritoneal shunt revision was carried out when a shunt malfunction was assessed at neuroradiological investigation. Hydromyelia shunting procedures were carried out only in cases of mainly unilocular and severely extended hydromyelic cavities. The spinal cord untethering procedure was carried out on a child with symptoms characterized by progressive weakness of the lower extremities and deterioration of bladder function, and with a low-lying spinal cord found by MRI to be associated with a moderately dilated lumbar hydromyelic cavity.

Many studies in the literature report the surgical results of different types of treatment for hydromyelia [6, 11, 12, 18, 19, 21, 23]. Although many of these treatments result in a good outcome, very few studies have specifically concentrated on the results obtained in patients with myelomeningocele and Chiari II malformation [2, 5, 8]. There was a significant correlation between the efficacy of treatment and the reduction in size of the hydromyelic cavity. In fact, all of the children who improved presented a reduction of the hydromyelia on MRI. Other authors have reported similar findings [3, 19]. However, it has never been proven that a significant reduction or the complete disappearance of the hydromyelic cavity is necessary to obtain postoperative clinical improvement. On the other hand, our study shows that a reduction of the cavity seen by postoperative MRI was also seen in the child who did not improve after surgery, although stabilization of the clinical status was obtained. Pain and pyramidal signs appeared to respond best to surgery, while scoliosis, worsening sensory deficit, and worsening bladder function responded less favorably.

Conclusions

The overall incidence of hydromyelia in the spina bifida population seems higher than that reported in the literature [15]. From our data, the overall radiological incidence of hydromyelia is higher than that calculated when considering only symptomatic hydromyelia (22.5% vs. 9.9%). The radiological picture (extension and dilation of the hydromyelia seen by MRI) seems to be an important, although not an absolute, indicator of clinical severity. Actually, symptoms and signs may vary greatly from one patient to the other. Worsening motor deficits in the lower limbs are the most common presenting symptoms in children. Progressive scoliosis also appears to be an important sign indicating deterioration of the muscle function due to hydromyelia. Generally, surgical treatment of hydromyelia is very rewarding. However, certain symptoms (pain, pyramidal signs, worsening motor deficits) respond to therapy better than others (scoliosis, worsening sensory deficit, worsening bladder function). The high incidence of hydro/syringomyelia in myelodysplastic patients, as well as the reversibility of the clinical manifestations after surgical treatment, suggest the need for a rigorous and continuous follow-up program with the use of regular cystometrograms, muscle testing, and spine MRI in all patients with spina bifida. Late deterioration is frequent in early childhood, and prompt intervention permits remission or stabilization of the clinical symptoms provided that treatment is carried out soon after their occurrence.

References

1. Caldarelli M, Di Rocco C, Colosimo C, Fariello G, Di Gennaro M (1995) Surgical treatment of late neurological deterioration in children with myelodysplasia. Acta Neurochir (Wien) 137:199–206
2. Caldarelli M, Di Rocco C, La Marca F (1998) Treatment of hydromyelia in spina bifida. Surg Neurol, 411–420
3. Firschung R, Sanker P (1993) MRI follow-up in syringomylia. Observations from twelve cases. Acta Neurochir 123:206–207
4. Gardner WJ (1965) Hydrodynamic mechanism of syringomyelia: its relationship to myelocele. J Neurol Neurosurg Psychiatr 28:247–259
5. Hardwidge C, Williams B (1992) Spina bifida and syringomyelia. Child's Nerv Syst 8:173
6. Hoffman HJ, Neill J, Crone KR, Hendrick B, Humphreys RP (1987) Hydrosyringomyelia and its management in childhood. Neurosurgery 21:347–351
7. Kokmen E, Marsh WR, Baker HL Jr (1985) Magnetic resonance imaging in syringomyelia and hydromyelia. Neurosurgery 17:267–270
8. La Marca F, Herman MD, Grant JA, McLone DG (1997) Presentation and management of hydromyelia in children with Chiari type II malformation. Pediatr Neurosurg 26:57–67
9. Lee BCP, Zimmerman RD, Manning JJ, Deck MD (1985) MR imaging of syringomyelia and hydromyelia. AJR 144:1149–1156
10. Maser H, Oberwittler C (1993) Syringomyelia in Chiari malformation: relation to extent of cerebellar tissue herniation. Neurosurgery 33:948–949
11. Matsumoto T, Symon L (1989) Surgical management of syringomyelia—current results. Surg Neurol 32:258–265
12. Milhorat TH, Johnson WD, Miller JI, Bergland RM, Hollenberg-Sher J (1992) Surgical treatment of syringomyelia based on magnetic resonance imaging criteria. Neurosurgery 31:231–245
13. Pillay PK, Awan IA, Little JR, Hahn JF (1991) Symptomatic Chiari malformation in adults: a new classification based on magnetic resonance imaging with clinical and prognostic significance. Neurosurgery 28:639–645
14. Pojunas K, Williams AL, Daniels DL, Haughton VM (1984) Syringomyelia and hydromyelia: magnetic resonance evaluation. Radiology 153:679–683
15. Schwartz M, Voth D, Just M, Ermert JA (1993) Form and incidence of hydro- and syringomyelia in spinal dysraphia in MRI. Acta Neurochir (Wien) 123:178–182
16. Sherman JL, Barkovich AL, Citrin CM (1991) The MR appearance of syringomyelia: new observations. AJNR 12:733–737
17. Sudo K, Doi S, Maruo D, Tashiro K, Terae S, Miyasaka K, Isu T (1990) Syringomyelia with spontaneous resolution. J Neurol Neurosurg Psychiatr 53:437–438
18. Tator CH, Meguro K, Rowed DW (1982) Favorable results with syringosubarachnoid shunts for the treatment of syringomyelia. J Neurosurg 56:517–523
19. Van Calenbergh F, Van den Bergh R (1993) Syringo-peritoneal shunting: results and problems in a consecutive series. Acta Neurochir (Wien) 123:203–205
20. Vaquero J, Martinez R, Arias A (1990) Syringomyelia–Chiari complex: magnetic resonance imaging and clinical evaluation of surgical treatment. J Neurosurg 73:64–68
21. Ventureyra ECG, Higgins MJ (1994) Syringomyelia and the Chiari type I malformation: new pathophysiologic concepts. Crit Rev Neurosurg 4:275–285
22. Williams B (1993) Pathogenesis of syringomyelia. Acta Neurochir (Wien) 123:159–165
23. Wisoff JH, Epstein F (1989) Management of hydromyelia. Neurosurgery 25:562–571

Pathogenesis of Syringomyelia

Toshiaki Abe, Yoshiji Okuda, Akira Isoshima, and Satoshi Tani

Introduction

Many theories have been proposed for the pathogenesis of syringomyelia. However, no one single theory succeeds in explaining all aspects of this disease state [13]. Recently, it was reported that the clinical and pathomorphological aspects of syringomyelia with spina bifida were different from those of syringomyelia with Chiari type I malformation [2, 9]. This suggests that the pathogenesis of these types of syringomyelia might differ. To investigate the differences in the pathogenesis of the two types of syringomyelia, 103 patients with syringomyelia were reviewed, with a focus on the role of the central canal in the formation of intraspinal syrinx.

Patients

One hundred and three patients with syringomyelia unrelated to tumor, who were surgically treated in our institution before the end of 1996, were evaluated. On the basis of magnetic resonance imaging (MRI) and intraoperative findings, cases of syringomyelia were classified into 6 types according to the associated lesions: type 1, Chiari type 1 malformation (70 cases); type 2, basal arachnoiditis (14 cases); type 3, congenital obstruction of the foramen Magendie (2 cases); type 4, spinal arachnoiditis (11 cases); type 5, spina bifida (3 cases); type 6, idiopathic (3 cases).

Methods

Pattern of Neurological Deterioration

The pattern of neurological deterioration was analyzed in patients with Chiari type 1 malformation, and the clinical grade of severity was determined. Neurologic deficits started with either a dissociated sensory loss (grade Ia) or a motor weakness (grade Ib) in an upper limb on one side. These symptoms were combined in a unilateral upper limb in grade II. A dissociated sensory loss or motor weakness then spread to the contralateral upper limb in

Department of Neurosurgery, Jikei University School of Medicine, 3-25-8 Nishi-shinbashi, Minato-ku, Tokyo 105, Japan

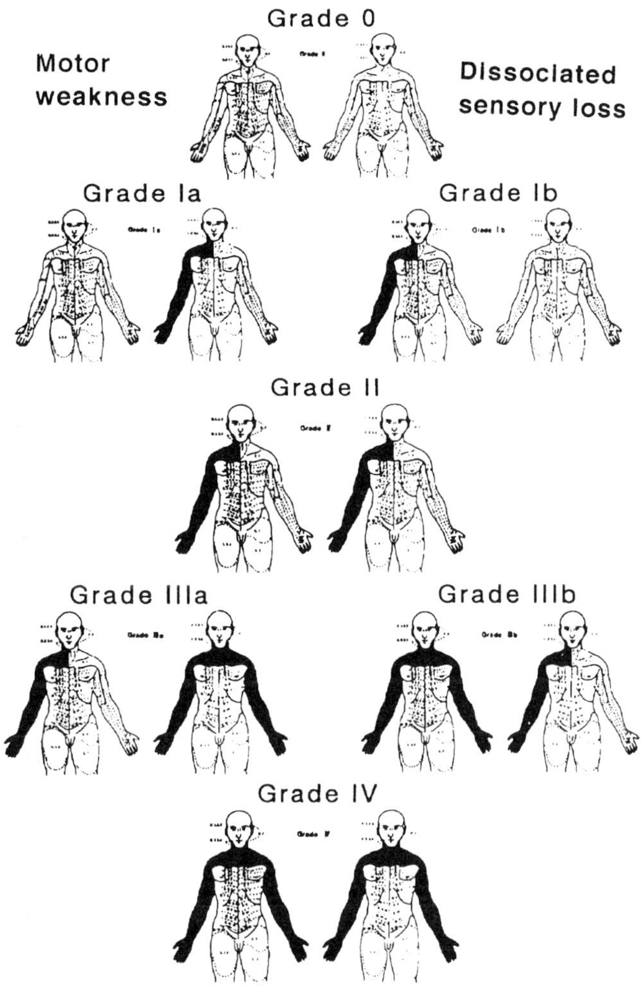

FIG. 1. Clinical grade of syringomyelia. *Grade 0*, no dissociated sensory loss (DSL) or motor weakness (MW); *Grade Ia*, DSL on one side of upper limb; *Grade Ib*, MW on one side of upper limb; *Grade II*, DSL and MW on one side of upper limb; *Grade IIIa*, DSL and MW on one side of upper limb and DSL on other side; *Grade IIIb*, DSL and MW on one side of upper limb and MW on other side; *Grade IV*, DSL and MW on both sides of upper limb with permission from [1]

grade IIIa or grade IIIb, respectively. Eventually, both dissociated sensory loss and motor weakness were present in both upper limbs in grade IV (Fig. 1) [1].

Eighty-seven patients with syringomyelia related to Chiari type 1 malformation were classified in this way, and the distribution of clinical severity was analyzed.

Neuroimaging Evaluation

Patients were examined with MRI before the operation and 1 month and 6 months after the operation. Patients were subsequently checked by MRI once or twice a year.

Pathological Examination

Case Presentation

The patient was a 65-year-old women with Crouzon disease who began to have a dissociated sensory disturbance of the left upper extremity 10 years before surgery. A weakness of the upper extremity on the same side then developed. MRI revealed syringomyelia with Chiari type 1 malformation. Foramen magnum decompression, laminectomy of the first cervical spine, obstruction of the central canal at the obex with Dacron fabric, and posterior fossa dura plasty were performed at the age of 65.

Postoperatively, the syrinx had collapsed and the neurological deficits were slightly improved. However, she died suddenly due to thalamic hemorrhage 4 years after the operation, at the age of 69.

It is important to investigate the role of the central canal in the pathogenesis of syringomyelia to determine whether the syrinx communicated with the fourth ventricle via a patent central canal. The brainstem and spinal cord from the obex to the upper end of the syrinx were histologically examined with 4-μm-thick serial axial sections stained with hematoxylin and eosin.

Results

Clinical Grade of Patients with Chiari Type 1 Malformation

Cases of syringomyelia with Chiari type 1 malformation were classified using the proposed clinical grading scale. We found that the severity of the clinical grade was well correlated with the average morbid period of the patients (Table 1). It is important to point out that 15 out of the 18 patients in grade I were grade Ia.

Neuroimaging Evaluation

The herniated tonsils were wedge-shaped and occupied the cisterna magna, the rostral end of the syrinx was conical, and the caudal part of the fourth ventricle was obliterated on typical MRIs of type 1 syringomyelia. These findings suggest that the herniated tonsils compressed the brainstem and spinal cord, and mechanically obstructed the flow of cerebrospinal fluid (CSF) at the foramen magnum (Fig. 2A). After foramen magnum decompression, the syrinx had collapsed. In addition, the tips of the herniated tonsils were rounded and shifted upward (Fig. 2B).

TABLE 1. Number of cases and average morbidity period in each grade

	No. of cases	Average morbid periods (years)
Grade 0	3	0
Grade Ia	15	3.1
Grade Ib	3	3.3
Grade II	24	6
Grade IIIa	6	8
Grade IIIb	2	8
Grade IV	10	15.3

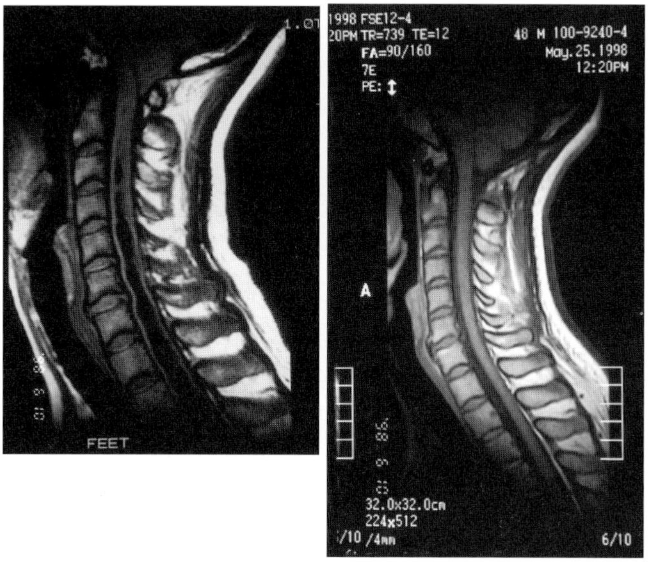

A B

FIG. 2. MRI of syringomyelia with Chiari type 1 malformation. **A** Before surgery; **B** after surgery

Postoperative upward displacement of the tonsils was identified in all cases of type 1 syringomyelia with collapse of the syrinx. However, direct communication between the fourth ventricle and the intraspinal syrinx was not identified in any case of type 1 syringomyelia. Axial MRI images of the spinal cord revealed the syrinx to be located on the symptomatic side in 80% of grade I and II patients.

Pathological Examination

Serial sections of the brain stem and the spinal cord revealed that the central canal was completely obstructed at the obex with Dacron fabric and surrounding scar tissue (Fig. 3, top right). The central canal was completely patent, with a fine lining of ependymal cells just below the obex (Fig. 3, bottom right). However, just above the syrinx, the central canal was completely obstructed with packed ependymal cells (Fig. 3, bottom left).

Discussion

The development of syringomyelia related to abnormalities in the posterior fossa is still incompletely understood. In 1965, Gardner [3] proposed his hydrodynamic theory of the pathogenesis of syringomyelia. In this theory, syringomyelia is attributed to arterial pulsations of CSF that are transmitted to the cervical cord via a patent central canal because of impaired outflow from the 4th ventricle. In 1969, Williams [12] attributed syringomyelia to craniospinal pressure dissociation owing to defective intracranial drainage partially obstructing free flow of CSF from the cranium into distensible spinal subarachnoid spaces.

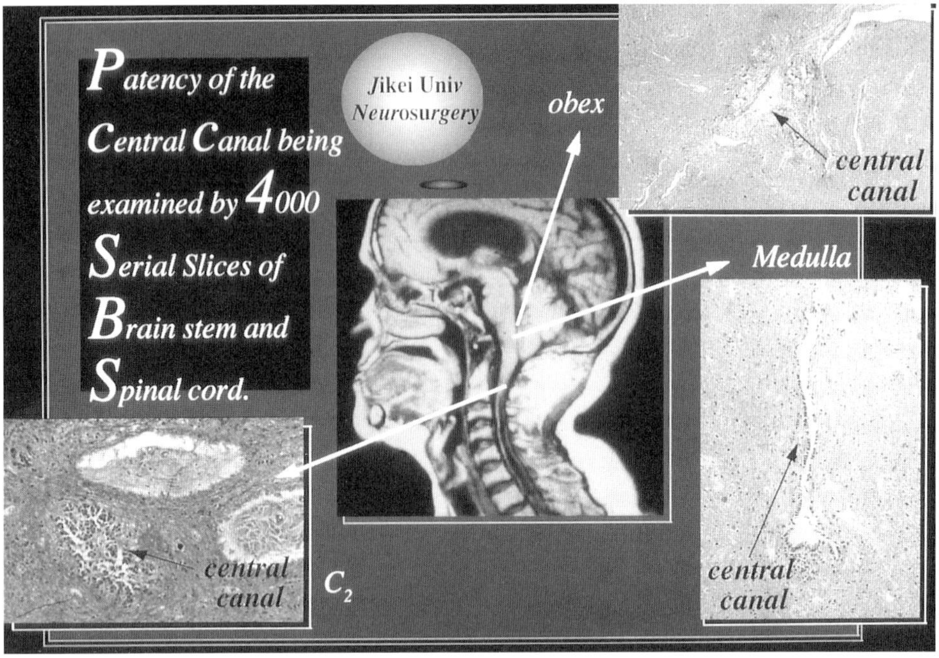

FIG. 3. Serial slices of the brainstem and spinal cord in a case of syringomyelia with Chiari type 1 malformation at the obex (*top right*), at the medulla (*bottom right*), and at the level of C2 (*bottom left*)

The pressure changes made CSF travel down the patent central canal from the floor of the 4th ventricle. The patency of the central canal between the 4th ventricle and the syrinx is an essential part of syrinx formation in these theories. However, MRI could not reveal such patency of the central canal in any of our cases of Chiari type 1-related syringomyelia. Pojunas et al. [10] and Sherman et al. [11] also reported similar MRI findings in their series. The central canal remaining patent under the condition of tonsillar descent blocking CSF flow at the craniovertebral junction is unreasonable [1]. Moreover, according to pathological examination, the central canal was completely obstructed with packed ependymal cells. These findings are not special features in Chiari type 1-related syringomyelia, but are commonly seen in normal persons older than 20 years [6, 8]. Milhorat [9] and Hinokuma et al. [4] also reported obstruction of the central canal in the same type of syringomyelia on postmortem examination. Based on these neuroimaging and pathomorphological findings, it is untenable that the syrinx related to Chiari type 1 malformation is formed by caudal flow of CSF from the 4th ventricle into the spinal cord via a patent central canal, as Gardner and Williams have proposed.

Syrinx related to spina bifida was commonly formed at the center of the spinal cord and connected with the 4th ventricle via a patent central canal, according a large series of pathomorphological examinations by Milhorat [9]. Therefore, syrinx with spina bifida can be formed by a caudal flow of CSF from the 4th ventricle into the spinal cord via a patent central canal.

Recently, Milhorat proposed a new theory. The central canal may function as a " sink" that is capable of removing substances from the parenchymal tissue of the spinal cord and delivering them into the 4th ventricle [7]. Chiari malformation disturbs this flow at the craniocervical junction and causes the central canal to dilate. However, this theory is inconsistent with our present autopsy case. The central canal was artificially plugged at the obex with Dacron fabric, but the central canal was collapsed rather than dilated. We estimated where the syrinx initially developed in the axial anatomical plain of the spinal cord by analyzing the symptoms and MRI findings.

The most common initial symptom was a dissociated sensory disturbance in the upper extremity on one side, whether or not the patients were aware of it. At this stage, MRI showed the syrinx to be located on the symptomatic side of the gray matter, commonly involving the posterior horn of the spinal cord. It is suggested that a loss of pain and thermal sensation is not caused by injuries of cruciate fibers of the intraspinal spinothalamic tract owing to the dilatation of the central canal, but by injuries of the dorsal horn neuron where the syrinx might develop initially. Studies of spinal somatosensory-evoked potentials by Kakigi et al. [5] found that the posterior horn neurons were damaged at the area of pain and thermal sensory disturbance.

In contrast, in cases of syringomyelia with Chiari type 2 malformation, Milhorat reported that the extension of the syrinx toward the posterior horn was not commonly seen on pathomorphological examination [9].

In conclusion, our data suggest that syringomyelia with Chiari type 1 malformation is caused by destruction of the gray matter starting from the posterior horn of the spinal cord, whereas syringomyelia with Chiari type 2 malformation and spina bifida is caused by a caudal flow of CSF from the fourth ventricle into the central canal of the spinal cord.

References

1. Abe T, Tanaka H, Nagashima H, Okuda Y, Ogawa T (1996) Role of the central canal in pathogenesis of syringomyelia with Chiari type 1 malformation. Nerv Syst Children 21: 299–306
2. Carmel PW (1991) Congenital syringomyelia. In: Batzdorf U (ed) Syringomyelia: current concepts in diagnosis and treatment. Williams & Wilkins, Baltimore, pp 140–150
3. Gardner WJ (1965) Hydrodynamic mechanism of syringomyelia: its relationship to myelocele. J Neurol Neurosurg Psychiatr 28:247–259
4. Hinokuma K, Ohama E, Oyanagi K, Kakita A, Kawai K, Ikuta F (1992) Syringomyelia. A neuropathological study of 18 autopsy cases. Acta Pathol Jpn 42:25–34
5. Kakigi R, Shibasaki H, Kuroda Y, Neshige R, Endo C, Tabuch K, Kishikawa T (1991) Pain-related somatosensory evoked potentials in syringomyelia. Brain 114:1871–1889
6. Kasantikul V, Netsky MG, James AE Jr (1979) Relation of age and cerebral ventricle size to central canal in man. J Neurosurg 51:85–93
7. Milhorat TH, Miller JI, Johnson WD, Adler DE, Heger IM (1993) Anatomical basis of syringomyelia occurring with hindbrain lesions. Neurosurgery 32:748–754
8. Milhorat TH, Kotzoen RM, Anzil AP (1994) Stenosis of central canal of spinal cord in man: incidence and pathological findings in 232 autopsy cases. J Neurosurg 80:716–722
9. Milhorat T, Capocelli AL Jr, Anzil AP, Kotzen RM, Milhorat RH (1995) Pathological basis of spinal cord cavitation in syringomyelia: analysis of 105 autopsy cases. J Neurosurg 82:802–812
10. Pojunas K, Williams AL, Daniels DL, Haughton VM (1984) Syringomyelia and hydromyelia: magnetic resonance evaluation. Radiology 153:679–683
11. Sherman JL, Barkovich AJ, Citrin CM (1986) The MR appearance of syringomyelia: new observations. AJNR 7:985–995

12. Williams B (1969) The distending force in the production of "communicating syringomyelia." Lancet II:189–193
13. Williams B (1991) Pathogenesis of syringomyelia. In: Batzdorf U (ed) Syringomyelia: current concepts in diagnosis and treatment. Williams & Wilkins, Baltimore, pp 59–90

Abstract

Treatment of Syringomyelia

Harold J. Hoffman

The term syringomyelia was coined by Ollivier in 1827. [3] The condition was regarded as a degenerative process of the spinal cord until relatively recent times. Gardner pointed out the developmental connection between syringomyelia and the physiological hydrocephalus and hydromyelia, evident in the fetus, that resolve after the outlets of the 4th ventricle become established. He postulated that the Chiari malformation associated with lack of opening of outlets of the 4th ventricle was the primary cause of cystic expansion of the central canal. [1]

Syringomyelia is detined as a condition marked by abnormal cavities filled with liquid in the substance of the spinal cord. We have used posterior fossa decompression with plugging of the obex in Chiari I's as well as Chiari II's. In some patients, we have used syrinx shunting into the pleural cavity. The Chiari II malformation is the commonest cause of syringomyelia in our patients, whereas the Chiari I malformation accounts for 25% of our patient population. Posterior fossa, decompression, and plugging of the obex will result in amelioration of symptoms in prevention of deterioration in the vast majority of patients with syringomyelia in childhood.

References

1. Gardner WJ (1965) Hydrodynamic mechanism of syringomyelia: Its relationship to myclocoele. J Neurol Neurosurg Psychiatry 28:247
2. Hall PV, Campbell RL, Kalsbeck JE (1975) Meningomyelocele and progressive hydromyelia. J Neurosurg 43:457–463
3. Ollivier CP (1827) *Traite de la Moelle Epiniere et de Ses Maladies.* Paris, Crevot, cd 2 vol 1
4. Turnbull FA (1933) Syringomyelie complications of spina bifida. Brain 56:304

Anatomy of the Spinal Cord with Meningomyelocele and Tethered Cord Symptoms

David B. Shurtleff[1], David Moskowitz[1], E. Weinberger[2], Sharon Duguay[1], and J. Loeser[3]

Summary. This chapter describes the anatomy of the spinal cord in children born with meningomyelocele, and reviews co-morbidities following the primary repair of meningomyeloceles. Data from 654 cases of meningomyelocele have been drawn from a computerized database, Patient Data Management System/fx [16]. We have also performed computer-assisted analysis of magnetic resonance imaging (MRI) studies of the spinal cord. This chapter describes the anatomy of the spinal cord of 41 patients examined by 67 MRI studies from a total of 83 patients. All cases were selected because they experienced symptoms compatible with a tethered cord and had had a neurosurgical procedure. An additional five were diagnosed with spinal cord hypoplasia. Tethered cord symptoms were related to local scarring, and improved following surgical release for 62 of the 83 postmeningomyelocele repair patients. Of the symptoms of the other 21 patients, 16 were relieved by other operations (e.g., CSF shunt repair) and five were not subjected to an untethering procedure because of a diagnosis of spinal cord hypoplasia. Etiologies other than, or in addition to, tethering included an obstructed cerebrospinal fluid shunt, syringohydromyelia, and benign tumor, as well as spinal cord hypoplasia. The areas of spinal cords were determined from axial MRI by digitized cross sections of 23 vertebral levels of the 41 patients and five normal controls. These studies differentiated very small, symptomatic spinal cords from the spinal cords of symptomatic and asymptomatic syringohydromyelia as well as from spinal cords of patients with spinal cord tethering. Collaborative, multicenter studies of larger numbers of patients are recommended.

Key words. Meningomyelocele, Tethered cord, Syringohydrobulbia, Spinal cord, Hypoplasia, Spina bifida aperta, Syringohydromyelia, Magnetic resonance imaging (MRI), Hydromyelia, Syringomyelia

Introduction

In 1973, Emery and Lendon [5] described a series of 100 infants and children born with meningomyelocele who had multiple cord abnormalities (Table 1). Four years later, Hoffman et al. [8] reported clinical signs and symptoms and operative observations that they attrib-

[1] Department of Pediatrics, Division of Congenital Defects,
[2] Department of Radiology,
[3] Department of Neurological Surgery, University of Washington School of Medicine, Seattle, WA, USA

TABLE 1. Differential diagnosis of tethered cord symptoms or pathologic anatomy

Type of study	Pathologic postmortem	MRI ±Sx	MRI Stable				
Authors	Emery and Lendon	Just et al.	McEnery et al.	Seattle			
Year	1972	1988	1992	1997[a]			
No. of patients	100	56	20	654			
%MM (%)	100	100	70	100			
Low-lying cord (%)	–	84	95	100			
Tc Sx post-MM repair	–	–	0%	83 (13%)[b,c,d]			
				TCR 48 (58%)	TCR+ other 14 (17%)[b]	Other pathology 21 (25%)	Sum other pathology ±TCR
Lipoma	1%	–	25%	0	0	0	0
Diastematomyelia	5%	–		0	0	0	0
Hydromyelia, syringomyelia	43%	7%	26%	0	7[f]	12[e]	19 (23%)
Dermoid/epidermoid	–	–		0	1	0	1 (1%)
Arachnoid cyst	6%	–		0			
Diplomyelia	26%	–		0			
Abnormal No. of central canals	18%	–		0			
Spinal cord hypoplasia	–	–	10%	0	4	5	9 (11%)
CFS shunt revision	–	–		0	1	4	5 (6%)
Normal	1%			0	0	0	0
Suboccipital decompression					1	2[e]	2 (2%)

Data drawn from Emery and Lendon [5], Just et al. [9], and McEnery et al. [12]. Percentages were calculated directly from data reported or derived from calculations from data reported.
Sx = symptoms.
Tc Sx post-MM repair = tethered cord symptoms postinitial meningomyelocele repair.
CSF shunt revision = cerebrospinal fluid shunt revision.
[a] Eliminate cases where CSF shunt provides relief.
[b] One patient had a composite of all 3 (therefore suspect 54% tethered cord alone).
[c] 83/654 (13%) = those with symptoms or signs; % below are of the 83 with presenting symptoms.
[d] Question whether low-lying or symptomatic or both.
[e] Two patients had both.
[f] Includes one myelocystocele.

uted to tension on the spinal cord or a "tethered spinal cord." In 1981, Yamada et al. [20] described the "tethered cord syndrome" (TCS), and later related this syndrome in cats and man to tension on the spinal cord. In 1991, Tani et al. [19] described changes in the length of the spinal canal upon flexion and extension of the back. In 1983, Reigel [15] described 102 cases of tethered spinal cord, most (88%) following prior meningomyelocele repair. The same year, McLone [13] cautioned that patients with repaired meningomyelocele should not be allowed to lose function; TCS is one of the correctable causes of loss of function. Eight years later, Herman et al. [7] divided 153 cases of TCS into those seen postmeningomyelocele repair (100 cases), and those following initial resection of lipomeningomyelocele (53 cases). Reigel

[15] reviewed cases with symptoms of tethered cord and emphasized that clinical symptoms and signs established the diagnosis, and that contrast studies defined only the pathologic anatomy. Throughout this period, many papers were published describing post-meningomyelocele repair in cohorts of patients, both with and without symptoms [1–4, 6, 9, 12, 18].

These clinical studies reported low-lying cords as either a finding in asymptomatic patients or as a symptomatic tethered cord. Hydromyelia and syringomyelia were reported by clinicians in 3–25% of cases, but the definition of what constitutes the difference between these two diagnoses, and their clinical significance compared with asymptomatic benign enlargement of the central canal [5] has not been discussed [1–4, 6, 7, 12, 15, 18]. In addition, diastematomyelia, thickened filum terminale, dermoid, epidermoid, spinal cord hypoplasia, and the need for excluding cerebrospinal fluid shunt obstruction or compression in the posterior fossa requiring a shunt revision or suboccipital decompression were all mentioned infrequently or not at all by these authors.

Only a few authors commented on the need for correction of multiple pathologic entities in a single individual. Herman and associates [7] cautioned against the diagnosis of TCS until the function of an associated cerebrospinal fluid shunt had been established. Reigel [15] mentioned three patients with acute shunt failure immediately following an untethering procedure, as well as acute posterior fossa compression as complications. Co-morbidities reported by most authors indicated a low-lying conus and other pathologic conditions which must have co-existed in some of their patients since the percentage of at least two conditions exceed 100% of their reported cases. Reported in abstract form [11] and as a finding in case descriptions [6], and presented before the International Symposium on Spina Bifida, Part 1, in Chicago in 1996, were several case examples by Byrd. These were cases where hypoplasia (atrophy or malacia) of the spinal cord in association with meningomyelocele as a cause for spasticity and apparent loss of function has not been distinguished from thin spinal cords in asymptomatic meningomyelocele patients or those with decreased viscoelastic attachment, causing symptoms as reported by Yamada et al. [20].

This study was therefore designed with two objectives in an attempt to clarify the anatomy of the spinal cord in these various conditions. These objectives include, in addition to those in our prior report [17],

1. to describe the quantitative significance of central canal enlargements, hydromyelia, or syringohydromyelia as defined by Rauzzino and Oakes [14];
2. to define the anatomy of spinal cord hypoplasia (atrophy or malacia) as distinct from normal spinal cords or those of children with meningomyelocele.

Methods

The world's literature was searched from 1859 to the present for pertinent citations. Only those few most closely related to this study have been included.

A data file commenced in 1957 and entered into a computer since 1968, labeled the Patient Data Management System (PDMS/fx) [16], was searched. We included in this search only those patients born since January 1965, and only those with a diagnosis of previously repaired meningomyelocele who were undergoing another neurosurgical procedure, lateral or fourth ventricle cerebrospinal fluid shunt revision or insertion, suboccipital decompression, syringohydromyelia (SHM) cavity drainage (this term includes hydromyelia and syrinx, often used interchangeably in the past), and any form of spinal exploration with laminectomy. *The absolute requirements for inclusion in this review were surgical indications that included symptoms compatible with TCS or spinal cord hypoplasia.* Magnetic resonance imaging, computerized tomography, and spinal contrast study data have not been entered into PDMS/fx files because they constitute their own permanent record. Spinal cord cross-sectional area data were collected for TCS patients and normal controls. Test–retest variations were determined.

Magnetic resonance image (MRI) scans of all of the patients with meningomyelocele seen in our center that are of sufficient clarity were included in this analysis. The axial cut nearest the center of the vertebral body was measured for the greatest lateral width of the central canal, syringohydromyelia (SHM), and the outer edge to the spinal cord to the nearest 1.0 mm using a translucent ruler and a hard copy of the MRI scan. The greatest lateral measurement of each was used to calculate the percentage of the width to the spinal cord represented by SHM.

The area of the cross section of the spinal cord at each vertebral level was determined by viewing the same axial cut for each vertebral body on an independent computer workstation. Motion or flow artifacts caused the axial MRI views of vertebral levels on some examinations to be uninterpretable because of indistinct borders to the spinal cord. The majority were sufficiently clear to provide reasonably accurate estimates of the cross-sectional areas of the cord (Figs. 1–3). The areas of the SHM and the spinal cord were automatically calculated by the computer after the borders of the SHM and the outer edges of the spinal cord were traced manually (Figs. 4 and 5). The first determinations were repeated after varying intervals of time to prevent possible effects of memory improving test–retest accuracy. The test–retest accuracy for the three measurements by the examiner (D.M.) was 1.7 mm ±2.3 of 1364 observations (95% confidence limits = 0.1 mm), and there were insignificant differences between the first and second, first and third, and second and third measurements.

The areas of cross sections of the cords of patients with symptoms and findings of TCS insufficient to warrant surgical exploration after correction of other causes were compared with those with untethering. Since there was no difference, these data were combined and, in the absence of SHM, were considered as meningomyelocele control cases.

Analyses for differences in proportions were tested by chi-square (χ^2) or Fisher's exact test. Differences in means were tested by Student's *T* test for unequal numbers, and spinal cord areas of patients with meningomyelocele were compared with those of age-matched normal controls by the paired *T* statistic.

Results

Of our 654 patients who experienced a primary meningomyelocele repair, 83 (13%) had developed tethered cord symptoms. These 83 postmeningomyelocele repair patients experienced 62 spinal cord untethering and 35 other neurosurgical procedures. Of these 35 other procedures, 21 were performed with resolution of the symptoms thought to be due to a tethered cord, and 14 were performed in addition to tethered cord release. Five were not operated on (Table 2). These five were patients who developed progressive spasticity in their legs and were noted to have spinal cords as thin and as undulant as four who did not respond to one or more untethering procedures. The youngest patient noted to have spinal cord hypoplasia was 7 days of age.

There were too few patients in the other groups of causes associated with TCS to analyze for significant differences in presenting symptoms and signs. Differences between the

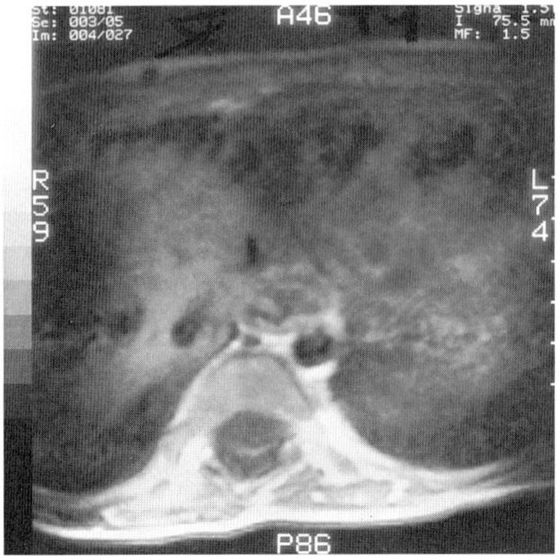

1

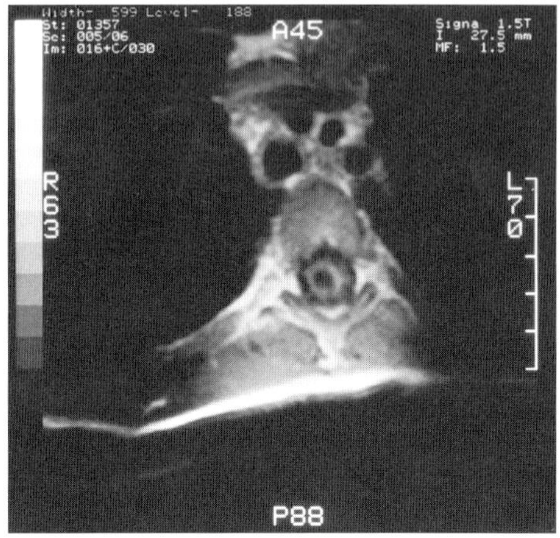

2

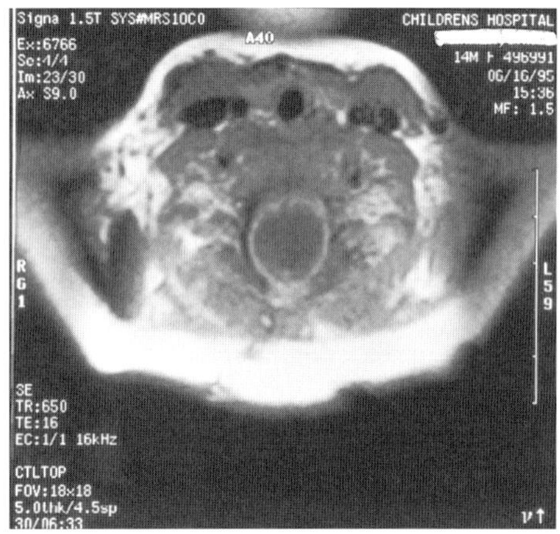

3

FIG. 1. Axial view of the thoracic cord of a meningomyelocele patient with a hypoplastic cord
FIG. 2. Axial view of the thoracic cord of a meningomyelocele patient with an enlarged central canal
FIG. 3. Axial view of the cervical cord of a meningomyelocele patient with SHM

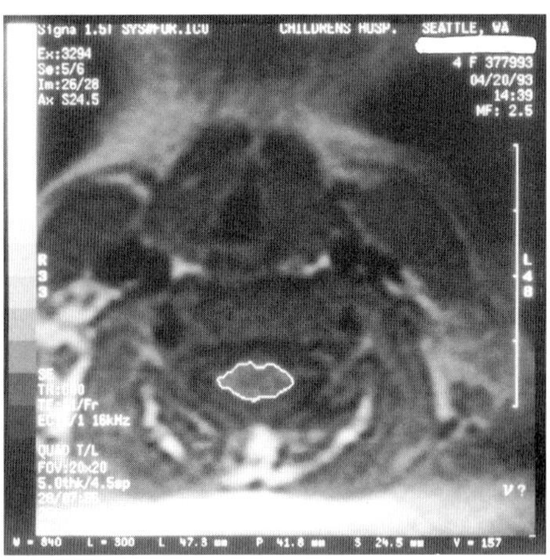

FIG. 4. Axial MRI scan with cord traced. No central canal visible

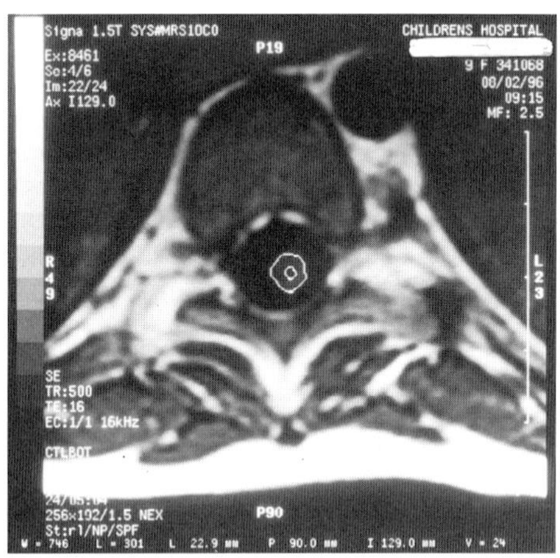

FIG. 5. Axial MRI scan with central canal and spinal cord traced

TABLE 2. Eighty-three cases with tethered cord symptoms

	Tethered cord release	Other cause and tethered cord release	Other cause
Untethering procedure	48	14[a]	–
SHM	–	6	10
SOD	–	1	2[c]
V-PSR	–	1	4
Dermoid removal	–	1	–
Myelocystocele drainage	–	1	–
SCH	–	4[b]	5[d]
TOTALS	48	14[a]	21

SHM, syringohydromyelia; SOD, suboccipital decompression; V-PSR, ventriculoperitoneal shunt revision; SCH, spinal cord hypoplasia.

[a] A total of 14 cases with at least two operations each (several had more than one untethering procedure).

[b] No relief from untethering procedures.

[c] Both SHM drainage and SOD.

[d] Not operated on; selected from symptom complex and MRI findings after the first four cases with axial cross-sectional areas less than 10 mm^2 did not respond to untethering procedures.

symptoms reported in the Seattle groups of patients and one other series [7] are insignificant except for the greater frequency in loss of urine continence in the Seattle group [17].

The number of operations for TCS with or without co-morbidities showed a significant increase, beginning in 1989, for patients with meningomyelocele [17].

The earliest age of operation for meningomyelocele patients postrepair, with tethered cord symptoms, was less than 1 year, with a distribution similar to that reported by Herman et al. [7, 17].

Spinal Cord Hypoplasia (Atrophy, Malacia)

The mean area of the cord at all vertebral levels for patients with and without SHM were remarkably similar and have been combined (Fig. 6). The mean areas of the spinal cord of patients with meningomyelocele were significantly smaller than normal in the thoracic vertebral levels ($T = 8$, df $= 1$, $P = 0.000002$) (Fig. 6, Table 3). Those patients with progressive spasticity and failure to develop useful function not stabilized by cord untethering usually developed symptoms as infants and had markedly small cord cross-sectional areas compared with age peers with meningomyelocele ($T = 11$, df $= 11$, $P < 0.000001$) (Table 3). The ages of patients with meningomyelocele and spinal cord hypoplasia were 7 days to 13 years.

Syringohydromyelia (SHM)

The majority of the patients with meningomyelocele and symptoms leading to an MRI of the neural axis had sufficient central canal enlargement to be visible and capable of being measured (42 of 67; Figs. 2, 3, and 5). However, only 7 of the 42 with measurable enlargement of the spinal cord central canal had symptoms sufficient to warrant surgical intervention. The 35 with symmetric, small SHM were all centrally placed and appeared to be enlarged spinal cord central canals. They ranged in lateral width from 1 to 18% of the spinal cord lateral width. None have become larger or symptomatic. The seven larger, symptomatic SHM were also all symmetric and centrally placed. They ranged in lateral width from 20 to 43% of the

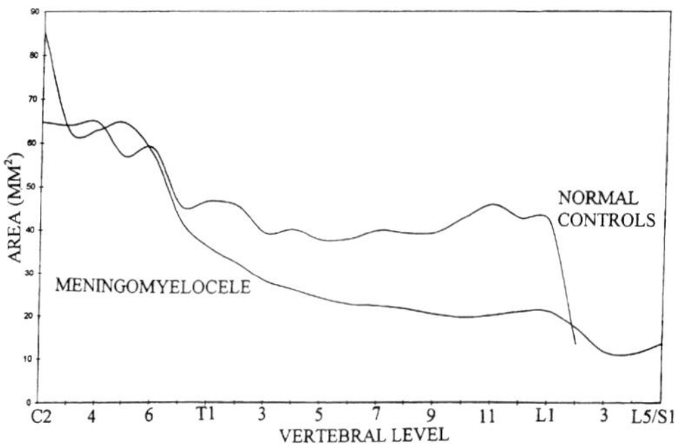

FIG. 6. Mean cord areas of meningomyelocele patients and normal controls

TABLE 3. Comparison of the mean cross section of the spinal cord for normal, meningomyelocele patients, and meningomyelocele patients with spinal cord hypoplasia

Level of axial MRI view	Normal	MM patients	MM patients with SCH
C2	64.0	82.8	117.3
C3	64.0	62.7	57.2
C4	64.7	62.4	52.0
C5	56.9	63.0	45.4
C6	58.8	56.4	47.4
C7	45.5	41.8	29.0
T1	46.6	34.4	19.2
T2	47.4	30.3	15.0
T3	41.7	30.3	12.2
T4	39.3	26.4	10.5
T5	37.3	24.3	10.6
T6	35.1	22.4	8.3
T7	37.3	21.9	7.7
T8	39.6	21.7	6.9
T9	43.6	20.6	6.7
T10	46.4	19.3	6.7
T11	43.0	19.0	5.7
T12	39.2	20.0	3.7
L1	42.0	20.3	7.9
L2	13.0	17.0	8.0
L3	–	12.0	9.0
L4	–	10.5	–
L5/S1	–	15.1	–

MM, meningomyelocele; SCH, spinal cord hypoplasia.
For statistical significance, see text.

spinal cord. These seven cases had maximum width in the C6–T3 and T10–T11 and, to a lesser extent, in the T5–T7 vertebral levels (Figs. 2, 3, 7, 8). All degrees of spinal canal enlargement were noted in some cases to be localized (Fig. 7), and if large and over a long segment, they were haustral in appearance (Fig. 8). These enlargements and relative constrictions do not conform to known anatomy or embryology. They are not consistent between or among cases except for the cervical and high thoracic cases exemplified by Figs. 3, 7, and 8.

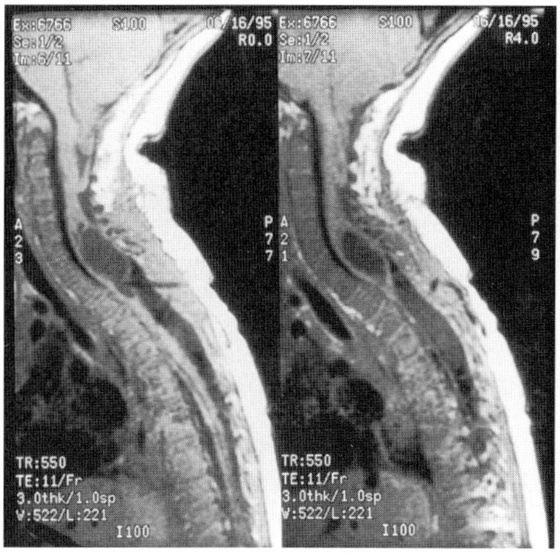

7

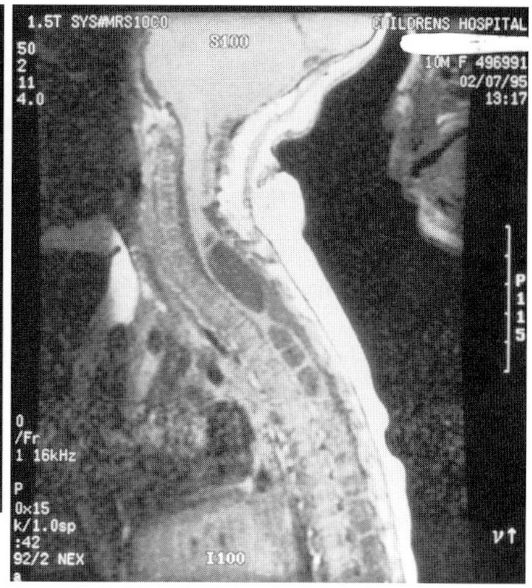

8

FIG. 7. MRI, sagittal view; localized symptomatic hydromyelia
FIG. 8. MRI, sagittal view; holocord symptomatic hydromyelia with haustral pattern

Discussion

This report follows one given in July 1997 [17] and is of an ongoing project that is both prospective (data from the PDMS file [16] including symptoms, surgical indications, operations, and findings at the time of surgery) and retrospective (primarily analyses of MRI studies). The selection of cases described in Methods and the small number of MRI studies performed on asymptomatic patients (because of the cost in our system of health care) introduce a bias. The findings of McEnery et al. [12], who studied neurologically stable children, suggest many of our asymptomatic meningomyelocele patients have the types of pathology described in our symptomatic patients and by Emery and Lendon [5]. The co-morbidities described further limit our conclusions at this time. We believe, however, that the following observations are valid.

Prevalence in the Population

As documented in our first report [17], the techniques for noninvasive anatomic definition, and awareness of the significance of symptoms and signs of TCS improved over the period of this study, favoring diagnosis earlier for those cared for in the later years of the study. We have demonstrated the onset of tethered cord symptoms throughout childhood without an increase in frequency during the adolescent growth spurt. This observation confirms Herman et al.'s [7] original description. Some of our young patients may yet develop TCS and alter our statistics.

Prevalence of Co-Morbidities

The large variation in the occurrence and type of co-morbidities and the inclusion of spina bifida occulta in some series, as well as the relatively low prevalence of each individual co-morbidity, decrease the ability of this report to define the significance of individual co-morbidities. The importance of eliminating a nonfunctional cerebrospinal fluid shunt as a cause for tethered cord-like symptoms, as recommended by the Chicago group [7], is supported by our findings (Table 2). Since virtually all asymptomatic, postrepair meningomyelocele patients have a low-lying conus with apparent adhesion of the cord dorsally (84–100%; Table 1), and since increased intracranial pressure can mimic tethered cord symptoms, the entire neural axis should be imaged if the patient has symptoms consistent with a tethered cord.

List of the Differential Diagnoses of Tethered Cord Syndrome

Table 1 provides a list of conditions that we believe may cause symptoms that can be mistaken for tethered cord.

Spinal Cord Hypoplasia (Atrophy or Malacia)

1. The greater cross-sectional area of the high cervical spinal cord in children with meningomyelocele compared with those of normal controls was expected because it probably represents caudally displaced medulla and cerebellum associated with the Arnold–Chiari II malformation (Fig. 6, Table 3).

2. The presence of spinal cord below L1 was also expected because of the many descriptions of caudally displaced lower spinal cord (Fig. 6, Table 3). We did not expect the areas of cross sections of cord distal to L1 to be so small, both because of the overgrowth theory, and because the dorsal curve of the distal spinal cord rendered our MRI cross sections as tangential to the axis of the cord rather than more nearly at right angles.

3. In addition, the smaller cross-sectional areas of the thoracic levels compared with normal spinal cords represent another feature of the multiple nervous system anomalies seen with meningomyelocele (Fig. 6, Table 3).

4. The markedly small cross-sectional areas of the undulant spinal cord of patients with progressive spasticity and failure to develop useful function, as well as failure to relieve symptoms by untethering procedures, were reported previously as spinal cord hypoplasia, atrophy, or malacia [11, 17]. These observations also suggest that stretching of the spinal cord, described by Tani et al. [19] and Yamada et al. [20], is not a likely cause for the symptoms. Such a thin spinal cord was noted in a 7-day-old patient, suggesting hypoplasia rather than postnatal atrophy or malacia secondary to a sterile inflammatory process as described by Emery and Lendon [5] McEnery et al. [12] described 10% of neurologically stable patients with meningomyelocele as having qualitatively small spinal cords. Our observations (Fig. 1, Table 3) suggest the need for further quantitative study of neurologically stable patients with meningomyelocele in order to be certain that our symptomatic patients with spinal cord hypoplasia constitute a clinically different subgroup. It is important to note that all our patients diagnosed with hypoplasia of the spinal cord had less than 30–50% of the comparable levels amongst other meningomyelocele patients. In fact, none of the spinal cord hypoplasia patients had cord cross sections exceeding 10 mm^2 below T5, and none of the normal controls or other meningomyelocele patients had cross-sectional areas below 10 mm^3. It is important to confirm or disprove this distinction, because prenatal ultrasound studies may soon be able to identify spinal cords small enough to allow clinicians to predict less favorable clinical outcomes. Secondly, if untethering is going to be ineffective, unnecessary surgery can be avoided.

Syringohydromyelia (Hydromyelia or Syrinx)

Our data clarify the definitions of these two words in cases of fluid collection in the spinal cords of patients with meningomyelocele. The symmetry and central location of the SHM strongly suggest that these lesions are central spinal cord canal enlargements (hydromyelia) and not syrinxes. We found the central canal in both symptomatic and asymptomatic post-meningomyelocele patients to be enlarged as well as duplicated both symmetrically and asymmetrically, as described by Emery and Lendon [5]. In addition, the noncircular cross sections of the cord of many of our patients required that we use the computerized digitation method for describing cross-sectional areas, normal cords, and both hydromyelic and nonhydromyelic cords of meningomyelocele patients.

We believe we have sufficent data to establish the vast majority of spinal cord fluid collections as enlargements of the central canal or hydromyelia, due to their symmetry and central location. The term syrinx should be used for asymmetric fluid collections either separate from, or contiguous with, the central canal.

A surprise was the more useful and simple comparison of the lateral widths of the fluid collections with spinal cord widths as identifying significant degrees of hydromyelia. We had expected the more time-consuming calculation of the areas of cross section to be more informative.

Conclusions

This study has suggested that other diagnoses and co-morbidities contribute to the clinical outcome of the treatment of meningomyelocele patients with tethered cord symptoms. In addition, there is a need to expand our quantitative studies of hypoplasia of the spinal cord and hydromyelia in order to better understand their contributions to the clinical outcome of the treatment of meningomyelocele. *Hence, there is need for multicenter, collaborative long-term studies with identical definition of data in order to address the unknowns identified to date in this study.* We invite potential collaborators to contact us.

Acknowledgments. Appreciation is expressed to Karen Sizemore, Elaine Smith, Katherine Stice, and Cynthia Shurtleff for their assistance in the preparation of this manuscript. Financial support was provided by the Birth Defects Research fund at the Children's Hospital and Medical Center, the Department of Neurological Surgery, University of Washington School of Medicine, and the March of Dimes Birth Defects Foundation.

References

1. Azimullah PC, Smit LM, Rietveld-Knol E, Valk J (1991) Malformations of the spinal cord in 53 patients with spina bifida studied by magnetic resource imaging. Child's Nerv Syst 7:63–66
2. Begeer JH, Wiertsma GP, Breukers SM, Mooy JJ, terWeeme CA (1989) Tethered cord syndrome: clinical signs and results of operation in 42 patients with spina bifida aperta and occulta. Z Kinderchir 44, Suppl 1:5–7
3. Bono R, Inverno M, Botteon G, Bruzzone MG, Vaghi MA, Solero CL, Perlasca E, Fedrizzi E (1993) Clinical features and MR imaging in children with repaired myelomeningocele. Ital J Neuro Sci 14:553–559
4. Carstans C, Fromm B, Ludwig B, Higer HP, Ermert J (1990) Intraspinale Anomalien bei der Myelomeningozele. Z Orthop Ihre Grenzgeb 128:559–563
5. Emery JL, Lendon RG (1973) The local cord lesion in neurospinal dysraphism (meningomyelocele). J Pathol 110:83–96
6. Hawnaur JM, Hughes D, Jenkins JP, Bannister CM, Isherwood I (1991) Investigation of children with suspected spinal dysraphism by magnetic resonance imaging. Eur J Pediatr Surg 1, Suppl 1:18–19

7. Herman JM, McLone DG, Storrs BB, Dauser RC (1993) Analysis of 153 patients with myelomeningocele or spinal lipoma reoperated upon for a tethered cord. Presentation, management and outcome. Pediatr Neurosurg 19:243–249
8. Hoffman JH, Hendrick EB, Humphreys RP (1976) The tethered spinal cord. Its protean manifestations, diagnoses and surgical correction. Child's Brain 2:145–155
9. Just M, Schwarz M, Ludwig B, Ermert J, Thelen M (1990) Cerebral and spinal MR-findings in patients with postrepair myelomeningocele. Pediatr Radiol 20:262–266
10. Lasser AM, Rasmussen GL (1938) A quantitative study of the newborn and adult spinal cords of man. J Comp Neurol 69:371–379
11. McDonald CM, Shurtleff DB, Weinberger E (1992) Diffuse spinal-cord atrophy/hypoplasia in myelomeningocele. Dev Med Child Neurol 34, Suppl 1:4
12. McEnery G, Borzyskowski M, Cox TCS, Nelville BGR (1992) The spinal cord in neurologically stable spina bifida: a clinical and MRI study. Dev Med Child Neurol 34:342–347
13. McLone DG (1983) Results of treatment of children born with a myelomeningocele. Clin Neurosurg 30:407–412
14. Rauzzino M, Oakes WJ (1995) Chiari II malformation and syringomyelia. Neurosurg Clin NA 6:293–309
15. Reigel DH (1983) Tethered spinal cord. Concepts Pediatr Neurosurg 4:142–164
16. Shurtleff DB (1991) Computer data bases for pediatric disability: clinical and research applications. Phys Med Rehabil Clin NA 2:665–687
17. Shurtleff DB, Duguay S, Duguay G, Moskowitz D, Weinberger E, Roberts T, Loeser J (1997) Epidemiology of tethered cord with meningomyelocele. Eur J Pediatr Surg 7, Suppl I:1–5
18. Tamaki N, Shirataki K, Kojima N, Shouse Y, Matsumoto S (1988) Tethered cord syndrome of delayed onset following repair of myelomeningocele. J Neurosurg 69:393–398
19. Tani S, Yamada S, Fuse T, Nakamura N (1991) Chances in lumbosacral canal length during flexion and extension—dynamic effect on the elongated spinal cord in the tethered cord. No to Shinkei—Brain & Nerve 43:1121–1125
20. Yamada S, Iacono RP, Andrade T, Mandybur G, Yamada BS (1995) Pathophysiology of tethered cord syndrome. Neuro Surg Clinics of NA 6:311–323

Abstract

The Tethered Spinal Cord

HAROLD J. HOFFMAN

The tethered spinal cord has been recognized for a long time. The neurologic deterioration which occurs as a result of traction on the conus medullaris by a thickened tight filum terminale was brought to the general attention by Anderson's article [1] in 1975, describing tethering as a result of intradural fibrous adhesions, diasternatomyelia, dermal sinus tracts, intradural lipomas, lipomyelomeningoceles, and adhesive arachnoiditis at the site of the previous neonatal myelomeningocele repair. Indeed, the term has been used as a very loose diagnosis to include all the previously mentioned surgical pathological entities.

The present symptoms and signs in this group of patients showed signs of motor or sensory loss in the lower extremities with bladder dysfunction. Scoliosis was associated with either lower limb involvement or bladder dysfunction. The results of operative treatment were dramatic in most cases. In all patients who had pain, there was either a total disappearance of their symptoms or a significant improvement. The tethered cord, which problably occurs more commonly than is recognized and whose diagnosis is dependent on an alert group of clinicians of various specialites, results in a reversible neurological deficit in most patients.

References

1. Anderson FM (1975) Occult spinal dysraphism: A series of 73 cases, Pediatrics 55:826–835
2. Fitz CR, and Harwood-Nash DC (1975) The tethered conus. Am J Radiol 125:515–523
3. Fukui J, and Kakizuki T (1980) Urodynamic evaluation of the tethered cord syndrome including tight filum terminale. Urology 15:539–552
4. Hoffman HJ, Hendrick EB, and Humphreys RP (1976) The tethered spinal cord: Its protean manifestations, diagnosis and surgical correction. Child's Brain 2:145–155
5. Pang D, and Wilberger JE (1982) Tethered cord syndrome in adults. J Neurosurg, 57:32–47
6. Yamada S, Zinke DE, and Sanders D (1981) Pathophysiology of tethered cord syndrome J Neurosurg 54:494–503

Department of Neurosurgery, The Hospital for Sick Children, 555 University Avenue, Toronto, Ontario, M5G 1X8, Canada

Abstract

Spina Bifida Occulta with Tethered Spinal Cord

Kuniyoshi Ohisuka

Spina bifida occulta is not a rare occurrence. But clinical evaluations, roentgenological findings, and neurological deficit about this disease have not been clarified enough. The author has studied 648 cases of spina bifida occulta from three points of view: radiological studies, clinical findings, and surgical explorations.

1. Radiological studies: The author has classified the degree of the laminal defect for three types using X-ray photographs: type A is the slightest one such as simple split, type B is a medium-size laminal defect, and type C the widest one. In this series, there are 411 cases of type A (63%), 193 of type B (30%), and 44 of type C (7%).

   Myelography has been done in 126 cases which have complained of severer disabilities: 61 cases in type A, 41 in type B, and 24 in type C. As a result, neurological abnormalities have been noted in 104 cases. The tight filum terminale has been shown in 76 cases: 53 cases in type A group (77%), 23 in type B (56%), and none in type C. On the other hand, low-placed conus medullaris has never been found in type A group, but it has been observed in 10 in type B (24%), and in all 24 in type C (100%). This fact indicates that the wider laminal defect is associated with the severer neurological abnormality.
2. Clinical features: The majority of this series were children and young adults aged between 5 months and 19 years. Various symptoms were observed in this series: low back pain with or without leg pain, urinary disturbance, neurological deficit, cutaneous manifestations on the back, and others. There are several cases without any symptoms instead of low-placed conus medullaris. Most of them have never showed any symptoms until maturity.

Nagano Prefectural Rehabilitation Center, 618-1 Yoko-cho, Shimokomazawa Nagano 381, Japan

Spinal Dysraphism—A Study of 119 Patients at AIIMS

Anupam Jindal and A.K. Mahapatra

Summary. Spinal dysraphism (SD) is a condition characterized by maldevelopment of the neural tube, notocord, mesoderm, and cutaneous ectoderm. The incidence of SD is 2–4/1000 live births. We studied 119 patients operated on from January 1991 to June 1996. Only 21 patients (17.6%) presented when they were less than 1 year old, and 17 patients came as adults (<16 years). The lumbar and lumbosacral regions were the most commonly involved site in 81 patients (74.7%). Weakness of the lower limbs (74%), difficulty in walking (54.6%), and muscle atrophy (41.2%) were the commonest indicators of motor system involvement. Loss of sensation, trophic ulcer, and backache were seen in 45, 14, and 10 patients, respectively. Cutaneous lipoma (26%), hypertrichiosis (20%), dermal sinus (13.4%), and middle dimple (7%) were the important cutaneous markers. Foot abnormality was seen in 25% of cases. Tethering of the cord, syringomyelia, and split cord malformation were the most common radiological findings. Only 10% of our patients had hydrocephalus which required a shunt. Out of 119 cases operated on, 43 showed an improvement. Twenty had sensory improvement and 18 showed motor improvement. Fifteen patients regained continence. Twelve patients were lost to follow-up. Sixty-seven patients had no change in neurological status postoperatively. Six cases deteriorated in terms of motor/sensory deficit, and one patient lost continence. CSF leak (8%) and wound infection (6%) were the most common complications. Six patients required further surgery in the form of a theroperitoneal (TP) shunt (four), a rotation flap (one), or reexploration and duraplasty (one).

Key words. Spinal dysraphism, Results, Complications

Introduction

Spinal dysraphism (SD) is a condition characterized by maldevelopment of the neural tube, notochord, mesoderm, cutaneous ectoderm, and rarely endoderm [1–8]. The incidence of SD is 2–4/1000 live births, and no epidemiological studies are available from India. The association of urological and orthopedic malformations complicates the management of these children. We present the outcome of 119 patient with SD operated on at the Department of Neurosurgery (AIIMS) from January 1991 to June 1996. This study was done to assess the results of our surgical treatment of spinal dysraphism.

Department of Neurosurgery, CN Centre, AIIMS, New Delhi 110029, India

TABLE 1. Age distribution of patients and site of spinal dysraphism

	No. of patients
Age group (years)	
0–1	21
1–5	40
5–16	41
>16	17
Site	
Cervical	2
Dorsal	16
Dorsolumbar	8
Lumbar	45
Lumbosacral	44
Sacral	4

Material and Methods

Between January 1991 and June 1996, 119 cases were on operated for SD and were analysed retrospectively. The age of the patients varied from 8 days to 47 years (mean 7.2 years) at the time of surgery. There were 73 male and 46 female patients. Only 21 patients were operated on at less than 1 year old, and 17 patients were over 16 years (Table 1). Twenty-nine patients required further surgery because of an incomplete operation carried out during first surgery elsewhere. All patients underwent detailed neurological examination, and were investigated to establish a diagnosis. Magnetic resonance imaging (MRI) was done routinely to delineate the underlying neural tube defect except in 12 cases. Twenty cases had computed tomography (CT) or a CT myelogram. Of these, 8 patients underwent MRI as well. The craniovertebral junction and the brain were evaluated by MRI whenever suggested by the clinical findings and permitted by the patient's financial status. Somatosensory evoked potentials (SSEPs) were found in 38 cases preoperatively and postoperatively as part of separate study carried out during same period. All patients had appropriate surgery (detethering, excision of bony/cartilaginous spur, intraspinal lipoma, etc.) depending on the underlying pathology. All patients with a neurological deficit or asymptomatic patients with a neural tube defect (on radiological investigations) underwent surgery. The patients were regularly followed up at the outpatients department.

Observations

Clinical Findings

Most of these patients presented with weakness of limbs (88), difficulty in walking (65), atrophy of muscles (49%), back swelling (31), or incontinence of urine and feces (Table 2). Trophic ulcer and autoamputation of toes were observed in 14 and 1 patients, respectively. Cutaneous abnormalities were observed in 66 patients, and included hypertrichiosis (Fig. 1) in 24, dermal sinus in 16, midline dimple in 9, naeves in 3, and hemangioma in 3 (Table 3). Orthopedic deformities were in common association, and as many as 28 of our

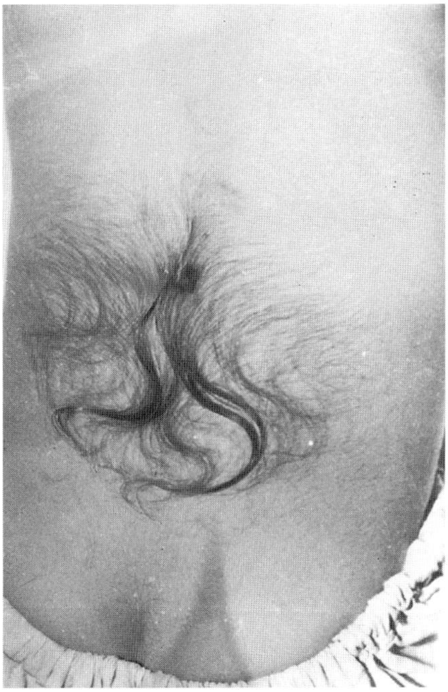

1

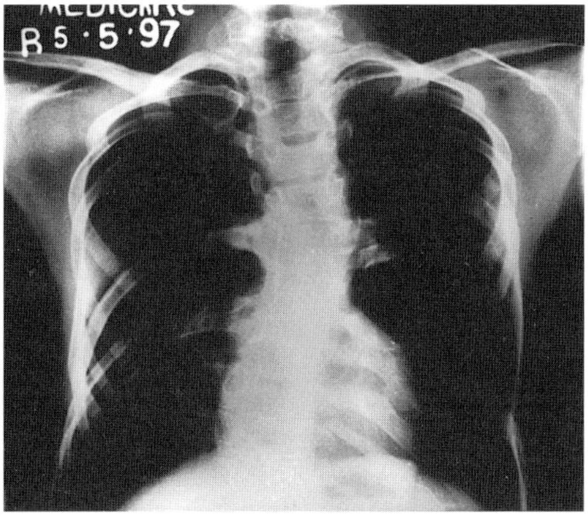

2

Fig. 1. Hypertrichiosis in a 12-year-old child with occult spinal dysraphism
Fig. 2. Chest X-ray of the child in Fig. 1 showing multiple fused ribs

Table 2. Clinical presentation

	Number
Motor system	
Weakness	88
Difficulty in walking	65
Muscle atrophy	49
Hyporeflexia	42
Flexor spasm	01
Hypertonia/hyperreflexia	06
Asymptomatic	16
Sensory system	
Loss of sensation	45
Trophic ulcer	14
Pain	10
Autoamputation	1
Autonomic disturbance	
Bladder and bowel	36
Bladder alone	17

TABLE 3. Cutaneous markers

Skin lesion	No. of patients
Cutaneous lipoma	31
Hypertrichiosis	24
Dermal sinus	16
Midline dimple	9
Naevus	3
Hemangioma	3
Gluteal asymmetry	3
Hypopigmented skin	1
Skin tag	1
Multiple neurofibroma	1

TABLE 4. Associated Pathology

	No. of cases
Skeletal deformity (X ray findings)	
Spina bifida	53
Scoliosis	22
Fused vertebra	7
Bifid sacrum	4
Kyphosis	4
Sacral dysgenesis	5
Hemivertebra	4
Fused lamina	2
Hemilamina	2
Scalloping	2
Lordosis	2
Absent/fused ribs	1
Foot/limb deformity	
Congenital Talipus equino varus (CTEV)	28
Short limb	10
Pes cavus	3
Flat foot	2
Congenital Dislocation of Hip (CDH)	1
CNA pathology	
Syrinx	30
Arnold Chiari Malformation (ACM)	16
Hydrocephalus	11
Aqueductal stenosis	2
Agenesis of corpus callosum	2
Nephrological abnormality	
Absent/small kidney	3
Horseshoe kidney	3
Cystic kidney	1
Hydronephrosis	1

patients had unilateral or bilateral Congenital Talipus equino varus (CTEV). Shortening of one limb was noticed 10 patients (Table 4). A total of 8 patients had urological abnormalities in the form of absent or small kidney, horseshoe kidney, or hydronephrosis (noticed incidentally on MRI). Syringomyelia was the most frequent associated central nervous system (CNS) abnormality, and was seen in 25% patients. The cavity size varied from a small terminal syrinx to large cavities. Chiari malformation was observed in 16 patients. Hydrocephalus had a very low incidence in our group (10%).

Radiological Findings

All patients were investigated to delineate the structural abnormality of the cord and for proper planning of the surgery. MRI scan was the most frequent investigation, and was performed on 107 patients, CT and CT myelogram was carried out on 13 and 7 patients, respectively. Tethered cord (76 patients) was the most frequent finding in our patients. Diastematomyelia/split cord malformation (Fig. 3) was noted in 38 patients and syringomyelia in 29 patients. Only 9 patients had simple meningocele, whereas meningomyelocele and lipomeningomyelocele were more frequent (Table 5). Plain X-rays (detailed information was available in 73 cases) of the spine and chest revealed several other defects of the vertebral column in the form of kyphosis, scoliosis, hemivertebra, sacral dysgenesis, and absent/fused ribs (see Table 4 and Fig. 2).

SSEP (Somatosensory Evoked Potentials)

SSEP were performed pre- and postoperatively in 38 patients. Most recordings were obtained by stimulating the posterior tibial nerve at the ankle. As sensory loss was a frequent finding, preoperative SSEP abnormalities were observed in 100% of children and 80% of adults (Fig. 4). Postoperatively, SSEPs were checked prior to discharge. Over 50% of patients showed SSEP improvement at the time of discharge (within 7–8 days of surgery).

TABLE 5. Radiological findings

	No. of cases
Tethering of cord	76
Syrinx	30
Diastematomyelia	38
Aruold-Chiari-Malformation (ACM)	16
Lipomeningomyelocele	22
Dermoid	15
Meningomyelocele	11
Intradural lipoma	15
Intraspinal lipoma	10
Thick filum	9
Meningocele	9
Diplomyelia	6
Dural band	2
Extradural cyst	1
Filum lipoma	2
Intradural dermoid	1

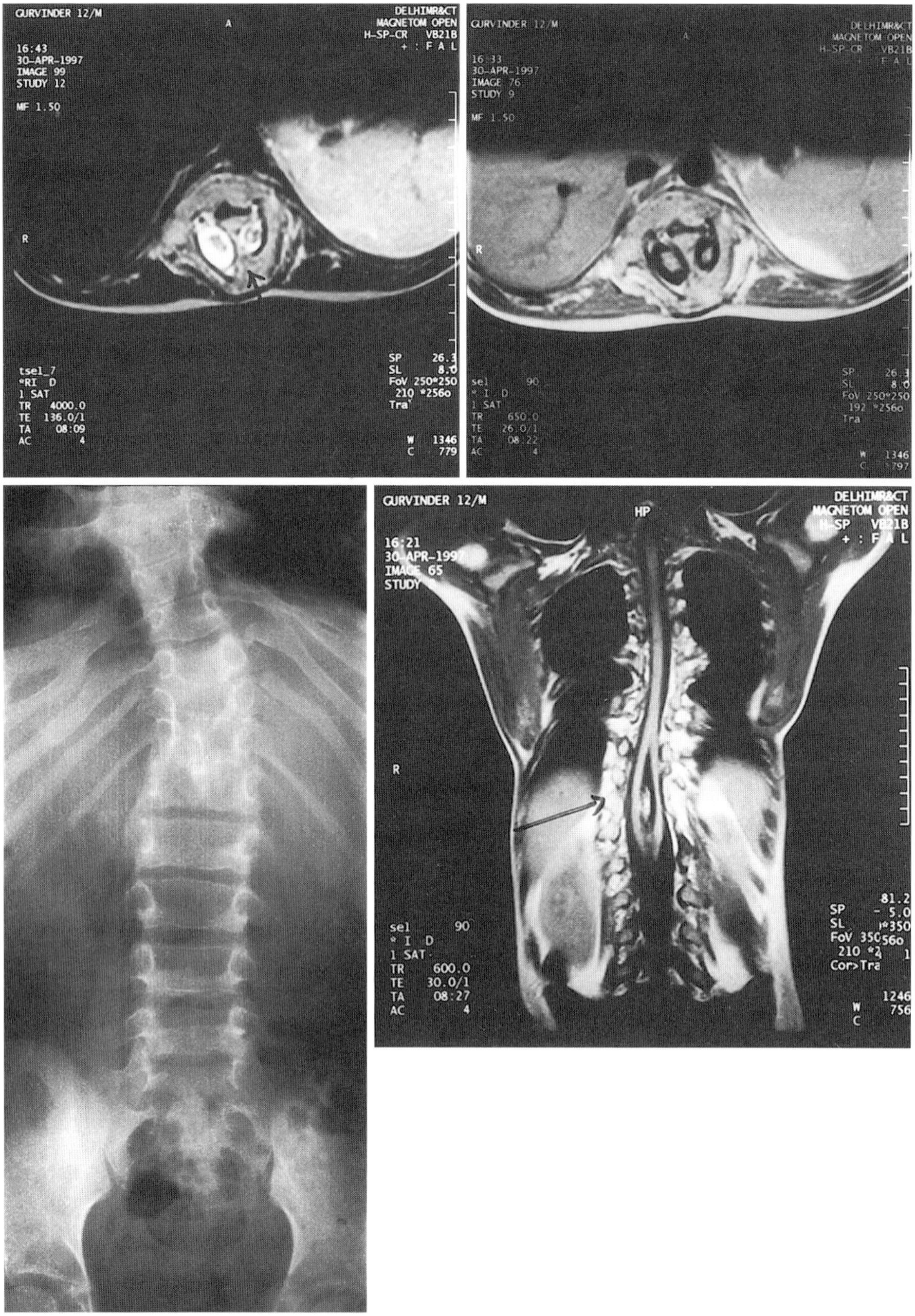

FIG. 3. The same patient as in Fig. 1. X-ray of the dorsolumbar spine, and magnetic resonance imaging showing a bony spur and diastematomyelia at the D12–L1 level

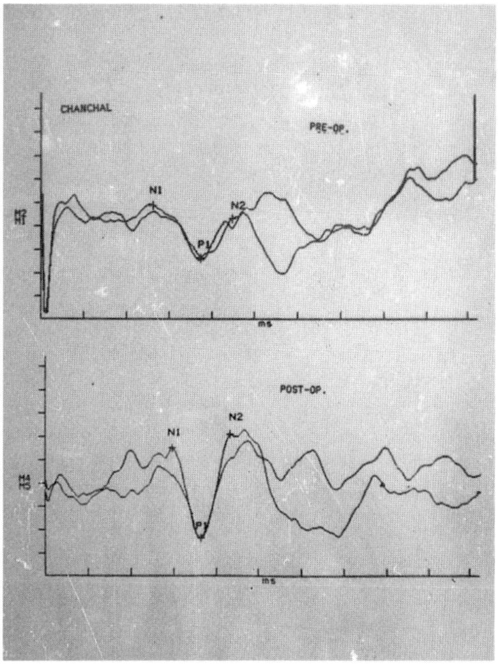

Fig. 4. Somatosensory evoked potentials a case of spinal dysraphism before and after surgery

Table 6. Surgical findings at this hospital[a]

Surgical findings	No. of cases
Tethering of cord	87
Intraspinal lipoma	22
Diastematomyelia and diplomyelia (SCM)	37
Dural band	15
Dermoid	13
Lipomeningomyelocele	22
Meningomyelocele	14
Tight/thick filum	16 (11 + 5)
Intradural lipoma	18
Meningocele	9
Dural ectasia	3
Thin conus	2
Intradural dermoid	1

[a] Primary surgery, 90 cases; reoperation, 29 cases.

Surgical Findings

Twenty-nine patients had their first surgery elsewhere and required a second operation because of either incomplete surgery or progressive neurological deficit. Tethering of the cord (87 patients) was the most frequently observed abnormality, followed by intraspinal lipoma (22) and split cord malformation (37). Dural bands causing tethering were seen in 15 patients,

TABLE 7. Results and complications

	No. of cases
Improvement	
Motor	18
Sensory	20
Bladder and bowel	15
Trophic ulcer	3
Neurological deterioration	
Motor	3
Sensory	3
Bladder and bowel	1
Complications	
CSF leak	15
Wound infection	7
Meningitis	1
Second surgery—shunt	4
—rotation flap	1
Reexploration and duraplasty	1
Death	1

a thick/tight filum was found in 16 patients (Table 6). The aim of surgery was to untether the cord and to preserve as much functional neural tissue as possible. In cases of intraspinal lipoma, as much of the lipoma as possible was removed and the conus was reconstructed. In cases of thick/tight filum terminale, the filum was divided. In the vast majority of cases the large dural defect was repaired using lumbar fascia. Over the last 2 years we have used laminotomy instead of laminectomy as and when possible. We are now using fascia lata routinely in cases of dural defect. The wound was closed in multiple layers to prevent CSF leak postoperatively.

Results

During the hospital stay and on follow-up, 43 patients showed an improvement in neurological status. The follow-up period ranged from 1 year to 5.5 years (mean 2.6 years), and 12 cases were lost to follow-up. Twenty patients had sensory improvement and 18 showed motor improvement. Continence was regained 15 of our patients. In 3 patients, trophic ulcers either healed completely or showed significant improvement (Table 7). Sixty-seven patients had no change in their neurological status postoperatively. There was a good correlation between SSEP and clinical outcome; wherever SSEP showed an improvement, clinical improvement followed. Neurological deterioration occurred in 6 patients. Motor and sensory deficits worsened in 2 patients each,and one patient had both. One of our patients deteriorated in both bladder and bowel function. One patient developed a fresh deficit during follow-up 2 years after surgery, and MRI revealed retethering of the cord. Fifteen of our patients had postoperative CSF leak. Four of these required thecoperitoneal shunt, and two patients underwent reexploration; one had a rotation flap from the erector spinae and the other had duraplasty to stop CSF leak. Wound infection occurred in 7 patients and one had meningitis. There was one operative mortality. The patient was a 6-month-old infant, a case of lipomeningomyelocele, who had a transfusion reaction during surgery and died.

Discussion

Spinal dysraphism is a common malformation of the nervous system reported in 200–400/100 000 live births [9–12]. Surprisingly there are very few publications from India on the subject. As the brain and spinal cord develop from the neural tube, defective neural tube formation also affects the brain [13–16]. Common associations are Arnold-Chiari-Malformation (ACM), syringomyelia, aqueductal abnormalities, and corpus callosum agenesis [15, 17, 18]. As the spina bifida aperta is apparent at birth, these neonates do present to pediatricians and neurosurgeons within a few days of birth. In India, where large numbers of deliveries are conducted at village level, at home or at the PHC (primary health center), these patients may reach tertiary referral hospitals very late. In our study, only 21 patients came to us when they were under 1 year of age; more surprisingly 17 patients were adults at the time of admission. Age has a special bearing on the outcome, as surgery done at an early age is more likely to prevent damage to neural tissue.

In the present study, 37 patients (31%) had split cord malformation. An incidence of 30% is reported by other authors [8, 18]. Among the cutaneous markers, hypertrichiosis was the commonest (20%), and the reported incidence varies from 20 to 56% [18–21]. The presence of hydrocephalus is reported in over 80% of unselected cases [15–17, 22, 23). Surprisingly, in our study only 10% of patients had hydrocephalus severe enough to require a VP shunt. The low incidence of hydrocephalus in our series is partly explained by the selection of cases, and probably represents a group of patients who had survived the neurological disorder. Mental retardation with SD is well known [11, 15, 17, 24, 25). Association with hydrocephalus and shunt infection and anomalies of the CNS are important reasons for subnormal mental function.

Urological abnormalities are not uncommon in spinal dysraphism. A recent publication by Warf et al. [26] reported MRI evidence of tethering in 40 among 76 patients treated for cloacal abnormalities. None of our patients had anorectal anomalies. In 1982, Reigal et al. established that the neural plaque contained functional neural tissue which should be meticulously preserved. SSEP were studied in 38 of our patients, and there was very good correlation between the SSEP finding and the clinical outcome; wherever SSEP showed an improvement, a clinical improvement followed [27]. Better postoperative care, improved anesthesia, and antibiotics have significantly reduced mortality. McLone [22] reported 2 deaths in a series of 100 patients, and we had one death among 119 patients.

During follow-up, clinical deterioration in the form of fresh deficits almost always have a treatable cause, hydrocephalus and rethering being the commonest [22]. However, of the 90 patients who had their first operation in our department, only one developed a fresh deficit in 2 years follow-up after surgery, and repeat MRI showed retethering of the spinal cord (more cases with a similar problem are likely on long-term follow-up, especially if routine postoperative MRI is done in all cases). Twenty-nine patients required repeat surgery, as the initial surgery was not adequate in correcting the underlying pathology. A proper radiological investigation is a must to delineate the underlying pathology. The overt meningocele is only the tip of the iceberg, and excision of a meningocele does not release the tethered cord. Today, MRI is the investigation of choice, and must be carried out in each case prior to surgery to avoid missed pathology and therefore to avoid repeated surgery [28]. A good rehabilitation service is necessary to help these children. Parents, teachers, nurses, and doctors need to participate actively in making each child an independent individual.

Conclusions

Our results indicate that surgery of SD, although difficult, can be carried out with fairly good results. Most complications can be managed conservatively. SSEPs, wherever available, are helpful in predicting the outcome of surgery. A thorough knowledge of the underlying pathology by proper imaging, meticulous surgery, and the use of an operating microscope are the keys to a good outcome.

References

1. Bell HH (1973) Anterior spina bifida and its relation to persistent neuroenteric canal. J Nerv Ment Dis 57:445–462
2. Bremer JL (1952) Dorsal intestinal fistula, accessory neuroenteric canal, diastematomyelia. Arch Pathol 54:53–54
3. Campbell LR, Dayton D, Sohal D (1987) Neural tube defect. A review of human and animal studies on aetiology of neural tube defect. Teratology 34:171–187
4. Cohen AR (1991) The mermaid malformation: cloacal extrophy and ocult spinal dysraphism. Neurosurgery 26:1001–1005
5. Dekaban AS, Barlelmez GW (1964) Complete dysraphism in 14 somite, human embryos. Am J Anat 1115:27–42
6. Herren RL, Edwards JE (1940) Diplomyelia (duplication of spinal cord). Arch Pathol 30:1203–1214
7. Lemire RJ (1966) Variation in development of caudal neural tube in human embryos (horizons XIV–XXI). Teratology 2: 361–370
8. Pang D, Dias MS, Anab-Barmade M (1992) Split cord syndrome malformation. Part 1. A unified theory of embryogenesis for double spinal cord malformation. Neurosurgery 31:451–480
9. O'Neill O (1995) Agenesis and dysgenesis of the sacrum: neurosurgical implications. Pediatr Neurosurg 22:20–28
10. Dabowitz V, Lober J, Zachary RB (1965) Lipoma of the cauda equina. Arch Dis Child 40:207–213
11. James HE, Oliff M, Mulcahy J (1978) Spinal dysraphism. A comprehensive diagnostic approach. Neurosurgery 2:15–21
12. Reigel DH (1982) Spina bifida. In: McLurin RL (eds) Pediatric neurosurgery. Grune and Strattaton, New York, pp 230–247
13. Gardner WJ (1964) Diastematomyelia and Klippel–Feil syndrome: relationship to hydrocephalus, syringomyelia and meningocele, meningomyelocele and anencephalus. Cleveland Clin Q 31:19–44
14. Gardner WJ (1973) The dysraphic state from syringomyelia to anencephaly. Excerpta Medica, Amsterdam
15. Lichteinstein BW (1959) Distant neuroanatomic complications of spina bifida (spinal dysraphism), hydrocephalus, Arnold–Chiari deformity, stenosis of the adueduct of Sylvius, etc. Pathogenesis and pathology. Arch Neurol Psychiatr 47:195–214
16. Gilmor RJ, Bathizlxy S (1978) Diastematomyelia: rare and unusual features. Neuroradiology 16:87–88
17. French BN (1982) Midline fusion defects and defects of formation. In: Youman JR (eds), Neurological surgery, 2nd edn. WB Saunders, Philadelphia, pp 1236–1380
18. Pang D (1992) Split cord malformation. Part II. Clinical syndrome. Neurosurgery 31:481–500
19. Guthkelch AN (1974) Diastematomyelia with median septum. Brain 97:729–744
20. James CCM, Lassman LP (1972) Spinal dysraphism. In: Spina bifida occulta. Appleton Century Croft, New York
21. James CCM, Lassman LP (1970) Diastematomyelia and tight filum terminale. J Neurol Sci 10:193–196

22. McLone DG, Dias L, Kaplan WB et al. (1985) Concepts in the management of spina bifida. In. Concepts in paediatric. Neurosurgery, vol 5. Humphery RP (ed) Karger, Basel, pp 97–106
23. Stark GD, Drummound M, Ponelrasert S et al. (1974) Primary ventriculoperitoneal shunts in treatment of hydrocephalus associated with myelomeningocele. Arch Dis Child 49:112–117
24. Laurence KM, Deresford A (1975) Incontinence, friends, marriage and children in 51 adults with spina bifida. Dev Med Child Neurol 123–128 vol 17
25. McLone DG, Czyzewski D, Raimondi AJ (1982) The central nervous system infection as a limiting factor in intelligence of children with spinal dysraphism. Paediatrics (Springer Field) 70:338–342
26. Warf BC, Scott RM, Harnes PD (1993) Tethered spinal cord in patients with anorectal and urogenital malformation. Pediatr Neurosurg 79:25–30
27. Kale SS, Mahapatra AK Pre- and postoperative somatosensory evoked potentials in spinal dysraphism (In press)
28. Mahapatra AK (1996) Spinal dysraphism. In: Ramani PS (ed) Textbook of spinal surgery. Bhooma Graphics, pp 487–500

Operative Treatment of Adult Spinal Cord Lipoma—Report of Six Cases

Yoshio Nakajima, Seishi Igarashi, and Tsunemaro Koyama

Summary. We report on a retrospective study of the operative results of adult spinal cord lipoma. The patients were three males and three females. The mean age was 42.8 years, ranging from 23 to 60 years. The term of illness ranged from 6 to 56 years, with a mean of 25.3 years. The most frequent complaints were leg weakness and urinary dysfunction. Other complaints were leg dysesthesia and bowel dysfunction. One patient was asymptomatic. All symptoms were progressive except in the asymptomatic case. Magnetic resonance imaging revealed lumbosacral spinal cord lipomas with tethered cord in all patients. Total or subtotal removal or debulking of the lipomas were done in all patients using an operative microscope and a cavitron ultrasonic surgical aspirator. Two patients improved in sensorimotor deficits and four remained unchanged. There was no operative morbidity. Our results suggest that adult patients with spinal cord lipoma have a chance to gain clinical improvement even though the term of illness is over 20 years.

Key words. Spinal cord lipoma, Tethered cord, Adult

Introduction

Spinal cord lipomas are complicated in approximately 30% of spina bifida occulta [1]. The majority of spinal cord lipomas are diagnosed in childhood because of their cutaneous manifestations, and adult spinal cord lipomas are rare [11]. In this report, we describe the operative results of 6 adult spinal cord lipomas, analysing their clinical symptoms and factors precipitating the symptoms. Surgical indication in this disease was discussed.

Materials and Methods

Six adult patients with spinal cord lipoma who were treated surgically at the Department of Neurosurgery, Ohtsu Municipal Hospital, during the last 18 years (1980–1997) were reviewed.

Diagnosis was based on physical, neurological, and neuroradiological examinations using plain X-P and magnetic resonance imaging (MRI). The spinal lipomas were finally proven during the operation in all cases.

Ohtsu Municipal Hospital, Department of Neurosurgery, 2-9-9 Motomiya, Ohtsu, Shiga 520-0804, Japan

Results

There were 3 males and 3 females. The age ranged from 23 to 60 years, with an average of 42.8 years. The mean term of illness was 25.3 years, ranging from 6 to 56 years. The most frequent complaints on admission were motor weakness in the lower extremities and urinary dysfunction, which were found in 4 cases. The other complaints were dysesthesia in the lower extremities in 2 cases, and bowel dysfunction in 1 case. In case 2, the lipoma was found incidentally on MRI. Four patients had spina bifida occulta (cases 1, 3, 4, 5) and 2 patients had associated anomalies of the skeletal system such as scoliosis and pes varus (Table 1). The symptoms of all patients except case 2 were progressive.

On neurological examination, motor weakness of the lower extremities was found in 4 cases, neurogenic bladder in 4 cases, changes of the deep tendon reflex in 3 cases (decreased ATR in 3 and decreased PTR in 2), and sensory disturbance in 3 (Table 2).

Plain lumbar or sacral X-ray films revealed spina bifida occulta in 4 cases (Fig. 1) and scoliosis in one case (Fig. 2).

MRI revealed lumbosacral spinal cord lipomas with tethered cord in all patients. The types of lipoma were classified into 3 groups after MRI. Lipomyelomeningocele, intradural lipoma, and filum lipoma was seen in 4 cases (Fig. 3), 1 case (Fig. 4), and 1 case (Fig. 5), respectively.

In the operation, we debulked lipoma with or without cutting of the filum terminale. All debulking and cutting procedures were done under the operative microscope. In the

1
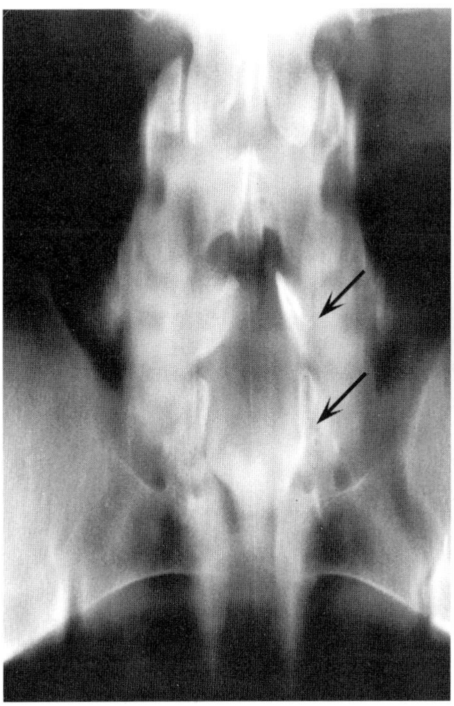
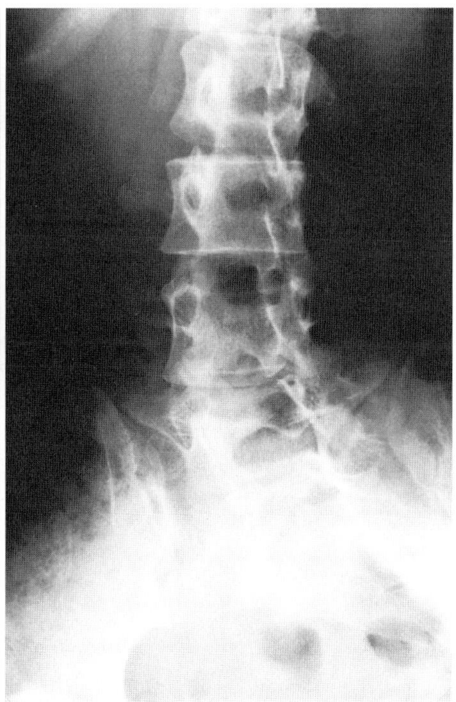
2

Fig. 1. Lumbosacral X-P shows spina bifida occulta in case 4. This finding was also seen in cases 1, 3, and 5

Fig. 2. Lumbosacral X-P shows scoliosis in case 1

TABLE 1. Clinical summary of cases

Patient No.	Age/sex	Diagnosis	Complaints	Associated anomaly	Surgical procedure	Result
1	31/F	Lipomyelomeningocele	Dysuria	Scoliosis Spina bifida	Total removal	Unchanged
2	56/F	Filum lipoma	–	–	Total removal filum terminale cut	Unchanged
3	38/F	Lipomyelomeningocele	R. leg weakness	Spina bifida	Subtotal removal	Unchanged
4	23/M	Lipomyelomeningocele	Bil. leg weakness Urinary incontinence Dimple at the buttock	Bil. pes varus Spina bifida	Debulking, filum terminale cut	Unchanged
5	60/M	Lipomyelomeningocele	L. leg dysesthesia L. leg weakness Urinary incontinence	Spina bifida	Subtotal removal, filum terminale cut	Improved
6	49/M	Intradural lipoma	L. leg dysesthesia Bil. leg weakness Urinary incontinence Constipation	–	Subtotal removal	Improved

Table 2. Neurological findings

	No. of cases	
Motor weakness in lower extremities		4
Unilateral	2	
Bilateral	2	
Sensory disturbance		3
Deep tendon reflex changes		3
Hyporeflexia of PTR	2	
Hyporeflexia of ATR	3	
Neurogenic bladder		4

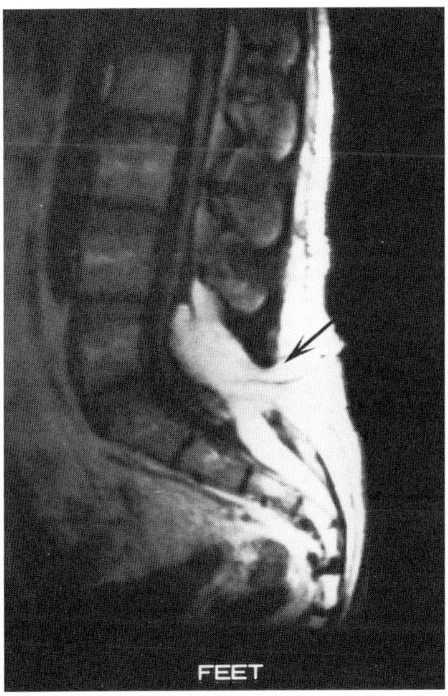

A

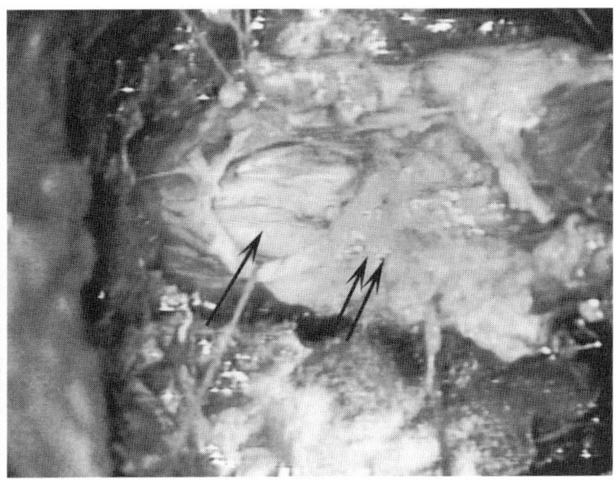

B

Fig. 3. **A** MRI shows lipomyelomeningocele in case 4. The *arrow* indicates lipoma. **B** In-operative photo. *Single arrow* shows low-set spinal cord, and *double arrows* show epidural lipoma in the sacral region

debulking procedure, we usually used a cavitron ultrasonic surgical aspirator, and for removal of the remaining fibrous tissue, we used a microsurgical technique. When we could not find the filum terminale, so cutting the filum terminale was not done.

On follow-up examination, motor weakness improved after surgery in 2 out of 4 cases, and sensory disturbance improved in 2 out of 3 cases. Although urinary dysfunction did not improve, further deterioration ceased after the operations. The asymptomatic patient (case 2) remained the same after surgery. Overall, 2 patients improved and 4 patients remained unchanged. The grade of excision (total, subtotal, debulking) and cutting the filum terminale did not affect the postoperative neurological status (Table 1). There was no operative morbidity.

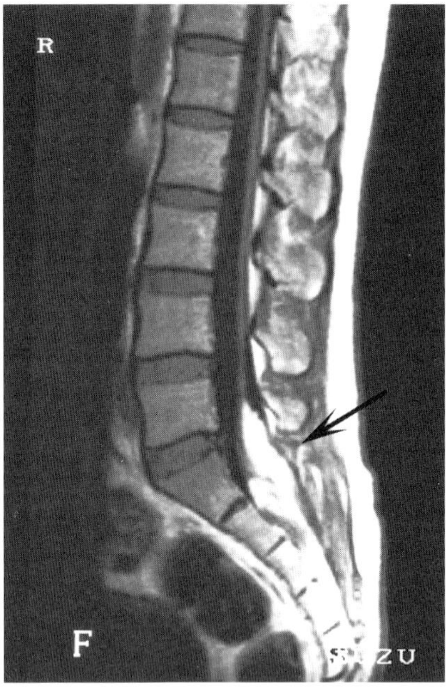

A

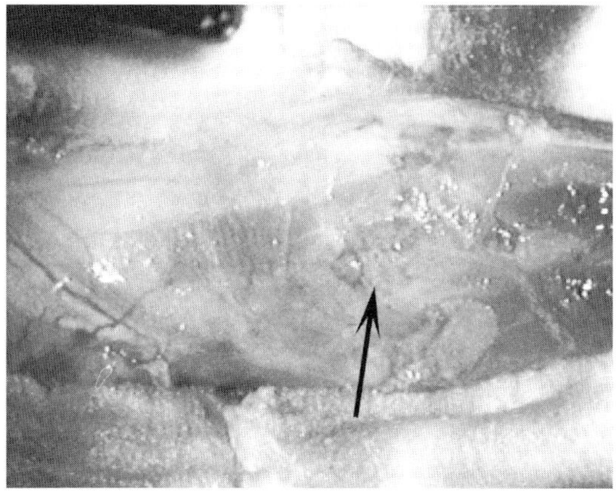

B

Fig. 4. **A** MRI shows intradural lipoma in case 6. The *arrow* indicates the lipoma. **B** In-operative photo. The *arrow* shows the intradural lipoma, which is seen through thinned dura mater

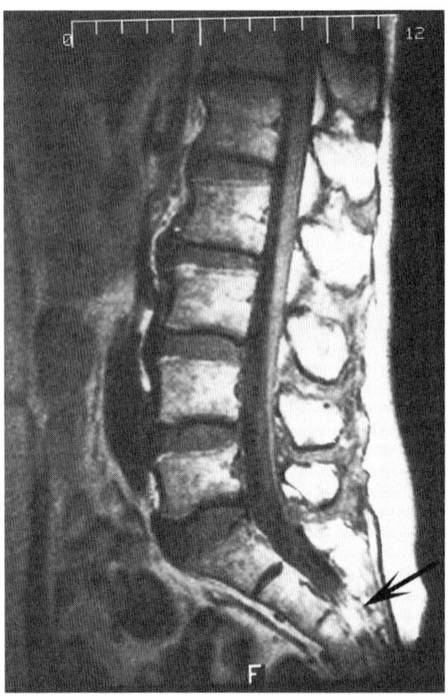

A

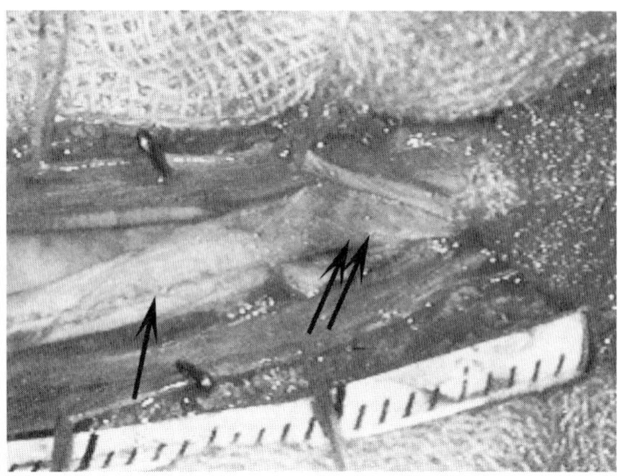

B

Fig. 5. **A** MRI shows filum lipoma in case 2. The *arrow* indicates the sacral lipoma. **B** In-operative photo. *Single arrow* shows the thickened filum terminale, and *double arrows* show a filum lipoma

Discussion

The embryological process of spinal cord lipoma is still unclear. Generally, the group of neural tube defects has been thought to occur after the completion of primary neurulation in this disease [8]. The theory put forward by McLone and Naidich [9] is that lumbosacral spinal lipoma develops as a result of a disjunction between the neural ectoderm and the cutaneous ectoderm at their common leading migrating edges, where they normally adhere to each other before meeting the corresponding neural or cutaneous ectodermal layer from the other side, fusing in the midline, and then separating with the fully formed neural tube below and the skin above. The early disjunction between the neural ectoderm and the cutaneous ectoderm before midline fusion allows mesenchymal cells to enter the neural tube before it is completely formed [9]. The degree and timing of the disjunction would reflect on the extent of the deformity, which could range from a filum terminale enlarged with fat to a massive lipoma covering most of the lumbosacral region [8].

The majority of spinal cord lipomas are diagnosed in the neonatal period or in infancy because of their cutaneous manifestations, such as subcutaneous lipoma, capillary hemangioma, dimple, bifurcating intergluteal cleft, and hairy patch [11]. However, if these cutaneous manifestations are lacking or overlooked, and patients have normal neurological findings in infancy, they do not draw clinical attention until adolescence or adulthood [8]. All lipomas produce neurologic deficits by virtue of the tethering effect on the cord [11]. Pang and Wilberger [12] suggested that the degree of traction on the conus determines the age of symptomatic onset. It is possible that in cases of marked tethering and severe stretching of the conus, neurological disturbance would appear in infancy or early childhood by growth spurts and developmental alterations in the spinal curvature [12]. A lesser degree of tethering might cause only minor and nonprogressive deficits at childhood [12]. In cases of the least amount of tethering, patients may remain subclinical in childhood until their condition is later aggravated by factors that upset the tenuous balance between abnormal tension and optimal cellular function [12]. Yamada et al. [13] showed that both acute and chronic tension applied to the spinal cord results in chronic cord ischemia, and that neurological dysfunction in patients with tethered cord correlates well with ischemia within the conus. Exacerbating circumstances in adults often include some form of trauma to the back and buttocks, or a maneuver that results in excessive stretching of the spine, such as childbirth in the lithotomy position, forced straight-leg flexion at the hips, and forward bending [8]. In our cases there was no specific incident immediately preceding their onset.

In the preoperative diagnosis of 2 out of the 6 patients, their anamneses reminded us of spinal lipoma. One patient (case 4) had noticed gait disturbance since 1 year old. He noticed bilateral pes varus at 9 years old and it was treated at 12 and 15 years old at different orthopedic clinics. He had a dimple on the buttock. Another patient (case 5) underwent removal of a lumbosacral mass at 5 years old. It is reported that cutaneous manifestations are present in 80–100% of children with spinal lipoma, but more than half of the adult patients have no history of external signs of spinal dysraphism [12]. Four of our 6 cases had no cutaneous manifestations. Pang and Wilberger [12] reported that characteristic symptoms in adults with spinal cord lipoma which compared with those of childhood were diffuse and nondermatomal leg pain, often referred to the ano-rectic region, progressive symmetrical sensorimotor deficits in the lower extremities, absence of progressive foot and spinal deformities, and common progressive neurogenic bladder. In our cases, progressive motor deficits in the lower extremities and neurogenic bladder were the most common features (4 of 6 cases), but symmetrical motor deficits were seen only in half the cases (2 of 4). Although 2 patients complained of unilateral leg dysesthesia, no patient complained of leg pain. Foot deformity was seen in one patient (case 4), but its progression ceased after puberty. Scoliosis was recognized in one patients (case 1). It was characteristic that neurological deficits of our cases were all progressive except in the asymptomatic case (case 2).

Some authors reported that plain X-rays of the spine are not necessary because an MRI scan is sufficient for diagnosis of spinal cord lipoma [8, 11]. However, as 5 out of 6 cases showed abnormal findings in X-ray films, such as spina bifida or scoliosis, we think the plain X-ray film is a useful screening aid when spinal cord lipoma is clinically suspected.

MRI offers many advantages, such as high contrast in the soft tissue, familiar anatomical scan planes, a large field of view, high tissue contrast, and complete noninvasiveness [1]. Our experiences in this series also suggested that operative findings had a pleasing conformity with those of MRIs.

Current literature and accumulating clinical experiences have shown that in patients with spinal cord lipoma who are not surgically repaired, about 90% will develop neurological deficits that are unlikely to be reserved, and that the chance of causing a neurological deficit with operative intervention is below 2%. Thus, all patients diagnosed as having spinal cord lipoma should undergo prophylactic surgical intervention [5, 7, 8]. This proposition justifies our surgical intervention on 5 progressive cases and 1 asymptomatic case.

The goal of surgical therapy is dissection of adhesions and section of the fatty stalk so that the conus medullaris and cauda equina are restored to normal unrestricted motion [2]. Colak et al. [2] advocated that the operative technique should be limited to decompressive laminectomy and subtotal resection, and a small portion of lipoma attached to the conus and spinal cord should be left in place because an attempt at complete removal would worsen the patient's clinical status. Lunardi et al. [6] reported that subtotal removal or simple decompression carries no higher risk of recurrence than total removal. In accordance with these reports, total or subtotal removal or simple debulking in our series did not worsen the patients' postoperative neurological status. Mapstone reported that the filum terminale should be identified and sectioned in all cases if it appears to be contributing to the tethering pathology [7]. We cut the filum terminale in 3 of 6 cases. Contrary to Mapstone's opinion, section of the filum terminale did not affect the surgical results compared with the results of patients whose filums were not cut. Mapstone stated that by surgical intervention, pain resolves in many patients, and those with sensorimotor symptoms have a roughly 50% chance of returning to their baseline, but those with bladder dysfunction rarely improve. He also reported that there is an excellent chance of preventing further deterioration in virtually all cases [7]. Our follow-up results coincide almost completely with this report.

Recently laser surgery has been able to facilitate the removal of a spinal cord lipoma because it facilitates the avoidance of dangerous traction on delicate neural structures [4, 10], and James et al. [4] reported that radical removal of spinal lipomas with a carbon dioxide laser was achieved in ten cases but was followed by paraplegia in one. According to our experiences and the literature, microsurgical dissection and the cavitron ultrasonic surgical aspirator are extremely helpful and safe in the removal of spinal cord lipoma [6].

In conclusion, our results suggest that adult patients with spinal cord lipoma have a chance to gain clinical improvement even though their term of illness is over 20 years. As surgical morbidity is very low and suddenly deteriorating cases have been reported previously [3], it is suggested that even asymptomatic patients are now candidates for surgery. Microsurgical dissection and the cavitron ultrasonic surgical aspirator are useful in that surgery.

References

1. Bajpai M (1994) Spina bifida and intraspinal lipomas. Aust N Z J Surg 64:177–179
2. Colak A, Tahta K, Ozcan OE, Eryilmaz M (1992) Congenital lumbosacral lipomas presenting as a form of occult spinal dysraphism. A report of 9 surgically treated cases. Zentralbl Neurochil 53:15–19
3. Fitnat D, Hamit ZG, Cumhur D, Ahmet Z (1991) Diagnosis and treatment of intraspinal lipomas. Turk J Pediatr 33:221–230
4. James HE, Williams J, Brock W, Kaplan GW, Hoi SU (1984) Radical removal of lipomas of the conus and cauda equina with laser microneurosurgery. Neurosurgery 15:340–343
5. Kanev PM, Lemire RJ, Loeser JD, Berger MS (1990) Management and long-term and follow-up review of children with lipomyelomeningocele, 1952–1987. J Neurosurg 73:48–52
6. Lunardi P, Missori P, Ferrante L, Fortuna A (1990) Long-term results of surgical treatment of spinal lipomas. Report of 18 cases. Acta Neurochir (Wien) 104:64–68
7. Mapstone TB (1994) Management of tethered spinal cord. Neurosurg Q 4:82–91
8. McComb JG, Chen TC (1996) Closed spinal neural tube defects. In: Tindall GT, Cooper PR, Barrow DL (eds) The practice of neurosurgery. Williams & Wilkins, Baltimore, pp 2753–2777
9. McLone DG, Naidich TP (1985) Spinal dysraphism: experimental and clinical. In: Holtzman RNN, Stein BM (eds) The tethered spinal cord. Thieme-Stratton, New York, pp 14–28
10. McLone DG, Naidich TP (1986) Laser resection of fifty spinal lipomas. Neurosurgery 18:611–615
11. Pang D (1995) Spinal cord lipomas. In: Pang D (ed) Disorders of the pediatric spine. Raven Press, New York, pp 175–201
12. Pang D, Wilberger JE (1982) Tethered cord syndrome in adult. J Neurosurg 57:32–47
13. Yamada S, Zinke DE, Sanders D (1981) Pathophysiology of "tethered cord syndrome". J Neurosurg 54:494–503

Curarino Syndrome and Related Conditions

Yasuo Yamanouchi[1], Takasumi Yasuda[1], Takayuki Inagaki[1], Keiji Kawamoto[1], Yoshinori Hamada[2], and You Kinoshita[3]

Summary. Currarino syndrome, with ano-rectal malformation, presacral mass, and sacral bony abnormality, is an uncommon condition. The embryogenesis of this anomalous complex is unclear, as is the question of whether this triad is one clinical entity. We present a case of the Currarino triad, and also a case with an imperforate anus, myelomeningocele at the lumbosacral area, and spinal bony anomaly. There are many combinations of anomalies around the sacrococcygeal area, including the gastrointestinal, urogenital, and neural systems. We suggest that the Currarino syndrome may be one of the special combinations of anomalous products of caudal eminence and a kind of caudal regression syndrome.

Key words. Currarino syndrome, Caudal eminence, Caudal regression syndrome

The Currarino triad is a unique complex of congenital caudal anomalies. These anomalies include ano-rectal malformation, sacral bony abnormality, and presacral mass [2]. This syndrome is considered to be a rare disease, and recently associated chromosomal abnormalities were reported [6, 7]. We report a case of this syndrome, and also the case of another patient with a disease apparently analogous to this syndrome. There is a question about whether this anomalous complex is one clinical entity. We suggest that this association of anomalies may be some special type of caudal repression syndrome.

Case 1

This is the case of a 5-month-old boy. At birth, he was found to have a bony protrusion in the sacral area. Since there were no abnormal neurological findings, he was merely followed up. However, sacral hypoplasia and a presacral mass lesion were identified by computed tomography (CT) and magnetic resonance imaging (MRI), and he was referred to our department for treatment. His mother's course of pregnancy had been uneventful and his family history was unremarkable. There were no abnormal neurological findings on admission.

Lumbo-sacral radiography revealed sacral hypoplasia, which was more clearly disclosed by 3D-CT (Fig. 1). Also the presence of spina bifida was clearly shown in the lower lumbar

[1]Department of Neurosurgery, [2]Department of Second Surgery, [3]Department of Pediatrics, Kansai Medical University, Osaka, Japan

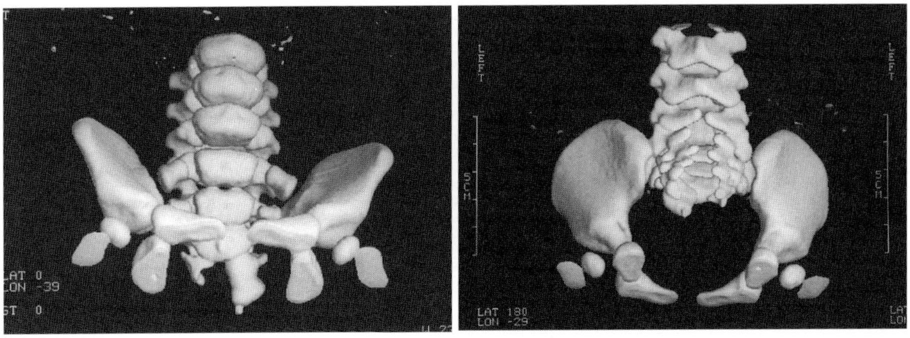

FIG. 1. 3D-computed tomographs (CTs)

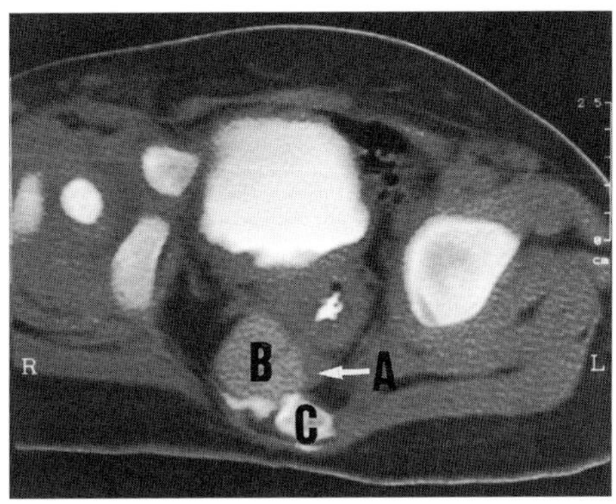

FIG. 2. CT myelogram. *A*, presacral mass lesion; *B*, anterior sacral meningocele; *C*, vertebral body

spine. Anterior sacral meningocele was shown by myelography, and a CT myelogram (Fig. 2) disclosed another presacral mass lesion adjacent to the meningocele.

MRI (Fig. 3) also confirmed the findings of sacral hypoplasia, anterior sacral meningocele, and presacral mass lesion. The presacral mass lesion was located in front of the meningocele, and identified as a relatively low-intensity area on the T1-weighted image and as a high-intensity area on the T2-weighted image.

This baby was referred to the division of pediatric surgery for examination, and a high-positioned anus was noted (Fig. 4). The severity of anal and rectal stenosis was in the lower limit of the normal range.

At surgery, a midline skin incision was made in the sacral region, and partial laminectomy was performed at the S3 level. After the midline dural incision was made, it was found that there was neither a tumor nor a tethering band in the dural sac. The dural sac was resected at the neck of the meningocele and sutured tightly.

Next, the remaining meningocele sac was removed and the elastic hard mass was removed totally without damaging the intestines.

Histologically, in this tumor smooth muscles, neural tissues with ganglion cells, peripheral nerves, mucus-producing glandular epithelia, transitional epithelia, and ependymal lining lumen were found. Because these were mature tissues with no malignant findings, the tumor was diagnosed as a mature teratoma. The patient's postoperative course has been uneventful.

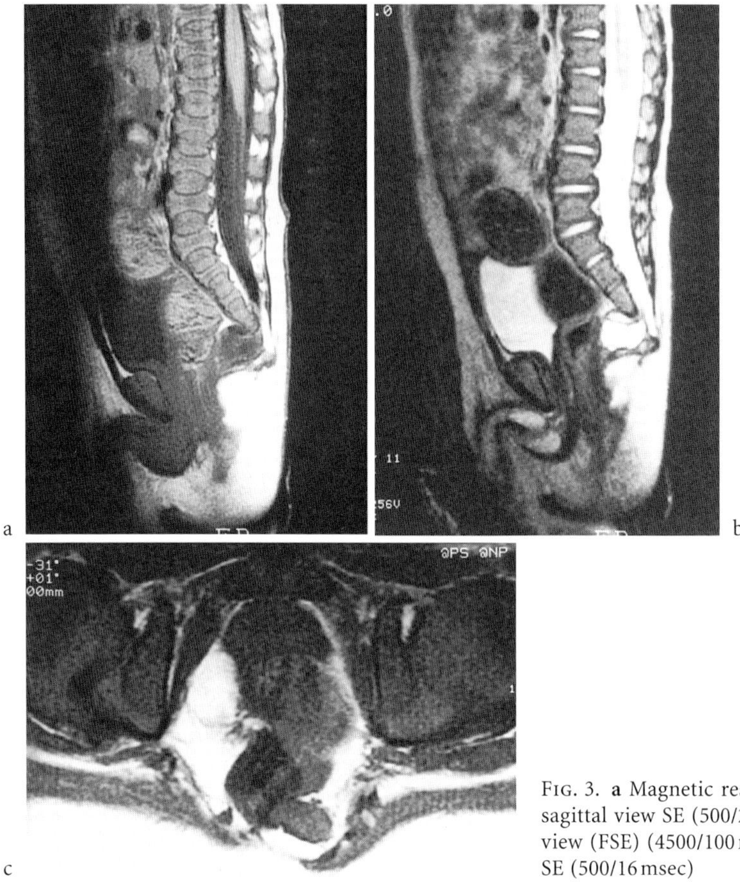

FIG. 3. **a** Magnetic resonance imaging (MRI) sagittal view SE (500/20 msec); **b** MRI sagittal view (FSE) (4500/100 msec); **c** MRI axial view SE (500/16 msec)

Case 2

A 1992-g male infant was born by Cesarean section to a 20-year-old gravida 1 para 0 woman. A ultrasound and MRI (Fig. 5) study at the 27th week of gestation revealed hydrocephalus and kyphosis, which suggested the presence of myelomeningocele.

The child had an Apgar score of 3 and intubated. The initial observation of the child revealed myelosclesis (Fig. 6a) and imperforate anus (Fig. 6b). He also had hydrocephalus and deformity of the right thorax and pulmonary dysplasia. In addition, although severe spinal scoliosis and partial spinal dysplasia were present, we evaluated that the baby was free from sacral dysgenesis.

Initially, the patient's parents refused any treatment. However, as the baby's abdominal swelling worsened day by day due to the imperforate anus, they reluctantly gave consent to proctostomy only, but refused any other surgical intervention. The baby died at 89 days after birth due to respiratory failure.

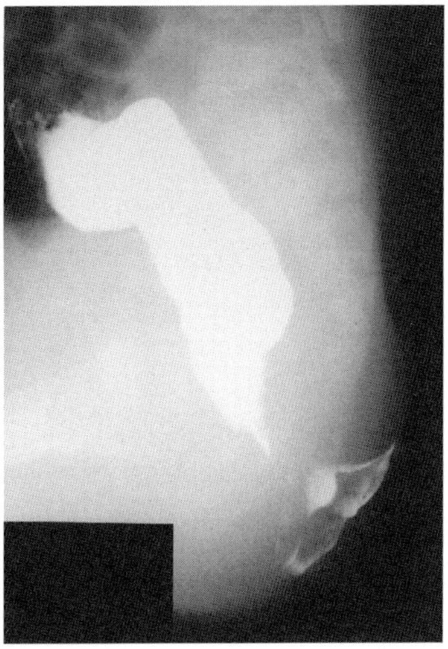

FIG. 4. Barium enema study

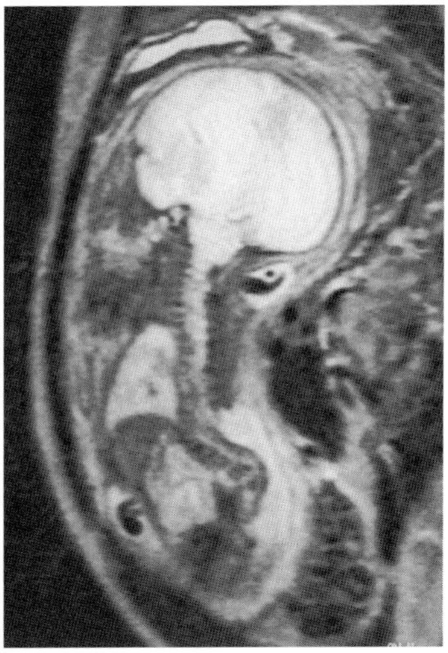

FIG. 5. MRI of the fetus FSE (4000/100 msec)

Discussion

Currarino triad is a congenital anomaly presenting with ano-rectal malformation (anal stenesis, anal ectopia, imperforate anus), sacral bony malformation (crescentric bony defect, malsegmentation), and presacral mass (anterior meningocele, teratoma, enteric cyst, any combination of these) [2]. It may relate to maternal diabetes which involves a diminished turnover of phosphoinositide or arachidonic acid, or an excess of free oxygen radicals [4]. Recently, chromosomal abnormalities (terminal deletion 7q35 [6] partial trisomy of 13q and 20p [7]) were reported in a Currarino triad case. In addition, incomplete cases who lack one or two of the three syndromes (triad) have been reported [2].

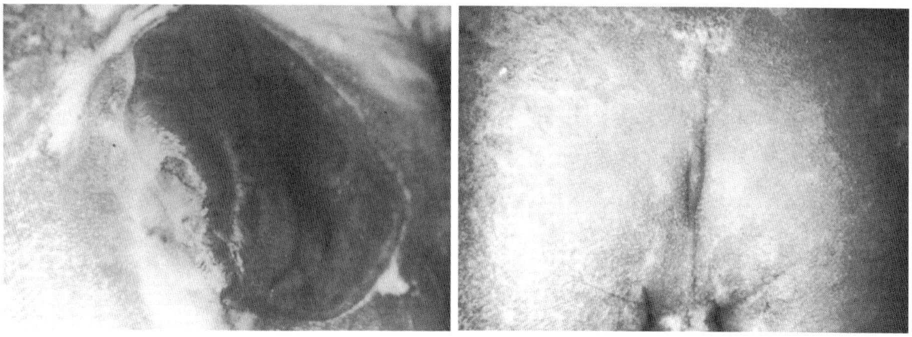

a b

FIG. 6. Photograph of the patient showing **a** the myeloschisis, and **b** imperforate anus

With regard to the embryogesis of this malformation complex, Currarino explained it in terms of an abnormal notochord [2]. According to his explanation, in normal notochordal development, the anterior wall of the spine develops by separating the neural tube from the intestinal tube. However, if some developmental anomaly occurs at an early fetal stage, the notochord is separated or deviated to one side, which results in unsuccessful fusion of the vertebral body, causing adhesion or formation of a fistula between the intestinal and neural tubes. Currarino states that ano-rectal anomaly is a consequence of the early abnormal adhesion of the hind gut and neural tube.

In Case 2 which we presented here, imperforate anus and myeloschisis were present. What is the correlation between this case and the Currarino syndrome? O'Neill et al. [8] reported various neuropathological findings such as low-lying conus, syringomyelia, and lipoma in sacral agenesis and dysgenesis. Pang [10] and Renshaw [11] reported the associated caudal anomalies in lumbosacral agenesis. There have also been reports of bony and spinal cord anomalies associated with ano-rectal anomalies [5, 12].

O'Rahilly et al. [9] postulated that sacral agenesis develops as an anomaly in the formation of the caudal eminence, and may arise as a faulty development of the primitive streak as early as Carnegie stage 8. The primitive streak probably persists until the caudal neuropore closes at stage 12, at which point it is replaced by the caudal eminence or end-bud. The caudal eminence appears at stage 9, and gives rise to the hindgut, notochord, caudal somites, neural cord, sacrum, and coccyx. Including our cases, there are many combinations of anomalies around this area [3, 5, 8, 10–12]. If these facts are also taken into account, the Currarino syndrome may be one of the special combinations of anomalous products of caudal eminence and a kind of caudal regression syndrome [1, 3]. It is necessary to be aware of the presence of such a syndrome clinically, and diagnose and treat it adequately.

References

1. Abraham E (1979) Sacral agenesis with associated anomalies (caudal regression syndrome): autopsy case report. Clin Orthop 145:168–171
2. Currarino G, Coln D, Votteler T (1981) Triad of anorectal, sacral, and presacral anomalies. AJR 137:395–398
3. Duhamel B (1961) From the mermaid to anal imperforation: the syndrome of caudal regression. Arch Dis Child 36:152–155
4. Goto MP, Goldman AS (1994) Diabetic embryopathy. Curr Opin Pediatr 6:486–491

5. Karrer FM, Flannery AM, Nelson MD, McLone DG, Raffensperger JG (1988) Anorectal malformations: evaluation of associated spinal dysraphic syndromes. J Pediatr Surg 23:45–48
6. Masuno M, Imaizumi K, Aida N, Tanaka Y, Sekido K, Ohhama Y, Nishi T, Kuroki Y (1996) Currarino triad with a terminal deletion 7q35 → qter. J Med Genet 33:877–878
7. Nagai T, Katoh R, Hasegawa T, Ohashi H, Fukushima Y (1994) Currarino triad (anorectal malformation, sacral bony abnormality and presacral mass) with partial trisomy of chromosomes 13q and 20p. Clin Genet 45:272–273
8. O'Neill OR, Piatt JH, Mitchell P, Roman-Goldstein S (1995) Agenesis and dysgenesis of the sacrum: neurosurgical implications. Pediatr Neurosurg 22:20–28
9. O'Rahilly R, Müller F, Meyer DB (1990) The human vertebral column at the end of the embryonic period proper. 4. The sacrococcygeal region. J Anat 168:95–111
10. Pang D (1993) Sacral agenesis and caudal spinal cord malformations. Neurosurgery 32:755–779
11. Renshaw TS (1978) Sacral agenesis: a classification and review of twenty-three cases. J Bone Joint Surg Br 60-A:373–383
12. Tunell WP, Austin JC, Barnes PD, Reynolds A (1987) Neuroradiologic evaluation of sacral abnormalities in imperforate anus complex. J Pediatr Surg 22:58–61

Congenital Spinal Hernia on First Thoracic Vertebral Level

G.I. Okladnikov

Congenital spinal hernias in children are malformations, and the severity of the symptoms depends on the degree of spinal cord involvement, association with hydrocephalus, or malformations of the brain or other parts of the body. The lesion is usually situated in the lumbar region, and in this connection we present a case of hernia with rare localization on the Th1 level. The patient was 2 months old and was mature at birth, and the delivery was without complications. While pregnant, his mother had had a respiratory infection, toxicosis, and pyelonephritis.

Immediately after delivery a soft tumor-like formation was detected about 3 cm × 3 cm × 2 cm in size. During the subsequment 2 months, this formation had increased to 6 cm × 6 cm × 4 cm.

On examination the general condition of the child was satisfactory, hydrocephalus was present, and the head circumference was 40 cm. The patient showed strabismus convergens from the left, there was no paresis of the extremities, the tendon reflexes were arc-normal, and there were no meningial symptoms. On the lower part of the cervical spine there was a tumor-like formation 6 cm × 6 cm × 4 cm, with skin atrophy and ulceration. X-ray examination of the soft tissue of the cervico-thoracic spine showed an oval malformation with clear, distinct borderlines, homogenous structure, situated on the dorsal surface of the vertebral column, and causing unclear visualization of the TH1 processus. On lumbar puncture, the cerebrospinal fluid was normal. Myelography with contrast emulsion was performed. A subarachnoid cavity was found which measured 4 cm × 4 cm × 3 cm, and which was connected to the hernia sac. The sac was not totally filled with the contrast substance, giving the impression of a multichamber construction.

Surgery was performed after puncture of the hernia sac and removal of 4 ml of xantochromous liquid. A multichamber construction was confirmed. Sac ligation and resection of the walls was performed using microsurgery and bipolar coagulation. The postoperative period was uneventful. There was no neurological deficit.

The main interest in this presentation is the rare localization of the spinal hernia. There are reports in the literature about sac-contrasting with oxygen or metrizamid. We used miodil emulsion to detect the size, sac construction, and its connection with the spinal canal, with good results.

Department of Neurosurgery, Medical Institute, Novosibirsk, Krasny Pr. 52 Novosibirsk 630091, Russia

Surgical Treatment of Lipomyelomeningocele for Prevention of Postoperative Retethering

Hiroaki Sakamoto[1], Shouhei Kitano[1], and Ken Fujitani[2]

Summary. We analyzed our refined surgical procedures to prevent the retethering of the spinal cord that is the main cause of late deterioration after surgery for lipomyelomeningocele. Out of 50 children with lipomyelomeningocele in whom, in operation, the dura had been repaired without Gore-Tex sheet, 6 had progressive deterioration due to retethering 1–12 years after surgery. Out of 15 children with lipomyelomeningocele in whom the dura had been repaired using this sheet, none had deteriorated in a period of 1–6 years after surgery. Application of the sheet for dural plasty brought less radical removal of the intradural lipoma with less incidence of neural injury, and involved neither technical difficulties nor significant complications. In conclusion, as well as various other procedures for maintaining the space of the cerebrospinal fluid around the cord, application of Gore-Tex sheet for dural plasty might possibly reduce the incidence of postoperative retethering.

Key words. Spinal dysraphism, Lipomyelomeningocele, Tethered cord, Retethering

Introduction

The goal of surgical treatment for lipomyelomeningocele is to untether the spinal cord from the anomalous lipoma fused to it. However, even if the spinal cord can be untethered during the operation, a tight adhesion between the cord and the surrounding dura may often develop after surgery [2, 3, 5, 9, 12, 13, 15] Magnetic resonance (MR) imaging showed such postoperative adhesion in most of the lipomyelomeningocele patients after surgery. Because the retethering of the spinal cord due to this postoperative adhesion has been recognized as the main cause of deterioration late after surgery, various surgical procedures have been proposed to keep the cord untethered, for example, debulking the intradural lipoma, reconstruction of the conus medullaris, and expansive dural plasty [2, 3, 9, 14]. We believe that maintaining the space of the cerebrospinal fluid (CSF) around the spinal cord can sufficiently prevent postoperative adhesion between the cord and the overlying dura. We have developed new procedures, such as repositioning of the spinal cord to the center of the dural sac and tacking the dura to the overlying solid structures, which are newly constructed laminae [15, 17]. These procedures are effective, but do not always prevent the postoperative adhesion of

[1] Department of Pediatric Neurosurgery, Osaka City General Hospital, 2-13-22 Miyakojima-hondori, Miyakojima-ku, Osaka 534, Japan
[2] Osaka Municipal Rehabilitation Center, Osaka, Japan

the cord to the surrounding dura. After clinical introduction of polytetrafluoroethylene (Gore-Tex), which is nonadhesive to adjacent vital tissues, we have applied Gore-Tex sheet in our surgical procedures with the hope of significantly reducing the incidence of adhesion [10]. Here, we describe our surgical treatment of lipomyelomeningocele using this material, and analyze the results.

Clinical Materials

We operated on 65 children (age at surgery less than 16 years) with lipomyelomeningocele in the lumbosacral region. In 50 of these children we did not use Gore-Tex sheet for dural plasty in the repair of the lipomyelomeningocele. After 1992, we did apply it for 15 patients with lipomyelomeningocele. We excluded patients with tethered cord due to fat filum or thickened filum, because such patients rarely require repair of the dysgenetic spinal cord or of the dural defect at surgery. The patients without the application of Gore-Tex sheet were followed up over a period of from 4 to 12 years, with a mean of 8 years, and those with application of the sheet were followed up over a period of from 1 to 6 years, with a mean of 3 years.

Methods

Table 1 shows a summary of our operative procedures for lipomyelomeningocele. The patient is placed in a prone position and a linear skin incision is performed. Osteoplastic laminotomy is carried out using a sagittal saw, and the laminar flap is reflected upward. The bleeding from the site of the laminotomy is controlled with bone wax. After the connection of the subcutaneous lipoma to the intradural space has been secured, the extradural lipoma is removed. The dura is incised at the cephalic portion next to the intradural lipoma and opened down to the top of the intradural lipoma. The underlying arachnoid is then tacked to the dura. The spinal cord is sharply dissected from the dura while preserving the cleavage

TABLE 1. Summary of the surgical procedures

Surgical procedures
Untethering and decompression
1. Laminotomy
2. Find the normal dura and cord
3. Dissect the cord from the dura
4. Untether the cord
5. Find the most caudal CSF space
6. Cut the abnormal filum
7. Debulk the subpial lipoma
8. Apply neuromonitoring
Prevention of retethering
1. Preserve the pial membrane
2. Reconstruct the conus medullaris
3. Reposition the shifted cord to the center of the dural sac
4. Dural plasty using Gore-Tex sheet
5. Laminoplasty
6. Tack the dura to the laminae

between the dura and the pial membrane of the spinal cord containing the subpial lipoma. If the nerve roots are involved in the intradural lipoma, the roots are carefully dissected from the lipoma with the help of neuromonitoring [16]. The dentate ligaments anchoring the cord to the dura are also cut. At the most caudal portion of the dural sac, the most caudal portion of the spinal cord and the sacral roots are dissected from the dura. If there is a thick filum, it is amputated. After the dissection of the spinal cord, whether or not it contains a subpial spinal lipoma, we have to confirm that no structures, except the normal nerve roots and/or the blood vessels, are anchoring the spinal cord to the surrounding dura. Then untethering of the spinal cord is completed.

After untethering, the subpial spinal lipoma is removed for decompression of the spinal cord. Preoperative MR imaging showed the thickness of the subpial lipoma behind the spinal cord. The pial layer of the spinal cord over the subpial lipoma is incised in such way that each pial fringe is preserved for reconstruction of the conus medullaris at a later stage of the operation. An ultrasonic surgical aspirator is applied at lower power for internal decompression of the subpial lipoma. The younger the patient is at the time of removal, the softer and less rich in blood vessels is the subpial lipoma. The dorsal nerve roots are good indicators for identification of the margin of the subpial spinal lipoma. No attempt is made to remove the subpial lipoma adjacent to the nerve roots or the spinal cord. When the volume of the spinal cord containing the subpial lipoma is satisfactorily reduced, a large portion of the subpial lipoma might be left behind. We have to confirm that the spinal cord containing the residual subpial lipoma is not too large for the dural sac. After removal of the subpial lipoma, the pial fringes are sutured for reconstruction of the conus medullaris. This is to reduce the volume of the conus medullaris (spinal cord) remaining in the dural sac. The reconstructed conus medullaris covered by the pial layer is less adhesive to the surrounding dura. Also, the pial layer shows a clear cleavage between the cord and the dura for the dissection of the cord from the adherent dura at the time of reoperation. In patients with a syrinx in the cord next to the intradural lipoma, the pial suturings for reconstruction of the conus should not be tight, but rather loose. Otherwise, such terminal syrinx might increased in size after surgery [6]. When the reconstructed conus is shifted toward one side of the dural sac, we perform the repositioning of the conus medullaris by pial stitches to the adjacent dura. Then the spinal cord is placed, without tethering or compression, at the center of the dural sac or is lying down on the bottom of the dural sac.

For dural plasty before 1990, lipophilized dura or paravertebral fascia was used for dural plasty. After 1991, dural plasty was performed using Gore-Tex sheet in patients who were likely to experience postoperative adhesion. Threads of 5–0 monofilament nylon were used for dural closure, and fibrin glue was used to supplement the seal of the dural closure. The layer of the paravertebral fascia was sutured. When the spinal cord containing the subpial lipoma was rather small for the dural sac, the dura was simply sutured and the Gore-Tex sheet (0.1 mm in thickness) was placed between the conus medullaris and the dural sac to prevent the dorsal or lateral surfaces of the cord, which were not covered by the normal pial membrane, from coming into contact with the inner surface of the dura.

The laminal flap was restored to approximately its original position. Nylon threads were used for the approximation of the lamina, but microplates were applied for more rigid fixing of the unstable laminae. The dura was tacked to the fixed laminar flap in order to expand the subarachnoid space behind the spinal cord. If necesary, the lamina was newly constructed using a bone graft obtained from the rib or iliac bone. No drain was placed in the operative wound. The patient was kept in a prone position (Matson's position) for at least 1 week [8].

We evaluated any patient presenting new symptoms, or signs such as motor weakness, foot deformity, sensory disturbance, pain, or deterioration in neurogenic bladder function, by close observation. Postoperative MR imaging was obtained every year. We recognized postoperative retethering as the cause of such deterioration when the patient showed progressive deterioration, and when MR imaging demonstrated no CSF space between the dorsal surface of the conus medullaris and the dura, which strongly indicated the adhesion of the cord to the dura [15].

Results

Table 2 shows the incidence of retethering after surgery in children with lipomyelomeningocele. Out of 50 patients with lipomyelomeningocele who underwent the initial operation without applying Gore-Tex sheet, 6 progressively deteriorated late after surgery. Their clinical symptoms and signs, such as motor weakness of the foot joints, leg pains or lumbago, hypalgesia in the lower part of the legs and/or the sacral region, and urinary or bowel incontinence, were progressive or newly developed. In these 6 patients with progressive deterioration, MR imaging showed both low-positioned conus and attachment of the cord on its dorsal or dorso-lateral surface to the inner surface of the surrounding dura. Neither formation nor enlargement of the syrinx was observed in these 6 patients. Clinical and radiological findings indicated that the deterioration in these 6 patients resulted from retethering of the cord. They all underwent reoperation to release the retethering. Out of 15 patients who underwent the initial operation using Gore-Tex sheet for dural plasty, none showed any deterioration late after surgery.

Case Presentation

The patient was a 2-year-old girl with lipomyelomeningocele, who had slight paresis of the left ankle. Sagittal MR imaging showed a large lipomatous tissue connected to the subcutaneous layer through the laminal, fascial, and muscular defect (Fig. 1A). Fat suppression MR imaging showed a CSF space at the most caudal portion of the dural sac (Fig. 1B). Axial computed tomography (CT) and MR imaging showed that a large lipoma compressed the spinal cord toward the ventral side of the spinal canal (Fig. 1C). At surgery, the spinal cord was sharply dissected from the dura while preserving the cleavage between the dura and the pial membrane of the spinal cord (Fig. 2A). If the nerve roots are involved in the intradural lipoma, the roots must be carefully dissected from the lipoma (Fig. 2B). In this patient,

TABLE 2. Incidence of retethering after initial surgery for lipomyelomeningocele

	Application of Gore-Tex sheet	
	No	Yes
Total number of patients	50	15
Patients with retethering	6	0
Follow-up period (mean)	4–12 years (8 years)	1–6 years (3 years)

Retethering was diagnosed by progressive deterioration and MR findings such as low-set conus and adhesion of the cord to the dura after surgery. In the present study, patients without clinical deterioration were not referred to as those with retethering.

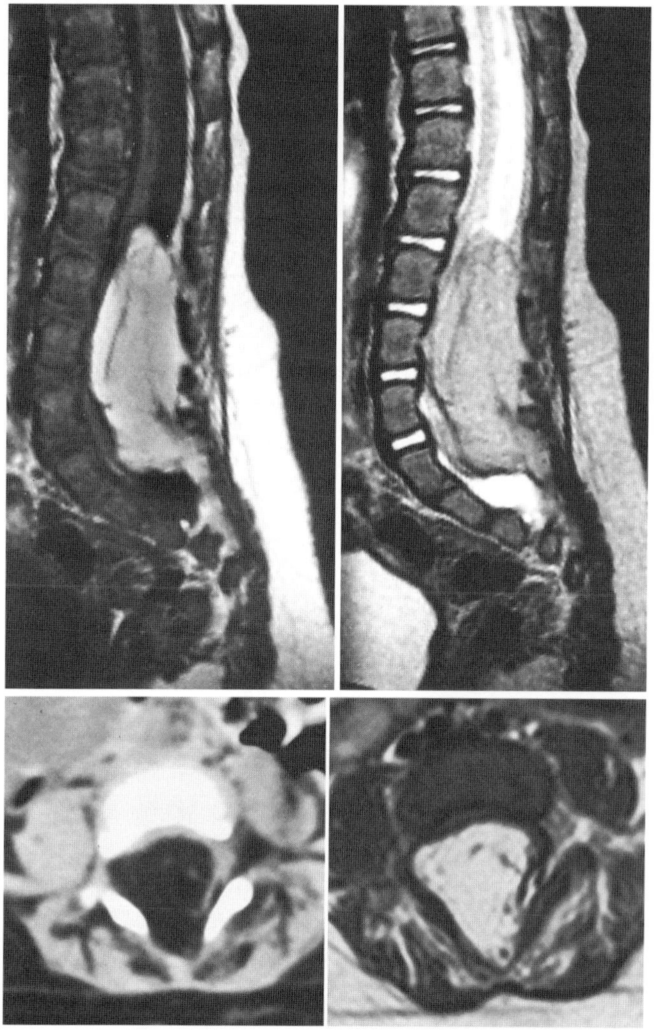

FIG. 1. Neuroimagings of a 2-year-old patient with lipomyelomeningocele. **A** Preoperative sagittal T1-weighted magnetic resonance (MR) image showing that a large spinal lipoma seems to compress the cord in the pinal canal. **B** Fat suppression MR image before surgery showing that the cerebrospinal fluid (CSF) space can be clearly differentiated from the lipoma. **C** Preoperative axial views of the T1-weighted MR image (*right*) and computed tomography (*left*) at L5 level demonstrating the relation between the spinal cord and the lipoma. **D** Postoperative sagittal MR images (*left*, T1-weighted image; *right*, T2-weighted image) showing that the CSF space between the spinal cord and the overlying dura indicates no evidence of adhesion between them

because the intradural lipoma was too large for the dissection of the cord from the dura, the intradural lipoma was partially removed before the complete dissection of the spinal cord (Fig. 2C). The whole spinal cord was completely dissected from the dura (Fig. 2D). After untethering of the spinal cord, the subpial lipoma was removed for decompression of the spinal cord. After removal of the subpial lipoma, the pial fringes were sutured for reconstruction of the conus medullaris. Dural plasty was performed using Gore-Tex sheet (Fig. 2E).

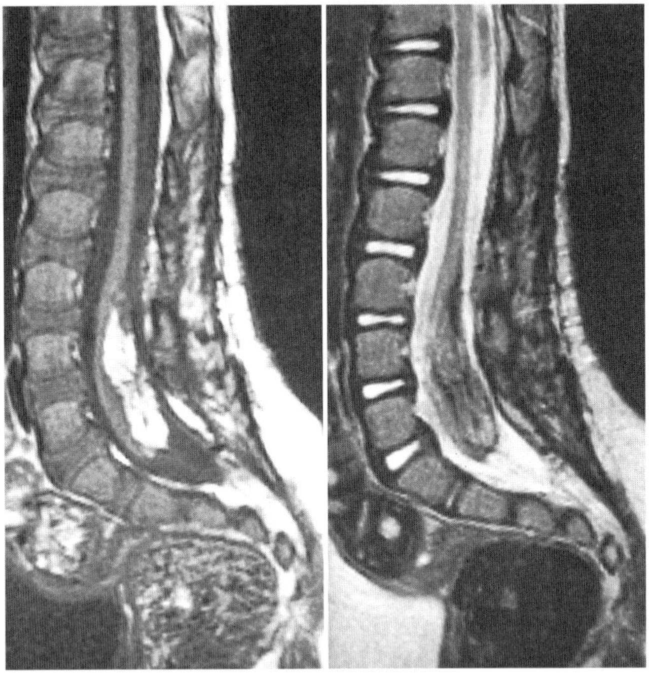

D

FIG. 1. *continued*

The weakness of the left foot improved over a follow-up period of 3 years. Postoperative MR imaging showed a CSF space around the cord (Fig. 1D).

Discussion

Retethering of the spinal cord and syrinx formation are the main causes of late deterioration after surgery for lipomyelomeningocele [4, 13]. Although MR imaging clearly shows the development of a syrinx and the size of the syrinx, it is unable to indicate the condition of retethering of the cord. To date, no neuroradiological imaging techniques are able to differentiate postoperative tethered cords from untethered low-positioned cords [11, 15]. Retethering requires re-untethering, but low-positioned cords do not. Only neurological examination can indicate the proper candidate for reoperation. Mechanical traction of the spinal cord by daily physical activities and/or dense adhesion of the neural structures are the possible cause of deterioration resulting from retethering [2]. Our clinical data concerning patients with retethering showed that progressive deterioration (which can be slow or rapid) due to retethering becomes irreducible [15]. We believe that once patients progressively deteriorate after their initial operation for lipomyelomeningocele, and when there are indications of postoperative adhesion on MR imaging, they should undergo reoperation for untethering as soon as possible.

After introduction of the Gore-Tex sheet in 15 patients with lipomyelomeningocele, not one developed late deterioration after surgery in a follow-up period from 1 to 6 years, with a mean of 3 years. Late deterioration develops most often in the period from 1 to 4 years [17].

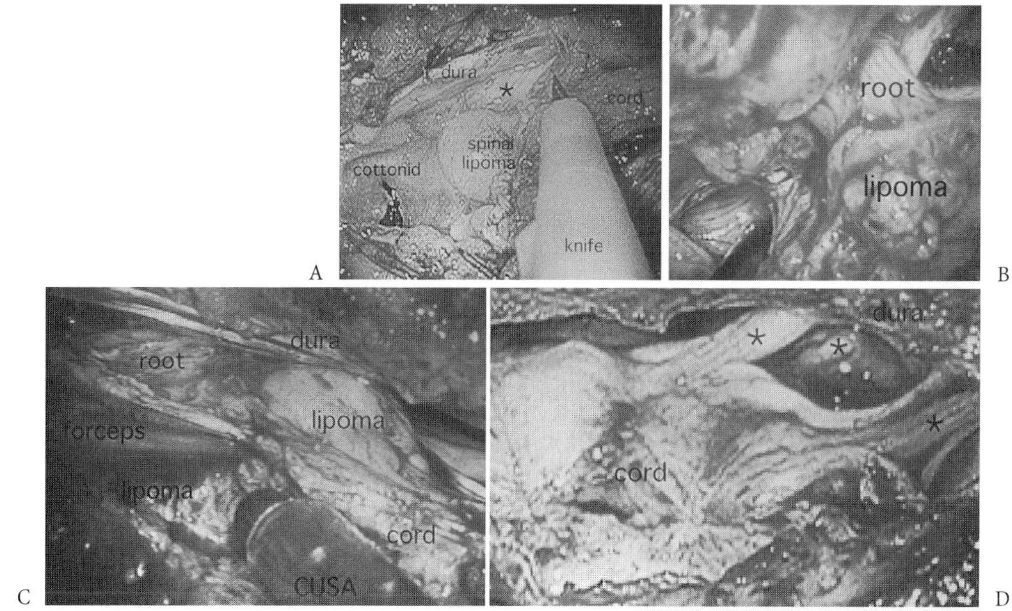

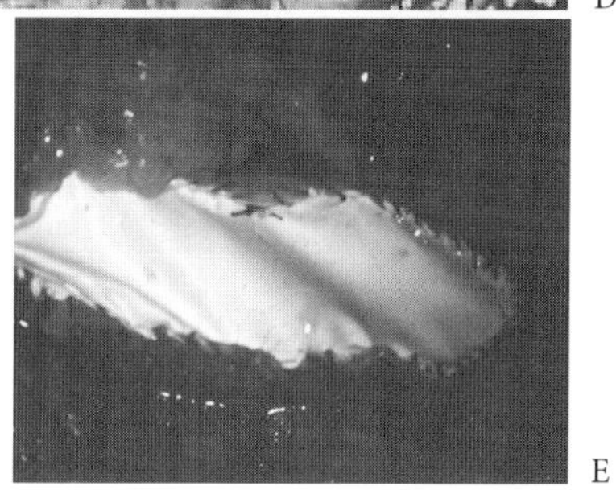

FIG. 2. Operative photographs. **A** Dissection of the spinal cord from the dura (*asterisk*, nerve root). **B** Dissection of the nerve root involved in the spinal lipoma. **C** Debulking of the subpial lipoma. **D** Dissection of the most caudal portion of the spinal cord (*asterisk*, nerve root). **E** Dural plasty with a Gore-Tex sheet

Although the follow-up period is not long enough to draw definite conclusions, the incidence of late deterioration with application of Gore-Tex sheet seems to be much lower than that without application of the sheet, or even than that in our newly developed surgical procedures. In addition to constructing the CSF space around the spinal cord by debulking the cord and complete untethering, application of the Gore-Tex sheet can possibly reduce the incidence of postoperative retethering in patients with lipomyelomeningocele. Although other materials, such as fascia, lypophilized dura, or even silastic membrane, may induce tight adhesion to the spinal cord, so far the Gore-Tex sheet has shown itself to be the best material for preventing postoperative adhesion [1, 7, 15, 18].

Postoperative adhesion as the main cause of retethering develops through contact of the spinal cord uncovered by normal pial membrane to the dorsally seated dura after surgery. To prevent contact of the cord with the dura, the subpial lipoma should be removed to reduce the volume of the spinal cord containing the subpial lipoma. Debulking of the subpial lipoma should be carried out to the extent that the spinal cord containing the subpial lipoma has no attachment to the surrounding dural sac. However, the removal of the subpial lipoma is often associated with the risk of cord or nerve injury if the neural structures are involved in the lipomatous tissue [3]. Even if the vital tissues are attached to this sheet, there is no (or minimum) adhesion between the sheet and surrounding tissues. Application of the Gore-Tex sheet for dural plasty could result in less radical removal of the subpial lipoma with less incidence of neural injury during its removal.

The possible disadvantages of the use of Gore-Tex sheet may be the risk of infection and the postoperative leakage of the CSF to the extradural space. We have encountered no meningitis or infection associated with application of this material. In 14 patient out of 15 receiving Gore-Tex sheet, the subcutaneous fluid collection in the lumbosacral region disappeared without significant intervention within 1 week after surgery. Prolonged subcutaneous fluid collection due to CSF leakage was observed only in one child. However, this patient was associated with subdural fluid collection even before surgery. We know that lipomyelomeningocele rarely accompanies a hydrocephalic condition. Therefore, special management of CSF leakage should be performed only in a child with the condition of hydrocephalus or increased intracranial pressure.

Myelomeningocele or myeloschisis as spina bifida apert is another main pathology inducing retethering of the cord after initial repair. Also the incidence of retethering associated during spina bifida aperta does not seem to be so high as that associated with lipomyelomeningocele [17]. We suggest that the Gore-Tex sheet should not be applied for the initial repair because it carryies a high risk of infection with operative application. When patients with spina bifida aperta demonstrate retethering of the cord late after the initial repair, we can then apply the Gore-Tex sheet to prevent future retethering with minimum risk of infection.

In conclusion, application of Gore-Tex sheet for dural plasty, as well as other procedures for maintaining the CSF space around the cord, can possibly reduce the incidence of postoperative retethering in the treatment of lipomyelomeningocele.

References

1. Boops FA, Chadduck WM (1991) Silastic duraplasty in pediatric patients. Neurosurgery 29:785–788
2. Bruce DA, Schut L (1979) Spinal lipomas in infancy and childhood. Child's Brain 5:192–201
3. Chapman PH (1982) Congenital intraspinal lipomas. Anatomic considerations and surgical treatment. Child's Brain 9:37–47
4. Chapman PH, Frim DM (1995) Symptomatic syringomyelia following surgery to treat retethering of lipomyelomeningoceles. J Neurosurg 82:752–755
5. Herman JM, McLone DG, Storrs BB, Dauser RC (1993) Analysis of 153 patients with myelomeningocele or spinal lipoma reoperated upon for a tethered cord. Presentation, management and outcome. Pediatr Neurosurg 19:243–249
6. Hoffman HJ, Taecholarn C, Hendrick EB, Humphreys RP (1985) Management of lipomyelomeningoceles. Experience at the Hospital for Sick Children, Toronto. J Neurosurg 62:1–8
7. Inoue HK, Kobayashi S, Ohbayashi K, Kohga H, Nakamura M (1994) Treatment and prevention of tethered and retethered spinal cord using a Gore-Tex surgical membrane. J Neurosurg 80:689–693
8. Matson DD (1969) Spina bifida and myelomeningocele. Neurosurgery of infancy and childhood, 2nd ed. Charles C Thomas, Springfield, pp 5–60
9. McLone DG, Mutluer S, Naidich TP (1983) Lipomeningoceles of the conus medullaris. Concepts Pediatr Neurosurg 3:170–177
10. Minale C, Nikol S, Hollweg G, Mittermayer C, Messmer BJ (1988) Clinical experience with expanded polytetrafluoroethylene Gore-Tex surgical membrane for pericardial closure:a study of 110 cases. J Cardiac Surg 3:193–201

11. Oi S, Yamada H, Mastumoto S (1990) Tethered cord syndrome versus low-placed conus medullaris in an over-distended spinal cord following initial repair for myelodysplasia. Child's Nerv Syst 6:264–269
12. Pierre-Kahn A, Lacombe J, Pichon J, Guidicelli Y, Reiner D, Saint-Rose C, Perrigot M, Hirsch JF (1986) Intraspinal lipomas with spina bifida. Prognosis and treatment in 73 cases. J Neurosurg 65:756–761
13. Pierre-Kahn A, Zerah M, Renier D, Cinalli G, Sainte-Rose C, Lellouch-Tubiana A, Brunelle F, Le Merrer M, Giudicelli Y, Pichon J, Kleinknecht B, Nataf F (1997) Congenital lumbosacral lipomas. Child's Nerv Syst 13:298–335
14. Reigel DH (1979) Kyphectomy and myelomeningocele repair. In: Ransohoff J (ed) Modern technics in surgery. Neurosurgery. chap 13. Mt Kisco, NY: Futura, pp 1–9
15. Sakamoto H, Hakuba A, Fujitani K, Nishimura S (1991) Surgical treatment of the retethered spinal cord after repair of lipomyelomeningocele. J Neurosurg 74:709–714
16. Sakamoto H, Hakuba K, Fujutani H, Hayashi M, Kiyama M, Nishimura S (1991) Anorectal pressure monitoring during surgery for reuntethering of the spinal cord in cases of lumbosacral lipomyelomeningocele. In: Shimoji K, Kurokawa T, Tamaki T, Willis WD Jr (eds) Spinal cord monitoring and electrodiagnosis. Springer, Berlin, pp 403–411
17. Sakamoto H, Fujitani K, Kitano S, Hakuba A (1992) Surgical treatment of lumbosacral lipoma to prevent postoperative tethered cord (in Japanese). Spinal Surg 6:103–110
18. Zide B, Constantini S, Epstein FJ (1995) Prevention of recurrent tethered spinal cord. Pediatr Neurosurg 22:111–114

Untethering Accompanied with Dural Plasty Using Gore-Tex Membrane

Toshiyuki Sugino, Takeo Gotoh, Mohammad Mouddul Haque, Yasuhiro Matsusaka, and Akira Hakuba

Introduction

An important aspect of untethering of lumbosacral lipoma is to prevent retethering of the spinal cord after the operation. In our department, we operate to prevent retethering by the following means: (1) reconstruction of the conus medullaris after the excision of the lipoma; (2) dural plasty using Gore-Tex membrane (WL Gore & Associates, Flagstaff, Aviz., U.S.A.); (3) performing expansive laminoplasty.

Case Demonstration

A 28-year-old male was admitted with the chief complaint of gait disturbance. In 1968, he had been delivered spontaneously at full term with a dimple and hair in the lumbosacral region. In 1984, at 16 years old, he had motor weakness in the right ankle and his gait was unstable. He was operated on in another hospital after the diagnosis of spina bifida from L5 down to S2 and lumbosacral lipoma. After the operation, he had a slight improvement of gait, but had disturbance in urination and bowel movement. In 1997, at 28 years old, he had motor weakness of both ankles and his gait was again unstable.

Neurological findings on admission showed motor weakness of both ankle joints, hyporeflexia of both patellar tendon reflex and achilles tendon reflex, and hypalgesia up to L5 level.

Magnetic resonance imaging (MRI) showed retethering due to a large residual lipoma at the L5 and S1 level (Fig. 1). He was operated on again in our institute on June 16, 1997.

The patient was placed in a prone position. Laminotomy of L4 was done, and the dura was opened in the midline. The dorsal portion of the lipoma had already been partially resected with the grafted dura mater. The bilateral nerve root was carefully separated from the lipoma. The lipoma was the dorsal type on the left side, and the intermediate type on the right side. That means type 3b on the left side and type 3a on the right side according to Hakuba's classification. The dorsal root on the right side was passing through the lipoma which existed ventral to the dorsal root. The lipoma was excised using a knife and a contact 4-watt YAG laser leaving 2 or 3 mm thickness of the lipoma. Because this laser can cut without bleeding, the cut surface is always dry. Then the conus medullaris was reconstracted using interrupted

Department of Neurosurgery, Osaka City University, 1-5-7 Asahi-wachi, Abeno, Osaka, Japan

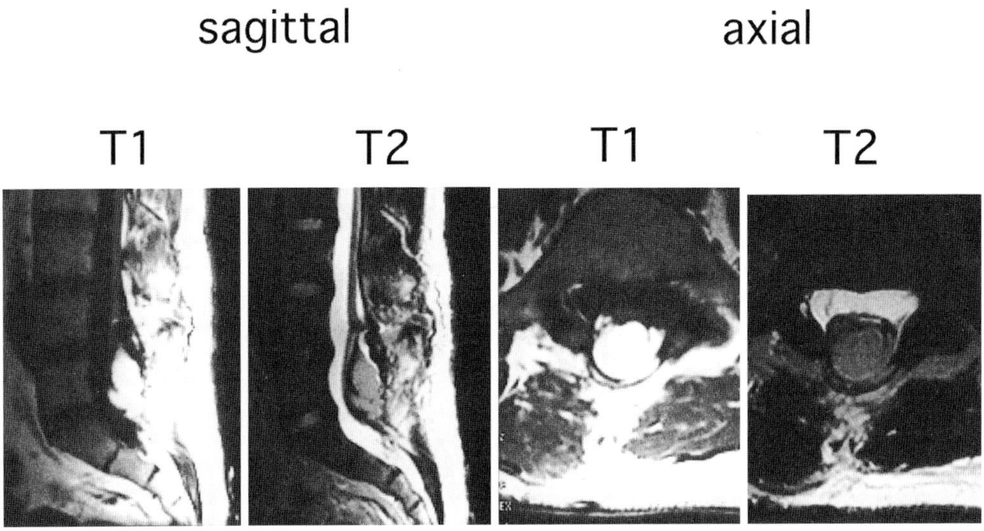

FIG. 1. Preoperative magnetic resonance imaging (MRI)

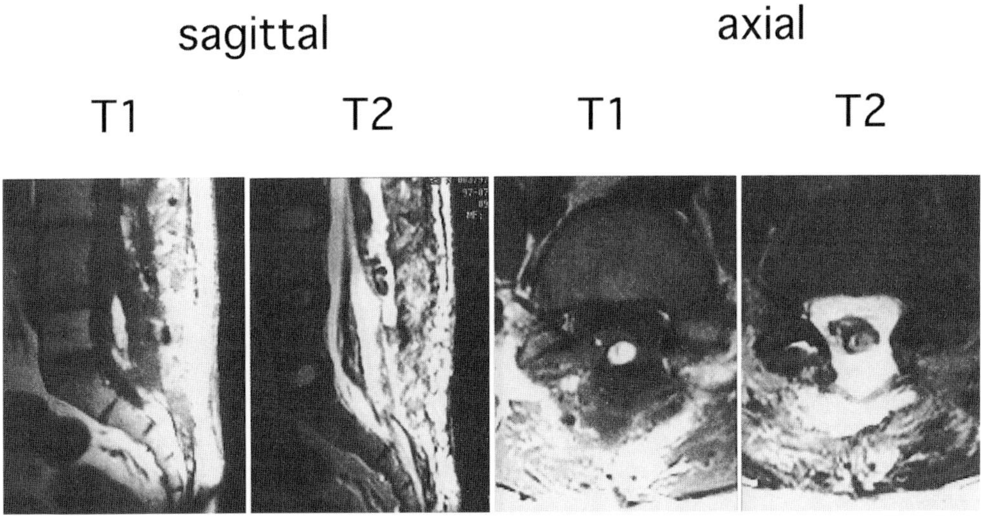

FIG. 2. Postoperative MRI

8-0 monofilament nylon. In order to prevent retethering of the conus medullaris, dural plasty using Gore-Tex membrane was performed. The suture line was covered with a collagen sheet soaked with fibrin glue. The expansive laminoplasty of L5 was done using the spinous process of L2 and L3.

Postoperative MRI showed minimum residual lipoma on the dorsum of the conus medullaris. Good CSF space around the conus medullaris was visible (Fig. 2).

The patient was discharged with improved muscle power in his feet, and his gait became stable.

Discussion

Gore-Tex membrane, which is one of the artificial dura mater, can prevent retethering of the conus. One of the complications when using this material is CSF leakage. Tight suturing with Gore-Tex sutures followed by covering with a collagen sheet soaked with fibrin glue reduce the chances of CSF leakage.

We have operated on 11 patients with lumbosacral lipoma by this means since 1992. None of the patients has developed retethering, although the follow-up period has not been very long.

Conclusion

Using Gore-Tex membrane in dural plasty of untethering prevent retethering. We will continue to follow-up all these patients.

Neurosurgical Treatment of Spasticity in Spina Bifida—Role of Rhizotomy and Its Limitations: Review

Nobuhito Morota and Hiroshi Nakagawa

Summary. The treatment of spasticity in patients with spina bifida, especially those with mylomeningocele (MMC), has been a challenge to all experts who are involved in taking care of these patients. Despite the fact that spacticity is not always present in patients with MMC, it is acknowledged that spasticity is one of the most predisposing factors to restricted locomotion function in their daily life.

The goal of this chapter is to reconfirm the impact of spacticity in these patients, and to discuss the way to relieve harmful spasticity through neurosurgical procedures. One issue here is the role of rhizotomy as a treatment for spasticity in MMC, which we studied though a review of the literature.

As is well known, functional posterior rhyzotomy (FPR) is effective in reducing spasticity in children with cerebral palsy. The efficacy of FPR to spasticity due to MMC has not been established, since the mechanism causing spasticity is different from the one causing to cerebral palsy. However, there may be a chance that rhizotomy could play a role in reducing spasticity in MMC if it were carried out to the ventral root instead of the dorsal root. Cordectomy at the level of the damaged spinal cord lesion would also be beneficial in cases where adhesion prevented ventral rhizotomy.

Although treatment with ventral rhizotomy and cordectomy seems more promising than FPR, further investigations and an accumulation of experience are needed to reach a conclusion about the neurosurgical treatment of spasticity.

Key words. Myelomeningocele, Spina bifida, Spasticity, Rhizotomy, Cordectomy

Introduction

Spasticity in patients with spina bifida, especially those with myelomeningocele (MMC), causes serious problems for their quality of life. Most treatment for spasticity in a patient with MMC has been aimed at correcting joint or muscular deformities by orthopedic procedures, since the direct regulation of spasticity in the central or peripheral nervous system was regarded as being very difficult. Neurophysiological treatment using electric stimulation to the cerebellum or spinal cord has been reported, but its usefulness in controlling spasticity has not been established.

Department of Neurological Surgery, Aichi Medical University, Nagakute-cho, Aichi-gun, Aichi 480-11, Japan

There has been a resurgence of functional posterior rhizotomy (FPR) as a treatment for spasticity caused by cerebral palsy [2, 7, 8, 15]. Despite the wide variety in surgical procedures and intraoperative neurophysiological criteria in lesioning the root/rootlets in FPR, its excellent results in reducing spasticity in patients with cerebral palsy has been widely accepted. Currently, FPR is regarded as a valuable neurosurgical treatment for spastic cerebral palsy [2, 14]. However, this procedure has seldom applied to spasticity in MMC.

Little attention has been given by neurosurgeons to controlling spasticity in patients with MMC. There have only been a few attempts, and these were not accepted with huge enthusiasm, as has been reported elsewhere [6, 13, 18]. In this chapter, we introduce FPR briefly, and review the literature about other neurosurgical procedures to reduce spasticity.

Functional Posterior Rhizotomy

Several surgical procedures have been proposed in FPR. Peacock modified Fasano's original procedure, and his surgery has been regarded as standard since then [2, 7, 8, 15]. In this surgery, a skin incision is made in the midline in the lumbo-sacral region. Osteoplastic laminotomy is carried out from Th12 to L5, and laminectomy is made from S1 to S3. The conus medullares and the whole cauda equina are observed when the dura is opened. After separating the dorsal root from the ventral one, the dorsal action potential of the pudendal nerve is mapped from S1 to the S3 root. The root is not included in lesioning if the pudendal action potential is confirmed on the mapping. This is the way to prevent postoperative urogenital dysfunction [5]. After mapping, the range of lesioning is decided and each root is electrically stimulated. Abnormal muscle responses are recorded by EMG. Those roots which are found to be abnormal are divided into 4–5 rootlets. Each rootlet is again stimulated, and is cut if abnormal responses are again recorded. The rate of root/rootlet cutting shows wide individual differences, but usually falls between 40% and 60% of the root/rootlet tested.

In patients with spastic cerebral palsy, extensive postoperative rehabilitation to regain motor control is mandatory. The success rate of surgery reported from major centers is excellent; most of them reported about 75%–90% [14].

Other Neurosurgical Procedures

Only a few neurosurgical procedures have been proposed to reduce spasticity [10, 16]. In patients with MMC, anterior rhizotomy is the simplest and most reliable procedure for achieving complete interruption of the spinal reflex arcs which produce spasticity [13]. Following the laminectomy/laminotomy of the lumbosacral region, the anterior root responsible for the harmful spasticity is cut after confirming muscle innervation by electrical stimulation. If the lesion is seriously anatomically distorted by a previous surgical repair or spinal cord/root injury due to MMC, and it is difficult to differentiate the anterior from the posterior root, total rhizotomy or spinal cordectomy would be the next surgical choice. Since the procedures are so invasive, the indications for surgery should be strict and limited. Candidates must be those who have no voluntary motor function of the lower extremities, and who suffer serious joint deformity due to spasticity which limits their activities in daily life.

Discussion

The initial neurosurgical treatment of MMC is aimed at protecting the neural tissue from further neural damage, since it is well known that the most significant factor affecting ambulatory status in patients with MMC is the level of neural damage [3]. The basic patterns of

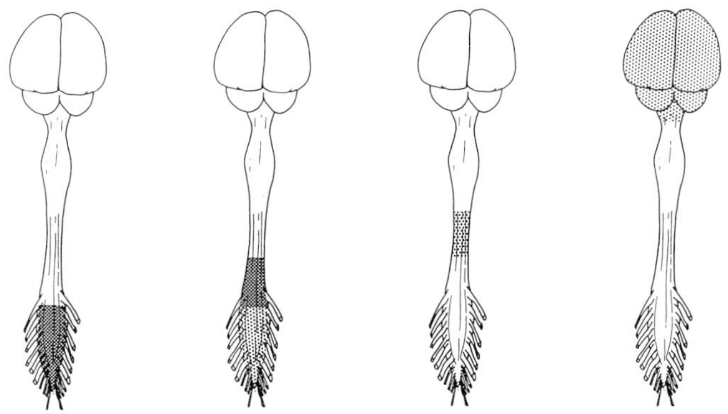

I II III IV

FIG. 1. Possible spinal cord lesions in myelomeningocele (modified from [4]). *Type I*: The lesion involves the terminal portion of the spinal cord. The patient is likely to have flaccid lower extremities. *Type II*: The lesion is above the terminal portion of the spinal cord. The spared terminal portion still has reflex function. The patient is likely to have spastic lower extremities. *Type III*: The spinal cord is incompletely damaged above the terminal portion, which remains intact. The patient would have spontaneous movement of the lower extremities with spasticity. *Type IV*: The lesion in the brain, including the brain stem, is the major source of neurological abnormality in the lower extremities

neural damage in MMC have been classified into four types by Stark and Baker [4] (Fig. 1). The lower extremities become flaccid and there would be no spasticity if the lesion locates on the caudal end of the spinal cord or cauda equina. If the lesion leaves a reflex or normal function of the spinal cord caudally, spasticity may be evoked by the exaggerated reflex circuit at the segment and may influence the ambulatory status of the patient [17]. Those patients with neural involvement at L5 or below will be community walkers, those with neural involvement at L4 will be functional walkers, while those with involvement at L3 and above cannot be community walkers [3]. Treatment of spasticity comes after the initial life-saving surgery. It plays an important role in improving or preventing functional deterioration of the lower extremities.

Spasticity may contribute to the development of foot deformity, which is another factor influencing the ambulatory status in patients with MMC. Spasticity in the lower limbs would most likely cause further musculoskeletal deformities, require more orthopedic procedures, and result in lower ambulatory status than in patients without spasticity [12]. Evaluation of the presence and degree of spasticity is important in predicting the functional outcome of patients with MMC.

The impact of spasticity on the quality of life of patients with MMC is more understandable when the relationship between the presence of spasticity and ambulatory status is examined. Mazur et al. [12] classified spasticity into four groups (Table 1). In his study, all 14 patients with sacral MMC belonged in group 1A, meaning flaccid paralysis. As the lesion goes up, the ratio of flaccid paralysis decreases and spastic paralysis (groups 2A and B) increases. Regarding ambulatory status, there were 51 community walkers (CW), 1 household walker (HW), and 7 nonwalkers (NW) among 59 patients with group 1A spasticity. As the degree of spasticity increased, the ratio of NW sharply increased. There were 5 NW among 10 group 1B patients, and 10 NW out of 26 group 2A patients. Among 14 patients in group 2B, there was

TABLE 1. Grade of spasticity (from [12])

Group 1A:	Complete flaccid paralysis below the lesion and normal upper limbs
Group 1B:	Flaccid lower limbs, spastic upper limbs
Group 2A:	Spastic lower limbs
Group 2B:	Spasticity in all four limbs

only 1 CW, 4 HW, and 9 NW. It is clear that the degree of spasticity, as well as the level of spinal cord lesion [12], seriously affects the quality of life in patients with MMC.

The pathogenesis of spasticity in MMC can be divided into two groups. Spasticity could be induced by organic lesions in the central nervous system associated with, or secondary to, MMC, such as tethered spinal cord, Chiari malformation, hydrocephalus, and hydro/syringomyelia (central spasticity). In this group, surgical treatment of spasticity must be based on the pathology. It should be differentiated from the type of spasticity in the second group. In the second group, spasticity is induced from functional lesions which could lead to an enhanced reflex function of the spinal cord below the lesion (functional spasticity). A spinal cord primarily damaged by MMC or functional abnormalities of the brain and brain stem would be a source of this type of spasticity. Spasticity caused in this manner must be treated in a functional way since there is no organic lesion responsible for the spasticity. Surgical ablation of the reflexly acting segments which cause harmful spasticity is strongly recommended by Smith et al. group [17].

The role of FPR in treating spasticity in MMC remains questionable. FPR is best indicated for spastic cerebral palsy. However, there is some doubt about its application to treat spasticity due to spinal cord injury or cerebrovascular disease. Even for a patient with cerebral palsy, the indications for FPR should be carefully examined if the patient has dystonia or athetosis [1, 9, 15]. Like severe spinal cord injury, spasticity following MMC might be different from that due to cerebral palsy in terms of its degree and mechanism. Storr [18] reported two patients with MMC whose spasticity was dramatically relieved after FPR. However, the effect of the surgery was only followed up for 6 months in both patients. The long-term result of the surgery is unknown. It would be safe to say that FPR can be applied for spasticity in patients with MMC if the motor function of the lower extremities remains useful for the patient.

Compared with FPR, ablation of reflexly acting segments by anterior rhizotomy or cordectomy seems the most promising surgical procedure to relieve spasticity in MMC if the lower extremities are completely useless (Fig. 2). Anterior rhizotomy to the root which contributes to spasticity would easily turn a spastic palsy into a flaccid one. Total rhizotomy or cordectomy at the level of scarred and functionless conus medullares will be recommended if anterior rhizotomy is technically difficult. McLaughlin et al. [13] reported that no spasticity was found in the lower extremities during the average follow-up period of 5.3 years in any patients who underwent either anterior rhizotomy or cordectomy for spasticity due to MMC. Patients with severe spasticity seem to benefit most from these procedures. Although cordectomy for the treatment for spasticity is not familiar, it has been a successful choice of treatment for spasticity due to spinal cord injury and other pathologies [6, 11]. These are reliable procedures for improving spasticity, but care must be taken when selecting candidates for surgery. Another concern about the procedure is postoperative bladder function, since the detrusor and sphincter muscles become flaccid. Adult patients may be able to use abdominal muscles for voiding [11]. Young children may have a problem in controlling abdominal pressure,

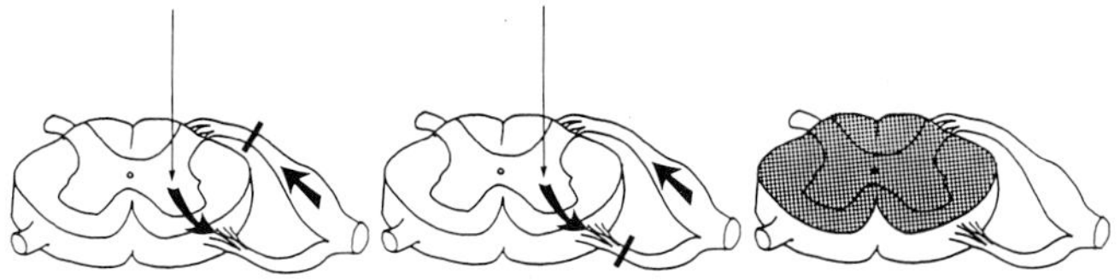

FIG. 2a–c. Surgical reduction of spasticity. **a** The abnormal segmental inflow impulse is eliminated by functional posterior rhizotomy. However, the excitatory impulse traveling through the spinal cord can be transmitted to the ventral root and cause spasticity. **b** All the outflow impulse is eliminated by anterior rhizotomy, which promises to eradicate spasticity as well as voluntary motor function. **c** Spinal cordectomy

which may result in worsened bladder function such as overflow incontinence. Combining posterior rhizotomy at the level of sacrum with the use of neurophysiological techniques will help avoid this complication [5].

Conclusions

Neurosurgical treatment of spasticity in patients with MMC has not received much attention in the past, and accumulated experience in this area is rather limited. However, a review of literature shows that recent advances in neurophysiology applied to FPR, and several procedures such as anterior/total rhizotomy, and cordectomy, are considered to be promising in relieving spasticity in patients with MMC. FPR, which is less invasive and does not compromise any residual motor function, may be applied in selected patients, although its long-term outcome in controlling spasticity in MMC is still unknown. Further study and more experience will be required in this challenging field before that question can be answered.

References

1. Abbott R (1991) Indication for surgery to treat children with spasticity due to cerebral palsy. In: Sindou M, Abbott R, Keravel Y (eds) Neurosurgery for spasticity. A multidisciplinary approach. Springer, Wien, New York, pp 215–217
2. Abbott R, Forem SL, Johann M (1989) Selective posterior rhizotomy for the treatment of spasticity. A review. Childs Nerv Syst 5:337–346
3. Asher M, Olson J (1983) Factors affecting the ambulatory status of patients with spina bifida cystica. J Bone Joint Surg (Am) 65A:350–356
4. Stark GD, Baker GCW (1967) The neurological involvement of the lower limbs in myelomeningocele. Dev Med Child Neurol 9:732–744
5. Deletis V, Vodusek D, Abbott R, Epstein F, Turndorff H (1992) Intraoperative monitoring of the dorsal roots. Minimizing the risk of iatrogenic micturation disorders. Neurosurgery 30:72–75
6. Durward QJ, Rice GP, Ball MJ, Gilbert JJ, Kaufmann JCE (1982) Selective spinal cordectomy. Clinicopathological correlation. J Neurosurg 56:359–367
7. Fasano V, Urciuoli R, Broggi G, Barolat-Romana G, Benech F, Ivaldi A, Sguazzi A (1977) New aspects in the surgical treatment of cerebral palsy. Acta Neurochir Suppl (Wien) 24:53–57
8. Fasano V, Barolat-Romana G, Zeme S, Sguazzi A (1979) Electrophysiological assessment of spinal circuits by direct dorsal root stimulation. Neurosurgery 4:146–151
9. Foerster O (1913) On the indications and results of the excision of posterior spinal nerve roots in men. Surg Gynecol Obstet 16:463–475

10. Gros C (1979) Spasticity. Clinical classification and surgical treatment. In: Krayenbuhl H (ed) Advances and technical standards in neurosurgery, 6. Springer, Wien, New York, pp 55–97
11. MacCarty CS (1954) The treatment of spastic paraplegia by selective spinal cordectomy. J Neurosurg 11:539–545
12. Mazur JM, Stillwell A, Menelaus M (1986) The significance of spasticity in the upper and lower limbs in myelomeningocele. J Bone Joint Surg (Br) 68B:213–217
13. McLaughlin TP, Banta JV, Gahm NH, Raycroft JF (1986) Intraspinal rhizotomy and distal cordectomy in patients with myelomeningocele. J Bone Joint Surg (Am) 68A:88–94
14. Morota N, Abbott R, Kofler M, Epstein FJ, Cohen H (1995) Residual spasticity after selective posterior rhizotomy. Childs Nerv Syst 11:161–165
15. Peacock WJ, Arens LJ, Berman B (1987) Cerebral palsy spasticity. Selective posterior rhizotomy. Pediatr Neurosci 13:61–66
16. Sindou M, Jeanmonod D, Mertens P (1991) Surgery in the dorsal root entry zone. Microsurgical DREZ-tomy (MDT) for the treatment of spasticity. In: Sindou M, Abbott R, Keravel Y (eds) Neurosurgery for spasticity. A multidisciplinary approach. Springer, Wien, New York, pp 165–182
17. Smith TWD, Duckworth T, Maltby B (1973) The importance of reflex function in myelomeningocele. Dev Med Child Neurol (Suppl) 15:46–54
18. Storr BB (1987) Selective posterior rhizotomy for treatment of progressive spasticity in patients with myelomeningocele. Preliminary report. Pediatr Neurosci 13:135–137

Abstract

Analysis of Patients with Spinal Lipoma Reoperated on for Retethering

Kaoru Ichihara, Yatsuo Itoh, and Kiyo Nakabayashi

After primary repair of spinal lipoma, late progressive neurological deterioration commonly occurs due to retethering. We report on 10 patients reoperated on following primary repair. Their ages ranged from 37 months to 196 months (average 91 months) at the time of surgery. The presenting symptoms were urinary disturbance, lower extremity weakness, deterioration in gait, pain, and orthopedic deformities. Four patients presented with severe neurological deficits, including deformity, and 6 patients with mild deficits. The operative procedures were untethering, reconstructive enlargement of the CSF pathway to prevent retethering (subtotal removal of lipoma, reconstruction of conus medullaris, and multiple dural tenting with dural plasty), and often terminal ventriculostomy for hydromyelia. All patients could be untethered. Follow-up from 4 months to 31 months (average 19 months) revealed that 7 patients had stabilization or improvement of their presenting symptoms, but 3 patients with severe neurological deficits had deterioration of their presenting symptoms. Our data suggest that early diagnosis and treatment are essential to provide the patients with the best possible chance of recovery, and that close follow-up and careful monitoring in patients with primary repair of spinal lipoma is important.

Department of Neurosurgery, Yokkaichi Municipal Hospital, Yokkaichi, Japan

Moderator's Comments on Sessions—Tethered Cord

Massimo Caldarelli

Subtle neurological deterioration in motor or bladder function, as well as progressive scoliosis or sensory loss, can be observed not only in misdiagnosed children or adolescents affected by occult spinal dysraphism, but also in those who were correctly diagnosed and adequately treated in their early infancy or childhood. While there is nowadays almost general agreement as to the modalities of treatment of "primary" tethered cord, discussion still continues about surgical indications for retethered spinal cord, and the appropriate surgical techniques to be adopted at the primary untethering procedure in order to avoid, or at least reduce, the risk of this "secondary" tethering.

The major interest in these problems is shown by the high number of contributions in this session devoted to the clinical and neurosurgical aspects of the tethered cord syndrome, and in particular to the problem of retethering.

The first report, by Dr. Yamanouchi and co-workers, is focused on a rare case of Currarino syndrome, which belongs to the group of the congenital "split notochord" syndromes. The case presented here showed an association of ano-rectal stenosis, presacral mass, and sacral bone abnormalities. From a pathological point of view the presacral mass consisted of an anterior meningocele associated with a mature teratoma. The malformation was dealt with surgically by means of excision of the presacral teratoma, closure of the communication between dural sac and meningocele, and spinal cord untethering. The authors comment on the embryological pattern of this rare malformative complex and on the possibilities of surgical treatment.

The following three reports focus on the problem of retethered spinal cord following surgical treatment of lipomyelomeningocele. That by Dr. Ichihara and co-workers analyzes ten cases of retethered spinal cord following primary treatment of lipomyelomeningocele, reoperated on 3–16 years after the first operation. The authors comment on the occurrence of this late complication and on the feasibility of a secondary untethering procedure, although weighted by an increased risk of postoperative neurological deterioration, compared with the low risk of the primary untethering procedure. For this reason, any surgical technique aimed at diminishing the incidence of this "secondary" tethering should be regarded with interest.

In this regard, the following two reports, by Dr. Sakamoto and co-workers and Dr. Sugino and co-workers, deserve particular attention as they suggest the use of a dural substitute (Gore-Tex) for dural repair to prevent secondary spinal cord tethering after surgery for

Department of Neurosurgery, Section of Pediatric Neurosurgery, Catholic University Medical School, Rome, Italy

lipomyeloschisis. In particular, Dr. Sakamoto and co-workers compare the results achieved using the traditional surgical techniques and those obtained using Gore-Tex for dural repair. It is well documented that even the low incidence of secondary tethering observed in the first group of patients (6 out of 50) is reduced to zero in the second one. However, the duration of follow-up in the two groups is not the same, and this fact imposes some caution before conclusive indications are taken. Similar results are shown in the report by Dr. Sugino and co-workers, who utilized Gore-Tex for dural repair in order to reduce the risk of secondary tethering.

The last contribution in this session, by Dr. Morata and co-workers, addresses a completely different topic, namely the surgical management of spasticity in spina bifida patients. Functional posterior rhizotomy for the treatment of spasticity related to cerebral palsy is well acknowledged nowadays. The interesting new aspect is the possibilities of treatment of spasticity in myelodysplastic patients. Actually, spasticity associated with spina bifida is a much more complex phenomenon than that associated with cerebral palsy. In fact, at least two pathogenetic mechanisms contribute to the pathogenesis of the former, namely spinal root and spinal cord damage. Moreover, the associated Chiari II malformation, hydro/syringomyelia, hydrocephalus, and tethered cord can further contribute, in varying combinations, to the occurrence of this phenomenon. Nevertheless, some patients, whose spasticity does not recognize any of the above-mentioned mechanisms as a causative factor, can benefit from functional posterior rhizotomy, especially those whose spinal defect is below the sacrum or who present spasticity above the spina bifida level.

Moderator's Comments on Sessions—Tethered Cord

Tsunemaro Koyama

The Currarino triad is a rare clinical entity. Dr. Y. Yamanouchi et al. presented one typical case of this syndrome. Although their case was a young baby, adult cases have been reported in the literature that presented persistent constipation due to presacral masses. We must keep this syndrome in mind, and if it is suspected, we should order sacral X-P, CT, and MRI.

A late complication of surgery on a lipomyelomeningocele is progressive neurological deficits after several years. This is due to retethering or syringomyelia. Dr. K. Ichihara et al. presented ten cases of retethering that were reoperated on following primary surgery for spinal lipoma. Their operative procedures were untethering, subtotal removal of the lipoma, reconstruction of the conus medullaris, and multiple dural tenting with dural plasty. If a syringomyelia existed, terminal ventriculostomy was also performed. Seven of ten patients had stabilization or improvement of symptoms, but there was deterioration in spite of retethering in three cases. As the authors suggest, early diagnosis and treatment are essentials to give patients the possibility of recovery. Although the authors performed terminal ventriculostomy on patients with syringomyelia, we would like to recommend syringosubarachnoid shunting for these cases to prevent the need for multiple operations.

Dr. H. Sakamoto et al. reported the advantages of Gore-Tex sheet to prevent postoperative retethering following primary surgery on lipomyelomeningocele. The operative procedures were untethering of the spinal cord from the subdural lipomatous tissue, debulking of the subpial lipoma, reconstruction of the conus medullaris, and dural plasty. For dural plasty, artificial dura or paravertebral fascia was used in 50 patients. Gore-Tex sheets were used in the latest 15 patients. Six patients (12%) deteriorated out of the 50, in all of whom the dura was repaired with artificial dura or paravertebral fascia, and retethering was confirmed on MRI and reoperation. On the other hand, none of the 15 patients deteriorated in whom the dura was repaired by Gore-Tex sheet, and retethering was needed less often compared with the patients for whom Gore-Tex sheet was not used. The authors' follow up period was 1–6 years after surgery with the application of Gore-Tex sheet. This report suggests that the application of Gore-Tex sheet for dural plasty is safe, and is useful for preventing complicated postoperative retethering.

Dr. T. Sugino et al. also reported the advantages of Gore-Tex sheet for dural plasty to prevent retethering of the spinal cord after an operation on lipomyelomeningocele. The authors report no patients with retethering after the use of Gore-Tex sheet. In Japan, the use of Lyodura, one of the artificial dura, has decreased in neurosurgical operations since 1996. In the future, the use of Gore-Tex sheet will be the standard technique for surgery on lipomyelomeningocele.

Currently, functional posterior rhizotomy, DREZ-otomy, intrathecal Baclofen, and peripheral neurotomy have been described as being effective for spasticity due to cerebral palsy. Dr. N. Morota et al. introduced the technique of the functional posterior rhizotomy to Japanese neurosurgeons, and reported good results (more than 90% effective) on 32 spastic patients with cerebral palsy. The author applied this technique to spastic patients with spina bifida, but their surgical results were not satisfactory. In Japan, intrathecal injection of Baclofen cannot be used, so functional surgery, including functional posterior rhizotomy, must be investigated for spastic patients.

Rightfulness of the Life-Saving Operation for Neural Tube Disorders: Long-Term Follow-Up Evaluation of Quality of Life

Yasushi Tsukamoto

Summary. Decision-making in selective nontreatment of severely handicapped newborns is a perplexing problem. We present the prognostic study of ten such patients who underwent operations for meningomyelocele or other neural tube defects. Five are already deceased, and of the remaining five, only two are enjoying a reasonable life. The difficulty of evaluating a patient's best interest at birth is that there is no way of knowing the intent of the patient, and someone must make a surrogate decision, and it is very difficult to assess the probable future quality of life of a neonate, as each patient will only develop within his or her own capacity.

Moreover, it is very difficult to obtain the usual informed consent, as parents are usually too upset to make a decision, and the burden of deciding to let the baby die is too heavy for them.

We believe it is preferable that the physician becomes the final decision-maker and bears that responsibility.

Key words. Meningomyelocele, Quality of life, Sanctity of life, Proxy consent

Decision-making in the selective nontreatment of a severely disabled newborn is one of the most difficult problems for medical professionals. There exist two main standpoints on this problem.

One stresses the sanctity of life: "Professional staff members of a health care facility . . . shall not deprive a handicapped infant of nutrition which is necessary to sustain life, or deprive a handicapped infant of medical treatment which is necessary to remedy or ameliorate a life-threatening condition" (USHR 6492) [1]. Judicial discussion is similar, as is describing this nontreatment as "involuntary euthanasia" [7].

The other viewpoint stresses the quality of life: "We withhold dialysis from an anencephalic infant girl precisely because she is so handicapped that she cannot experience any benefit from the treatment. Handicap, therefore, is a morally valid reason for withholding treatment in some cases . . . " [2].

The latter position seems more popular nowadays, but the definition of "some cases" is not easy. Being a neurosurgeon, I have a great concern with this problem, especially about decision-making for meningo-myelocele patients.

In this report, I present my own experiences in the management of these cases and make some comments.

Kantoh Central Hospital, 6-25-1 Kamiyoga, Setagaya-ku, Tokyo 158-8531, Japan

Our Experiences

Meningomyelocele is a situation involving the midline of the osseous spine, and patients usually have an external saccular lesion on the back which contains neural elements of the spinal cord. Newborns with myelocele present severe clinical problems. First, without surgical intervention, over 90% of patients will die of meningitis from the rupture of the sac within a year. Even with an operation on the sac, the patient will continue to have paraplegia of the legs and urinary and fecal incontinence and usually be unable to stand up or walk throughout life.

Many (80–90%) of these patients also have or develop hydrocephalus, which results in mental retardation or, without a ventricular shunt operation, death. Consequently, they usually need to undergo at least two operations to enoure their survival, and nearly half of them die as infants. Even for those who survive, paraplegia of the lower extremities and some mental retardation is inevitable.

For the past 15 years I have participated in the decision-making and the operation for ten meningomyelocele or similar cases. Of these, five had a typical meningomyelocele with secondary hydrocephalus, two had hydroencephalo-dysplasia, and three had miscellaneous neural tube anomalies with hydrocephalus. These cases are listed in Table 1. Two typical cases are described below.

TABLE 1. Prognosis of severely disabled neural tube disorder newborns

Dates of birth and death (years. month. day)	Disorders	Operations	Remarks
1. 1969.3.4 1972.3.25	Encephalocele, sec. hydrocephalus	Plasty 1, shunt 1	Father's consent, mother was upset
2. 1972.4.2 1974.3.21	Hydroencephalo- dysplasia	Shunt 1	Nasogastric tube feeding, hospitalized whole life
3. 1974.6.2 ?	Meningomyelocele, sec. hydrocephalus	Plasty 1, shunt 3	Sac ruptured, meningitis cured, fairly good mental ability
4. 1974.11.27 15 years old	Hydrocephalus	Shunt 13	Sitting only, no speech, being looked after by father
5. 1976.4.15 1979.8.21	Meningomyelocele, sec. hydrocephalus	Plasty 1, shunt 4	Admitted 6 times, death from meningitis
6. 1977.9.8 1980.11.19	Down's syndrome, heart failure, meningitis	Shunt 1	Mental retardation, hemiplegia, heart failure
7. 1980.4.27 10 years old	Meningomyelocele, hydrocephalus	Plasty 1, shunt 5	Wheelchair, mentally well
8. 1984.5.14 6 years old	Hydroencephalo-dysplasia	Shunt 3, hematoma 1	Unable to walk, few words, epilepsy, getting worse
9. 1985.3.26 1986.8.25	Sacral teratoma, hydrocephalus	Removal 1, shunt 6, hematoma 1	Hematoma due to shunt sepsis
10. 1985.10.16 5 years old	Meningomyelocele, sec. hydrocephalus	Plasty 1, shunt 3	Sitting only, epilepsy, unable to speak

A girl (case 5) was born with meningomyelocele. Her legs were completely paralyzed and the cyst on her back was nearly rupturing. To avoid meningitis from the rupture, an emergent plastic operation on the cyst was done on the day of birth. Consent for the operation was given by the young father. On that occasion he was told about the emergency and the possible paraplegia. At that time the baby's head looked normal, and there was little expectation of mental retardation. About 1 week after the operation she developed gradual hydrocephalus. A shunt operation was indicated. The parents and grandmother were reluctant to consent to it, but finally agreed. The patient was discharged 4 months after birth with paralyzed legs and mental retardation. Later she was hospitalized five times because of shunt failure or meningitis, and underwent five operations. She died of meningitis 3 years later.

A baby (case 6) was born with Down's syndrome and heart failure. A cardiac operation was scheduled 2–3 years later. After cardiac catheterization to define the abnormality, the patient developed right hemiplegia, probably due to the embolization in the brain, and was unable even to sit down. Later he also developed meningitis followed by hydrocephalus. Despite his multiple handicaps, his parents wanted the shunt operation and the patient was refered to our department. He was operated on, but succumbed to meningitis at 3 years old. In this case, the mental retardation due to Down's syndrome did not affect the parents's decision-making.

Of the ten patients mentioned above, five are already deceased. Their life spans were 17–40 months, with an average of 31 months. They each underwent 1–8 operations.

The other five patients are still alive, and are from 5 to 15 years old, with an average of 9 years. They underwent 4–13 operations, with an average of six.

We operated on all these cases, but with hindsight, one could say that in some of the cases we should not have done so. Although the death of a patient does not necessarily mean that the operation was meaningless, considering that all the dead infants had died within 4 years of birth, and nearly half of their life was spent in the hospital (case 2 was hospitalized for the whole of his life), I cannot help feeling they might have been happier if they had died just after birth without surgical intervention.

To evaluate the quality of life of the living patients is rather difficult, because to ask them such a question directly may be harmful. However, judging from my own viewpoint or that of the parents, which means judging mainly by the patient's mental capacity, two of them are in good condition. For example, case 7 (10 years old), who is mentally well after seven operations and is attending school in a wheelchair, can be seen to be enjoying a good quality of life. However, case 4 (15 years old), who underwent 13 operations but still has no verbal connection with his parents at all, can hardly be said to be enjoying a good quality of life.

Our fundamental attitude has been to try to save these babies, as can be seen by the fact that we have operated on all these neural tube disorder patients, although of the ten cases considered only two have a reasonable quality of life. It is easy to say that one should have operated only on these two cases, but to foretell the long-term prognosis on the day of birth is very difficult, or I would say almost impossible, even for the most experienced pediatric surgeons. These patients develop within their own capacity, which is very different from adult cases. Because of this difficulty and the possibility (even though it is as low as 20%) of having a reasonable quality of life, we are still inclined to continue these operations.

According to Dr. Todres of Neonate intensive care unit (NICU) of Massachúsetts General Hospital (MGH), United States [8], 142 (67%) of 222 American pediatricians do not recommend surgical intervention for a baby with severe meningomyelocele, which is very different from the Japanese attitude.

Informed Consent

It is necessary to obtain the informed consent of parents to operate on these babies, or to forego treatment and let them die. Judging from papers on judicial cases in Western countries, it is not unusual that the opinion of the doctor and the parents are different. In Japan, such a conflict is very rare. Parents are usually too upset to have an opinion. When such a deformed baby is born, we usually tell the father, but even a father finds it very difficult to accept. He usually asks us to act in the best interests of the baby and lets us choose among the alternatives. The mother and other relatives should also be involved in the decision-making, but as the plastic operation on the sac must be done on the first or second day after birth, there is usually no time to wait for their opinions. Of course, some parents are very intelligent and understand the situation and can be relied on completely, as in a court case in Illinois. On this occasion the couple were a physician and a nurse, but such parents are very rare. Usually we are forced to make our own decision and then to get their consent.

Besides the possible prognosis for the baby, it is necessary to consider the intellectual and financial situation of the parents before making this decision, as it is essential for the baby's good quality of life to have a reasonable and loving family. As we have only a few good institutions for handicapped children, it is very difficult for a handicapped child to live without the support of the parents. Finance is also important. Even if parents are eager to raise their handicapped child, it is almost impossible to provide a good quality of life if the mother needs to work and thus has little time to look after her child. In such a case the baby is left in the hospital for a long time, sometimes for all its life, as in case 2.

Our attitude might be interpreted as being too paternalistic, but this is usually forced upon us. As well as the fact that the parents are too upset to make their own decision, it is very hard for them to say that their own child should die. If they selected that option, as the final decision-maker, they would have to bear the burden of their baby's death for their whole lives. In such a sorrowful case, the final decision-makers must be the physicians, and the burden of responsibility must be endured by the physicians [6].

Conclusion

In 1968, Prof. Matson, a neurosurgeon in USA, wrote that it is unethical to do the plastic operation on a baby with meningomyelocele who has typical paraplegia and incontinentia urinae and albi [5]. In 1971, after evaluating the prognosis of 524 such patients, Lorber [3] concluded that we should not operate on patients with total paraplegia and possible hydrocephalus, as their future quality of life would be miserable. According to his data, among 116 such patients, only 19% had a nearly normal IQ and not one was living a reasonable life.

I am afraid that after 30 years of major developements in medical technology, the situation has not changed very much. Athough prenatal diagnosis has made great progress and the number of disabled children born has decreased, prenatal decision-making is still the same problem. To admit the selective nontreatment of severely disabled children, one must admit the assumption that "there is a point at which death is preferable to life" [4].

However, there is a wide range of opinion among doctors as to when this point has been reached. Such discrepancies are not a good thing. I believe that we should now be able to be more precise about the prognosis (our following up is based on only 10 patients), and should have many more discussions about this difficult problem.

References

1. Dotson ML (1982) Notice to healing providers. Department of Health and Human Service, HR 6492, se 202, 206. 3
2. Fost N (1982) Putting hospitals on notice. Hasting Center Report 12:7
3. Lorber J (1971) Results of treatment of meningomyelocele. Dev Med Child Neurol 13:279–303
4. Mason JK, McC Smith RA (1994) Law and medical ethics. Butterworths, London
5. Matson D (1968) Surgical treatment of meningomyelocele. Pediatrics 42:225–227
6. Nishida H et al. (1987) The medical decision making in neonate in the ethical perspective (in Japanese). J Jpn Assoc Neonate 23:337–341
7. Robertson JA (1975) Involuntary euthanasia of defective newborns: legal analysis. Stanford Law Rev 27:213–269
8. Todres D et al. (1977) Pediatrician's attitudes affecting decision-making in defective newborns. Pediatrics 60:197–201

Preoperative Symptomatic Progression of Lumbosacral Lipoma Operated on After Age One

Kyu-Chang Wang and Byung-Kyu Cho

Summary. The clinical course of lipoma patients who had been treated conservatively for a period reveals some aspects of the natural course of this disease. Of 68 lipoma patients who were managed during the last 4 years, 34 underwent surgery after age 1. Of those, 12 showed a progression of symptoms. The median age of detection of progression was 5 years (0–11 years). Six showed progressive foot weakness/deformity, three were found to have symptoms of progressive neurogenic bladder, two were diagnosed to have hydronephrosis, and one revealed a contracted kidney. Two infants presented with symptoms of progressive neurogenic bladder (in one case) and foot weakness (in the other case) while they were waiting for surgery (both at age 2 months). The results show that the natural course of lumbosacral lipoma is progressive in the majority of patients, which supports the use of prophylactic surgery.

Key words. Lumbosacral lipoma, Progression, Prophylactic surgery

Introduction

Lumbosacral lipoma is the most frequent occult spinal dysraphism, and usually presents with neurogenic bowel/bladder, foot weakness/deformity, or skin stigmata. It is believed by many investigators [1–3, 5, 6, 10] to be a progressive lesion. However, descriptions of the detailed pattern of neurological progression are seldom available. The clinical course of lipoma patients who were treated conservatively for a period reveals certain aspects of the natural course of this disease. We investigated the cases of 34 children for whom surgery was delayed due to neglect by parents or primary medical care personnel, or other nonmedical reasons. The preoperative clinical courses of these cases provided features of the natural history of the lesion, although the information was obtained retrospectively and some details were from the parents' memory. To investigate the pattern of preoperative symptomatic progression, the 34 patients were reviewed and the results were compared with those of patients who underwent surgery before the age of 1 year.

Division of Pediatric Neurosurgery, Seoul National University Children's Hospital, 28 Yongon-dong, Chongno-gu, Seoul 110-744, Korea

Clinical Material and Methods

We have a management protocol to operate on lumbosacral lipoma patients at the age of 2 or 3 months. If a patient shows progressive neurological deficits while waiting for surgery, we operate earlier. However, many patients visit our hospital after the age of 3 months, especially when the lower back mass is small. Frequently, symptoms of neurogenic bladder and mild foot deformities are neglected until the time of toilet training or walking. Sixty-eight children with lumbosacral lipoma (excluding filar lipoma) were managed at our Myelomeningocele Clinic during the period from March 1993 to December 1996. Of these 68 patients, 34 underwent neurosurgical operations for untethering after the age of 1 year (11 between the ages of 1 and 2 years, 9 between the ages of 2 and 5 years, 10 between the ages of 5 and 10 years, and 4 after the age of 10 years). Of the 68 patients, 19 were asymptomatic, 38 showed urological symptoms, 34 had orthopedic problems, and 30 complained of difficulties in bowel control when they underwent neurosurgical operations. Surgery was delayed until the age of 2 years, mainly owing to the parents' neglect of the problems. In contrast, among the 23 patients who underwent surgery after the age of 2 years, 20 had delayed operations owing to the neglect or ignorance of the primary medical care personnel.

To investigate the pattern of preoperative spontaneous symptomatic progression in patients with lumbosacral lipoma, age at deterioration, type of deficits, and outcome after surgery were analyzed. The proportions of patients who had symptoms preoperatively (regardless of the presence of progression) were calculated according to age at surgery. Rates of preoperative symptomatic progression were compared between the groups who underwent surgery before and after the age of 1 year. Using the Kaplan–Meier method, the progression-free rate curve was obtained.

In the present study, progression of symptoms means newly apparent symptoms, a worsening of pre-existing symptoms, or detection of damage which could have been prevented by proper management, e.g., hydronephrosis or contracted kidney. Progressive foot deformity caused by skeletal maturation which did not accompany neurological deterioration was excluded. Symptoms which seemed to be pre-existing and stable, but which had only recently been found, were also excluded. In this respect, information on the patient's earlier neurological status from watchful parents was necessary in order to classify a symptom as a progressive one.

Results

The symptom-positive rate (excluding "skin lesion only") in patients who underwent surgery before the age of 1 year was 65%, and this increased as the age at surgery increased (Table 1).

TABLE 1. Age and preoperative presence of symptoms

Age at surgery (years)	No. of cases	No. of symptomatic patients
<1	34	22 (65%)
1–<2	11	8 (73%)
2–<5	9	7 (78%)
5–<10	10	8 (80%)
>10	4	4 (100%)
Total	68	49 (72%)

Among the 34 patients who underwent surgery after the age of 1 year, 12 showed preoperative symptomatic progression up to the age of 11. The median age of deterioration or detection of the progressing deficits was 5 years (birth to 11 years). Six had progressive foot deformity at the ages up to 7 years (median 4.5 years), three showed progression of neurogenic bladder at the ages of 9 months, and 8 and 9 years, respectively. Two revealed hydronephrosis at the ages of 1 and 5 years, respectively. One was found to have a unilateral contracted kidney at the age of 11 years.

After a follow-up period of 1–10 years (mean 5 years), all six patients with progressive foot weakness/deformity were stable. Three had orthopedic operations (Table 2). After a follow-up period of 3–9 years, three patients with progressive symptoms of neurogenic bladder were on clean intermittent catheterization, and one had augmentation cystoplasty (Table 3). Of the two patients who were found to have hydronephrosis, one underwent ureteroneocystostomy and had no further renal damage after a follow-up period of 8 years. In the other patient, hydronephrosis disappeared after treatment (Table 4). No further renal damage was noted in the patient with a unilateral contracted kidney during the follow-up period of 2 years (Table 5).

On the other hand, two of 34 patients below the age of 1 year showed progression of neurogenic bladder and foot weakness, respectively, at the age of 2 months while they were waiting for elective prophylactic surgery. After surgery, one had improvement of neurogenic bladder, while the other showed stable bilateral foot weakness (Table 6). The rates of preop-

TABLE 2. Cases with progressive foot weakness/deformity

Case No.	Age at detection	Age at surgery	F/U duration (years)	Results
1	7	9	6	Stable, OS op
2	To 6 months[a]	1	10	Stable, OS op, retethering op
3	5	5	7	Stable
4	To 2[a]	2	4	Stable
5	5	9	2	Stable, OS op
6	To 4[a]	5	1	Stable

F/U, follow-up; OS, orthopedic; op, operation.
[a] Gradual progression to the age recorded.

TABLE 3. Cases with progressive neurogenic bladder

Case No.	Age at detection	Age at surgery	F/U duration (years)	Results
1	To 9 months[a]	1	9	CIC
2	8	8	4	Augmentation cystoplasty, CIC
3	9	10	3	CIC

F/U, follow-up; CIC, clean intermittent catheterization.
[a] Gradual progression to the age recorded.

TABLE 4. Cases with hydronephrosis

Case No.	Age at detection	Age at surgery	F/U duration (years)	Results
1	5	5	8	Ureteroneocystostormy, stable
2	1	2	2	Disappeared hydronephrosis

F/U, follow-up.

TABLE 5. A case with a contracted kidney

Case No.	Age at detection	Age at surgery	F/U duration (years)	Results
1	11	13	2	Stable

F/U, follow-up.

TABLE 6. Cases with preoperative neurological progression who were younger than 1 year

Case No.	Symptom	Age at detection	Age at surgery	F/U duration	Results
1	NB	2 months	6 months	3 years	No NB
2	Foot weakness	2 months	3 months	9 months	Stable

F/U, follow-up; NB, neurogenic bladder.

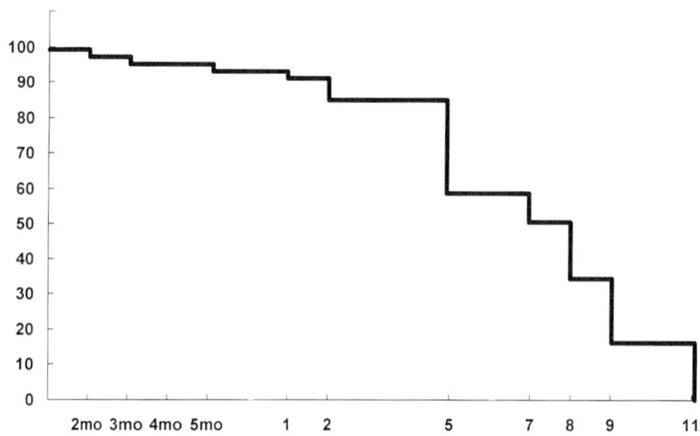

FIG. 1. Progression-free rate of 68 patients with lumbosacral lipoma. The rates are 93%, 90%, and 85% at ages 6 months, 1 year, and 2 years, respectively

erative symptomatic progression of the groups which were older or younger than 1 year were 12/34 (35%) and 2/34 (6%), respectively. The difference was statistically significant ($P = 0.006$, Fisher's exact test).

The decaying curve of the progression-free rate of the 68 patients is shown in Fig. 1. The progression-free rates at the ages of 6 months, 1 year, and 2 years were 93%, 90%, and 85%, respectively. The rates at 5 years and 10 years, i.e., 60% and 17%, respectively, were less reliable owing to the small number of patients. At the age of 5 years, there was a sharp drop from 85% to 60%, which was caused by progression in three patients.

Discussion

Although the modern concept of lumbosacral lipoma was introduced in the early 1980s, many patients did not receive adequate medical care because of neglect by their parents and the ignorance of the primary medical care personnel. When the back mass was sizable, the parents usually sought medical attention early. On the other hand, if the mass was small and the symptoms were not evident, the lesions were frequently neglected. Patients who had abnormalities in urodynamic studies often appeared to void normally. Sometimes abnormal voiding patterns were overlooked as "the voiding pattern in infancy," especially when the patients were first babies. Delayed toilet training or late appearance of symptoms of neurogenic bladder made their parents seek medical attention. Ankle weakness and deformity had similar aspects. Some parents took their children to hospital when the foot weakness or deformity became evident at the age of standing or walking. Some patients were referred by pediatricians who had a chance to see the skin stigmata of the lipoma incidentally. In the majority of patients, parents noticed the problems before the child was 2 years old. After the age of 2, neglect or ignorance by the primary medical care personnel was the main reason for delayed surgery. Lack of knowledge about the proper management of the lesion led primary medical care personnel to remove the subcutaneous portion only, or to give parents information about myelomeningocele which was very negative. Some recommended conservative management owing to the lack of neurological symptoms, or to their own lack of knowledge about the role of surgery even for symptomatic patients.

Prophylactic surgery for lumbosacral lipoma is widely accepted because the lesion is progressive, and even though surgery does not reverse significant neurological deficits, it is relatively safe [2, 4, 5, 7–10]. Although the data were from nonrandomized, retrospective studies with selection bias (not a community population-based study, but a study on hospitalized patients), many investigators agreed that the lesion is progressive and the patients tend to be symptomatic as they get older [1–3, 5, 6, 10]. Even Pierre-Kahn et al. [10], who insisted that the natural course of the lesion, the operative risk, and the long-term effects of surgery should all be considered carefully before deciding to operate, supported the idea that the lesion is progressive. However, detailed reports on the period of neurological deterioration, the pattern of progression, and results after untethering are seldom available. In addition, the wide acceptance of prophylactic surgery for lumbosacral lipoma patients does not justify conservative management and the randomization of patients at the level of current standard neurosurgical practice. In this respect, the 34 patients who underwent surgery after the age of 1 year gave us a good chance to investigate the natural course of lumbosacral lipoma.

In the present study, neurological symptom-positive rates increased as the patients became older. Pierre-Kahn et al. [10] reviewed the literature and calculated the percentage of symptomatic patients according to age. At 1 year it was less than 45%, and increased to about 85% at age 20. Although the rates of symptomatic patients were higher in the present study, the pattern of increase according to the age of the patients coincided with that reported in the literature [10].

The 34 patients who underwent surgery after the age of 1 year provided us with a good chance to study the natural course of the lesion, although we could not obtain an exact figure for preoperative symptomatic progression because this study is retrospective and not randomized. Like previous studies, this is not a community population-based study, but a study on hospitalized patients. The randomization of the patients to surgery and nonsurgery groups to investigate the natural course of the lesion could not be justified in our opinion. Another important limitation of the present study is the fact that a significant amount of information was from the parents. If the information seemed unreliable, we did not count the patient as a case with symptomatic progression. Although information was only taken from watchful parents, their reliability is still in question, at least to some extent. It was difficult to differentiate foot deformity with progressive neurological deterioration from deformity merely caused by skeletal maturation. A definite progression of weakness and the age of the patient were helpful for differentiation. However, a comparison of the ankle motor power before and after standing/walking was not easy, and could be inaccurate. Although the hydronephrosis and contracted kidney could have been congenital and stable for a long time, they were regarded as progressive lesions because they are frequently preventable or reversible with adequate urological management. Data from preoperative serial urodynamic studies were necessary to answer this question.

The majority of the progressed symptoms were stabilized by untethering. One case with hydronephrosis and one with neurogenic bladder showed cures. They were operated on at the early ages of 2 years and 6 months, respectively. Most of the patients who showed stabilization but no recovery were operated on at older ages. This supports the importance of early surgery for prevention of further damage and possible recovery in cases with symptomatic progression.

Many investigators reported that the natural course of lumbosacral lipoma is poor [1–3, 5, 6, 10]. Chapman and Davis [3] stated that neurological status deteriorated in 65% of patients. Hoffman et al. [5] compared the proportion of asymptomatic patients in groups below and above the age of 6 months, which was 35/56 vs. 12/41, to demonstrate the progressive nature of the lesion. Bruce and Schut [1] reported that 48% of patients showed spontaneous neurological deterioration. Kanev and Bierbrauer [6] also described the declining pattern of symptom-free rates with increasing age. According to the literature review by Pierre-Kahn et al. [9], the rate of progression was 56%. Spontaneous neurological deterioration was found in 36% of patients in their series. In the article by the same group in 1997 [10], the rate of spontaneous neurological progression was reported to be 11% when they counted only "definitely progressive" lesions confirmed by themselves. Despite the limitations of the present study, it has shown a chronological pattern of symptomatic deterioration which revealed the progressive nature of the lesion.

To evaluate the role of surgery in lumbosacral lipoma, the surgical risk and long-term results of untethering should be considered, as well as the natural course of the lesion. In the literature, neurological deterioration by surgical insult has been reported in 0–4% of cases [2, 4, 10]. The postoperative long-term results are generally better than the natural course of the lesion. Byrne et al. [2] stated that 93% of asymptomatic infants remained symptom-free after a mean follow-up period of 44 months. Koyanagi et al. [8] reported similar postoperative long-term results. The long-term outcome is less favorable in the series reported by Pierre-Kahn et al. [10]. Only 53% of asymptomatic patients stayed free of symptoms, and 60% of symptomatic patients remained in an improved state after a follow-up period of more than 5 years. Although Pierre-Kahn et al. [10] emphasized the decay of the beneficial effects of untethering surgery, it is generally accepted that the long-term outcome after untethering is better than the natural course of the lesion. The high probability of spontaneous symptomatic progression shown in the present study also supports prophylactic surgery.

Acknowledgment. This study is partly supported by a Seoul National University Hospital Research Grant.

References

1. Bruce DA, Schut L (1979) Spinal lipomas in infancy and childhood. Child's Brain 5:192–203
2. Byrne RW, Hayes EA, George TM, McLone DG (1995) Operative resection of 100 spinal lipomas in infants less than 1 year of age. Pediatr Neurosurg 23:182–186
3. Chapman PH, Davis KR (1983) Surgical treatment of spinal lipomas in childhood. In: Raimondi AJ (ed) Concepts in pediatric neurosurgery, vol 3. Karger, Basel, pp 178–190
4. Harrison MJ, Mitnick RJ, Rosenblum BR, Rothman AS (1990) Leptomyelolipoma: analysis of 20 cases. J Neurosurg 73:360–367
5. Hoffman HJ, Taecholarn C, Hendrick EB, Humphreys RP (1985) Management of lipomyelomeningoceles: experience at the Hospital for Sick Children, Toronto. J Neurosurg 62:1–8

6. Kanev PM, Bierbrauer KS (1995) Reflections on the natural history of lipomyelomeningocele. Pediatr Neurosurg 22:137–140
7. Kanev PM, Lemire RJ, Loeser JD, Berger MS (1990) Management and long term follow-up review of children with lipomyelomeningocele, 1952–1987. J Neurosurg 73:48–52
8. Koyanagi I, Iwasaki Y, Hida K, Abe H, Isu T, Akino M (1997) Surgical treatment supposed natural history of the tethered cord with occult spinal dysraphism. Child's Nerv Syst 13:268–274
9. Pierre-Kahn A, Lacombe J, Pichon J, Giudicelli Y, Renier D, Sainte-Rose C, Perrigot M, Hirsch JF (1986) Intraspinal lipomas with spinal bifida: prognosis and treatment in 73 cases. J Neurosurg 65:756–761
10. Pierre-Kahn A, Zerah M, Renier D, Cinalli G, Sainte-Rose C, Lellouch-Tubiana A, Brunelle F, Le Merrer M, Giudicelli Y, Pichon J, Kleinknecht B, Nataf F (1997) Congenital lumbosacral lipomas. Child's Nerv Syst 13:298–334

Management of Spinal Lipoma in Children—Comparison of Neurological Status Between Surgical and Nonsurgical Cases

Hiroaki Date[1], Chiaki Ito[1], and Akira Yamaura[2]

Summary. The clinical course of 27 patients with spinal lipoma is reviewed. Nearly 70% of such infants will present some signs or symptoms and deteriorate during the first 10 years, and this is caused mainly by tethering of the cord. Untethering surgery is effective, and is recommended to relieve the symptoms of older patients who present a worsening of symptoms. Although this study suggests that prophylactic surgery in early infancy will prevent later deterioration, we need to study the natural evolution of lipoma by following whole lipoma patients, including asymptomatic nonhospitalized ones, for a period of over 10 years. To clarify the efficacy of prophylactic surgery, bladder and bowel functions should be assessed objectively with the use of scoring even in early infancy.

Key words. Spinal lipoma, Surgery, Natural history

Introduction

Lumbosacral spinal lipoma is a very common congenital spinal dysraphic state, but its natural history is not well known. While some patients exhibit progressive neurological deterioration, others remain asymptomatic even at school age or in adolescence [11]. We have studied the change in neurological scores of children with spinal lipoma during the period of their growth, and assessed the effects of surgery on very young patients with lipoma.

Materials and Methods

This study included 27 patients (13 females and 14 males) with ages ranging from 3 to 23 years. All patients were followed for 3 years or longer at Chiba Children's Hospital in Japan. In this study, spinal lipomas are limited to those of the conus medullaris, and filar types of lipoma or lipomyelomeningoceles are excluded.

Lipomyelomeningoceles are defined as a lipoma in which a dysplastic spinal cord is located outside of the spinal canal with lipoma, and are usually associated with complex or severe abnormality of the cord itself. Lipoma of the filum, on the other hand, is a very simple one and can be treated without any deterioration. The most common but controversial one is a lipoma of the conus.

[1] Department of Neurosurgery, Chiba Children's Hospital, 579-1 Heta-cho, Midori-ku, Chiba 266, Japan
[2] Department of Neurosurgery, Chiba University School of Medicine, Chiba, Japan

TABLE 1. Spina bifida neurological scale (SBNS) [9]

Motor (M)	Sensation (S)	Bladder/bowel (B/B)
6. S1 intact	4. S3 intact	5. Normal
5. L5 intact	3. S1 intact	4. B/B +, ±
4. L4 intact	2. L4 intact	3. B/B ±, ±
3. L3 intact	1. No sensation below L4	2. B/B −, ±
2. L2 intact		1. No control
1. L1 intact		

SBNS = sum of (M + S + B/B).
+, intact; ±, incomplete; −, no control.

TABLE 2. Neurological scores of 11 nonoperated patients

Case	Age/sex	SBNS		
1.	6 ♀	M6S4B5	15	No symptoms
2.	11 ♀	M6S4B4	14	Mild incontinence
3.	11 ♂	M5S3B3	11	Club foot/residual urine
4.	16 ♂	M5S3B5	13	Calcaneus foot
5.	15 ♂	M6S3B5	14	Scoliosis since 11 years old
6.	14 ♀	M4S3B3	10	Varus deformity since 11 years old
7.	9 ♂	M4S2B4	10	Varus deformity since 7 years old
8.	11 ♀	M3S2B4	9	Varus deformity/incontinence
9.	16 ♂	M4S3B4	11	Equinus since 11 years old
10.	14 ♀	M4S3B5	12	Club foot since 10 years old
11.	5 ♀	M6S3B2	11	Incontinence

Mean age 11.6 years; mean SBNS 11.8.

The patients were divided into two groups, 11 nonoperated and 16 operated. Nonoperated patients were those whose parents rejected surgery, or whose home doctor did not recommend surgery. Operated patients were further divided into two subgroups: (a) five who presented obvious neurological deterioration before surgery, and (b) 11 who underwent surgery in early infancy for prophylaxis purposes.

Neurological status was evaluated with the spina bifida neurological scale (SBNS) proposed by Oi and Matsumoto [9] (Table 1). This scale is expressed by the sum of three neurological functional scores; motor, sensory, and bladder and bowel functions. There are 15 points on the scale, and the more disabling the handicap is, the lower the score.

Results

Eleven Nonoperated Patients

The mean SBNS of the 11 nonoperated patients was 11.8 (Table 2). Their mean age was 11.6 years. Only one patient remained asymptomatic at age 6. Of the other ten symptomatic patients, four patients (cases 2–5) presented some neurological defictis but remained stable. The mean SBNS of these patients was 13. The other six patients (cases 6–11) showed progressive neurological deterioration with age, and their mean SBNS was 10.5. Neurological deterioration began when they were from 7 to 11 years old.

TABLE 3. Neurological scores of five operated group A patients before surgery

Case	Age/sex	SBNS before operation		
1.	10 ♂	M4S2B2	8	Incontinence since 9 years old
2.	18 ♂	M6S2B2	10	Lumbago since 14 years old
3.	8 ♂	M4S2B3	9	Club foot, incontinence since 6 years old
4.	3 ♀	M6S3B3	12	Progressed incontinence
5.	17 ♀	M5S2B3	10	Incontinence since 14 years old

Mean age 11.2 years; mean SBNS 9.8.

TABLE 4. Changes of neurological status after surgery in group A operated patients

Case	Age/sex	SBNS after surgery		
1.	12 ♂	M4S2B2	8	Decreased incontinence, increased power in toes
2.	22 ♂	M6S2B2	10	Pain relief
3.	9 ♂	M4S2B3	9	Improved walking
4.	7 ♀	M6S3B4	13	Decreased incontinence
5.	18 ♀	M5S3B3	11	Decreased incontinence

Mean age 13.6 years; mean SBNS 10.2.

Sixteen Operated Patients

Five patients, who were operated upon when neurological worsening was manifested, showed a much lower SBNS (mean 9.8) when they were operated on at 11.2 years (Table 3). The progressively worsening signs were incontinence, low back pain, and foot deformity, and the symptoms were aggravated when they were 9, 14, 6, and 14 years old, respectively. Table 4 shows the changes in neurological status of these five patients after surgery. All patients showed an improvement in their symptoms after surgery, and none experienced neurological deterioration. Precise SBNS of the other 11 patients of group B, who underwent prophylactic removal of lipoma in early infancy, was impossible before surgery because bladder and bowel functions could not be evaluated in this age group, especially in patients younger than 3 years of age (Table 5). Varus deformity of the ankle and persistent incontinence were manifest signs in this age group, and were found in 6 of 11 infants (cases 6–11). Table 6 shows changes in the neurological status of these infants after surgery. Their mean SBNS was 12.7 when they were 4.4 years old.

Sixteen Nonprophylactic Surgery Patients (Tables 2 and 3)

Five operated patients of group A and 11 nonoperated patients can be regarded as the patients who had no prophylactic surgical treatment in infancy. Of these 16 patients, only one grew up without any neurological signs and symptoms, while four showed some neurological deficits, although these did not progress. Eleven of the 16 (cases 6–11 of the nonoperated patients and five operated group A patients), nearly 70%, showed some neurological deficits which progressively worsened with growth.

TABLE 5. Neurological scores of 11 operated group B patients before surgery

Case	Age at surgery/sex	SBNS before surgery		
1.	4 yr 8 mo ♂	M6S3B5	14	
2.	11 mo ♂	M6S3?		
3.	1 mo ♂	M6S4?		
4.	9 mo ♂	M6S3?		
5.	4 mo ♀	M6S3?		
6.	4 mo ♀	M4S3?		Varus deformity
7.	11 mo ♂	M5S3?		Varus deformity
8.	4 mo ♀	M5S4?		Varus deformity
9.	1 yr 6 mo ♀	M5S3?		Varus deformity
10.	3 yr 2 mo ♀	M6S3B3	12	Incontinence
11.	3 mo ♂	M4S3?		Varus deformity

Mean age 1 year 2 months.

TABLE 6. Changes of neurological status after surgery in group B operated patients

Case	Age/sex	SBNS after surgery		
1.	7 ♂	M6S3B5	14	
2.	5 ♂	M6S3B5	14	
3.	3 ♂	M6S3B4	13	Incontinence (+)/CIC
4.	3 ♂	M6S3B4	13	
5.	3 ♀	M6S3B4	13	Incontinence (+)
6.	5 ♀	M6S3B4	13	Residual urine (+)/incontinence (−)
7.	4 ♂	M6S3B4	13	Residual urine (+)/incontinence (−)
8.	5 ♀	M5S3B5	13	Varus unchanged
9.	6 ♀	M5S3B4	12	Varus unchanged/incontinence (+)
10.	4 ♀	M6S3B5	14	
11.	3 ♂	M4S2B2	8	Varus unchanged/incontinence (+)

Mean age 4.4 years; mean SBNS 12.7.

Discussion

Natural History

Children with spinal lipoma most frequently have an intact neurological status at birth, but later can progress to various degrees of bladder, bowel, and foot dysfunction. The most common cause of such neurological deterioration is thought to be spinal cord tethering by the lipoma [13], and progressive deterioration is reported to be linked to the patient's increasing age in a logarithmic relationship [5]. Many doctors recommend early preventive surgery such as debulking the lipoma and releasing the spinal cord from the lipoma [4, 7]. On the other hand, there are some patients who showed no deterioration even at school age or as adults, and controversy still exists regarding the management and timing of surgery [1].

Hoffman et al. [4] reported that by the age of 4 years, all children with spinal lipomma would neurologically deteriorate and become symptomatic. Herman et al. [3] also reported that the age of presentation of tethered cord patients varied from 6 to 9 years in the spinal lipoma group. Our results in this study indicate that nearly 70% of infants would develope some neurological deficits during the first 10 years of life. In one-third of the patients, aggravation began after 9 years of age. Of course, we must keep in mind that a number of asymptomatic lipoma patients do not visit the hospital, and this figure would be much lower in a "true" natural history of spinal lipoma [11].

Symptoms and Signs

Neurological aggravation and/or improvement can be recognized only when the precise neurological status of the patient is followed chronologically. SBNS [9] is a useful scoring system for this purpose, and the natural evolution of spinal lipoma and/or the result of surgical management can be objectively assessed. However, neurological status in early infancy is difficult to assess, especially that of bladder and bowel functions, even by SBSN. If the patients are infants, we can hardly make a diagnosis of "on" symptoms. Although the word "asymptomatic" is usually used when we cannot find any symptoms or signs in young infants, it does not always mean they are neurologically normal.

Effects of Surgery

The benefits of prophylactic surgery have been widely reported [1, 2, 6, 7, 10], but many papers report that 50–70% of the motor deficits caused by spinal lipomas are not reversed by surgery [6, 8, 12]. Postoperative neurological deterioration is reported as ranging from 0 to 4% [1, 4, 5, 8]. In our group A patients, in which surgery was undertaken only when the signs and symptoms progressed, surgery had the effect of stabilizing the symptoms or improving them. However, this improvement was mainly subjective or minimal, e.g., pain relief, improvement in walking, and decreased incontinence, and was not reflected in neurological scores. The change of SBNS was minimal (from 9.8 to 10.2). Postoperative magnetic resonance imaging of these five patients showed an elevation of the conus, and tethering of the cord is the most usual cause of deterioration.

In the case of group B patients, who underwent prophylactic surgery, it was difficult to evaluate the neurological improvement after surgery because precise evaluation before surgery is nearly impossible for small infants. Some patients who had been assessed as normal before surgery developed some deterioration later, and vice versa. A mean SBNS of 12.7 at the age of 4.4 years is a better score than that of the nonoperated and of group A operated patients. Although this result might indicate the efficacy of early prophylactic surgery, we know that neurological aggravation could start much later. Five years is still a short period for evaluating the efficacy of prophylactic surgery.

In conclusion, nearly 70% of infants with spinal lipoma will deteriorate during the first 10 years of life, and this aggravation is caused mainly by tethering of the cord. Untethering is effective, and is recommended to relieve symptoms for older patients who present a worsening of symptoms. Although it seems feasible that prophylactic surgery in early infancy may prevent later deterioration, we cannot be sure of that at the moment. To clarify the efficacy of prophylactic surgery, bladder and bowel functions should be assessed objectively by some system of scoring, even in early infancy. We also need to know the natural evolution of lipoma by following lipoma patients, including asymptomatic nonhospitalized ones, for a period of at least 10 years.

References

1. Bruce DA, Schut L (1979) Spinal lipomas in infancy and childhood. Child's Brain 5:192–203
2. Byrne RW, Hayes EA, George TM, McLone DG (1995) Operative resection of 100 spinal lipomas in infants less than 1 years of age. Pediatr Neurosurg 23:182–187
3. Herman JM, McLone DG, Storrs BB, Dauser RC (1993) Analysis of 153 patients with myelomeningocele or spinal lipoma reoperated upon for a tethered cord. Pediatr Neurosurg 19:243–249
4. Hoffman HJ, Taecholarn C, Hendrick EB, Humphreys RP (1985) Management of lipomyelomeningoceles. Experience at the Hospital for Sick Children, Toronto. J Neurosurg 62:1–8
5. Kanev PM, Bierbrauer KS (1995) Reflections on the natural history of lipomyelomeningocele. Pediatr Neurosurg 22:137–140
6. Kanev PM, Lemire RJ, Loeser JD, Berger MS (1990) Management and long-term follow-up review of children with lipomyelomeningocele, 1952–1987. J Neurosurg 73:48–52.
7. La Marca F, Grant JA, Tomita T, McLone DG (1997) Spinal lipomas in children: outcome of 270 procedures. Pediatr Neurosurg 26:8–16
8. McLone DG, Naidich TP (1986) Laser resection of fifty spinal lipomas. Neurosurgery 18:611–615
9. Oi S, Matsumoto S (1992) A proposed grading and scoring system for spina bifida: spina bifida neurological scale (SBNS). Child's Nerv Syst 8:337–342
10. Pierre-Kahn A, Lacombe J, Pichon J, Giudicelli Y, Renier D, Sainte-Rose C, Perrigot M, Hirsch JF (1986) Intraspinal lipomas with spina bifida. Prognosis and treatment in 73 cases. J Neurosurg 65:756–761
11. Pierre-Kahn A, Zerah M, Renier D, Cinalli G, Sainte-Rose C, Lellouch-Tubiana A, Brunelle F, Le Merrer M, Giudicelli Y, Pichon J, Kleinknecht B, Nataf F (1997) Congenital lumbosacral lipomas. Child's Nerv Syst 13:298–335
12. Schut L, Bruce DA, Sutton LN (1983) The management of the child with a lipomyelomeningocele. Clin Neurosurg 30:464–476
13. Yamada S, Zinke D, Saunders D (1981) Pathophysiology of tethered cord syndrome. J Neurosurg 54:494–503

Treatment of Tethered Spinal Cord

Nobuko Yamashita, Ken Kamiya, and Kazuo Yamada

Summary. Thirty-four children with lumbosacral spinal dysraphism were followed up in our hospital by magnetic resonance imaging (MRI). There were 18 patients with lumbosacral lipoma, 15 with myelomeningocele, and 1 with congenital dermal sinus. All patients except for one case of lumbosacral lipoma received surgical treatment. Sixteen children with lumbosacral lipoma and 12 with myelomeningocele showed tethered spinal cord on MRI. After surgery for lumbosacral lipoma, three of these patients suffered tethered cord syndrome. The incidence of tethered cord syndrome was three out of 34 patients with tethered spinal cord. A 14-year-old girl with apparent of urinary incontinence and a 14-year-old boy with progressive urinary incontinence received surgery for untethering. Tethered spinal cord after surgery for spinal dysraphism is frequently detected by MRI, but not all cases suffer from neurological deterioration. Careful periodic follow-up is thought to be the best way to select patients for surgery, and cine-MRI might help to predict the onset of tethered cord syndrome.

Key words. Spinal dysraphism, Tethered cord syndrome, Cine-MRI

Introduction

Tethered cord syndrome is a well known pathologic condition which involves progressive neurological deterioration due to tethering of the spinal cord. Most patients present symptoms such as back pain, gait disturbance, urinary incontinence, bowel dysfunction, scoliosis, and foot deformities during the period of rapid growth. Tethered spinal cord after surgery for spinal dysraphism is commonly detected by magnetic resonance imaging (MRI), and some of these cases suffer from tethered cord syndrome. Its incidence has been reported to be from 3 to 19% [6, 9–12]. A timely operation for untethering and release of the spinal cord is needed to improve or stabilize the neurological problems of the syndrome. It is important to determine which patients should receive this surgical treatment after surgery for spinal dysraphism. We reviewed our experience of patients with spinal dysraphism and studied their MRI findings in order to attempt to predict the presentation of tethered cord syndrome.

Department of Neurosurgery, Nagoya City University, 1 Kawasumi Mizuho-cho, Mizuho-ku, Nagoya 467-8602, Japan

Material and Methods

We investigated 48 patients with spinal dysraphism from 1979 to 1997, and were able to follow up 34 of them in our hospital by MRI. The follow-up period was from 4 months to 15 years, and the mean was 7 years. The original lesions were lumbosacral lipoma in 18 patients, myelomeningocele in 15, and congenital dermal sinus in one (Table 1). Thirty-three of these patients had received surgical treatment, the exeption being a case with lumbosacral lipoma. This patient was referred to us when he was 10 years old, and did not show any neurological deterioration in the follow-up period. The repair of myelomeningocele was performed 2 days after birth. The lumbosacral lipomas had been treated from 4 days to 12 years of age. The patient with congenital dermal sinus was operated on at 7 months of age. All patients were followed up as out-patients with MRI. Some of them were also examined by cine-MRI in order to study pulsatile movements of the CSF and spinal cord in the lumbar area. The studies were performed on a 1.0-tesla MRI system.

Results

MRI revealed tethered spinal cord in 17 cases of lumbosacral lipoma and 13 cases of myelomeningocele (Table 1). In three of these patients, neurological function deteriorated late after repair of the lumbosacral lipoma, and we diagnosed them as having tethered cord syndrome (Table 2). The incidence of tethered cord syndrome was three out of 34 patients.

Case 1 was a 14-year-old girl who had received an operation for lumbosacral lipoma at 12 months of age and presented urinary incontinence. The MRI revealed tethering of the spinal cord at the level of L5 and S1 and residual lipoma (Fig. 1). Surgery for untethering was performed and the symptoms gradually improved. Case 2 was a 14-year-old boy with deterioration of bladder function. He had been treated surgically at 11 months old. His MRI showed tethering of the cord to the lipoma at the level of L5 and S1, and he received an operation for untethering. His symptoms were stabilized. Case 3 was a 12-year-old boy who showed gait

TABLE 1. Lumbosacral spinal dysraphism

	No. of patients followed up	Tethered spinal cord
Lumbosacral lipoma	18 (1)	17
Myelomeningocele	15	13
Congenital dermal sinus	1	0

TABLE 2. Three cases of tethered cord syndrome

Age/sex	Neurological deterioration
14 y, F	Urinary incontinence
14 y, M	Urinary incontinence
11 y, M	Gait disturbance

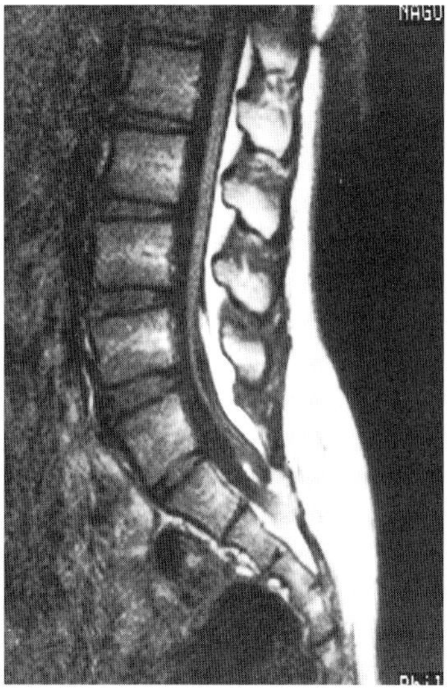

FIG. 1. A 14-year-old girl with tethered cord syndrome. Magnetic resonance imaging (MRI) revealed tethering of the spinal cord at the level of L5 and S1 and residual lipoma

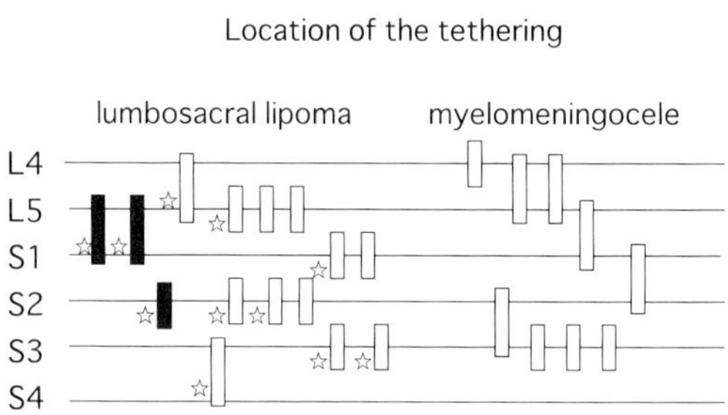

FIG. 2. Sites of the adhesion shown by MRI. There was no difference in level between patients presenting tethered cord syndrome (*solid bars*) and those who did not (*open bars*): *stars*, lipoma

disturbance. He had been operated on for lumbosacral lipoma when he was 4 days old. MRI revealed tethering of the cord at the level of S1 and S2, residual lipoma and syrinx at the lumbar area. We recommended surgical treatment for him.

The site of the tethering was reviewed by MRI (Fig. 2). There was no difference of level between the patients presenting tethered cord syndrome and those who did not. Whether lipoma remained or not was also unrelated.

Three patients were examined by cine-MRI: a child after surgery for lumbosacral lipoma and two children after surgery for myelomeningocele. After an operation for lumbosacral lipoma, a 2-year-old boy had no neurological problems and his cine-MRI showed pulsatile movements of CSF and spinal cord in the lumbar area with ECG (Fig. 3). The same finding was observed in the other two cases.

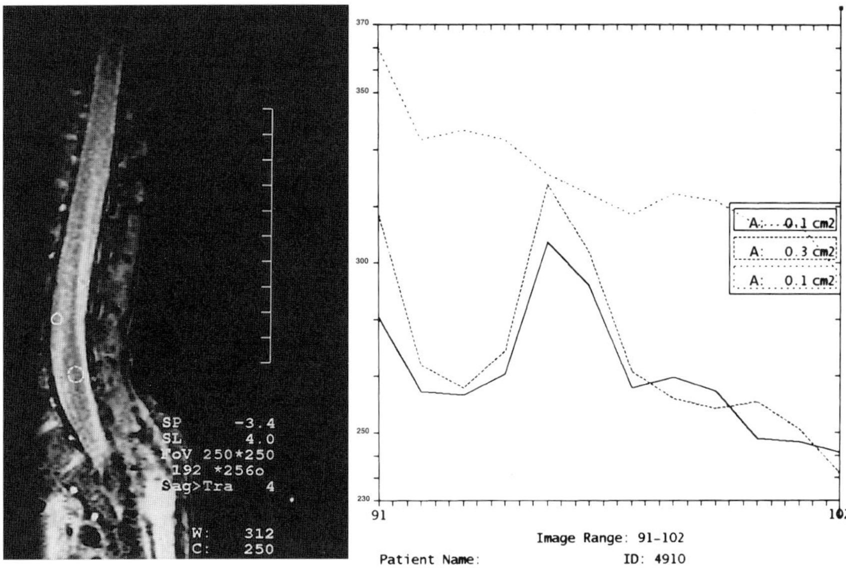

FIG. 3. Cine-MRI of a 2-year-old boy after surgery for lumbosacral lipoma. Cine-MRI showed pulsatile movements of the spinal cord and CSF

Discussion

Tethered cord syndrome can be caused by various types of spinal dysraphism. In particular, tethered cord syndrome after surgery for spinal dysraphism, as with lumbosacral lipoma and myelomeningocele, has become a problem. Many patients have been followed up by MRI, and tethering of the spinal cord to the site of the previous operation is a common finding in these cases [2, 12]. However, it is also well known that not all of the patients with such findings suffer from progressive neurological deterioration or tethered cord syndrome. Its incidence has been reported to be from 3 to 19% [6, 9–12]. Our own experience corresponded with these reports. The symptoms of tethered cord syndrome can be improved or stabilized by surgical treatment, and the timing of the operation is thought to be crucial. Early diagnosis is important to prevent further neurological impairment [4].

At present, tethered cord syndrome is mainly diagnosed from clinical findings. The patients are followed up radiologically as well as neurologically, and MRI gives us detailed information about anatomical structure. Tamaki et al. [12] reported that a large proportion of patients with tethered cord syndrome showed tethering at the last laminae in addition to the site of previous repair on MRI. We could not find such a correlation in our small sample of patients. In our study, there was no difference in the level of tethering between patients with tethered cord syndrome and those without. Whether lipoma remained or not was also unrelated. We thought that it was difficult to predict which patients would show tethered cord syndrome in the future merely from the findings on MRI.

A few other procedures have been combined with neurological observations to attempt the early diagnosis of tethered cord syndrome. Boor et al. [2] found posterior tibial nerve somatosensory evoked potentials (SSEP) to be a sensitive indicator of tethered cord syndrome, and reported that its decline slowed after untethering. SSEP has the capacity to reflect early functional change. Spinal cord movements can be evaluated using ultrasonography [1, 3]. The absence of spinal cord movements has been described as a characteristic finding of tethered cord, but ultrasonography is available only for patients with large dysraphic laminae, and postoperative scarring often disturbs clear imaging.

We examined patients with cine-MRI in order to catch pulsatile movements of the spinal cord and CSF with ECG in the lumbar area. The mechanism of pulsatile movements of the brain and spinal cord is not completely understood. It is generally believed that transmission of the arterial pulse into the brain and spinal cord causes the phenomenon. In our preliminary study, cine-MRI demonstrated pulsatile movements of the spinal cord and CSF in children after surgery for spinal dysraphism. We thought that the pulsatile movements of the spinal cord might signify untethering of the spinal cord. Assessment of spinal cord motion in the patients with spinal dysraphism using MRI has been reported [5, 7, 8]. The investigation dealt with longitudinal motion of the cord in the cervical region. Only patients with signs and symptoms of tethered cord syndrome as well as decreased cord motion on MRI were operated on, but children with a marked decrease in those symptoms did not improve after surgery. In those studies, cord pulsations were best observed in the cervical region, but we thought it reasonable to observe the lumbar area, taking clinical symptoms into consideration.

We managed cine-MRI as a prolongation of the usual static MRI, although it took slightly longer. The examination is not invasive. The patient does not need to attend the hospital for another examination, and the entire procedure is convenient for them.

The patients we examined were young children, and their follow-up period was short. We would like to gather data from more cases, including preoperative ones, and follow up the findings. We would also like to confirm the correlation between tethered cord syndrome and a decrease in pulsatile movements. We thought that pulsatile movements of the spinal cord and CSF on cine-MRI might offer some promise of predicting tethered cord syndrome.

References

1. Balasubramanian C, Laurent JP, McCluggage C, Oshman D, Cheek WR (1990) Tethered-cord syndrome after repair of meningomyelocele. Child's Nerv Syst 6:208–211
2. Boor R, Schwarz M, Reitter B, Voth D (1993) Tethered cord after spina bifida aperta: a longitudinal study of somatosensory evoked potentials. Child's Nerv Syst 9:328–330
3. Hall WA, Albright AL, Brunberg JA (1988) Diagnosis of tethered cord by magnetic resonance imaging. Surg Neurol 30:60–64
4. Herman JM, McLone DG, Storrs BB, Dauser RC (1993) Analysis of 153 patients with myelomeningocele or spinal lipoma reoperated upon for a tethered cord. Pediatr Neurosurg 19:243–249
5. Johnson DL, Levy LM (1995) Predicting outcome in the tethered cord syndrome: a study of cord motion. Pediatr Neurosurg 22:115–119
6. Kanev PM, Lemire RJ, Loeser JD, Berger MS (1990) Management and long-term follow-up review of children with lipomyelomeningocele, 1952–1987. J Neurosurg 73:48–52
7. Levy LM, DiChiro G, McCullough DC, Dwyer AJ, Johnson DL, Yang SSL (1988) Fixed spinal cord: diagnosis with MR imaging. Radiology 169:773–778
8. McCullough DC, Levy LM, DiChiro G, Johnson DL (1990–1991) Toward the prediction of neurological injury from tethered spinal cord: investigation of cord motion with magnetic resonance. Pediatr Neurosurg 16:3–7

9. Oi S, Yamada H, Matsumoto S (1990) Tethered cord syndrome versus low-placed conus medullaris in an over-distended spinal cord following initial repair of myelodysplasia. Child's Nerv Syst 6:264–269
10. Sakamoto H, Hakuba A, Fujitani K, Nishimura S (1991) Surgical treatment of the retethered spinal cord after repair of lipomyelomeningocele. J Neurosurg 74:709–714
11. Steinbok P, Irvine B, Douglas Cochrane D, Irwin BJ (1992) Long-term outcome and complications of children born with meningomyelocele. Child's Nerv Syst 8:92–96
12. Tamaki N, Shirataki K, Kojima N, Shouse Y, Matsumoto S (1988) Tethered cord syndrome of delayed onset following repair of myelomeningocele. J Neurosurg 69:393–398

Abstract

Surgical Treatment for Delayed Tethered Cord Syndrome After Repair of Myelomeningocele

Reizo Shirane and Takashi Yoshimoto

We present a series of 16 patients who underwent surgery at our institute between 1990 and 1993 for delayed tethered cord syndrome after repair of myelomeningocele. The patients' ages ranged from 3 to 16 years. Presenting symptoms included leg pain, back pain, progressive lower limb weakness and deformity, and incontinence. Time of onset and the speed of progression of symptoms cannot usually be predicted on follow-up with neuroimaging techniques. In order to detect this disease at any stage, examination starting from early childhood is indispensable. However, the range of clinical examinations by the neurosurgeon alone is limited, and collaboration with urologists and orthopedic experts is essential.

In addition, all patients underwent untethering with intraoperative monitoring of evoked electromyographic potentials around the anal sphincter and gastrocnemius muscles. The surgical goal is to perform complete untethering, prevent retethering, and protect patients from developing new symptoms after the operation. Duroplasty was performed using PTFE membrane to prevent postoperative adhesions of the spinal conus. Follow-up duration ranged from 3 to 6 years. The outcome was excellent in younger children, particularly in improvement in gait disturbance and elimination of pain. However, improvements of the symptoms were disappointing in older patients. Reappearance of the symptoms was found in two patients, in whom duroplasty had been performed without using PTFE membrane. We conclude that patients with tethered cord syndrome after repair of myelomeningocele who present with progressive neurological compromise have a relatively good prognosis with regard to neurological function, and exhibit improvement following complete untethering.

Department of Neurosurgery, Tohoku University School of Medicine, Sendai, Japan

Moderator's Comments on Sessions—Tethered Cord

Joong Uhn Choi

In this session, five papers on tethered cord syndrome were presented.

Dr. Tsukamoto examined the results of ten operations for severely disabling meningomyelocele. Only two out of ten were enjoying a reasonable life. Considering the expected quality of life of such patients, the decision to undertake surgery is a very difficult problem, and the ethical, socioeconomic, and religious positions of the parents also have to be considered.

Dr. Wang et al. and Dr. Date et al. presented the progression of symptoms in spinal lipoma. More than 35% over the age of 1, and 75% over the age of 3 showed progression of their neurological status. These two papers strongly supported prophylactic surgery for spinal lipoma.

Dr. Shirane et al. and Dr. Yamashita et al. considered retethering after an operation for meningomyelocele or lumbosacral lipoma. Decision making for reoperation is not an easy task. Collaboration with urologists and orthopedic experts is essential. In addition to magnetic resonance imaging (MRI), cine-MRI and other noninvasive methods might help to predict the onset of tethered cord syndrome. Intraoperative electrophysiological monitoring and duroplasty using poly tetra fluoro ethylene membrane were recommended to improve the outcome for patients with a retethered cord.

Department of Neurosurgery, Yonsei University College of Medicine, Seoul, Korea

Tethered Cord Syndrome in Low Motor Level Children with Myelomeningocele

John F. Sarwark, Daniel T. Weber, Ana Paula Gabrieli, David G. McLone, and Luciano Dias

Summary. The clinical presentation of tethered spinal cord and the results of tethered cord release were examined in a group of 30 low motor level (L3 and below) children with a history of myelomeningocele without concomitant central nervous system (CNS) complications. Changes in orthopedic and/or neurologic status formed the basis for consideration for tethered cord release.

Tethered cord release in symptomatic low lumbar and sacral level children with myelomeningocele appears to be of benefit, especially with respect to stabilization of scoliosis in selected patients, back pain resolution at the site of closure, and stabilization of prior decline of motor function. Results in cases with spasticity were more equivocal.

Key words. Tethered cord, Myelomeningocele, Spine

Introduction

Symptomatic retethering of the spinal cord following primary myelomeningocele repair occurs in 11%–27% of cases [2, 4, 8, 12]. Although the conus medullaris is frequently found to be low-lying in children with a myelomeningocele in general [8], and may even appear adherent to the dorsal dura in the majority of cases [12], the significance of this finding depends on its association with clinical signs and symptoms of tethered cord syndrome [1, 12].

Symptomatic retethering of the spinal cord in children with myelomeningocele is most frequently due to scarring, or adhesive arachnoiditis involving the neural placode or spinal cord with resultant adherence to the overlying dura or skin [7, 10–14].

This study retrospectively examined the clinical outcomes of a select group of 30 low motor level, pediatric myelomeningocele patients who all underwent tethered cord release after developing signs of symptomatic tethered cord.

Materials and Methods

The selected group of 30 patients consisted of 17 females and 13 males. The average age at the time of tethered cord release was 7 years. The range of ages was from 1 year, 1 month to 14 years, 5 months. The focus was then restricted to patients who had been functioning as L3 motor level or better (community ambulation).

Northwestern University Medical School, Children's Memorial Hospital, 2300 Children's Plaza, No. 69 Chicago, IL 60614, USA

Sixteen (53.3%) of the patients were low lumbar motor level (L3–L5), and fourteen (46.7%) were sacral motor level.

Thirty-three cases were ultimately analyzed in this study for their clinical presentations. The areas of clinical evaluation in this study included: 1, new or rapidly progressive scoliosis in patients with no primary vertebral anomalies; 2, deterioration of motor function; 3, spasticity (frequently seen in the hamstring muscles, ankle dorsiflexors/evertors); 4, back pain at the site of closure.

Observations and Results

Clinically, these patients presented with a new onset or recently progressing scoliosis, spasticity with or without contractures, decrease in motor function, and low back pain at the site of closure. One or more of these findings was present in all cases, and led to the suspicion of tethered spinal cord. The anatomic site of tethered cord was confirmed in all cases by magnetic resonance imaging (MRI) or computed tomography–myelography [7]. In order to isolate tethering as the etiology for the patients' clinical deterioration, patients with concomitant CNS complications, e.g., shunt dysfunction or hydromyelia, were excluded from the study. Twenty-nine such patients who would otherwise have been considered were excluded on the basis of this criterion of concomitant CNS complications.

The results of release 1 year after the procedure were as follows. Regarding scoliosis, in 75% of cases the curve either remained stable or decreased by more than 10 degrees, with 25% experiencing curve progression greater than 10 degrees. The most recent follow up in this group revealed that 11.8% experienced a decrease in curvature >10 degrees, 47.1% remained stable, and 41.2% ultimately progressed >10 degrees.

In the group with spasticity, 43.8% improved, 56.3% remained stable, and none worsened. Most (78.6%) of the children who had experienced a decline in motor function improved postoperatively, and all those with back pain experienced complete resolution.

Discussion and Results

Debate continues as to the significance of, and approach to, symptomatic tethered spinal cord in children with a myelomeningocele [1].

There is recent literature which supports tethered cord as a causal factor in developmental scoliosis in myelomeningocele patients, and which seems to indicate that tethered cord release is beneficial for many patients [3, 6, 10, 11]. McLone and co-workers [3–6] reviewed 30 myelomeningocele patients with developmental scoliosis and tethered cord, and found that of the 24 in whom the curvature was less than 45 degrees at the time of release, all either stabilized or improved in the first year, and 63% ultimately stabilized or improved. They concluded that tethered cord contributes to developmental scoliosis, and that release of the tethered cord is of benefit in those cases where intervention occurred before the curve became greater than 50 degrees.

Symptomatic retethering after secondary release in 13% of our patients is concerning. However, this number is similar to pathologic adhesion of the spinal cord after primary closure [2, 4, 9, 13] for MM.

In conclusion, this study supports the release of a tethered spinal cord in low motor level children with myelomeningocele who are showing signs/symptoms of tethered spinal cord and who have MRI findings consistent with tethered spinal cord.

References

1. Banta JV (1991) The tethered cord in myelomeningocele: should it be untethered? Dev Med Child Neurol 33:173–176
2. Barson AJ (1970) The vertebral level of termination of the spinal cord during normal and abnormal development. J Anat 106:489–497
3. Herman JM, McLone D, Storrs B, Dauser R (1993) Analysis of 153 patients with myelomeningocele or spinal lipoma reoperated upon for a tethered cord. Pediatr Neurosurg 19:243–249
4. McLone DG (1992) Continuing concepts in management of children with spina bifida. Pediatr Neurosurg 18(5–6):254–256
5. McLone D, Naidich T (1989): The tethered spinal cord. In: McLaurin RL, Schut L, Venes JL, Epstein F (eds) Pediatric neurosurgery, 2nd edn. Saunders, Philadelphia, pp 71–97
6. McLone DG, Herman JM, Gabrieli AP, Dias L (1990–1991) Tethered cord as a cause of scoliosis in children with myelomeningocele. Pediatr Neurosurg 16:8–13
7. Moufarrij NA, Palmer JM, Hahn JF, Weinstein MA (1989) Correlation between magnetic resonance imaging and surgical findings in the tethered spinal cord. Neurosurgery 25:341–346
8. Oi S, Yamada H, Matsumoto S (1990) Tethered cord syndrome versus low-placed conus medullaris in an over distended spinal cord following initial repair for myelodysplasia. Child's Nerv Syst 6:264–269
9. Peterson MC (1992) Tethered cord syndrome in myelodysplasia: correlation between level of lesion and height at time of presentation. Dev Med Child Neurol 34:604–610
10. Reigel DH (1983) Tethered spinal cord. Concepts in pediatric neurosurgery, vol 4. In: Humphreys RP (ed) Karger, Basel, pp 142–164
11. Reigel DH, Tchernoukha K, Bazmi B, Kortyna R, Rotenstein D (1994) Change in spinal curvature following release of tethered spinal cord associated with spina bifida. Pediatr Neurosurg 20:30–42
12. Rekate HL (1991) Neurosurgical management of the child with spina bifida. Comprehensive management of spina bifida. In: Rekate HL (ed) CRC Press, Boston, pp 93–112
13. Tamaki N, Shirataki K, Kojima N, Shouse Y, Matsumoto S (1988) Tethered cord syndrome of delayed onset following repair of myelomeningocele. J Neurosurg 69:393–398
14. Venes JL, Stevens EA (1983) Surgical pathology in tethered cord secondary to myelomeningocele repair. In: Humphreys RP (ed) Concepts in pediatric neurosurgery, vol 4. Karger, Basel, pp 165–185

Intraspinal Lipoma Associated with Tethered Cord Syndrome in School-Age and Adolescent Patients: Surgical Management and Prognosis

Joon Ki Kang, Byung Chul Son, Sin Soo Jeun, Yong Kil Hong, Chun Kun Park, Chul Ku Jung, and Moon Chan Kim

Summary. From 1980 to 1996, 60 patients with lipomyelomeningocele were treated at the Kangnam St. Mary's Hospital. Of these patients, 20 school-aged and adolescent patients with tethered cord syndrome (TCS) were studied with respect to the clinical, radiological, and pathological features and surgical management of this syndrome. Specific circumstances involving additional tugging of the already tight conus, and direct trauma to the back or buttocks precipitated symptomatic onset in 50% of patients. Diffuse and nondermatomal leg pain, often referred to the anorectal region, was the most common presenting symptom. Progressive sensorimotor deficits in the lower extremities, as well as bladder and bowel dysfunction, were also common findings, but progressive foot and spinal deformities were not seen. The most common tethered lesions were thickened filum, fibrous band adhesion into the placode sac, and intradural lipoma. The surgical outcome was gratifying in relation to pain and motor weakness, but disappointing in the resolution of bowel and bladder dysfunction. Of these 20 patients with TCS, preoperative deficits improved after surgery in 11 patients (55%), remained stable in 7 (35%), and worsened in 2 (10%).

Key words. Intraspinal lipoma, Tethered cord, Adult onset, Surgical outcome

Introduction

Tethered cord syndrome (TCS) is a developmental abnormality of the neuroaxis, usually diagnosed in childhood. Adults with TCS are arguably the most neglected individuals in the population with a neurosurgical disease. The actual tethering has been attributed to a variety of pathological entities, including a thickened, tight filum terminale [1, 7, 11], intradural lipomas with or without a connecting extradural component [1, 4], intradural fibrous adhesion [2, 16], diastematomyelia [5, 8], and adherence of the neural placode following previous closure of a myelomeningocele [9]. However, sufficient differences in the mode of onset, clinical manifestations, and outcome exist between pediatric and adolescent patients with tethered cord to warrant a more detailed analysis of the adult syndrome [13]. The most problematic technical consideration in surgery for the release of the tethered cord in school-age and adolescent patients is how to preserve functioning neural elements and rebuild the dural sac to maintain normal CSF circulation. The purpose of this chapter is to review some unique fea-

Department of Neurosurgery, Kangnam St. Mary's Hospital, The Catholic University of Korea, College of Medicine, 505 Banpodong, Seocho Ku, Seoul 137-040, Korea

tures in clinical presentation, factors precipitating onset of symptoms, diagnostic clues, pathological entities, and surgical outcome in adolescent patients with TCS.

Materials and Methods

From 1980 to 1996, 60 patients with lipomyelomeningocele were treated at the Kangnam St. Mary's Hospital. Of these patients, 20 school-age and adolescent patients with TCS were studied with respect to the clinical, radiological, and pathological features and surgical outcome of this syndrome. The age distribution and type of lesions of the lipomyelomeningocele (type I, dorsal; type II, transitional; type III, mixed) are shown in Table 1. Their ages ranged from 7 to 25 years, with a mean of 16.5 years. The mean age of onset was 16 years, and none of the patients had onset of symptoms before 7 years of age. Among the 20 patients with TCS, there were 7 with type I, 5 with type II, and 8 with type III. The presenting complaints that led to neurosurgical consultation in adulthood are listed in Table 2. Pain was the most common presenting symptom, and was a prominent complaint in 18 patients (90%). Fifteen patients (75%) presented with progressive leg weakness or walking difficulties, and most commonly revealed saddle anesthesia or hypesthesia. Thirteen patients (65%) had

TABLE 1. Age distribution and type of lesion in 60 patients with intraspinal lipoma

Age	No. of patients	Type of lesions		
		I	II	III
Birth–1 month	8	1	6	1
2–6 months	14	5	5	4
7–12 months	7	3	3	1
13 months–3 years	8	3	3	2
4–6 years	3	1	1	1
7–10 years	7	5	1	1
11–16 years	8	2	2	4
17–25 years	5		2	3
Total	60 (100)	20 (33.3)	23 (38.4)	17 (28.3)

TABLE 2. Presenting signs and symptoms in 20 patients

Signs and symptoms	No. of patients (%)
Pain	18 (90)
Sensorimotor deficits	15 (75)
Bladder dysfunction	13 (65)
Spastic	3 (15)
Hypotonic	5 (25)
Nonspecific	12 (60)
Bowel dysfunction	5 (25)
Trophic ulceration	3 (15)
Deformity of foot	11 (55)
Scoliosis	4 (20)
Back lesions	20 (100)

bladder symptoms, 3 had spastic symptoms, and 5 had hypotonic symptoms. Five patients had bowel dysfunction and 11 patients had foot deformity. Radiological investigations were performed on the 20 patients with TCS with metrizamide myelography and computerized tomography (CT). Since 1987, magnetic resonance imaging (MRI) has been used for most patients with a suspected diagnosis of TCS. Intradural mass associated extradural mass was found in 20 patients, a low level of the conus was found in 17 patients, and a tethering band was identified in 13 patients with the CT myelography and MRI studies.

Results

Twenty patients underwent surgery for release of tethered conus. Four different tethering entities were encountered at operation. Twenty patients had various combinations of two or more types of pathology (Table 3); each was thought to contribute to the tethering process. Each entity was individually treated using an intraoperative monitoring system (somatosensory evoked potential (SEP), urodynamic study). All intradural lipomas were either densely adherent to the thecal wall or were connected with an extradural component through a dural defect, where the conus was in effect anchored. The portions adherent to the dura were sharply dissected away, leaving the rest of the mass gliding freely within the dural sac. All dural defects were closed with lumbodorsal fascial grafts. The surgical outcome for the 20 patients is shown in Table 4. The relief of pain was most gratifying: 18 (90%) of patients with significant pain became asymptomatic following surgery. The next best results were obtained with resolution of sensorimotor deficits, and 10 patients enjoyed a significant improvement. Only 5 patients were unchanged by surgery. The results for sphincter dysfunction were disappointing. Only 5 of 18 patients (27.8%) with this problem were helped by surgery.

TABLE 3. Pathological entities in 20 patients with tethered cord syndrome

Pathological entities	No. of cases (%)
Lipomyelomeningocele/tight filum	3 (15)
Lipoma/tight filum, placode	10 (50)
Lipoma/adhesion	4 (20)
Lipomyelomeningocele/adhesion	3 (15)

TABLE 4. Surgical outcome in 20 patients with intraspinal lipoma with tethered cord syndrome

Preoperative complaints or deficits	No. of cases	Outcome			
		Normal	Improved	Unchanged	Regressed
Pain	18	13	5	0	0
Sensorimotor deficits	15	2	8	5	0
Sphincter dysfunction	18	0	5	12	1
Trophic ulceration	3	0	2	1	0
Scoliosis	4	0	1	3	0
Foot deformities	11	0	1	9	1

Discussion

The difference in growth rate between the spinal cord and musculoskeletal elements accounts for the fact that the normal conus medullaris may terminate anywhere from T12 to the L2–L3 interspace [3]. A conus below the L2–L3 interspace in an adult is abnormal, and has been termed a "tethered conus" [7]. The syndrome is usually diagnosed in childhood, and although the presentation is variable and may be insidious, tethered conus should be suspected in patients with an unexpected spastic gait, a neurogenic bladder, bowel dysfunction, lower-extremity weakness, scoliosis, or foot deformity [7]. These symptoms and signs may be related to traction upon the conus and cauda equina by an intradural mass and tethering band, and may grow worse with age owing to accelerated skeletal growth in relation to the neuroaxis during puberty.

After experimental tethering in growing cats, Kang et al. [12] reported a reduction in spinal cord blood flow (SCBF) in the distal spinal cord close to the tethering of 32% of the normal flow in 2 weeks. Untethering of the cord 2 weeks after tethering resulted in an increase in SCBF, and it returned to the normal level (Fig. 1). This study supports the hypothesis that spinal cord dysfunction in the early stage of tethering results from mechanical and vascular damage to a spinal cord segment, which results in widespread ischemic involvement of the cord in a prolonged tethering effect during growth.

There are several reported cases of adult presentation of a tethered conus, and it is unclear why these patients should have been symptom-free and the diagnosis overlooked for so long. Sostrin et al. [15] described three patients with acquired spinal stenosis and a tethered conus, and suggested that the stenosis made the primary tethered conus symptomatic. Pool [14] theorized that a tethered conus eventually became symptomatic in one patient because local stretching and ischemia occurred from the repetitive and insidious low back trauma associated with the patient's occupation. The description of spinal vasculature in patients with scoliosis given by Hilal and Keim [10] supports this hypothesis, since they demonstrated that tension on the conus caused arterial stretching and ischemia, with resultant cord damage.

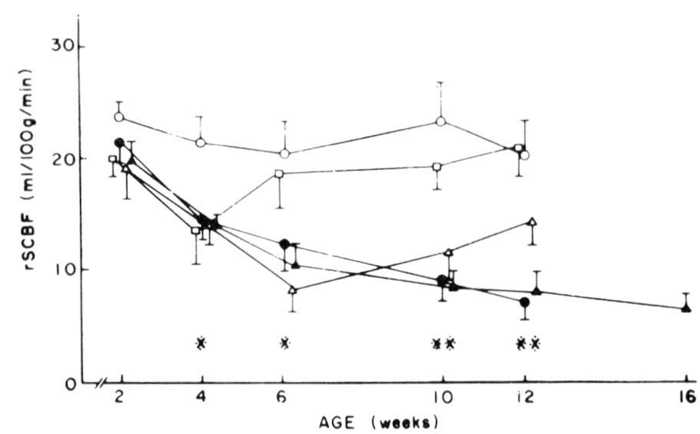

FIG. 1. Tethered growing animals showed progressive reduction of regional spinal cord blood flow (rSCBF); similar findings were made in growing animals untethered after 8 weeks. However, growing animals untethered after 2 weeks showed progressive increase of rSCBF (L3) to normal control level. *Open circles*, normal control growing animals; *closed circles*, tethered growing animals; *open squares*, 2 weeks-untethered growing animals; *open triangles*, 4 weeks-untethered growing animals; *closed triangles*, 8 weeks-untethered growing animals. *$P < 0.05$; **$P < 0.01$ (from [12], with permission)

TABLE 5. Comparison between childhood and adolescence tethered cord syndrome

Parameter	Childhood (0–6 years)	Adolescence (7–25 years)
Pain	Uncommon	Common, localized anorectal, diffuse, bilat
Sensorimotor deficits	Common early signs: walking difficulty, abnormal gait	Common, frank, leg weakness
Sphincter disturbance	Common, incontinence, dribbling, delayed toilet training	Common, urinary frequency, urgency, incontinence
Trophic ulcerations of the legs foot deformities	Relatively common. Common early signs: neuromuscular	Uncommon
Back lesions	Common	Uncommon
Spine deformity	Common, worsening scoliosis	Uncommon
Aggravating factors	Growth spurts	Precipitating factors: trauma, stretching of conus, lumbar spondylosis, disc hem, herniation

Experimental studies [2] also indicate that the damage from local cord stretching is absorbed within a short distance above or below the level of the insult, and this may explain the causal relationship of these patients' symptoms. These clinical and experimental reports, indicating a delicate balance between skeletal maturation and traction upon the tethered conus, may explain why some patients remain symptom-free until adulthood.

The childhood and adult versions of TCS are compared in Table 5. Pain is an uncommon presenting complaint in children with TCS [1, 11], as opposed to a 90% incidence in our group of adolescents. In a large number of children with TCS, the pain, when present, is located in the lumbosacral region, with variable radiation down both legs. The anal and perineal pain described by 12 of our adolescent patients has not been noted in children. Progressive foot deformity is one of the most common presenting features in children with TCS [1]. None of our patients who did not have preexisting foot deformity developed this problem with the adult onset of neurological dysfunction. This suggests that insults to the adult conus cause frank sensorimotor deficits or even atrophy, but do not result in any type of muscle imbalance. Progressive scoliosis was seen in 33% of a series of children with TCS [11], but progressive spinal deformity has not been described in reports of adult TCS. The incidence of urological symptoms appears to be similar in the childhood and adult syndromes [1, 4, 6]. Unlike adults, however, children rarely admit to urgency, incomplete voiding, or stress incontinence.

In the management of an adult patient with TCS, three questions should be considered. Should it be treated aggressively? Should it be studied and operated on as soon as is reasonably possible? Would it be reasonable to operate on patients who are neurologically intact prophylactically? In general, we do not agree with aggressive treatment of adults with TCS because they have relatively advanced neurological deficits, and the functional zone they have retained is very narrow, which means that it is necessary to maintain the balance between skeletal maturation and conus traction upon the TC. If aggressive treatment is tried, it could result in a worsening of their neurological deficits. Preoperative studies are necessary to plan the treatment in order to avoid operative morbidity or complications. However, if adult patients with TCS have impending neurological deficits and/or progression of their existing neurological deficits, it is reasonable to operate as soon as possible.

There are various controversial opinions about operating on patients who are neurologically intact or for prophylatic purposes. However, if tethering pathology is confirmed by radiological investigation, and the patient will not be able to do much exercise or work, an operation should be performed and the spinal cord released prophylactically. The operative results for pain are most gratifying [15]. Most of our patients had no pain after surgery, and sensorimotor deficits also responded favorably with surgical release of the conus. Many authors with experience of childhood TCS have commented on the poor operative results in terms of urinary dysfunction [6, 11]. Our results for bladder dysfunction in adult TCS patients are equally disappointing. Of the 20 patients with TCS, preoperative deficits improved after surgery in 11 patients (55%), remained stable in 7 (35%), and worsened in 2 (10%). Early diagnosis, adequate release of the tethered cord, and reforming the dural sac are the keys to successful management.

Conclusions

We have reviewed the clinical, radiological, and pathological records of 20 patients with adolescent TCS, and have reached the following conclusions.

1. The majority of adolescent patients with TCS have precipitated symptomatic onset or aggravated existing complaints. Pain is the most common presenting feature; it is usually bilateral, and often involves the anorectal region.
2. The pathological lesions causing tethering are intradural lipoma and tight filum.
3. In the pathogenesis of adult TCS, it was suspected that the degree of cord traction resulted in neurological dysfunction in later life due to the abnormal tension, aggravated by trauma or repeated tugging of the conus during exercise.
4. The surgical outcome is excellent for the resolution of pain and sensorimotor deficits, but disappointing for bladder dysfunction.
5. To preserve the functioning neural elements during the untethering procedure, an intraoperative monitoring system (SEP, urodynamic studies) should be applied. Early diagnosis and adequate surgical release are the keys to a successful outcome.

References

1. Anderson FM (1975) Occult spinal dysraphism: a series of 73 cases. Pediatrics 55:826–835
2. Barry A, Patten BM, Stewart BH (1957) Possible factors in the development of the Arnold–Chiari malformation. J Neurosurg 14:285–301
3. Basson AJ (1970) The vertebral level of termination of the spinal cord during normal and abnormal development. J Anat 106:489–497
4. Bruce DA, Shut L (1979) Spinal lipomas in infancy and childhood. Childs Brain 5:192–203
5. Dale AJD (1969) Diastematomyelia. Arch Neurol 20:309–317
6. Dubowitz V, Lorber J, Zachary RB (1965) Lipoma of the cauda equina. Arch Dis Child 40:207–213
7. Fitz CR, Harwood-Nash DC (1975) The tethered conus. AJR 125:515–523
8. Gilmor RL, Batnitzky S (1979) Diastematomyelia: rare and unusual features. J Indiana State Med Assoc 72:274–278
9. Heinz ER, Rosenbaum AE, Scraft TB (1979) Tethered spinal cord following meningomyelocele repair. Radiology 131:153–160

10. Hilal SK, Keim HA (1972) Selective spinal angiography in adolescent scoliosis. Radiology 102:349–359
11. Hoffman HJ, Mendrick EB, Humphreys RP (1976) The tethered spinal cord: its protean manifestations, diagnosis and surgical correction. Childs Brain 2:145–155
12. Kang JK, Kim MC, Kim DS, Song JU (1987) Effects of tethering on regional spinal cord blood flow and sensory-evoked potentials in growing cats. Childs Nerv Syst 3:35–39
13. Pang D, Wilberger JE (1982) Tethered cord syndrome in adults. J Neurosurg 57:32–47
14. Pool JL (1952) Spinal cord and local signs secondary to occult sacral meningoceles in adults. Bull NY Acad Med 28:655–663
15. Sostrin RD, Thompson JR, Rouhe SA (1977) Occult spinal dysraphism in the geriatric patient. Radiology 125:165–169
16. Yashon D, Beatty RA (1966) Tethering of the conus medullaris within the sacrum. J Neurol Neurosurg Psychiatr 29:244–250

Importance of Morphological Classification for Surgical Treatment of Lumbosacral Lipoma

Kenji Ohata, Toshihiro Takami, Moududul Haque, Takeo Gotou, and Akira Hakuba

Summary. We examined the surgical outcome of lumbosacral lipoma in order to clarify the risk factors of postoperative retethering of the spinal cord. Fifty-four patients with lumbosacral lipoma underwent surgery during the last 23 years. Age at operation, preoperative neurological findings, morphological type of lipoma, and operative findings were evaluated for two groups of patients, those with or without reoperation for postoperative retethering. Morphological classification was performed based on radiological and operative findings according to Hakuba's classification. The morphological type of lipoma and the timing of the operation were closely related to the occurrence of postoperative retethering. All type IIb, IIc (extraspinal variant), and IIIa (intraspinal variant) patients underwent reoperation. For patients operated on before 1 year of age, the surgical results were satisfactory. Morphological classification of lipoma is helpful in determining operative strategy and surgical prognosis.

Key words. Lumbosacral lipoma, Retethering, Morphological classification, Tethered cord

Introduction

Lumbosacral lipomas are associated with spina bifida occulta and usually cause serious neurological deficits during the period of growth, making early surgical treatment to untether the cord mandatory [4, 6, 11]. The goal of surgical treatment is to prevent neurological deterioration due to tethering of the spinal cord. However, retethering of the spinal cord is occasionally observed after surgical treatment, with delayed neurological deterioration [8, 9].

We examined 54 surgically treated cases of lumbosacral lipoma in order to clarify the factors related to postoperative retethering of the spinal cord, focusing in particular on the morphological type of lipoma.

Clinical Materials and Methods

Patients

Fifty-four patients with lumbosacral lipoma underwent surgery in our institute between 1975 and 1998. There were 24 males and 30 females. The age of patients at surgery was less

Department of Neurosurgery, Osaka City University Medical School, 1-4-3 Asahi-machi, Abeno-ku, Osaka 545-8586, Japan

than 1 year in 26 cases, between 1 and 20 years in 26 cases, and adult in 2 cases. Preoperative neurological examination revealed no deficits in 28 patients, urinary and bowel dysfunction in 22 patients, motor weakness of the lower extremities in 16 patients, and sensory disturbance in 9 patients.

Radiological Study

Radiological study included myelography and computed tomography scanning until 1984, and thereafter consisted exclusively of magnetic resonance (MR) imaging. Sagittal MR imaging provided diagnostic radiological findings for tethered cord of a low-lying spinal cord running along the dorsal portion of the spinal canal attached to the lipoma, and lack of a cerebrospinal fluid space behind the dorsal surface of the conus medullaris (Fig. 1).

Evaluation of Factors Related to Postoperative Retethering

Age at first surgery, preoperative neurological findings, morphological type of lipoma, and operative findings were evaluated to clarify factors related to postoperative retethering. Morphological type was classified according to Hakuba's classification depending on radiological and operative findings (Tables 1 and 2) [4]. Six patients who had their first operation in other institutions were not included in the evaluation of age at first operation.

Operative Technique

A detailed description of the procedure for tumor resection and cord untethering has been published previously [3, 10]. The basic procedure is described here.

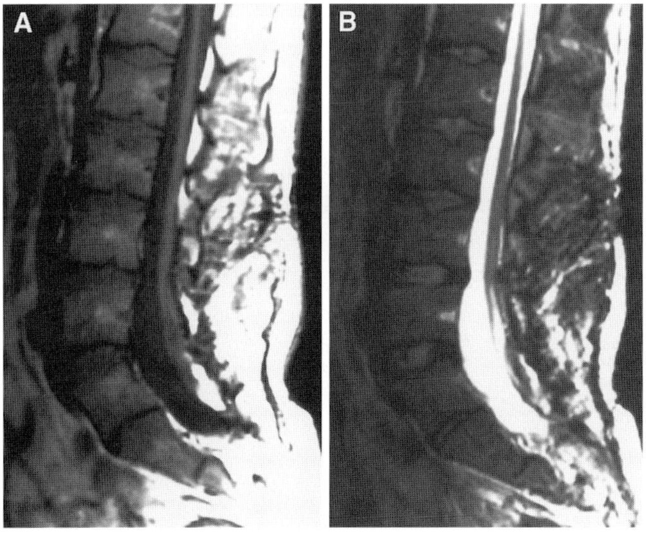

Fig. 1. Cases of morphological types IIIa and IIIb. Magnetic resonance imaging demonstrated the retethering of the conus medullaris during postoperative follow-up. **A** T1-weighted image revealed a low-lying spinal cord and residual lipomatous tissue at S1 level. **B** T2-weighted image revealed no cerebrospinal fluid space behind the low-lying spinal cord

TABLE 1. Hakuba's morphological classification scheme

Type	Subtype	Description
I		Most anomalous type, accompanied by severe malformations such as diastematomyelia
II		Extraspinal type, characterized by prolapse of the lower spinal cord outside the spinal canal through the spina bifida
	IIa	Kyphotic type, in which the spinal cord protrudes out of the spinal canal through spinal bifida accompanied by its dural tube, and the dorsal part of the prolapsed spinal cord and its pia-arachnoid as well as the dura mater are blended into a fibrofatty structure in the subcutaneous lipoma
	IIb	The conus medullaris protrudes out of the spinal canal through the spina bifida and dorsocaudal defects of the dural tube, and fuses with the lipoma outside the spinal canal
	IIc	The conus medullaris protrudes out of the spinal canal accompanied by its dural tube and ending in a fibrolipomatous structure in the extraspinal lipoma
III		Intraspinal type, characterized by the fact that the spinal cord stays entirely within the spinal canal
	IIIa	The spinal cord is fused with the intraspinal lipoma through a defect of either the dorsocaudal or dorsolateral dural sac
	IIIb	A broad-based type, characterized by the fact that the lipoma inserts broadly into the lower spinal cord dorsally to the dorsal nerve roots through a broad dorsal dural defect
	IIIc	A stalk type, in which a fibrolipomatous stalk enters into the subarachnoid space through a small dorsal dural defect and attaches either directly to the conus or to the subpial lipoma of the conus medullaris
IV		Epidural lipoma

TABLE 2. Morphological classification in 54 cases of lumbosacral lipomas

Single type		No.	Combined type	No.
Type I		1	Type IIb + IIc	2
Type II	IIa	3	Type IIc + IIIc	1
	IIb	2	Type IIIa + IIIb	11
	IIc	7		
Type III	IIIa	7		
	IIIb	11		
	IIIc	6		
Type IV		3		

After osteoplastic laminotomy, durotomy was performed from the upper margin of the lipoma down to the lower margin. Resection of the lipoma was performed close to the fibrotic interface between lipoma and cord, avoiding injury to the cord and nerve roots. We usually monitored sphincter function with the electromyogram (EMG) and rectal pressure. After untethering of the conus medullaris, the dural defect was reconstructed with the paravertebral fascia or fascia lata until 1993, and thereafter with Gore-tex membrane (polytetrafluoroethylene, Gore-Tex, Flagstaff, AZ, USA). The suture lines were reinforced by application of fibrin-glue-soaked collagen sponge (Helistat, Cola-Tec, Kansas City, MO, USA), followed by an expansive laminoplasty. In older patients, the lipoma was fibrotic, hard, and well vascularized.

Results

Of the 48 patients who underwent the initial operation in our institution, 22 were operated on at less than 1 year of age. Two of these 22 patients underwent reoperation for retethered cord. Eleven patients underwent operation between 1 and 5 years of age, and 2 of them underwent reoperation for retethered conus. Types IIb, IIc, and IIIa patients underwent reoperation due to retethered conus more often than did other patients (Table 3).

After the first surgery, neurological status remained intact in 24 of 28 patients without preoperative neurological deficits, and was improved in 3 of 26 patients with preoperative neurological deficits. Seven of 26 patients with preoperative neurological deficits and 4 of the 28 patients without preoperative neurological deficits underwent reoperation due to retethered cord. Of the 26 patients with preoperative neurological deficits, retethering of the spinal cord occurred in 3 of 16 patients with paraparesis, 1 of 9 patients with sensory disturbance, and 4 of 22 patients with urinary and bowel dysfunction. There was no correlation between preoperative neurological findings and the occurrence of retethering.

The lipoma was much softer and less vascular in patients operated on at less than 6 months of age, and therefore resection of the lipoma was much easier and less traumatic. For patients with morphological types IIb, IIc, or IIIa disease, resection of the lipoma was not easy since neural structures were extensively involved by lipoma. Identification of the cord–lipoma interface was difficult in type IIb and type IIc patients, and dissection of the nerve roots from the lipoma was very difficult in type IIIa patients.

TABLE 3. Morphological types in cases with reoperation

Single type		No.	Combined type	No.
Type I		0	Type IIb + IIc	1
Type II	IIa	0	Type IIc + IIIc	1
	IIb	1	Type IIIa + IIIb	3
	IIc	2		
Type III	IIIa	2		
	IIIb	0		
	IIIc	1		
Type IV		0		

Discussion

Neurological dysfunction caused by lumbosacral lipoma is usually absent or mild in infants. Accordingly, the purpose of surgical treatment in infancy is to prevent the neurological deterioration caused by tethering of the spinal cord as the patient grows. Surgery for untethering of the cord in infancy can prevent critical neurological dysfunction for a long period of time [4–9]. Schut et al. [11] noted that if children with lumbosacral lipoma are not operated on in infancy, all will suffer some neurological, urological, or orthopedic complications. In patients with neurological deficit before surgery, surgery can prevent progression of deformity or deficit but rarely improve neurological condition [11].

Chapman [2] originally divided lumbosacral lipomas into three types (dorsal, caudal, and transitional) based on the site of attachment of the lipoma to the conus medullaris. Hakuba et al. [4] developed a classification scheme with four types and six subtypes of lumbosacral lipomas. Type IIb is the caudal variant, type IIIa the transitional variant, and type IIIb the dorsal variant of Chapman's classification. In patients with types IIb, IIc, or IIIa disease, postoperative retethering of the spinal cord occurred more commonly than in patients with other types. These findings suggest that the risk of postoperative retethering can be determined based on morphological type using Hakuba's classification. Preoperative morphological evaluation and classification will be useful for surgical strategy and prediction of long-term surgical outcome. Careful surgical technique and close postoperative follow-up are required, especially for types IIb, IIc, and IIIa patients.

A retrospective analysis of 100 children who underwent surgery for spinal lipoma indicated that untethering of the spinal cord and debulking of the lipoma in the first year of life were safe and effective [1]. We were relatively easily able to resect the lipoma, especially in patients less than 6 months of age. Our findings showed that the surgical outcome was better when the operation was performed at less than 1 year of age than when it was performed between 1 and 5 years of age. We therefore believe that untethering surgery should be performed in younger infants, ideally at less than 1 year of age, before the neurological dysfunction is manifest.

Conclusions

Classification of lumbosacral lipoma using Hakuba's morphological scheme is well correlated with the difficulty of surgery to untether the spinal cord and debulk the lipoma, and with surgical prognosis. Treatment to prevent cord tethering is best indicated for younger infants before the neurological dysfunction is manifest or becomes severe.

References

1. Byrne RW, Hayes EA, George TM, McLone DG (1995) Operative resection of 100 spinal lipomas in infants less than 1 year of age. Pediatr Neurosurg 23:182–186
2. Champman PH (1982) Congenital intraspinal lipomas. Anatomic considerations and surgical treatment. Childs Brain 9:34–47
3. Hakuba A (1990) Lumbosacral lipoma. In: Kikuchi H, Hakuba A (eds) Illustrated techniques in microneurosurgery. Igaku-Shoin, Tokyo, New York, pp 239–248
4. Hakuba A, Fujitani K, Hoda K, Inoue Y, Nishimura S (1986) Lumbosacral lipoma, the timing of the operation and morphological classification. Neuro-Orthopedics 2:34–42

5. Herman JM, McLone DG, Storrs BB, Dauser RC (1993) Analysis of 153 patients with myelomeningocele or spinal lipoma reoperated upon for a tethered cord. Pediatr Neurosurg 19:243–249
6. Hoffman HJ, Taecholarn C, Hendrick EB, Humphreys RP (1985) Management of lipomyelomeningoceles. J Neurosurg 62:1–8
7. Kanev PM, Bierbrauer KS (1995) Reflections on the natural history of lipomyelomeningocele. Pediatr Neurosurg 22:137–140
8. Kanev PM, Lemire RJ, Loeser JD, Berger MS (1990) Management and long-term follow up review of children with lipomyelomeningocele, 1952–1987. J Neurosurg 73:48–52
9. Pierre-Kahn A, Lacombe J, Pichon J, Giudicelli Y, Renier D, Saint-Rose C, Perrigot M, Hirsch JF (1986) Intraspinal lipomas with spina bifida. Prognosis and treatment in 73 cases. J Neurosurg 65:756–761
10. Sakamoto H, Hakuba A, Fujitani K, Nishimura S (1991) Surgical treatment of the retethered cord after repair of lipomyelomeningocele. J Neurosurg 74:709–714
11. Schut L, Bruce DA, Sutton LN (1982) The management of the child with a lipomyelomeningocele. Clin Neurosurg 30:464–476

Clinical Analysis of Congenital Dermal Sinus in the Sacrococcygeal Region—Experience of Five Cases

Kouzo Moritake and Seiichi Ando

Introduction

A congenital dermal sinus (CDS)—an anomalous communication between the surface of the skin and deeper structures—is the result of developmental abnormalities in the separation of the neuroectoderm and the cutaneous ectoderm [1]. During the past 3 years, we have had experience of five cases of sacrococcygeal CDSs, and have found two clinical characteristics which these cases have in common.

Summary of the Cases

Four cases which had a dermal dimple with a pinpoint hole at its center were diagnosed as CDS within 3 months after birth (Table 1). One case demonstrated symptoms of repeated local infection at the age of 14 (Table 1). Other preoperative clinical and magnetic resonance imaging (MRI) findings are also shown (Table 1). Table 2 gives the surgical and pathological findings and the clinical outcomes.

Results and Discussion

The configuration of CDS cannot always be delineated on MRI (Table 1), but MRI is capable of visualizing surrounding structures and complicated lesions.

During surgery, we found two clinical characteristics of the sacrococcygeal CDS. First, the sacrococcygeal CDS tends to extend caudally (3 cases of 5, Table 2). Wang et al. [2] found the same tendency, and they said that since the embryology of the sacrococcygeal region is different from that of the regions above it, the sacrococcygeal CDS is a different entity from the CDS situated above. Second, the sacrococcygeal CDS is apt to attach to a pathological prominence of the sacral or coccygeal bone (4 cases out of 5, Table 2). This prominence was demonstrated in 2 cases by MRI. The embryological significance of this prominence is yet to be studied, since there has been no mention of it in the literature to date.

In order to prevent serious infection, the sacrococcygeal CDS should be removed as soon as it is detected. Case 3 supports this view, because of the pathological evidence of inflammation in the asymptomatic stage (Table 2).

Department of Neurosurgery, Shimane Medical University, 89-1 Enya-cho, Izumo, Shimane 693-8501, Japan

TABLE 1. Summary of five cases of congenital dermal sinus

Case No.	Sex	Age: Diagnosis	Age: Operation	Site	Symptoms	MRI
1	F	14 years	17 years	Sacrococcygeal	Repeated infections	Dermal sinus (Gd-enhanced)
2	F	At birth	4 years	Sacrococcygeal	Pain on sitting	Enlarged coccygeal bone (high intensity in T1 with fat suppression)
3	F	At birth	4 years	Sacrococcygeal	None	1. Dermal sinus (T1) 2. Slightly enlarged coccygeal bone
4	F	3 months	2 years	Sacrococcygeal	None	n.p.
5	F	At birth	2 years	Sacrococcygeal	None	1. Subcutaneous lipoma 2. Tethered cord

TABLE 2. Operative findings and outcome

	Findings		Histology			Outcome
Case No.	Direction of the sinus	Prominence of the sacral or coccygeal bone	Dermal sinus	Inflammation	Other	
1	Rostral and caudal (bifurcated)	(+)	(+)	(+)	(−)	Excellent
2	Caudal	(+)	(+)	(−)	(−)	Excellent
3	Caudal	(+)	(+)	(+)	(−)	Excellent
4	Caudal	(+)	(+)	(−)	(−)	Excellent
5	Unconfirmed	Unconfirmed	(+)	(−)	Subcutaneous lipoma	Excellent

References

1. Juan F, Martiez-Lage, Juan A. Esteban, Máximo Poza, Carlos Casas (1995) Congenital dermal sinus associated with an abscessed intramedullary epidermoid cyct in a child: case report and review of the literature. Child's Nerv Syst 11:301–305
2. Kyu-Chang Wang, Hee Jin Yang, Chang Wan Oh, Hyun Jib Kim, Byung-Kyu Cho (1993) Spinal congenital dermal sinus. Journal of Korean Medical Science 8:341–347

The Cause of the Chiari Malformation

David G. McLone

It is the Chiari malformation that makes the child with spina bifida different from all the other children that we see in our myelomeningocele clinic. The child with traumatic paraplegia or the child with a lipoma usually has problems restricted to the bladder and bowel or weakness in the lower extremities. I am not trying to minimize those, and I know that they present significant problems in society, but the Chiari malformation inflicts additional significant difficulties on the child. The Chiari malformation will kill 15–20% of the children who have it before they reach the age of 20. It will render some 25% of afflicted children permanently dependent, and 90% of them will have hydrocephalus and all of the associated complications and revisions. Almost all of these children have abnormal respiratory problems and their blood gasses are not normal. Vocal cord paralysis is present in one-third of the children. They have gastric reflux, apnea, and swallowing and learning disabilities. As we work with these children, we find that the majority have some degree of attention deficit disorder (ADD).

For many years people from different disciplines, both pathologists and anatomists, have attempted to link the myelomeningocele to this hindbrain malformation [1, 7, 13, 14]. Many theories have been postulated, the simplest of which is that because the spinal cord is tethered at the bottom, it pulls the hindbrain out of the back of the skull [7]. There are others who postulated that the embryo has hydrocephalus, and the hydrocephalus blows open the back so that the back actually reopens instead of never closing [13, 14] and the force of the hydrocephalus pushes the posterior fossa content down into the upper cervical spine.

The amazing thing about this deformity is that in our series of 100 cases, which have been followed since 1975, in spite of the pan cerebral abnormality, many children have normal intelligence [9, 10], participate normally in society, and in a high percentage of patients we anticipate independence. As everyone is aware, in a Chiari malformation, a portion of the cerebellum, usually the vermis but sometimes also the tonsils, is herniated through the foramen magnum down into the cervical spine (Fig. 1). What they often do not realize is that there is also upward herniation [2, 3]. The cerebellum is herniating upward out of the posterior fossa into the middle fossa (Fig. 2). In fact, we are talking not about a simple herniation through the foramen magnum, but about a pan cranial abnormality of the skull and brain: there is *lükenschadel* of the skull; there are too many gyri, and there is ectopic gray matter; there are degrees of dysgenesis and in some cases agenesis of the corpus callosum;

Northwestern University Medical School, Children's Memorial Hospital, 2300 Children's Plaza No. 28, Chicago, IL 60614, USA

1 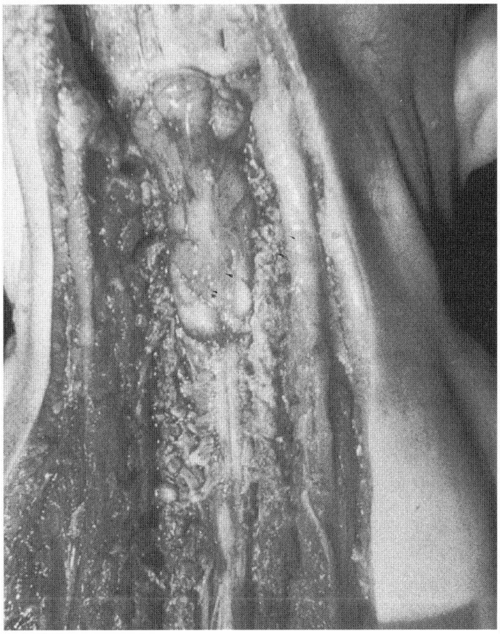

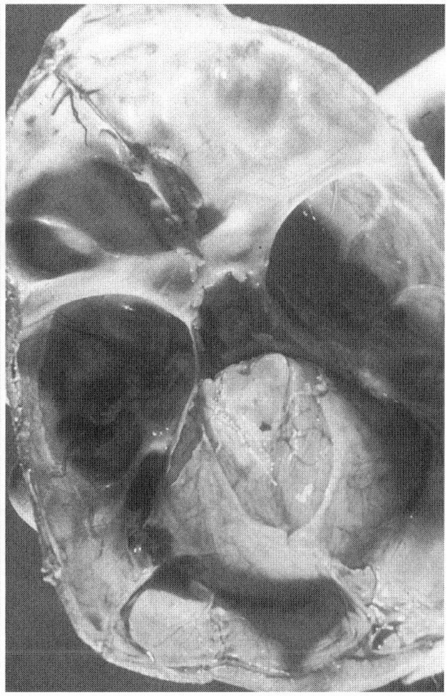 2

FIG. 1. The cerebellar vermis and tonsils are herniated with the brain stem into the cervical canal
FIG. 2. A short tentorium with the cerebellum herniating into the middle fossa is typical of the Chiari II malformation

the massa intermedia located in the third ventricle is huge; there is a deficit in the tentorium; in some of these children, the tentorium is almost absent; there is an extremely small posterior fossa, and in some children there is almost no posterior fossa; there is scalping at the base of the skull and a very enlarged foramen magnum. In spite of this gross deformity, the brain generates normal intelligence and is compatible with independent living for the majority of these children. Now with the miracle of magnetic resonance imaging (MRI), we can look at these deformities, determine where the fourth ventricle is and the extent of this deformity, and know that there are many other things that can occur. For example, Fig. 3 shows cysts in the fourth ventricle and cysts in the brain stem. What are they? Are they related to the myelomeningocele, or are they caused by some genetic defect, or by some metabolic defect in the embryo that affects the entire nervous system? This is a possibility, but it would have to affect all of the germ layers because we know that the skull is abnormal and the nervous system is abnormal so it would be a very unusual defect.

Fortunately, we have the splotch mouse in our laboratory, and these mice develop a myelomeningocele at the lumbosacral junction [11]. The affected mouse has abnormal feet. When it is examined with a scanning electron microscope and the image is maginfied to the size of a human, they look amazing similar. The myelomeningocele of the mouse is essentially the same as a myelomeningocele that occurs in the human. Occasionally the mouse, instead of developing a myelomeningocele, will develop anencephaly (the same thing can happen in a human), with a herniated brain and open skull with brain herniating out as in a child with anencephaly. So this mouse, at least anatomically, is an excellent example of what occurs in the human. What about genetically? The defect in this mouse is in the PAX3 gene.

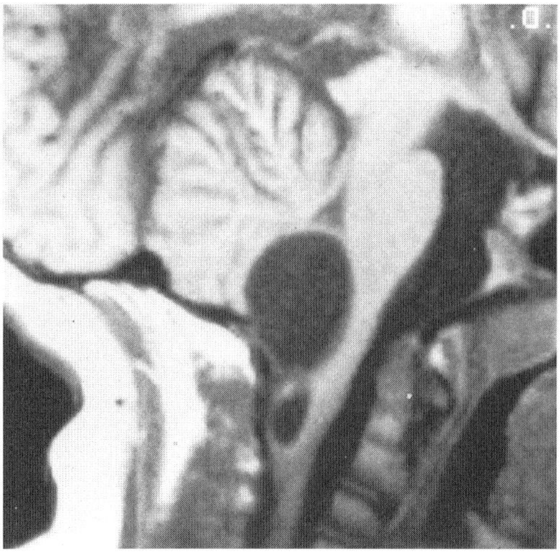

FIG. 3. Sagittal MRI of Chiari II malformation. Note cysts in the brain stem and leaking of the quadrigeminal plate

The PAX3 gene is a transcription factor; that is a gene that generates a protein that goes back into the nucleus and turns on and off a whole cascade of events which lead to neurulation. Using this information, we went to our clinic to look for children who potentially had a PAX3 defect.

Theories about the cause of this malformation have been advanced by several people including Marin-Padilla and Marin-Padilla [8], Penfield and Coburn [15], and Daniel and Strich [4]. I have had discussions bordering on arguments with many of these people because there are problems with almost all these theories. The one which is accepted by most people is that of Padget [13, 14]. The problem with Padget's theory is that hydrocephalus is necessary to generate the force to push the brain down into the brain stem. However, we know that there is not just downward herniation, but also upward herniation, and that makes it unlikely that hydrocephalus is the generating force. Figure 4 is an example of a midtrimester spontaneously aborted fetus. This fetus has a marked Chiari malformation in the posterior fossa and absolutely no hydrocephalus. A very good piece of work done by Japanese neurosurgeons Osaka et al. [12] looked at a group of aborted fetuses and showed quite clearly that the Chiari malformation was present in spite of the fact that there was no evidence of hydrocephalus. The Chiari malformation precedes hydrocephalus, and we will show quite clearly that hydrocephalus is the result of the Chiari malformation, not the cause.

An interesting experiment was done by Desmond and Schoenwolf [5], in which they looked at developing chick embryos and showed that the hollow neural tube, the myelocele, goes from the head end of the embryo all the way to the posterior portion. If this tube is filled with a dye, it can be seen that it closes spontaneously from the cervical to the spinal portion. This is called occlusion. I have seen this in the laboratory, and some of these central canals were closed in our embryos, but I always thought it was an artifact, when in fact it occurs in chickens and in all mammals, including humans. There is a period of time of about 48h, during which the central canal is occluded (Fig. 5). Why would this happen? Schoenwolf and Desmond [16] vented the fluid out of the cephalic portion and found the developing cerebral hemispheres to be markedly deformed. Therefore, a distended ventricular system is essential for normal development; it is the scaffolding that supports the normal development of the cerebral hemisphere. Had they examined the posterior fossa, they would have seen that the

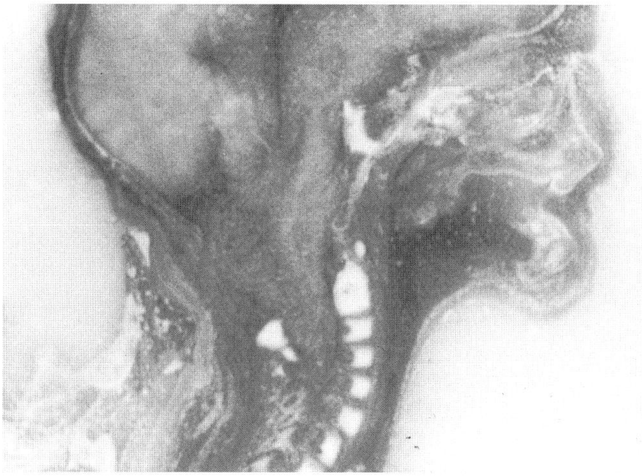

Fig. 4. Midtrimester fetus with a myelomeningocele and severe Chiari II malformation without hydrocephalus

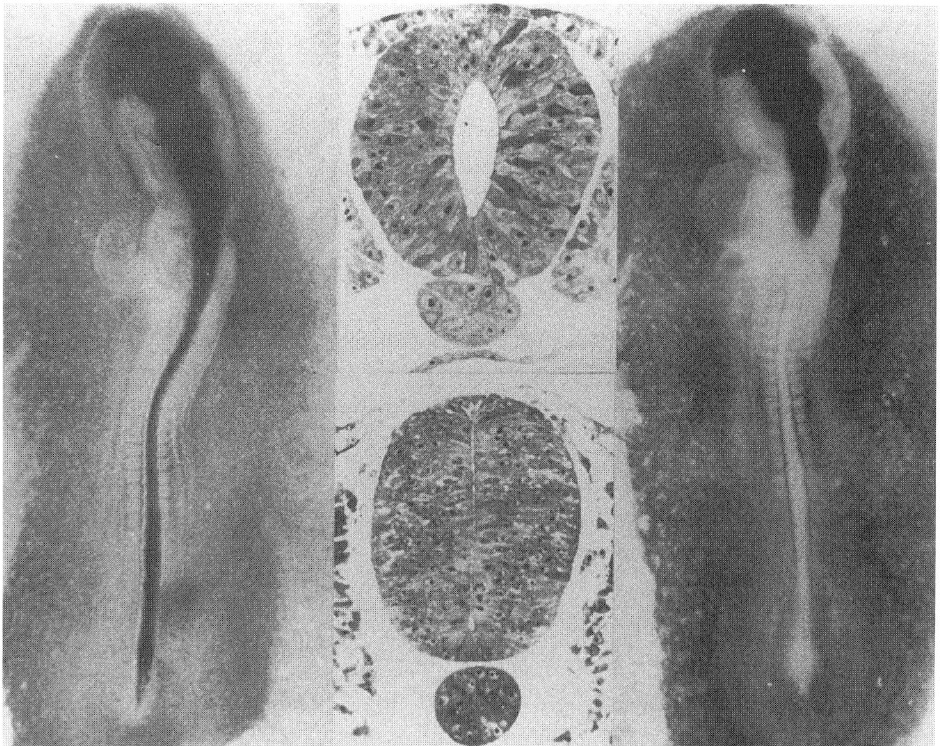

Fig. 5. An embryo with dye in the myelocele. *Left* and *upper middle*, prior to occlusion; *right* and *bottom middle*, after occlusion

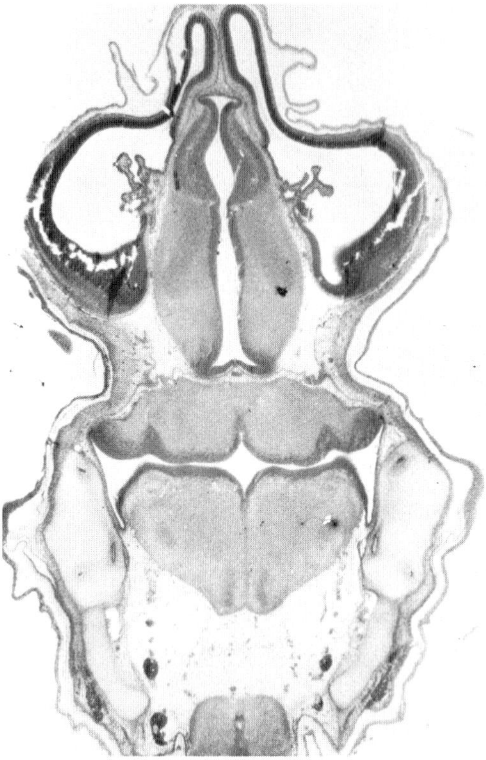

FIG. 6. Human embryo at about 35 days shows the large space surrounding the brain stem, no cerebellum, and the posterior fossa enclosed in cartilage

embryos were developing a Chiari malformation. In our laboratory, Inagaki [6] and Wang (personal communication) examined the posterior fossa of the chick in the same experiment and showed that there were early Chiari malformations. This occlusion is a critical event that allows the cerebral hemispheres to distend. However, if there is an open myelomeningocele at the bottom when occlusion is over, after about 48h, and the neural tube reopens, all the fluid runs out through the open myelomeningocele, and the cerebral hemispheres are decompressed. This leads to the development of the Chiari malformation. Figure 6 shows a 34-day-old human embryo. It can be seen from the posterior fossa that there is as yet no cerebellum. There is a significant amount of room in the posterior fossa because the spaces have been distended by the fluid. It is important to note that these is cartilage on either side, surrounding the posterior fossa. The posterior fossa is already determined and is solid; it is already in a cartilaginous box. What determines the size of this box is the distending force which occurs during occlusion. If that force is not there, the posterior fossa will be small. There will be not only cerebral deformities from the collapse of the mantle, but also a very small posterior fossa which will lead to the Chiari malformation. So it is the decompression of these vesicles (the embryonic ventricles, if you will) during primary neurulation that leads to the Chiari malformation. The neural tube is left open so that the fluid can pass out and decompress the head of the embryo. In the embryo, the telencephalic hemispheres are beginning to develop, and as is shown in the embryo with a myelomeningocele (Fig. 7), everything has collapsed (Wang, personal communication). In a normal embryo without a myelomeningocele, there is adequate space in the posterior fossa; only the choroid plexus is present. The generation

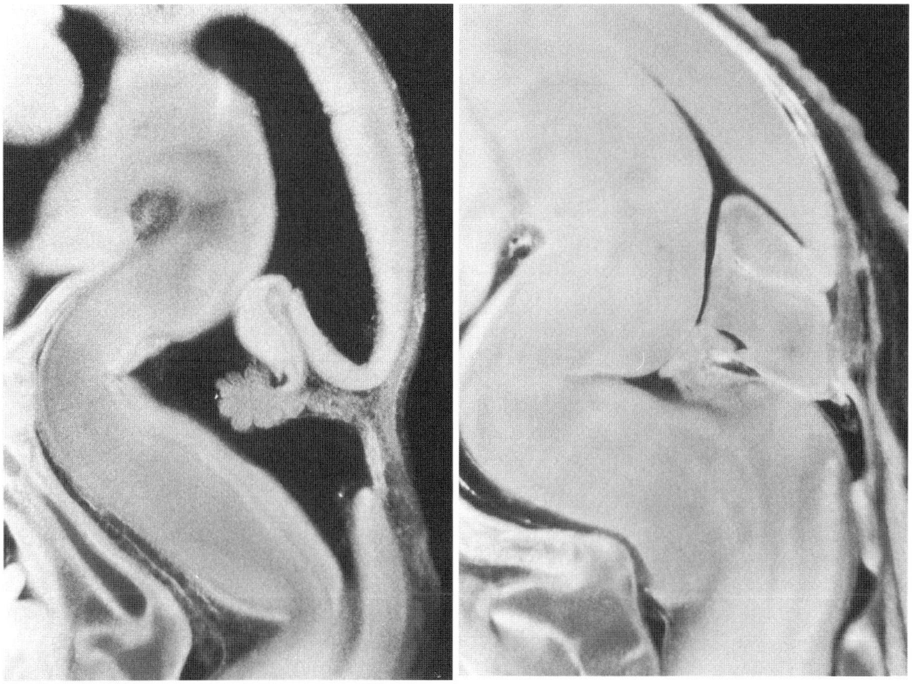

A B

FIG. 7. **A** The emryonic hindbrain with a large fluid-filled space into which the cerebellum will develop. **B** An embryo with a myelomeningocele which shows the collapse of the fluid spaces

of the cerebellum will occur here, but it will balloon into and fill the space. The opening at the base of the skull, the foramen magnum, shows that the hindbrain is well within the skull. In the embryo with a myelomeningocele, there is no room for the anticipated cerebellum and already there is some herniation of the contents of the posterior fossa into the upper cervical spine. So even before the cerebellum has developed there are signs of herniation. The critical step is the loss of the volumetric expansion that the embryo needs to anticipate the development of the elements in the posterior fossa.

If we take the embryo, strip off the mesenchyme, and look in the posterior fossa, it can be seen that this overcrowding is already there and it is impossible for the embryo to develop a subarachnoid space. If the subarachnoid space in the posterior fossa is inadequate or is missing, this will lead to hydrocephalus. The severity of this compaction will determine how severe the hydrocephalus is and how rapidly it will progress. Because everything falls in on itself, instead of having a large third ventricle with a tiny massa intermedia, we find a large massa intermedia and a small third ventricle. In the newborn, this makes it difficult to determine where one can perform a third ventriculostomy to treat the hydrocephalus. In a normal skull, the skull plate, the parietal plate, and the collagen bundles stream out as the brain expands and pulls them out. In the child with a myelomeningocele, because of a collapse of the mantle, they stream out but they turn back on themselves and cannot be pulled out; this leads to *lükenschadel* of the skull. When an ultrasound is performed, we see that the parietal plates have caved in instead of being rounded externally because the open myelomeningocele is decompressing the intracranial compartment, producing a child with a Chiari II malformation. The myelomeningocele is linked to the formation of the Chiari malformation because it is the myelomeningocele which allows the escape of cerebral spinal fluid, and decompression of the embryonic vesicles, leading to the Chiari malformation. However, in a child with a lipoma a Chiari malformation does not develop because the lipoma plugs the hole and prevents the escape of fluid.

References

1. Barry A, Patten BM, Stewart BH (1957) Possible factors in the development of the Arnold–Chiari malformation. J Neurosurg 14:285–301
2. Chiari H (1891) Uber Veranderungen des Kleinhirns infolge von Hydrocephalie des Grosshirns. Dtsch Med Wochenschr 17:1172
3. Chiari H (1895) Uber Veranderungen des Kleinhirns, der Pons und der Medulla oblongata infolge von congenitaler Hydrocephalie des Grosshirns. Denkschr Akad Wiss 63:71
4. Daniel PM, Strich SJ (1958) Some observations on the congenital deformity of the central nervous system known as the Arnold–Chiari malformation. J Neuropathol Exp Neurol 17:255
5. Desmond ME, Schoenwolf G (1985) Timing and positioning of occlusion of the spinal neurocele in the chick embryo. J Comp Neurol 235:479
6. Inagaki T, Schoenwolf GC, Walker ML (1997) Experimental model: change in the posterior fossa with surgically induced spina bifida aperta in mouse. Pediatr Neurosurg
7. Lichtenstein BW (1942) Distant neuroanatomic complications of spina bifida (spinal dysraphism): hydrocephalus, Arnold–Chiari deformity, stenosis of the aqueduct of Sylvius, etc., pathogenesis and pathology. Arch Neurl Psychiatr 47:195
8. Marin-Padilla M, Marin-Padilla TM (1981) Morphogenesis of experimentally induced Arnold–Chiari malformation. J Neurol Sci 50:29
9. McLone DG, Knepper PA (1989) The cause of Chiari II malformation: a unified theory. Pediatr Neurosurg 15:1
10. McLone DG, Raimondi AJ, Sommers MW (1981) The results of early treatment of 100 consecutive newborns with myelomeningocele. Proceedings of the VII Congress of the European Society for Paediatric Neurosurgery. Z Kinder Chir 2:115
11. McLone DG, Dias MS, Goossens W, et al. (1997) Pathological changes in exposed neural tissue of fetal delayed splotch (Spd) mice. Childs Nerv Syst 13:1
12. Osaka K, Matsumoto S, Tanimura T (1978) Myeloschisis in early human embryos. Childs Brain 4:347
13. Padget DH (1972) Development of so-called dysraphism, with embryologic evidence of clinical Arnold–Chiari and Dandy–Walker malformations. Johns Hopkins Med J 130:127
14. Padget DH, Lindenberg R (1972) Inverse cerebellum morphogenetically related to Dandy–Walker and Arnold–Chiari syndromes: bizarre malformed brain with occipital encephalocele. Johns Hopkins Med J 131:228
15. Penfield W, Coburn DF (1935) Arnold–Chiari malformation and its operative treatment. Arch Neurol Psychiatr 40:328
16. Schoenwolf G, Desmond ME (1984) Neural tube oclusion precedes rapid brain enlargement. J Exp Zool 30:405

Nonneoplastic Retrocerebellar Cystic Lesions—with Special References to Dandy–Walker Syndrome (DWS)

Kiyoshi Sato and Hajime Arai

Summary. This paper presents a redefinition of Dandy–Walker syndrome (DWS) diagnostic criteria through a review of the neuroimaging features of nonneoplastic retrocerebellar cyst cases experienced by the authors, and classical descriptions of DWS by previous investigators.

Pediatric Patients and Methods of Neuroimaging Investigations

When one of the authors (KS) was a neurosurgical resident at the Children's Memorial Hospital in Chicago, he had occasion to conduct a retrospective analysis of 37 pediatric cases of Dandy–Walker syndrome (DWS) treated at Cook County and Children's Memorial Hospitals by Prof. A.J. Raimondi and his associates during the period from 1963 to 1977 [21–23, 26]. Between 1978 and 1997, we had experience of 38 pediatric cases of nonneoplastic retrocerebellar cyst diagnosed and treated at Juntendo University Hospital in Tokyo [3].

Various neuroimaging methods were utilized to diagnose DWS and other retrocerebellar cystic lesions. Cisternal pneumoencephalography and cerebral angiography were the main methods used for diagnosis in the Chicago cases [20]. Computed tomography (CT) scanning of the head, CT cisternography via the lumbar route using a water-soluble contrast medium or radio-isotope, and cerebral angiography were used for the Juntendo cases treated prior to 1995 [2]. Cases were investigated by either or both CT and magnetic resonance (MR) imaging of the head, and CT cisternography was limited to cases where diagnosis of an intra-arachnoid cyst of the posterior fossa was established.

Results

Diagnosis of DWS by Pneumoencephalography and Cerebral Angiography

Cisternal pneumoencephalography offered findings specific to DWS where enormously strong cystic dilatation of the fourth ventricle which extended into a retrocerebellar region, severe anterior rotation of a maldeveloped cerebellar vermis with and without aqueductal

Department of Neurosurgery, Juntendo University Hospital, Hongo, Tokyo 113-0033, Japan

a,b c d,e f

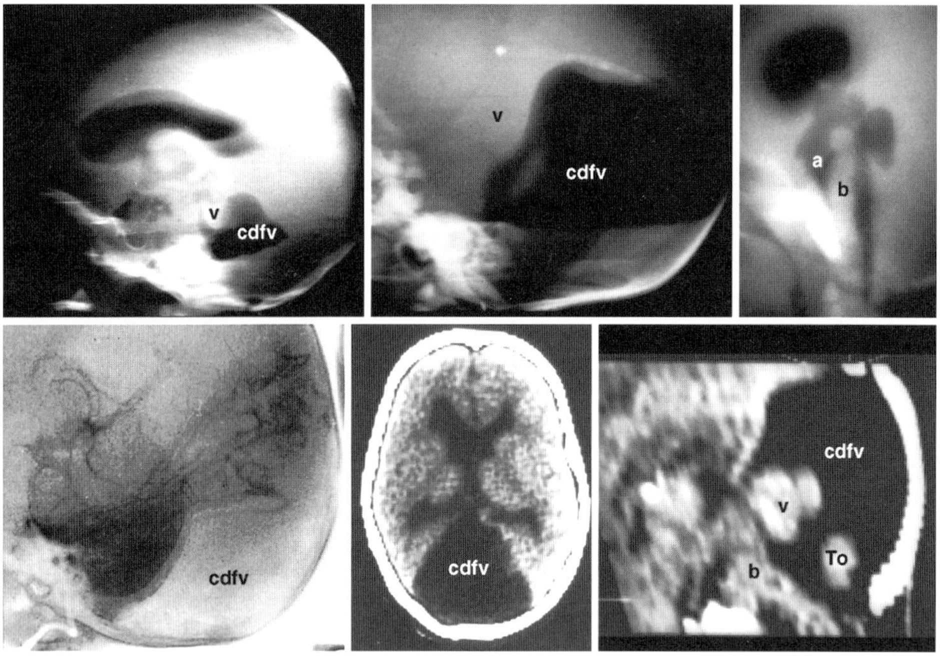

FIG. 1. Diagnosis of Dandy–Walker syndrome (DWS) by **a–c** pneumoencephalography, **b** cerebral angiography, and **e**, **f** CT scanning of head. *v*, malformed cerebellar vermis with anterior rotation; *cdfv*, cystic dilatation of fourth ventricle with its extension to retrocerebellar region; *b*, maldeveloped brain stem; *a*, air around the brain stem. **e** and **f**, axial and sagittal reconstruction views, respectively, of the posterior fossa by CT scanning of the head obtained from a 5-year-old male with DWS

compression, an underdeveloped brain stem, and abnormally high insertion of the tentorium with upward bulging were consistently observed. It was also frequently observed that air introduced into the cisterna magna and/or fourth ventricular cavity migrated to the subarachnoid space around the brain stem, suggesting patency of the fouth ventricle's outlet foramia (Fig. 1a–c). Cisternal pneumoencephalograms appeared to us to resemble the pneumoventriculogram (Fig. 2a) and macro- and microscopic findings of the midsagittal section of the posterior fossa obtained in a postmortem investigation of a case of DWS published by Brodal and Hauglie-Hanssen in 1959 [8] (Fig. 2b,c).

Angiography of DWS cases, the final diagnoses of which were confirmed by pneumocisternography, revealed the existence of retrocerebellar cystic lesions in association with cerebellar hypoplasia. These findings were disclosed specifically in lateral views of the capillary and early venous phases (Fig. 1d). Lateral displacement of the left and right posterior cerebral arteries and hypoplastic superior cerebellar artery crossing over the posterior cerebral artery might frequently be observed. However, a maldeveloped cerebellar vermis with anterior rotation due to the effect of pressure of a huge fourth ventricular cyst, which appeared to us to be a pathognomonic feature in DWS-case pneumoencephalograms, could not be identified by angiography. This was attributed to the unusually poor opacification of the posterior inferior cerebellar arteries running along the inferior

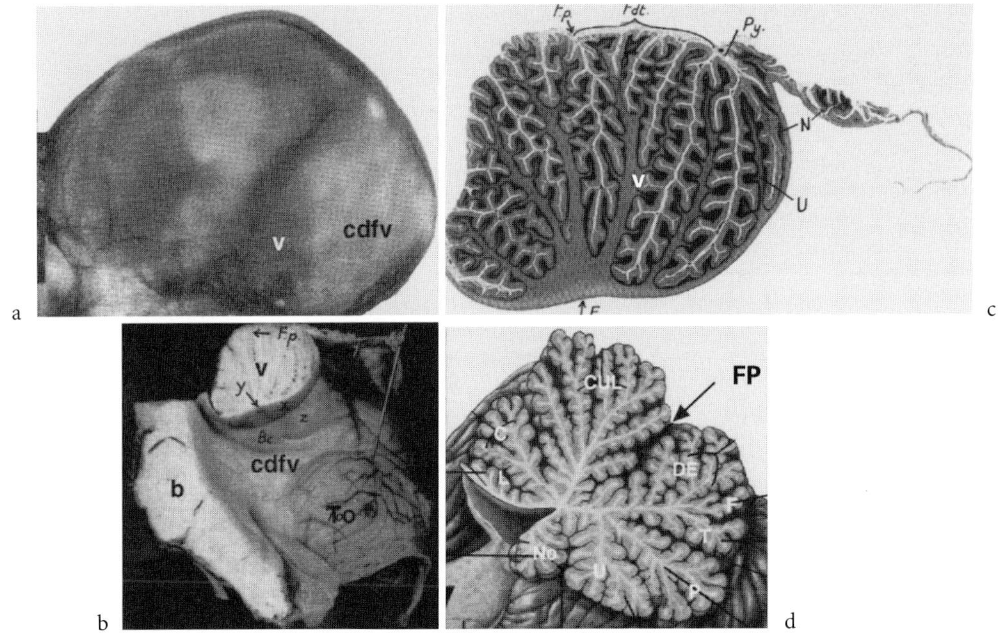

FIG. 2. **a** Pneumoventriculogram. **b** Midsagittal section of the posterior fossa obtained in a postmortem investigation of a case with DWS. **c** Microscopic finding of an underdeveloped cerebellar vermis. Note the defective development of the cerebellar vermis, especially the inferior vermis. Adapted from [8]. **d** Microscopic image of the midsagittal section of a normal cerebellar vermis. (Adapted from [33].) *b*, underdeveloped brain stem; *v*, maldeveloped cerebellar vermis with anterior rotation; *cdfv*, cystic dilatation of fourth ventricle with its extension to retrocerebellar region; *Fp*, primary fissure; *y* and *f*, fastigium; *Fdt*, Folium-declive-tuber; *p* or *Py*, pyramis; *N* or *No*, nodule; *U*, uvula; *To*, tonsilla

surface of the inferior vermis, probably due to hypoplasia of the arteries in cases with DWS (Fig. 1d).

Diagnosis of Retrocerebellar Cystic Lesions by CT-Cisternography and CT and MR Imaging of the Head

Thirty-eight cases with retrocerebellar cystic lesions were investigated by various neuroimaging methods, and the results were retrospectively analyzed to facilitate differential diagnosis and clarify indications for surgery [2]. The retrocerebellar lesions were divided into subtypes A and B depending on whether or not maldevelopment of the rhombencephalic roof was involved in pathogenesis of the retrocerebellar cysts [24, 27] (Table 1). Subtype A included intra-arachnoid cysts with and without communication (see Fig. 5c) with the surrounding subarachnoid space [2, 16] in six and two cases, respectively, glioependymal cyst [32] in one case, enlarged cisterna magna with communicating hydrocephalus [24] in one case, and mega cisterna magna [18] in 10 cases (Fig. 5b). Subtype B included classic DWS [5] in four cases (Fig. 3), persistent Blake's pouch [27] or arachnoid pouch of cisterna magna [24] in one case (Fig. 4a), Dandy–Walker variant [18] in three cases (Fig. 4b,c and Fig. 5a), DWS with occipital meningocele [6, 29, 30] in one case (Fig. 4d), and Dandy–Warburg syndrome [19] in one case (Fig. 4e).

Table 1. Nonneoplastic retrocerebellar cysts (1978–1997)

Subtype A: without a maldeveloped rhombencephalic roof	
Intraarachnoid cyst [28]	8
Communicating [16]	6
Noncommunicating [16]	2
Glioependymal cyst	1
Enlarged cisterna magna with communicating hydrocephalus [32]	1
Mega cisterna magna [18]	10
Subtype B: with a maldeveloped rhombencephalic roof	
Dandy-Walker malformation (DWM) [23]	4
DWM with occipital meningocele [6]	1
Dandy-Walker variant [18]	3
Persistent Blake's pouch [27] or arachnoid pouch of cisterna magna [24]	1
Dandy-Warburg syndrome	1
Total no. of cases	38

a,b c d,e f

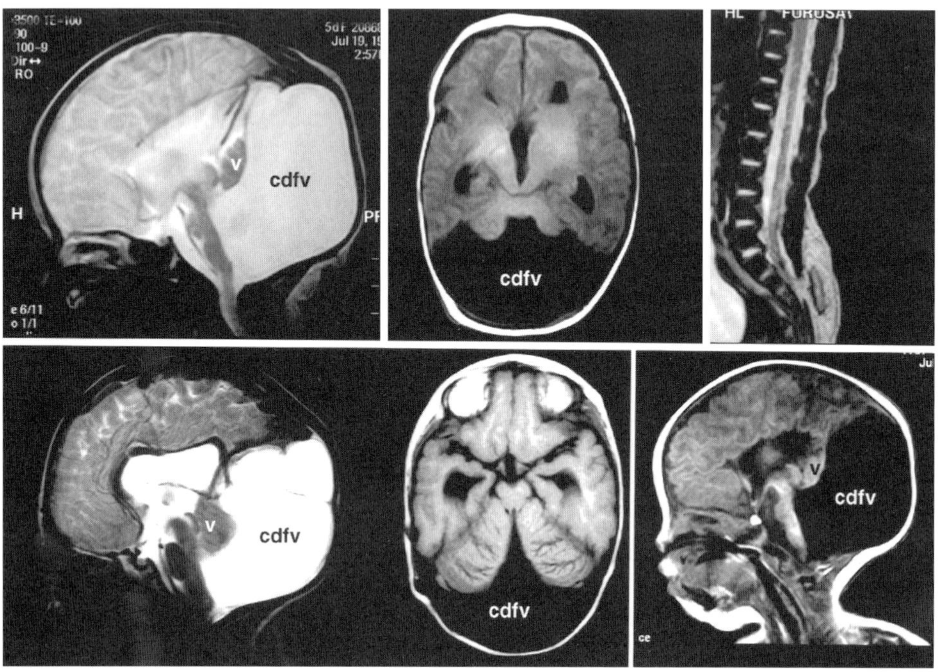

Fig. 3. **a** Mid-sagittal, and **b** axial magnetic resonance image (MRI) of the head of a 1-month-old male with classic DWS. Associated anomalies in this case included agenesis of the corpus callosum, hypoplastic brain stem, spina bifida occulta, intraspinal lipoma with tethered cord (**c**), persistence of duct of Botallo, and Meckel's diverticulum. **d** Midsagittal and **e** axial MRI of the head of a 3-year-old male with classic DWS associated with hypospadia. **f** Midsagittal MRI of the head of a 2-year-old male with classic DWS

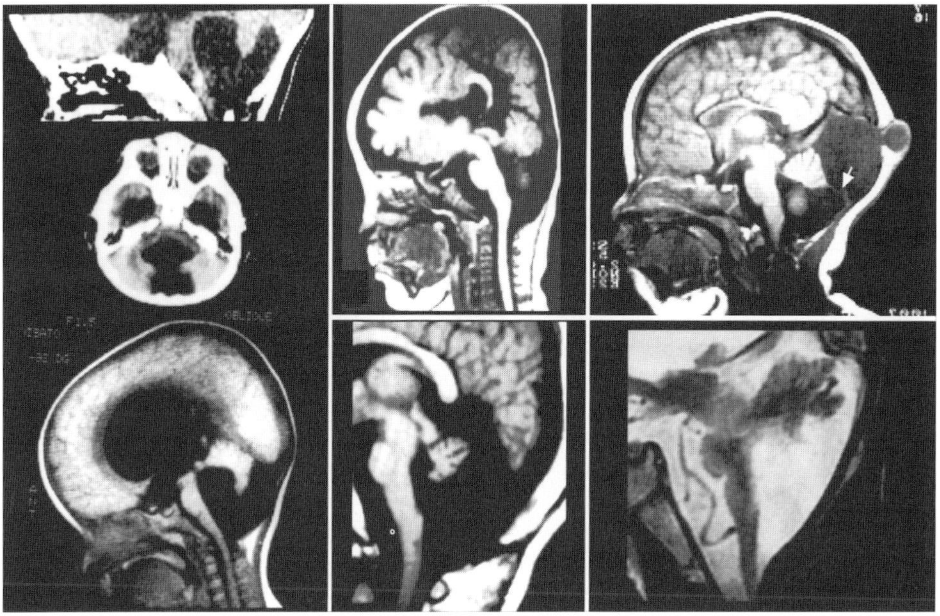

a b,d c,e

FIG. 4. **a** Persistent Blake's pouch. A retrocerebellar cyst with direct communication to the cystic fourth ventricle and hypoplastic or atrophic cerebellum are prominent features, but neither enlargement of the posterior fossa nor high insertion of tentorium was observed in this 2-year-old female case (*upper*, midsagittal reconstruction CT; *middle*, axial CT scanning of the head of a 2-year-old female with hydrocephalus. **b**, **c** Midsagittal MRI of the posterior fossa in cases tentatively diagnosed as Dandy–Walker variant (please read the Discussion section in the text). **d** MRI in a case with Dandy–Walker malformation with occipital meningocele. The arrow indicates a membranous structure which appears to divide the retrocerebellar cyst into two compartments which include the occipital meningocele and the prominent cisterna magna. **e** Maldeveloped cerebellum in a 10-year-old male with Dandy–Warburg syndrome

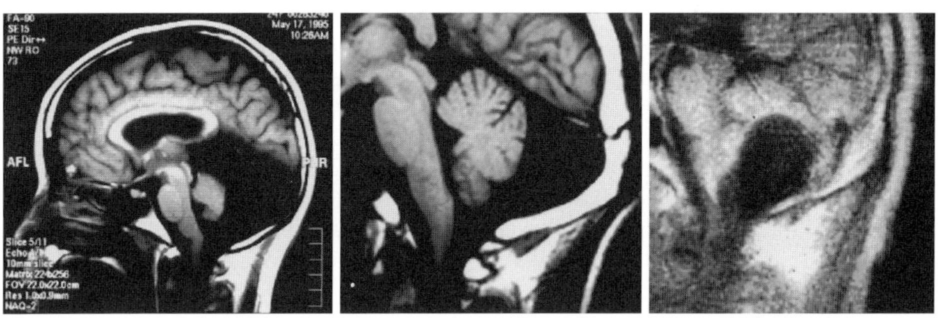

a b,c

FIG. 5. **a** Dandy–Walker variant. **b** Mega cisterna magna. **c** Noncommunicatingintraarachnoid cyst, the diagnosis of which was confirmed by CT cisternography

Discussion

The following short review of DWS-related publications will be useful when we define the morphological criteria of DWS. In 1914, Dandy and Blackfan [11] described a 13-month-old girl with severe supratentorial hydrocephalus associated with cystic dilatation of the fourth ventricle, hypoplasia of the cerebellar vermis, and absence of the foramina of Luschka and Magendie. The authors concluded from clinicopathological findings that atresia of the outlet foramina of the fourth ventricle to the subarachnoid space had caused hydrocephalus in this patient (Atresia theory). In 1942, Taggart and Walker [31] reported three infants in whom hydrocephalus was assumed to have resulted from a congenital defect in the foramina of Magendie and Luschka. In 1941, Sahs [25] reported a case of congenital anomaly of the cerebellar vermis without hydrocephalus, but the structural abnormality of the posterior fossa closely resembled cases with a congenital type of hydrocephalus reported by Dandy in 1914 and 1921 [11, 12], although the foramina of Luschka was patent.

In 1954, Benda [5] suggested, after pathological investigation of six hydrocephalus patients, that cystic dilatation of the fourth ventricle is not always induced by the occlusion of the foramina of Magendie and Luschka, and that congenital malformation of the cerebellar vermis itself might be related to the pathogenesis of this type of hydrocephalus. This theory apparently conflicted with the atresia theory proposed by Dandy and Blackfan, and Taggart and Walker. However, Benda praised their achievements and proposed naming the type of hydrocephalus associated with cerebellar vermis hypoplasia and cystic dilatation of the fourth ventricle the Dandy–Walker syndrome.

In 1959, Brodal and Hauglie-Hanssen [8] reported on the pathological study of two DWS patients. They compared histopathological findings of cystic dilatation of the fourth ventricle in these cases with the 1943 histopathological findings of Bonnevie [7] in murine hydrocephalus (Hy-1). They found that the findings in human cases resembled those of Hy-1, and assumed that this anomaly of the posterior fossa had developed before the formation of the area membranacea posterior (AMP) in which the foramen Magendie is later opened. In considering Bonnevie's work, Brodal and Hauglie-Hanssen believed that dorsal bulging of the area membranacea anterior (AMA) occured from unknown causes, and this abnormal bulging of the AMA has been considered to arrest development of the cerebellar vermis, although pathogenesis of the AMA bulging has itself never been explained. Brodal and Hauglie-Hanssen therefore concluded that occlusion of the foramina of Magendie and Luschka is not directly involved in the maldevelopment of the cerebellar vermis in DWS.

Since 1960, D'Agostino et al. [10], Hart et al. [17], Gardner et al. [14] and many other investigators have introduced new ideas about the cause of DWS. Nevertheless, it is generally agreed that the basic picture of DWS is as a maldevelopment of the inferior vemis associated with cystic dilatation of the fourth ventricle. However, its cause is still unknown. Because, in DWS patients, associated anomalies are found not only in the central nervous system [15] but also in other organs [17], and because family and hereditary backgrounds [5, 26] are likely to be relevant in connection with the disease, we are of the opinion that more complicated and unknown teratogenic factors are involved in DWS etiology.

In reviewing DWS cases treated at Cook County and Children's Memorial Hospitals and nonneoplastic retrocerebellar cases at the Juntendo University Hospital, we have considerable difficulty in differentiating DWS from other nonneoplastic retrocerebellar lesions, especially when MRI and CT imaging of the head have been considered as acceptable noninvasive diagnostic techniques for infants and children with this problem. In the past, various diagnostic methods such as pneumoencephalography and CT cisternography, in addition to MR and CT imaging, were utilized in combinations to arrive at an appropriate diagnosis for cystic lesions in the posterior fossa [2]. Accordingly, the variety of retrocerebellar cystic lesions as listed in Table 1 could reasonably have been designated.

The difficulty and confusion in diagnosing retrocerebellar cystic lesions has been augmented by the application of a variety of terminologies, such as Dandy–Walker variant [15], persistent Blake's pouch [27], arachnoid pouch of the cisterna magna [24], and Dandy–Walker complex [4], to a variety of retrocerebellar lesions. The term Dandy–Walker variant originated with axial CT scanning of the posterior fossa in cases with retrocerebellar cysts where the roof and lateral wall of the fourth ventricle were recognized, although the cerebellar vermis was hypoplastic [18]. The anterior rotation of the hypoplastic cerebellum was not as prominent as in the case of DWS. Rayboud [24] roughly classified retrocerebellar cystic lesions as true Dandy–Walker malformation, Dandy–Walker variant, or arachnoid pouch of the cisterna magna. He described the first and second types as being associated with cerebellar vermis hypoplasia, but not the third.

In 1989, Barkovich et al. [4] proposed a revised classification of posterior fossa cysts and cyst-like malformations, based on the results of MR imaging, where the retrocerebellar cystic lesions are divided into Dandy–Walker complex, posterior fossa cyst, and prominent cisterna magna. These three diagnostic categories were considered to represent a continuum of development anomalies of the posterior fossa. The Dandy–Walker complex was further divided into two subgroups, type A and type B, based on the presence or absence of the vermis in an axial image of the mid-fourth ventricle. That is a difference which depends on the degree of anterior rotation of the vermis. In other words, in Dandy–Walker complex type A, the vermis was absent on axial images at the level of the fourth ventricle because of extreme anterior rotation and/or hypoplasia or aplasia of the vermis. As described by Barkovich et al., type A appeared to correspond to what had been diagnosed as Dandy–Walker syndrome since the introduction of the terminology by Benda in 1954. In contrast with this, Dandy–Walker complex type B differed from type A by the interposition of a portion of the cerebellar vermis between the mid-fourth ventricle and the enlarged cisterna magna in axial images. Traditionally, type B would be considered as mega cisterna magna. Posterior fossa cysts are characterized by discrete posterior fossa cerebrospinal fluid collections that did not directly communicate with the fourth ventricle. The vermis and cerebellar hemisphere are complete and of normal size. Finally, a prominent cisterna magna is an enlarged cisterna magana without enlargement of the posterior fossa where the vermis and cerebellar hemisphere are atrophic.

In the present retrospective study, the case illustrated in Fig. 1e,f and the three cases illustrated in Fig. 3 undoubtedly represent cases of classic DWS or Dandy–Walker malformation which appear to correspond with the findings reported by Brodal and Hauglie-Hanssen [8] and also with MRI of the Dandy–Walker complex type A published by Barkovich et al. [4]. It should be noted, however, that there is great difficulty in diagnosing the cases of various types of retrocerebellar cysts other than classic DWS by MRI alone. Axial CT findings of the case illustrated in Fig. 4a correspond to the Dandy–Walker variant because the lateral wall of the fourth ventricle can be appreciated in CT axial views of the posterior fossa, but midsagittal MRI findings may indicate a possible diagnosis of either persistent Blake's pouch or prominent cisterna magna associated with surpatentorial hydrocephalus. The cases illustrated in Fig. 4b,c, where no supratentorial hydrocephalus was involved, are characterized by posterior fossa pathologies including cystic dilatation of the fourth ventricle and severely atrophic cerebellar vermis. Since the fastigium and inferior medullary velum are well recognized, although the cerebellum is extremely hypoplastic, a diagnosis of Dandy—Walker variant is plausible. However, these cases could also be diagnosed as Chiari IV malformation or prominent cisterna magna, respectively, by the definition of Barkovich et al. based on the absence of an enlarged posterior fossa. The case illustrated in Fig. 4d was diagnosed as Dandy–Walker variant with occipital meningocele [5, 29, 30]. However, this would be occipital meningocele associated with prominent cisterna magna, because the membranous structure indicated by the arrow in the picture appears to divide the fourth ventricular cyst into two compartments, or prominent cisterna magna and occipital encephalocele. The case illustrated in Fig. 5b appears to be a case of prominent cisterna magna, although the possibility of posterior fossa cyst should be considered. The case illustrated in Fig. 5c could correspond with the Barkovich et al. definition of a posterior fossa cyst. To arrive at an appropriate diagnosis of these cases, however, CT cisternography in addition to CT and MR imaging would appear to be necessary.

Conclusion

From the present study, we conclude that classification of retrocerebellar cysts still is very difficult when the investigating diagnostic procedure is limited to CT and MRI. Nevertheless, among nonneoplastic retrocerebellar lesions, classic DWS is a pathognomonic disease which undoubtedly can be diagnosed by either CT or MRI of the head alone. That is, severe anterior rotation of a malformed cerebellar vermis due to cystic dilatation of the fourth ventricle, enlargement of the posterior fossa, abnormally high insertion of the tentorium with its upward bulge, and underdevelped brain stem are uniformly observed. The frequent coexistence of associated anomalies not only in the central nervous system, but also in other systemic organs appears to be a clue supporting a diagnosis of DWS. It is our impression that such invasive diagnostic technology as CT cisternography is still mandatory, in addition to CT scanning and MRI of the head when an appropriate classification of various retrocerebellar lesions is required.

References

1. Adam R, Greenberg JO (1978) The mega cisterna magna. J Neurosurg 48:190–192
2. Arai H, Sato K (1991) Posterior fossa cysts: clinical, neuroradiological and surgical features. Child's Nerv Syst 7:156–164
3. Arai H, Sato K, Raimondi AJ (1993) Dandy–Walker syndrome. In: Raimondi AJ et al. (eds) Intracranial cyst lesions. Springer-Verlag, New York, chap 13, pp 183–200
4. Barkovich AJ, Kjos BO, Norman D, Edwards MS (1989) Revised classification of posterior fossa cysts and cystlike malformations based on the results of multiplanar MR imaging. AJNR 10:977–988
5. Benda CE (1954) The Dandy–Walker syndrome or the so-called atresia of the foramen Magendie. J Neuropathol Exp Neurol 13:14–29
6. Bindal AK, Storrs BB, McLone DG (1991) Occipital meningoceles in patients with the Dandy–Walker syndrome. Neurosurgery 28:844–847
7. Bonnevie K (1943) Hereditary hydrocephalus in the house mouse. 1. Manifestation of the hy-mutation after birth and in embryos 12 days old or more. Skr Norske Vidensk Akad l. Mat-Nat KI No 4
8. Brodal A, Hauglie-Hanssen E (1959) Congenital hydrocephalus with defective development of the cerebellar vermis (Dandy–Walker syndrome). Clinical and anatomical findings in two cases with particular reference to the so-called atresia of the foramen of Magendie and Luschka. J Neurol Neurosurg Psychiatry 22:99–108
9. Cinalli G, Vinikoff L, Zerah M, Renier D, Kahn AP (1997) Dandy–Walker malformation associated with syringomyelia. J Neurosurg 86:871

10. D'Agostino AN, Kernohan JW, Brown JR (1963) Dandy–Walker syndrome. J Neuropathol Exp Neurol 22:450–470
11. Dandy WE, Blackfan KD (1914) Internal hydrocephalus: an experimental, clinical and pathological study. Am J Dis Child 8:406–482
12. Dandy WE (1921) The diagnosis and treatment of hydrocephalus due to occlusion of the foramina of Magendie and Luschka. Surg Gynecol Obstet 32:112–124
13. Domingo Z, Peter J (1996) Midline developmental abnormalities of the posterior fossa: correlation of classification with outcome. Pediatr Neurosurg 24:111–118
14. Gardner E, O'Rahilly R, Prolo D (1975) The Dandy–Walker and Arnold–Chiari malformations. Arch Neurol 32:393–407
15. Golden JA, Rorke LB, Bruce DA (1987) Dandy–Walker syndrome and associated anomalies. Pediatr Neurosci 13:38–44
16. Handa J, Nakano Y, Aii H (1977) CT-cisternography with intracranial arachnoid cysts. Surg Neurol 8:451–454
17. Hart MN, Malamud N, Ellis WG (1972) The Dandy–Walker syndrome. A clinicopathological study based on 28 cases. Neurology 22:771–780
18. Harwood-Nash DC, Fitz CR (1976) Neuroradiology in infants and children. Mosby, St. Louis
19. Pagon RA, Claren SK, Milam DF, Hendrickson AE (1983) Autosomal recessive eye and brain anomalies: Warburg syndrome. J Pediatr 102:542–546
20. Raimondi AJ (1972) Pediatric neuroradiology. Saunders, Philadelphia, London, Toronto
21. Raimondi AJ, Soare P (1974) Intellectual development in shunted hydrocephalic children. Am J Dis Child 127:664–671
22. Raimondi AJ, Samuelson GS, Yarzagaray L, Norton T (1969) Atresia of the foramina of Luschka and Magnesia. The Dandy–Walker cyst. J Neurosurg 31:202–216
23. Raimondi AJ, Sato K, Shimoji T (1984) The Dandy–Walker syndrome. Karger, Basel
24. Raybaud C (1982) Cystic malformations of the posterior fossa. J Neuroradiol 9:103–133
25. Sahs AL (1941) Congenital anomaly of the cerebellar vermis. Arch Pathol 32:52–63
26. Sato K, Shimoji T, McLone DG et al. (1981) Phenotypic frequencies of H.L.A. antigens among patients with Dandy–Walker syndrome and other congenital malformations in the central nervous system. Afr J Clin Exp Immunol 2:145–150
27. Shaw CM, Alvord EC Jr (1977) Congenital arachnoid cysts and their differential diagnosis. In: Vinken PJ, Bruyn GW (eds) Handbook of clinical neurology, vol 31. North-Holland, Amsterdam, pp 75–135
28. Starkman SP, Brown TC, Linell EA (1958) Cerebral arachnoid cysts. J Neuropathol Exp Neurol 17:484–500
29. Suzuki Y, Mimaki T, Tagawa T et al. (1988) Dandy–Walker cyst associated with occipital meningocele. Pediatr Neurol 4:236–240
30. Tachi N, Tachi M, Sasaki K et al. (1988) Walker–Warburg syndrome in a Japanese patient. Pediatr Neurol 4:236–240
31. Taggart J, Walker AE (1942) Congenital atresia of the foramens of Luschka and Magendie. Arch Neurol Psychiatr 48:583–612
32. Wolpert SM, Scott RM (1981) The value of metrizamide CT cisternography in the management of cerebral arachnoid cysts. AJNR 2:29–35
33. Carpenter MB (1991) Core text of neuroanatomy, 4th edn. Williams & Wilkins, Baltimore, p 55, Fig. 2.36

Discussion and Moderators' Comments on Sessions—Hind-Brain Anomalies

Kintomo Takakura

D. McLone: Several years ago, you did a study on HLA typing looking for a genetic factor in the Dandy–Walker syndrome, and it is possible you have found some correlation. Have you found any genetic component?

K. Sato: When I was in Chicago, I collected blood from Dandy–Walker syndrome cases and I reported the results of this HLA study to a journal. However, I was unable to arrive at any conclusion in this study. Since my return from Chicago, I have tried to find cases of Dandy–Walker syndrome but, as I have mentioned, I am confused as to just what constitues Dandy–Walker syndrome. During the past 15 years, I have collected only two cases of what can be categorized as the classic type. Also, there are many similar anomalies of the posterior fossa, so I did not continue the HLA typing study. However, you have so many cases of Dandy–Walker syndrome that you can couduct a study. A scientist who analyzed the results in Chicago told me he could not arrive at any conclusion.

K. Mori: Allow me to ask a couple of questions concerning the Dandy–Walker syndrome. Thank you for your very good presentation, but you did not mention treatment. What is your choice of treatment? I feel that it is dependent on the pathogenesis of the disease. In general, do you treat this condition? Secondly, in Dandy–Walker syndrome we often see the association of agenesis of the corpus callosum. Do you have any idea why there is such frequent association embryologically? We often see a Dandy–Walker syndrome variant, and a third question would be, is this a subtype of the Dandy–Walker cyst?

K. Sato: Treatment of Dandy–Walker syndrome is probably a double shunt; a ventriculo-peritoneal shunt and a cyst–peritoneal shunt connected by a Y-tube, as suggested by Dr. David McLone. I always utilize this mode of treatment, and the results appear to be very good. I think that a ventriculo-peritoneal shunt is sufficient if the aqueduct is open, and I do not believe a double shunt is essential in such cases. In regard to the association of agenesis of the corpus callosum, many say this might be the result of hydrocephalus, but I do not agree. As you know, in cases of hydrocephalus, we see the coexistence of a posterior fossa cyst and agenesis of the corpus collosum, and I do not believe this is a result of the hydrocephalus. The variant is unclear. Dr. Valcovitch classified Dandy–Walker syndrome in accordance with the degree of anterior rotation of the hypoplastic vermis, but it probably depends on how much anterior rotation progresses, and then this finding may be changed. My feeling is that the variant and the classic types are essentially the same.

H. Hoffman: If you see that the aqueduct is open on the MRI, why not just put a shunt in the fourth ventricle?

K. Sato: Theoretically, as you mention, the cyst–peritoneal shunt should be sufficient. However, we usually see both supratentorial and infratentorial hydrocephalus simultaneously. In that case, I do not see any effective reduction in ventricular size after a cyst–peritoneal shunt.

H. Hoffman: I have seen hydrocephalus disappear with a shunt to the fourth ventricle.

K. Sato: I see. I think such cases exist, but after reduction of the pressure of the posterior fossa, the aqueduct often collapses, after which no communication is found between the supra- and infratentorial ventricular systems. In such a case, a double shunt is required, but if, as you said, the posterior shunt is sufficient, the simple, single shunt is best. It therefore depends on the case, but in my cases a double shunt was required in all cases.

W. Chiu: You did not mention anything about the size of the posterior fossa when you classified those multiple cysts or cyst-like lesions. I understand that a Dandy–Walker cyst or arachnoid cyst tends to present a large posterior fossa, yet the so-called Chiari Type IV is a very small posterior fossa, and magnetic resonance imaging (MRI) becomes more valuable and gives much more information. I think the size of the posterior fossa will indicate the diagnostic method.

K. Sato: I think that point is also mentioned by Dr. Valkovitch. A case which can be diagnosed as Dandy–Walker malformation or Dandy–Walker cyst should have a large posterior fossa, and scalloping of the bony structure of the posterior fossa and elevation of the tentorium should exist. If, for some reason, hydrocephalus does not exist, what has happened? This is my question. Also, if the hydrocephalus process exists, then the typical findings of Dandy–Walker syndrome would be produced, but if for some reason hydrocephalus does not occur, then such secondary changes of the posterior fossa could not be produced.

W. Chiu: Most arachnoid cysts present hydrocephalus, yet maybe only 60% of Dandy–Walker cysts present hydrocephalus. I also think we can state that the size of the posterior fossa itself can provide some idea of the disease patients have, or what else may be present in addition to the morphological change in the cerebellum or brainstem structures.

K. Sato: Perhaps Prof. Maurice Choux could explain to us the idea of passes and breakthrough pouch?

M. Choux: My question is a little bit different. Contrary to what we read in many textbooks or papers, we never see significant cases of Dandy–Walker syndrome without hydrocephalus. My question is: Do you ever have examples of children with Dandy–Walker syndrome without hydrocephalus during the first month of life and, secondarily, would your management be different for small babies and older patients, or not?

K. Sato: In the last three cases I described, which were all treated by cyst–peritoneal shunt soon after birth, I did not see any change in the size of the cerebellum and I did not see any clinical improvement in those cases. I would probably prefer to diagnose these three cases as Chiari Type IV, but I am not certain. Some papers state that if you recognize Chiari Type IV in a case, myelomeningoceles should also be present, as well as changes in the posterior fossa. I am just confused. The only classic type of Dandy–Walker syndrome should be referred to as Dandy–Walker cyst or syndrome.

M. Choux: You mentioned cases of Dandy–Walker syndrome with tethered cord. How many cases do you have in your material?

K. Sato: I have nine cases, only one of which is with tethered cord.

M. Choux: It really is uncommon?

K. Sato: Since the introduction of MRI, we have been able to see a variety of associated anomalies in these cases.

Kim: I agree with your double shunt for a Dandy–Walker cyst with hydrocephalus. I should also like to know (if there is) a big difference in pressure, supratentorial pressure and infratentorial pressure, for example, in Dandy–Walker cyst pressure and ventricular pressure. You mentioned the necessity for a connector. In my experience, a pressure difference sometimes exists, and so ventricle is enlarged and the cyst is not decreased in size. What do you think about the pressure difference pertaining to a Dandy–Walker cyst? It is supratentorial or infratentorial? I mean, the double shunt is a separated entity and is better than a Y-connected shunt.

K. Sato: A double shunt should probably be connected because intracystic pressure and intraventricular pressure should be the smae. Otherwise a brain stem shift may be caused by the pressure difference which could also induce aqueductal stenosis. The point of importance is a double shunt with a Y-connector. Also, a small baby with 2 or 3 tubes is not unusual. I think simpler is better, and therefore I just connect both tubes with a Y-connector.

Kim: The cerebral aqueduct is sometimes open and sometimes closed. We do not definitely know in the case of the Dandy–Walker cyst. We conducted a detailed radiological study and found the aqueduct sometimes open and sometimes closed. I have experienced several cases in which a double shunt with a Y-connector was utilized, but there was no decrease in hydrocephalus. That is why I made the comment.

K. Sato: Thank you very much.

K. Takakura: Professor Sato, what is the general long-term outcome for patients?

K. Sato: There are nine patients living with us. It has been reported that Dandy–Walker syndrome cases have a very high mortality rate. I should probably direct this question to Professor Choux or Professor McLone. Probably one-third of patients die quite early, but in my series, as shown here, nine patients still survive.

D. McLone: In all forms of hydrocephalus, the mortality rate is significantly higher than we anticipated. In our institution, it is 20% with shunt in 20 years. This is a significant problem.

One thing impressed me in the Dandy–Walker group. In the true Dandy–Walker syndrome there is a level of mental retardation. In fact, in my experience, a child having true Dandy–Walker syndrome and normal intelligence is quite unusual.

K. Takakura: Thank you very much Professor Sato and all participants. I now close this session.

Studies on Natural Development of Brainstem Function with Asymptomatic Myelomeningocele from School-Age to Adolescence Using Brainstem Auditory Evoked Potentials (BAEPs)

Motoharu Fujii[1], Tadanori Tomita[2], David G. McLone[2], and Koreaki Mori[1]

Summary. We studied the brainstem auditory evoked potentials (BAEPs) in 48 patients with asymptomatic myelomeningocele (MMC) from school age to adolescence, except for patients with symptomatic Chiari II malformation. The brainstem function of asymptomatic patients with MMC from school age to adolescence was still maturing based on the result of this BAEP study. In particular, III–V interpeak latency (IPL), which basically represented intrinsic function in the brainstem, was gradually becoming shorter and closer to the normal range with growth, although each of the wave latencies and IPLs were still much prolonged compared with the normal ranges of BAEPs in the literature. We found that the maturation of the brainstem function was delayed even in asymptomatic patients with MMC according to this study. These data indicated that it was very important to study the BAEPs consecutively on each patient with growth to predict the "delayed-onset" type of symptomatic Chiari II malformation.

Key words. Adolescence, Brainstem auditory evoked potentials (BAEPs), Chiari II malformation, Children, Myelomeningocele

Introduction

Brainstem dysfunction resulting from Chiari II malformation has emerged as the leading cause of death among infants and young children with myelomeningocele (MMC). Most of the early-onset type of symptomatic Chiari II malformation occurs during the first year of life, but some cases of symptomatic Chiari II malformation appear as clinical symptoms in school-aged children, and this should be called "delayed-onset" symptomatic Chiari II malformation, although death is less likely to occur during the period from school age to adolescence. On the other hand, it is very difficult to give an accurate prediction of the onset of clinical symptoms resulting from Chiari II malformation or to prevent clinical deterioration, especially in young children. It is also very difficult to assess the current status of brainstem functioning objectively during clinical deterioration.

The study of brainstem auditory evoked potentials (BAEPs) is thought to be a useful objective indicator to understand the function of brainstem maturation in patients of all ages. Some articles have been published in relation to the use of BAEPs in patients with MMC.

[1] Department of Neurosurgery, Kochi Medical School, Kohasu, Okoh-cho, Nankoku, Kochi 783-8505, Japan

[2] Division of Pediatric Neurosurgery, Children's Memorial Hospital, Chicago, IL, USA

However, there has been very little systematic information about the developmental function in the brainstem of asymptomatic patients with MMC. In this series, we tried to evaluate the natural developmental course of brainstem function in asymptomatic patients with MMC, from school age to adolescence, using the method of BAEPs.

Patients and Methods

We examined 86 BAEPs in 48 patients with clinically asymptomatic MMC from school age to adolescence. There were 16 males (33%) and 32 females (67%), whose ages ranged from 1 year 2 months to 25 years.

In this series, BAEPs were recorded through silver electrodes. Pick-up electrodes were placed on the vertex (Cz), reference electrodes on the earlobe of the stimulated side, and the ground electrode on the forehead (Fz). Electrode impedance was kept below 3 kilo-aum. Mono-aural auditory stimuli consisted of rarefaction at a rate of 10–13 Hz and an intensity of 75–90 dB. A minimum of 1.032 responses were averaged. At least two trials were evaluated, and responses were superimposed to demonstrate any consistency. Differential input was filtered for a bandpass of 50 Hz to 3 kHz. Masking was 45 dB. Analysis time was 10 ms. The instruments used to measure BAEPs in this series were the Neuropack 4 or 4-mini by Nihon Koden Co., Tokyo. All IPLs were plotted on graphs.

Results

Each interpeak latency (IPL) tended to become gradually shorter with age, but most of them were still prolonged compared with normal ranges in other series of BAEP studies in the literature (Figs. 1 and 2). From the results in this series, brainstem function in asymptomatic patients with MMC still seemed to be maldeveloped and delayed even in the period from school age to adoles cence. In particular, the III–V IPL, which represents intrinsic function in the brainstem, was gradually maturing and coming closer to the normal range of BAEPs with age (Figs. 3 and 4). The BAEP graphs in this series indicate a separation into two age

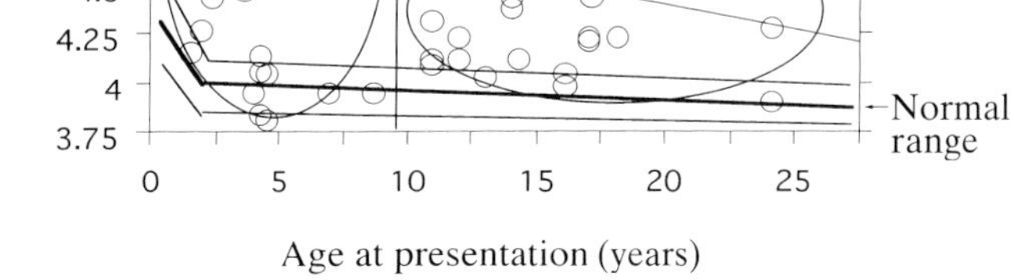

FIG. 1. I–V interpeak latencies (IPLs) in brainstem auditory evoked potentials (BAEPs) in asymptomatic patients with myelomeningocele (MMC) from school age to adolescence with right-side ear stimuli. $Y = 4.89 - 0.025X$; $R^2 = 0.098$

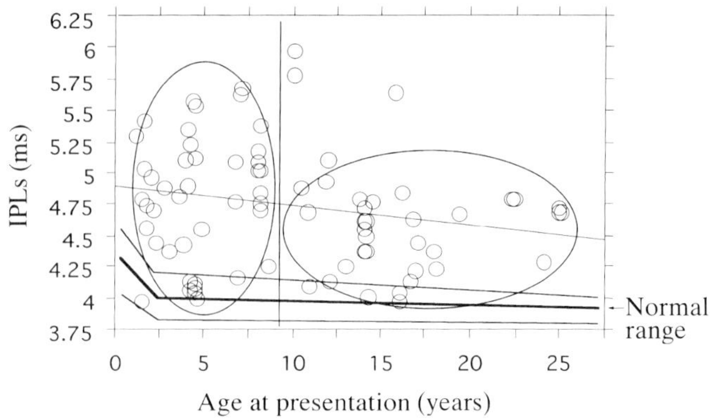

FIG. 2. I–V IPLs in BAEPs in the same patients with left-side ear stimuli. $Y = 4.893 - 0.016X$; $R^2 = 0.045$

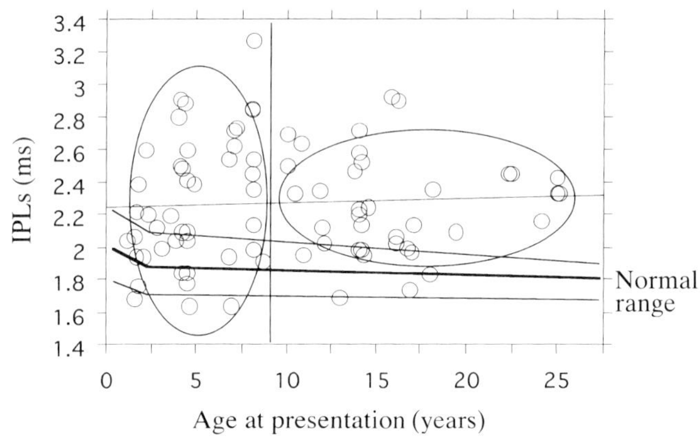

FIG. 3. III–V IPLs in BAEPs in the same patients with right-side ear stimuli. $Y = 2.252 - 0.002X$; $R^2 = 0.001$

groups, one of children less than 10 years old, and the another of children more than 10 years old. Among the patients younger than 10 years old, the plotted data tend to be much more scattered than the data of patients over 10 years old. These findings suggested that the natural developmental course of brainstem function might be much more flexible in children less than 10 years old than in children more than 10 years old among patients with MMC.

Discussions

Some abnormalities in BAEPs have already been reported in patients with MMC in the period from young childhood to adolescence [1, 6–9, 11]. Holliday et al. [5] reported that there were abnormalities in 50–86% of BAEPs in children with MMC. Recordings of BAEPs in patients with MMC, and particularly those with the asymptomatic status of Chiari II malformation, have been studied in "older" children [6, 7, 9, 11]. However, there have been few on-going

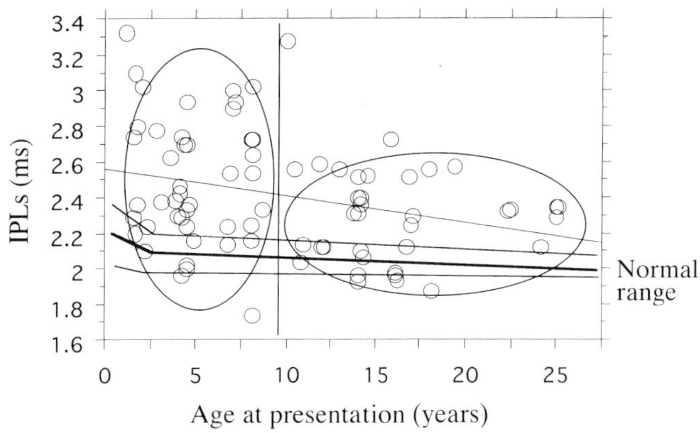

FIG. 4. III–V IPLs in BAEPs in the same patients with left-side ear stimuli. $Y = 2.563 - 0.015X$; $R^2 = 0.078$

studies of BAEPs during growth, particularly in asymptomatic patients with MMC from school age to adolescence. Therefore, in this series, we tried to evaluate the natural developmental course of brainstem function in asymptomatic patients with MMC in this period, using the method of BAEPs.

From the results in this series, almost all parameters of IPLs in these patients showed delayed maturational changes compared with normal maturational changes reported in the literature. These findings suggested that even the natural maturation of intrinsic brainstem function in patients in this age range was delayed compared with that of normal subjects.

The report by Docherty et al. [2] showed some abnormal BAEPs in clinically asymptomatic patients with Chiari II malformation, although these authors concluded that the usefulness of BAEPs for predicting the subsequent development of symptomatic Chiari II malformation was questionable. However, as we have already reported elsewhere [3, 4, 10, 12], we believe that recordings of BAEPs are of value in predicting the development of the "early-onset" type of symptomatic Chiari II malformation among patients with these anomalies. We should also recognize the value of the study of BAEPs in increasing our understanding of how the present status of brainstem functioning in individual patients with these anomalies can predict the "delayed-onset" type of Chiari II malformation [13]. We should recognize deviations from the maturational baseline in brainstem function shown by BAEP recordings from patients with asymptomatic MMC from school age to adolescence, in whom development is delayed.

Another finding from this series is that the developmental course of brainstem function in patients with MMC tended to vary considerably between patients during their growth. However, in patients over 10 years old, the developmental course of brainstem function had a tendency to become close to the normal range of BAEP studies, although brainstem function was still undeveloped compared with that of normal subjects. Consequently, according to these results, we should consider different types of natural developmental course of brainstem function before and after about 10 years old. Therefore, we should monitor patients with MMC more carefully before they are 10 years old than after 10 years old in attempts to predict the "delayed-onset" type of symptomatic Chiari II malformation.

In conclusion, the first thing we would like to emphasize is that we should recognize the differences in maturational baseline between MMC patients and normal subjects in relation to brainstem function indicated by BAEP recordings in the period from school age to adolescence. Secondly, we believe we should pay great attention to patients around 10 years of age, although this point has not previously been discussed in any reports of BAEP studies. This study has shown the significance of the "delayed-onset" type of symptomatic Chiari II malformation, and in delayed-onset-type symptomatic cases, we should carefully follow up all patients, particularly around 10 years of age. (Unfortunately, these data have not yet been analyzed mathematically.) Finally, we strongly reassert that it is extremely important to know the developmental course of each IPL in BAEPs in asymptomatic patients with MMC, from school age to adolescence, to allow a prediction of the subsequent brainstem dysfunction, the so-called "delayed-onset" type, that can result from Chiari II malformation. If it were possible to confirm that maturational changes in the IPLs of BAEPs in patients with asymptomatic MMC differ according to the severity of the clinical manifestation of symptomatic Chiari II malformation, subsequent recordings of BAEPs could aid in predicting the development of symptomatic Chiari II malformation, and might be a valuable indicator of prognosis with growth.

References

1. Barnet AB, Weiss IP, Shaer C (1993) Evoked potentials in infant brainstem syndrome associated with Arnold–Chiari malformation. Dev Med Child Neurol 35:42–48
2. Docherty TB, Herbaut AG, Sedgwick EM (1987) Brainstem auditory evoked potential abnormalities in myelomeningocele in the older child. J Neurol Neurosurg Psychiatr 50:1318–1322
3. Fujii M, Tomita T, McLone DG, Grant JA, Mori K (1996) Natural course of brainstem auditory evoked potentials in infants less than 6 months old with asymptomatic meningomyelocele. Pediatr Neurosurg 25:227–232
4. Fujii M, Tomita T, McLone DG, Grant JA, Stack CV, Mori K (1997) Developmental normomaturation of brainstem auditory evoked potentials in children with asymptomatic meningomyelocele during the first year of life. Child's Nerv Syst 13:147–153
5. Holliday PO, Pillsbury D, Kelly DL Jr, Dillard R (1985) Brainstem auditory evoked potentials in Arnold–Chiari malformation: possible prognostic value and changes with surgical decompression. Neurosurgery 16:48–53
6. Lutschg J, Meyer E, Jeanneret-Iseli C (1985) Brainstem auditory evoked potentials in meningomyelocele. Neuropediatrics 16:202–204
7. Mori K, Nishimura T (1995) Electrophysiological studies on brainstem function in patients with myelomeningocele. Pediatr Neurosurg 22:120–131
8. Mori K, Uchida Y, Nishimura T, Eghwrudjakpor P (1988) Brainstem auditory evoked potentials in Chiari II malformation. Child's Nerv Syst 4:154–157
9. Nishimura T, Mori K, Uchida Y, Ohira T, Tamura K (1991) Brain stem auditory evoked potentials in myelomeningocele: natural history of Chiari II malformations. Child's Nerv Syst 7:316–326
10. Nishimura T, Mori K, Sada Y, Fujii M (1995) Apneic spells in a patient with myelomeningocele without Chiari II malformation. Neurol Med Chir (Tokyo) 35:876–881
11. Stone JL, Bouffard A, Morris R (1983) Clinical and electrophysiological recovery in Arnold–Chiari malformation. Surg Neurol 20:313–317
12. Taylor MJ, Boor R, Keenan NK, Rutka JT, Drake JM (1996) Brainstem auditory and visual evoked potentials in infants with myelomeningocele. Brain Dev 18:99–104
13. Worley G, Erwin CW, Schuster JM, Park Y, Boyko OB, Griebel ML, Weidman ER, Radtke RA, Oakes WJ (1994) BAEPs in infants with myelomeningocele and later development of Chiari II malformation-related brainstem dysfunction. Dev Med Child Neurol 36:707–715

Respiratory Disturbance in Type II Chiari Malformation

Yutaka Otsubo[1], Hiroshi Ito[1], and Ken'nichi Sekido[2]

Summary. We report on four patients who had Chiari malformation associated with spina bifida and who died of respiratory disturbance, and discuss their pathogenesis. Of the four patients, two died within 1 year after birth. They still showed severe Chiari malformation on magnetic resonance imaging (MRI) after treatment of the myelomeningocele and hydrocephalus. One case died from the absence of spontaneous respiration, and the other died of recurrent pneumonia of resistant bacteria based on tracheomalacia and ataxic respiration. The other two patients died several years after untethering of the myelomeningocele and ventriculo-peritoneal shunting (V-P shunt). When shunt malfunction was accompanied by sudden development of brainstem disorder, the patients died. The pathogenesis in these two cases was considered to be suddenly increased intracranial pressure altering the compensatory conformation of the brainstem and Chiari malformation, which caused the sudden brainstem disorder.

Key words. Chiari malformation, Respiratory disturbance, V–P shunt

Introduction

The factor of greatest importance threatening the life of a patient with myelomeningocele is brainstem disorder, chiefly characterized by respiratory disturbance evoked in association with Chiari malformation [1, 2, 4, 5]. Since the advent of magnetic resonance imaging (MRI), we have experienced four fatal cases of myelomeningocele with Chiari malformation after respiratory disturbance. Actually, these cases account for only a small percentage of our all cases, but apart from one case of death due to ventriculitis from shunt infection, there has been no other death from myelomeningocele due to any other causes.

We report and discuss the pathogenesis of death due to respiratory disturbance with myelomeningocele, hydrocephalus, and Chiari malformation in these four cases.

Case 1

The patient was a male infant who had been delivered spontaneously after a 40-week gestation to healthy parents.

[1] Department of Neurosurgery, Tokyo Medical University Hospital, 6-7-1 Nishi-shinjuku, Shinjuku-ku, Tokyo 160, Japan
[2] Department of Neurosurgery, Kanagawa Children's Medical Center, Yokohama, Japan

He had thoracolumbar myelomeningocele. As there was no systemically complicating anomaly despite the spinal cord lesion being at a high level, a closure and untethering of the myelomeningocele was performed 9h after birth. Two days postoperatively, an increase in head circumference and stridor and attacks of apnea developed; the patient underwent ventriculo-peritoneal (V-P) shunt on the 12th day. In response to the V-P shunt, the stridor disappeared for a time, but the apnea attacks continued to occur. Decompression of the posterior fossa and arachnoidal adhesiotomy was performed 2 months later, but no clear improvement in the apnea attacks followed. The patient was placed on assisted ventilation under tracheotomy with nasogastric tube feeding, but he developed tracheomalacia and repeatedly had pneumonia. He died at 9 months.

Case 2

The patient was a male infant with lumbar myeloschisis with marked kyphosis (Fig. 1). Spontaneous movement of the extremities was weak, and spontaneous respiration was occasionally ataxic. A closure and untethering was performed at 6h after birth. MRI was carried out the next day. It revealed an extremely small and shallow posterior fossa with a deformity of the brainstem (Fig. 2). With mechanical ventilation, the patient's spontaneous breathing gradually became weaker and bradyarrhythmia appeared. The infant died on the 14th day. Autopsy revealed that the inferior end of the cerebellar tonsil was herniated down to the upper thoracic level, and the brainstem was markedly compressed and showed hemorrhagic foci on the medulla oblongata.

Case 3

The patient was a female infant with lumbosacral myelomeningocele. Closure and untethering was performed 8h after birth. Postoperatively, an increase in head circumference, pseudomeningocele, stridor, and apnea attacks appeared. V-P shunt was performed on the 7th day. Chiari malformation was evident on MRI (Fig. 3). The stridor and apnea attacks disappeared after the shunting, and the patient was discharged home. The patient had an uncom-

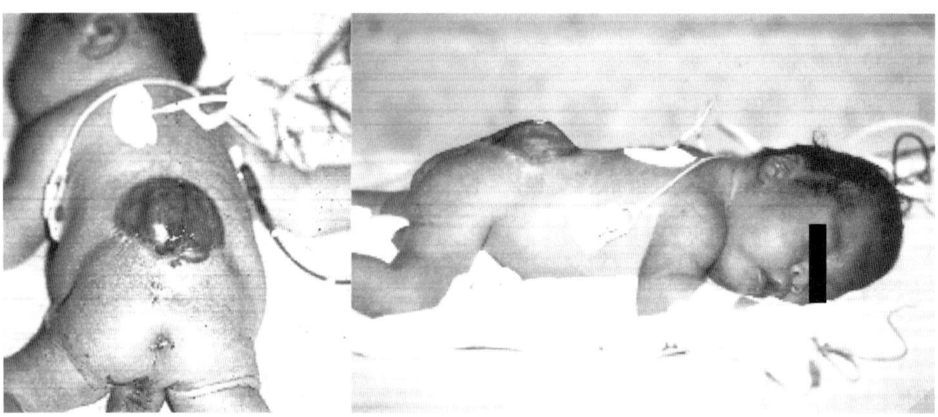

Fig. 1. Case 2. Lumbar myeloschisis with marked kyphosis

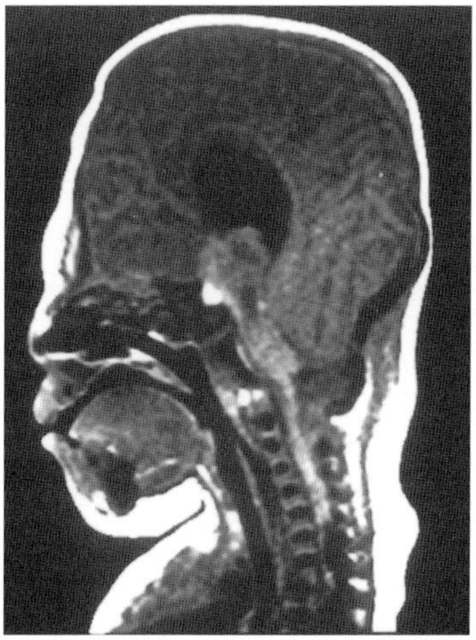

FIG. 2. Magnetic resonance image (MRI) of case 2 at 2 days after birth

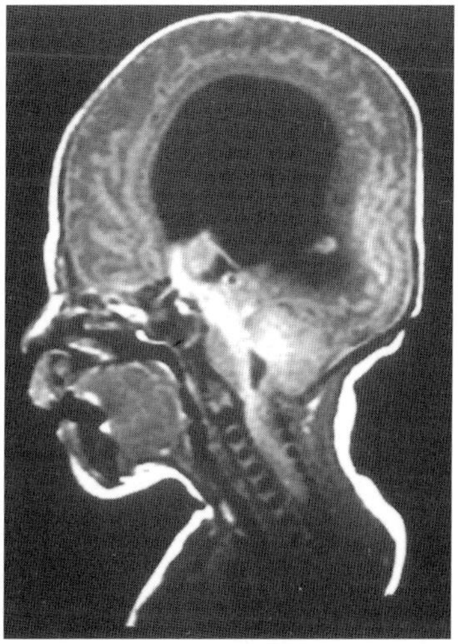

FIG. 3. MRI of case 3 at 6 days after birth

plicated course thereafter. Figure 4 showed a CT scan at the age of 4 years, when she was capable of walking by herself with the aid of short lower limb braces. She practiced urinary autocatheterism, and her IQ was 98. When she was 4 years and 10 months, she developed a headache and vomiting that lasted for 2 days. Subsequently posterior cervical pain and opisthotonous posture developed. A diagnosis of shunt malfunction was made at another hospital. While in the ambulance on the way to our hospital, she suddenly developed apnea with bradycardia. Cardiac arrest followed, and she died.

Case 4

The patient was a female infant with sacral myelomeningocele. Closure and untethering was performed 12h after birth. Postoperatively, stridor and seizure-like activity appeared with

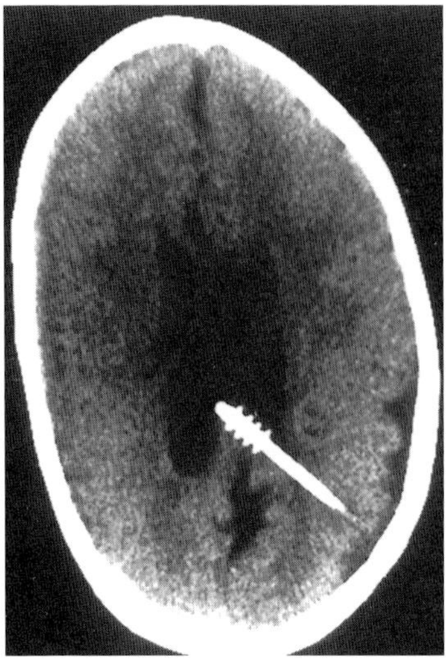

FIG. 4. Computed tomography (CT) scan of case 3 at the age of 4 years

hydrocephalus; V-P shunt was performed on the 8th postnatal day. After the shunting, respiratory disturbance disappeared and she took food well. She was therefore discharged home. At the age of 12 months, she was able to walk by herself, and followed an uneventful course. When she was 2 years and 4 months old, she had anorexia and vomiting over a few days, and she became sleepy. She was examined at a nearby clinic and then transferred to our hospital. During shuntgraphy because of a suspicion of shunt malfunction, apnea and bradyarrhythmia developed suddenly and she died. The shuntgraphy demonstrated occlusion of the shunt tube on the ventricular side.

Discussion

Our current protocol for the treatment of myelomeningocele is shown in Fig. 5. As can be seen, closure and untethering is undertaken as early as practicable. The patient undergoes CSF shunting where symptoms of intracranial hypertension or brainstem symptoms develop with ventriculomegaly on computed tomography (CT). Patients with a disappearance of respiratory disturbance after shunting are discharged home, with regular attendance at other departments. Posterior fossa decompression is considered in patients with residual symptoms of respiratory disturbances even after shunting. The cases presented here can be divided into two types (Fig. 6). In the first type, the symptoms of Chiari malformation are already severe at birth. These symptoms can not be improved despite CSF shunting and posterior fossa decompression. Death results from respiratory disturbance or a complicating infection. This type of patient may have an embryological abnormality or immaturity of the brainstem and cerebellum, so they have a surgically irreversible factor in terms of current treatment. We have had a few other cases with a clinical course of tracheomalacia or prolonged expiratory apnea with cyanosis, thus requiring tracheotomy and long-term respiratory management.

The other type of case consists of those cases where respiratory disturbance developed following closure and untethering, but disappeared in response to V-P shunting. After a long period, when shunt malfunction suddenly occurred, the symptoms of Chiari malformation

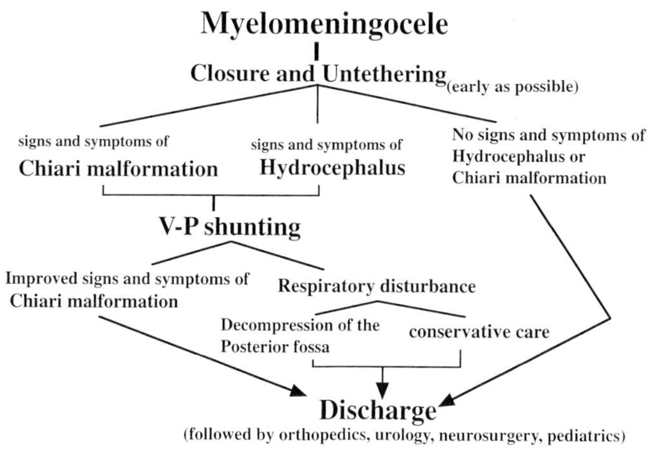

FIG. 5. Our current protocol for myelomeningocele

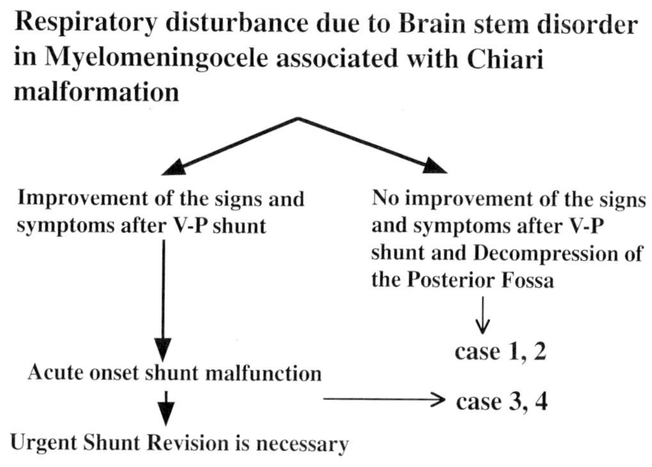

FIG. 6. Schematic presentation of our cases

which had been compensated for by shunting became progressively manifest. That is, a rapidly increasing intracranial pressure converges as a pressure directed downward to the small posterior fossa through the widely opening tentorial incisula. This converging pressure may give rise to brainstem ischemia or hemorrhage [3]. Tomita and McLone [6] reported three cases of acute respiratory arrest in myelomeningocele which occurred with shunt malfunction. While their cases were saved by appropriate treatment, situations requiring time for shunt revision, or the development of complicating bradycardia, must be potentially fatal.

The affect on the brainstem of decompression of the posterior fossa, including arachnoid adhesiotomy and resection of abnormal tissues, still varies case by case, and has not necessarily produced a clearly favorable outcome in all cases treated. However, decompression of the posterior fossa may be effective in assuaging the acute development of brainstem disorder in cases of a rapid increase in intracranial pressure related to chance shunt malfunction occurring several years later. Should this hold, we may have to be more positive in undertaking this surgical approach.

Conclusions

1. Patients with fatal respiratory disturbance in type II Chiari malformation can be divided into two types.
2. In the first type, the symptoms of Chiari malformation are already intractable in the postnatal period.
3. The other type is seen after a long period. When a rapid increase in intracranial pressure develops, symptoms of Chiari malformation, which have been compensated for by V-P shunt, become progressively manifest.

References

1. Cochrane DD, Adderley R, White CP, Norman M, Steinbok P (1990) Apnea in patients with myelomeningocele. Pediatr Neurosurg 16:232–239
2. Holinger PC, Holinger LD, Reichert TJ, Holinger PH (1978) Respiratory obstruction and apnea in infants with bilateral abductor vocal cord paralysis, meningomyelocele, hydrocephalus, and Arnold-Chiari malformation. J Pediatr 92:368–373
3. Ito H, Kawakami H, Maruyama H, Miwa T (1982) Clinicopathological considerations of late death in cases of treated congenital hydrocephalus. Neurol Med Chir (Tokyo) 22:51–58
4. Oren J, Kelly DH, Todres ID, Shannon DC (1986) Respiratory complications in patients with myelodysplasia and Arnold-Chiari malformation. Am J Dis Child 140:221–224
5. Papasozomenos S, Roessmann U (1981) Respiratory distress and Arnold-Chiari malformation. Neurology 31:97–100
6. Tomita T, McLone DG (1983) Acute respiratory arrest. A complication of malformation of the shunt in children with myelomeningocele and Arnold-Chiari malformation. Am J Dis Child 137:142–144

Hydrocephalus Associated with Spina Bifida: Specific Pathophysiology and Therapeutic Problems

Shizuo Oi

Summary. The critical period for hydrocephalus associated with spina bifida ranges widely from the beginning of the fetal period to the postnatal stages, as in the other form of congenital hydrocephalus. In the author's experience, the earliest diagnosis of fetal hydrocephalus in spina bifida was made at 13 weeks gestational age in 61 cases. The specific forms of hydrocephalus which occur in spina bifida include: progressive/overt hydrocephalus in the fetus; a postshunt isolated cerebrospinal fluid (CSF) compartment in infantile hydrocephalus; slit ventricle syndrome in the late stage of shunted hydrocephalus; hydromyelic hydrocephalus; holoneural canal dilatation (HNCD) and its unique isolation of the CSF compartment (i.e., isolated central canal dilatation (ICCD) or isolated rhombencephalic ventricle (IRV); long-standing overt ventriculomegaly in the adult (LOVA). The pathophysiology of hydrocephalus is unique, and therapeutic regimes differ. They require the delicate shunt CSF flow regulation applicable to characteristic intracranial pressure (ICP) dynamics and/or superb neuroendoscopic technique to normalize the CSF circulation.

Introduction

The management of hydrocephalus is a major part of the total care of spina bifida patients. The characteristics of the pathophysiology of hydrocephalus associated with spina bifida are varied, and differ from the fetal period to adulthood.

Table 1 [15] summarizes the major critical disorders relating to the central nervous system (CNS), along with the development and aging of spina bifida patients. Based on the usual patterns in each age group, the pathophysiology of hydrocephalus is characterized along with its chronological changes. The treatment modalities are also complex and differ from one to the other. These include fetal surgery, shunt selection in the postnatal chronological changes of neonatal/infantile hydrocephalus, treatment for slit ventricle syndrome/isolated compartments in long-standing shunt-dependent hydrocephalus, and long-standing overt ventriculomegaly in adult (LOVA)/arrested/slowly progressive hydrocephalus in adulthood.

Department of Neurosurgery, Tokai University, School of Medicine, Isehara-City, Kanagawa 259-11, Japan

TABLE 1. Chronological aspects of neurological problems in the management of patients with spina bifida in different periods of their lives [15]

I.	Fetal period	Intrauterine diagnosis, prenatal decision making
II.	Neonatal period	Morphological/pathophysiological evaluation and treatments for spina bifida and hydrocephalus
III.	Infancy	Treatment for symptomatic Chiari malformation and management of hydrocephalus
IV.	Pre-school/school-age period	Evaluation/treatment for tethered cord syndrome and syringomyelia, and management of hydrocephalus
V.	Adolescence/adulthood	Progression of spinal neuro-deficits, psychological/psychiatric problems, management for hydrocephalus: LOVA/delicate shunt dependence, Medico-social problems

This chapter deals with these specific areas of pathophysiology and the therapeutic problems encountered in individual clinical examples of hydrocephalus associated with spina bifida.

Spina Bifida in the Fetus and the Development of Hydrocephalus during Fetal Life

Prenatal Diagnosis in Utero [1, 11–13, 16]

The morphology of the fetal brain and spinal cord may be reliably evaluated by recently developed diagnostic imaging, including real-time ultrasonography and magnetic resonance imaging (MRI). Ultrasonography was the first imaging technique used to screen or regularly monitor fetal CNS malformation. The biparietal diameter (BPD) and the size of the lateral ventricle are repeatedly evaluated, and if these are found to be abnormal, the brain morphology is further analyzed. In my studies, MRI was used to evaluate fetal brain and spinal cord morphology, and recently the heavily T_2-weighted spin-echo sequence with reversal imaging (TR 4300 ms, TE 130 ms) has been used.

The quality of ultrasonography is adequate to delineate the severity of ventriculomegaly and the ventricular configuration, especially with continuous morphological detection by the real-time cine-mode technique. Magnetic resonance imaging is also useful for investigating underlying disease in dysgenetic fetal hydrocephalus and secondary hydrocephalus. In fetuses with spina bifida aperta (myeloschisis), heavily T_2-weighted images demonstrate the cystic change in the primary lesion (myeloschisis), deformed legs and feet, Chiari malformation, and the specific configuration of ventricular dilatation. Magnetic resonance imaging may be superior to ultrasonography in demonstrating the CNS structures in one slice, such as a midline sagittal slice of the entire brain and spinal cord, whereas ultrasonography is preferable for delineating these structures on continuous images in real time. For this reason, the motion of the fetus is not a practical problem in ultrasonography, but it is necessary to piece together separate findings to demonstrate anatomical relationships or the overall state of the CNS. It is particularly useful to perform such imaging in patients with midline anomalies associated with hydrocephalus, such as spina bifida with Chiari malformation. Our method of using heavily T_2-weighted imaging with a superconducting magnet is extremely useful both technically and practically. The total imaging time less than 90 s, and sedation of the fetus is not necessary.

Perspective Classification and the Development of Hydrocephalus in a Fetus with Spina Bifida (Table 2) [16]

In our recent publications, a new classification of congenital and infantile hydrocephalus was proposed in the hope of establishing a correlation with the expected prognosis, namely, "Perspective classification of congenital and infantile hydrocephalus" (PCCH). This classification is based on the multifactorial aspects affecting the prognosis of congenital hydrocephalus. Three major concepts are included: clinico-embryological stage (Stages I–V); clinico-pathological type (Type P, primary; Type D, dysgenetic; Type S, secondary); clinico-chronological category (Category F, fetal; Category N, neonatal; Category I, infantile).

This newly proposed classification may be valuable in discussions of the controversial problems involved in prenatal/postnatal therapeutic management of hydrocephalus, and of patients who have spina bifida as well, offering a more clearly identified hydrocephalic state together with the anticipated postnatal outcome.

The clinico-embryological stages are listed below.

Stage I occurs between 8 and 21 weeks of gestation, which is the period of legal permissible termination of pregnancy in Japan. Cell proliferation is the main process in neuronal maturation.

Stage II extends from 22 to 31 weeks of gestation, the period of intrauterine preservation of the fetus before pulmonary maturation is completed. Cell differentiation and migration are the main processes in neuronal maturation.

Stage III extends from 32 to 40 weeks of gestation, a period of possible premature/preterm neonatal hydrocephalus if delivery occurs. Axonal maturation is the main process in neuronal maturation.

Stage IV occurs between 0 and 4 weeks postnatal age, the period of neonatal hydrocephalus. Dendritic maturation is the main process in neuronal maturation.

Stage V extends from 5 to 50 weeks postnatal age, the period of infantile hydrocephalus. Myelination is the main process in neuronal maturation.

In our experience of 61 fetuses with hydrocephalus, there were 19 cases (31.1%) of primary, 34 cases (55.7%) of dysgenetic, and eight cases (13.1%) of secondary hydrocephalus. Hydrocephalus was diagnosed in two fetuses (dysgenetic) at PCCH Stage I, in 28 fetuses (nine

Table 2. Postnatal outcome in patients with fetal hydrocephalus according to PCCH stage and type[a] [16]

	Outcome (postnatal DQ/IQ) by clinico-embryological stage			
Type of hydrocephalus	I	II	III	Total
Primary	–	67.5 (35–100)	76.6 (20–132)	74.2 (20–132)
Dysgenetic	20	49.5 (20–114)	59.4 (20–120)	52.4 (20–120)
With spina bifida aperta (myeloschisis)	–	45.0 (20–80)[b]	81.3 (60–120)[b]	63.1 (20–120)
Secondary	–	70, 15, 20	5, 20	26 (5–70)

[a] Individual DQ/IQ values are given for patients whose secondary hydrocephalus was diagnosed in Stages II or III. Other values in the table reflect the mean DQ/IQ values with ranges provided parenthetically. –, not applicable.

[b] Postnatal outcome in patients with myeloschisis at Stage II was significantly poorer than that of patients with myeloschisis at Stage III ($P < 0.1$).

with primary, 16 with dysgenetic, and three with secondary hydrocephalus) at Stage II, and in 31 fetuses (10 with primary, 16 with dysgenetic, and five with secondary hydrocephalus) at Stage III. Among the 34 fetuses with dysgenetic hydrocephalus, only two were found to show hydrocephalus at PCCH Stage I; 16 cases exhibited hydrocephalus at Stages II or III. There were 14 fetuses with spina bifida. Even within the category of dysgenetic hydrocephalus, the time of onset of fetal hydrocephalus differed from case to case. The time of intrauterine diagnosis of fetal hydrocephalus made by ultrasonography ranged from 17 to 38 weeks (mean 30.7 weeks) in 14 cases of spina bifida aperta (myeloschisis). Regarding the postnatal outcomes of these fetuses with hydrocephalus, among patients who had exhibited dysgenetic hydrocephalus at PCCH Stages I or II, only one had an acceptable postnatal outcome. The average of intelligence quotient (IQ) or development quotient (DQ) in the subtypes of dysgenetic hydrocephalus varied, ranging from 20 to 120 (mean 63.1) in spina bifida aperta (myeloschisis). The IQ or DQ of the patients in whom myeloschisis was diagnosed at PCCH Stage III (range 60–120, mean 81.3) was significantly higher than that of the patients whose myeloschisis was diagnosed at Stage II (range 20–80, mean 45.0. The analysis revealed that the only significant factor affecting the mean) ($P < 0.1$). This study revealed that the only significant factor affecting outcome was the length of the fetal period after the diagnosis of hydrocephalus. These data may support the concept that the results of an on-going hydrocephalic state may become irreversible during the fetal period.

Shunt-Dependent Hydrocephalus and CSF Overdrainage Syndrome

Immediately after, or sometimes at the same time as, repair of myeloschisis in newborn patients with spina bifida operta, they undergo ventriculo-peritoneal (V–P) shunt. The goal of this treatment is to reach the status of "shunt-dependent arrested hydrocephalus". However, it has recently been recognized that overdrainage of cerebrospinal fluid (CSF) is often associated with some harmful, and occasionally life-threatening, events for children with shunted hydrocephalus. We have previously analyzed the pathophysiology of this clinical entity in 164 patients with pediatric hydrocephalus treated with ventriculo-peritoneal shunts. In some cases, the overdrainage was felt to be a causative factor of postshunt isolated ventricles, such as isolated IV ventricle and isolated unilateral hydrocephalus, as well as being a causative factor in a severe form of slit-ventricle syndrome [2–9, 14]. Then various forms of ventricular system isolation may develop, along with overdrainage of CSF via the shunt. Functional occlusion of the foramen of Monro may result in progressive unilateral dilatation of the lateral ventricle (Type I = isolated unilateral hydrocephalus (IUH)). If the aqueduct of Sylvius is involved in cases with obstruction of the fourth ventricular outlets to the cistern, isolation and expansion of the fourth ventricle will occur (Type II = isolated fourth ventricle (IFV)). In more advanced cases, dilatation of both the fourth ventricle and the central canal of the spinal cord can develop, forming an expanded primary rhombencephalic ventricle including the metencephalon and myelencephalon (Type III = isolated rhombencephalic ventricle (IRCV)). However, this type may involve only the central canal of the spinal cord without dilating the fourth ventricle (Type IV = isolated central canal dilatation (ICCD)) [14].

In a previous publication (Table 3), we analyzed the clinical features and pathophysiology of specific forms of hydromyelia together with the chronological changes of associated hydrocephalus [14]. Nine patients were studied; all had hydromyelia with varying degrees of associated hydrocephalus. Clinically applicable classification systems were used to evaluate the progression of the hydrocephalus (Stages I–IV) and to define the compartment isolated after

Table 3. Clinical summary of nine patients with hydromyelia associated with hydrocephalus[a] [14]

Case No.	Sex, age (yrs)	Underlying conditions	Stage of Hydrocephalus	Initial shunt (age at placement)	Signs and symptoms suggestive of hydromyelia (age, yrs)	Level of Hydromyelia	Postshunt compartment		Outcome (follow-up period)	
							Type	Treatment	Syrinx size	Symptoms
Cases not associated with Chiari malformation										
1	M, 17	None	IV	VP (14 yrs)	Scoliosis (8), muscle atrophy (13), sensory dissociation/UE weakness (17)	C6–T1	–	VP revision	Decreased (1 yr)	All improved
2	M, 10	Premature birth	I	VP (1 mo) VA (10 yrs)	Scoliosis (3), UE weakness (7)	C1–6	III	Fourth VP shunt	Collapsed (3 mos)	All improved
3	F, 4	Myeloschisis	I	VP (3 days), fourth VP (4 yrs)	Scoliosis (4), progressive quadriparesis/sensory dissociation (4)	Holocord	III	Fourth VP revision	Collapsed (1 mo)	All improved
4	F, 56	None	IV	VP (56 yrs)	Quadriparesis (56)	C2–7	–	–	Collapsed (1 mo)	Improved
Cases associated with Chiari malformation										
5	M, 6	Myeloschisis, Chiari Type II	IV → I	VP (4 mos)	Unclear	Medulla–C4	IV	VP revision	Unchanged (1 mo)	Unclear
6	M, 7	Myeloschisis, Chiari Type II	I	VP (2 wks)	None	Medulla–C2	IV	None	Unchanged (2 wks)	None
7	M, 6	Myeloschisis, Chiari Type II	I → IV	VP (4 mos)	Progressive quadriparesis (1)	C2–4	IV	VP revision (decompression pending)	Unchanged (1 mo)	Unchanged
8	F, 1	Myeloschisis, Chiari Type II	I	VP (1 mo)	Unclear	C3–5	IV	VP revision	Unchanged (1 mo)	Unclear
9	F, 23	Trauma, Chiari Type I	II	VP (9 yrs)	Progressive quadriparesis (21)	C2–T9	IV	Posterior fossa decompression	Decreased (1 yr)	Improved

[a]Classifications of stages of hydrocephalus and types of postshunt compartment are described in the text. VP, ventriculoperitoneal; VA, ventriculoatrial; UE, upper extremity.

shunting in the previously communicating cerebral ventricles (Types I–IV). Four patients had Stage IV disease (holoneural canal dilatation), one had Stage II and four had Stage I disease (holoneural canal dilatation), and one had Stage II and four had Stage I disease (both Stages I and II with supratentorial hydrocephalus). All patients were initially treated by ventriculo-peritoneal shunting at an average age of 9.9 years. Five patients had progressive spinal symptoms before or after treatment of their hydrocephalus. Two patients had Type III isolation (an isolated rhombencephalic ventricle) with a functioning ventricular shunt; ventriculography confirmed a communication between the fourth ventricle and the hydromyelia, and both patients improved after placement of a shunt in the fourth ventricle. The remaining patients had Type IV isolation (isolated central canal dilatation) with a functioning ventricular shunt [14].

Clinical Problems and Management of Hydrocephalus in Adulthood

Clinical problems in the management of spina bifida patients differ according to age (Table 4). However, little has been said about the specific problems of spina bifida patients in adulthood. In our previous publication, a series of follow-up cases of spina bifida, of both open and occult forms, was analyzed, with the main focus being on chronological changes in neurological condition as assessed using the spina bifida neurological scale (SBNS) [10]. In our series of 141 cases of spina bifida, 18 patients (13.5%) were over 16 years of age. These included nine cases each of spina bifida aperta (myeloschisis) and spina bifida occulta (spinal lipoma). The age range was from 16 to 47 years (mean 23.5 years) in the former group and from 16 to 57 years (mean 29.2 years) in the latter group. During the long-term follow-up with quantitative analysis of the spinal neurological changes using the SBNS, the final outcomes appeared very grave. Except for one case in each group—one Grade III in the spina bifida aperta group and one Grade II in the spina bifida occulta group—all patients over the age of 27 years were classed as having Grade IV disease. There were two patients with spina bifida aperta in whom postoperative paraplegia appeared after delayed radical repair (at the ages of 3 years and 18 years) and three patients with spina bifida occulta in whom obvious neurological deterioration was observed, with ongoing paraparesis at the spinal level or late onset of sexual problems. The other group included two patients with spinal lipoma in whom late neurological deterioration was observed and who were obliged to undergo a second operation in spite of aggressive early procedures performed during infancy. Among the patients with spina bifida aperta, two had marked ventriculomegaly as a form of long-standing overt ventriculomegaly in the adult (LOVA). After the CSF shunt procedure, both these patients had problems with delicate shunt dependence and requested fine shunt flow regulation. Two patients in this group also suffered from severe depression. These clinical features are typical of LOVA. The common underlying condition in LOVA in aqueductal stenosis may be congenital, but this study suggests that it could be one of the specific forms of hydrocephalus associated with spina bifida aperta (myeloschisis) [10].

Conclusion

The analysis in this study shows that the major neurological problems in spina bifida aperta patients in adulthood are mainly related to management of the hydrocephalus. The pathophysiology of hydrocephalus changes along with the patient's development and age. The

TABLE 4. Clinical features, score/grade on SBNS, specific neurological problems and medico-social problems in patients with spina bifida aperta (myeloschisis) in adolescence and adulthood (age range 16–47 years, mean 23.3 years) [15]

Case No.	Age (years)	Sex	Age at operation/ reoperation	Spina bifida neurological scale Total	M	R	BB	Grade	Specific neurological problem	Medico-social problem
1	47	F	18 years	3	1	1	1	IV	Postoperative paraplegia	–
2	30	M	3 years	5	3	1	1	III	Postoperative paraplegia	–
3	27	M	5 months	4	2	1	1	IV	LOVA: occult (not shunted)	Depression, severe
4	20	F	0 days	5	3	1	1	III	–	–
5	18	F	4 days	6	4	1	1	III	–	–
6	18	M	3 days	7	4	2	1	III	–	Convulsions at school
7	17	F	0 days	4	2	1	1	IV	LOVA: delicate shunt dependency	Depression, severe
8	17	M	0 days/17 years	7	5	1	1	III	–	–
9	16	F	2 days			?		III	LOVA: delicate shunt dependency	IQ change (108 → 81)

M, motor (1–6); R, reflex (1–4); BB, bladder and bowel (1–5); LOVA, long-standing overt ventriculomegaly in adult (Oi et al, 1996).

underlying physiological changes are based on the hydrodynamic changes with or without shunt placement. The specific clinical entities of fetal hydrocephalus, "shunt-dependent arrested hydrocephalus", isolated compartments after shunt, and LOVA were discussed.

References

1. Oi S (1992) Is the hydrocephalic state progressive to become irreversible during fetal life? Surg Neurol 37:66–68
2. Oi S, Matsumoto S (1985) Slit ventricles as a cause of isolated ventricles after shunting. Nerv Syst Child 1:189–193
3. Oi S, Matsumoto S (1985) Pathophysiology of nonneoplastic obstruction of the foramen of Monro and progressive unilateral hydrocephalus. Neurosurgery 17:891–896
4. Oi S, Matsumoto S (1986) Pathophysiology of aqueductal obstruction in isolated IV ventricle after shunting. Nerv Syst Child 2:282–286
5. Oi S, Matsumoto S (1986) Isolated fourth ventricle. J Pediatr Neurosci 2:125–133
6. Oi S, Matsumoto S (1986) Morphological findings of post-shunt slit ventricle in experimental canine hydrocephalus. Aspects of causative factors of isolated ventricles and slit ventricle syndrome. Nerv Syst Child 2:179–184
7. Oi S, Matsumoto S (1986) Dynamic change in intracranial pressure in slit-like ventricles and isolated ventricles in childhood hydrocephalus after shunt placement. In: Ishii S (ed) Hydrocephalus. Excerpta Medica, Amsterdam, pp 135–147
8. Oi S, Matsumoto S (1987) Infantile hydrocephalus and slit ventricle syndrome in early infancy. Nerv Syst Child 3:145–150
9. Oi S, Matsumoto S (1989) Hydrocephalus in premature infants—characteristics and therapeutic problems. Nerv Syst Child 5:76–82
10. Oi S, Matsumoto S (1992) A proposed grading and scoring system for spina bifida: spina bifida neurological scale (SBNS). Child's Nerv Syst 8:337–342
11. Oi S, Matsumoto S, Katayama K, et al. (1990) Pathophysiology and postnatal outcome of fetal hydrocephalus. Child's Nerv Syst 6:338–345
12. Oi S, Matsumoto S, Katayama K, et al. (1990) Prenatal neuroimagings in fetal dysraphism. Neurosonology 3:90–96
13. Oi S, Yamada H, Kimura M, et al. (1990) Factors affecting prognosis of intrauterine hydrocephalus diagnosed in the third trimester: computerized data analysis on controversies in fetal surgery. Neurol Med Chir 30:456–461
14. Oi S, Matsumoto S, Kudo H, et al. (1991) Hydromyelic hydrocephalus—correlation of hydromyelia with various stages of hydrocephalus in post-shunt isolated hydrocephalus. J Neurosurg 74:371–379
15. Oi S, Sato O, Matsumoto S (1996) Neurological and medico-social problems of spina bifida patients in adolescence and adulthood. Child's Nerv Syst 12:181–187
16. Oi S, Honda Y, Hidaka M, Sato O, Matsumoto S (1998) Intrauterine high resolution MR imaging in fetal hydrocephalus and prenatal estimation of the postnatal outcomes with perspective classification. J Neurosurg 88:685–694

Endoscopic Surgery for Obstructive Hydrocephalus

Joong-Uhn Choi and Dong-Seok Kim

Summary. Endoscopic surgery is popular in the neurosurgical field. In the last 7 years we have performed 60 endoscopic procedures for the treatment of noncommunicating hydrocephalus, 57 endoscopic third ventriculostomies, and 3 septostomies. The age distribution of patients varied from 2 months to 62 years. Forty-seven out of 57 operations were performed with endoscopic third ventriculostomy alone, and 10 patients had endoscopic third ventriculostomy and ventriculoperitoneal shunt simultaneously. The most common cause of noncommunicating hydrocephalus is aqueductal stenosis, and we treated 27 cases. Other causes were tectal tumors (9), posterior fossa tumors (10), pineal tumors (4), thalamic tumor (1), arachnoid cysts (4), and obstructions of the fourth ventricular exit (2). Forty-one out of 47 patients who were treated by endoscopic third ventriculostomy alone showed a successful result (87%). However, six patients had unsatisfactory results, and these needed a ventriculoperitoneal shunt. Three of the six unsuccessful cases were below 1 year of age.

There were some complications with endoscopic third ventriculostomy: two cases of transient diabetes insipidus, one epidural hematoma, one delayed intraventricular hemorrhage, two obstructions of the fenestration site, and one injury to the fornix.

Two patients showed a thick third ventricular floor, through which we failed to make fenestration during endoscopy. These two cases were excluded from our series. Technical points and treatment protocol are discussed.

Key words. Endoscopic third ventriculostomy, Endoscopic surgery, Obstructive hydrocephalus

Introduction

In the era before the shunting of cerebrospinal fluid, the most common operation for the relief of obstructive hydrocephalus was third ventriculostomy [7, 17–19, 26, 27, 30]. Third ventriculostomy was first performed by Dandy [5] in 1922. Unfortunately, this operation had a high failure rate when the hydrocephalus was congenital [6, 21]. Third ventriculostomy also had a significant surgical morbidity rate [4, 6, 22, 28]. The development of the valved shunt by Nulsen and Spitz in 1951 revolutionized the management of hydrocephalus. However, in the long term, shunting for hydrocephalus still has numerous drawbacks related to shunt mal-

Department of Neurosurgery, Brain Research Institute, Severance Hospital, Yonsei University College of Medicine, C.P.O. Box 8044, Seoul, Korea

function and infection. In part, the report by Guiot [10] that third ventriculostomy using stereotactic methods could be safe and easy stimulated our interest [3]. Interest was further stimulated by the report by Sayers and Kosnik [25] that third ventriculostomy was effective for the control of congenital hydrocephalus if it was preceded by a period of low-pressure shunting.

Mixter [20] had actually done endoscopic third ventriculostomy as early as 1923, but the procedure never became popular because of the large diameters and poor illumination of the existing instrumentation. This situation changed in the 1960s with the development of fiberoptic technology. The incorporation of this technology into endoscopic equipment permitted the construction of small-diameter endoscopes with high-intensity external light sources [8, 9, 31–33]. This chapter describes a simple technique for third ventriculostomy using modern endoscopes. The author has performed endoscopic third ventriculostomy in 57 patients with noncommunicating hydrocephalus since 1989, and now reports the results of this procedure with a review of literature.

Method

Patient Selection

Noncommunicating hydrocephalus is a primary indication for endoscopic third ventriculostomy. Our selection criteria include aqueductal stenosis and noncommunicating hydrocephalus due to tumor or cyst. This method is not suitable for patients who have had meningitis or subarachnoid hemorrhage, or who have congenital hydrocephalus. Routine preoperative work-ups were brain computed tomography (CT), radio-isotope cisternography, CSF flow study with phase contrast MR and cine MR.

Instrumentation

The instrumentation for endoscopic third ventriculostomy consists of a 30° Hopkins pediatric telescope with an outside diameter 2.7 mm, a sheath for the telescope with an outside diameter 3.8 mm, a stylet, coagulating electrodes (Karl Stortz, Tuttlingen Germany), a fiberoptic light guide, a Xenon light source, and an endovision system. We used the rigid type of endoscope only for third ventriculostomy, but a steerable type can be used, which has the advantage of being able to change the direction of view when manipulating the intraventricular structures. To perforate the third ventricle floor, a monopolar coagulating electrode was applied via a working channel.

Operative Technique

Third ventriculostomy is performed under general anesthesia. The patient is positioned supine, and routine skin preparations and draping are used for a burr hole. A burr hole is made 1 cm in front of the coronal suture and 2–3 cm lateral to the midline. The right lateral ventricle is tapped using a ventricular catheter through the burr hole, and a peelaway catheter is placed via a tract. The tip of the tapping catheter is directed to the glabella and tragus of the right ear. The telescope with sheath is then advanced into the lateral ventricle through the peelaway catheter. The foramen of Monro is identified, and the telescope is now advanced through the foramen to visualize the floor of the third ventricle.

The site for third ventriculostomy is located half-way along the midline between the infundifular recess and the mamillary body. In some cases of severe hydrocephalus, the dome of

a,b 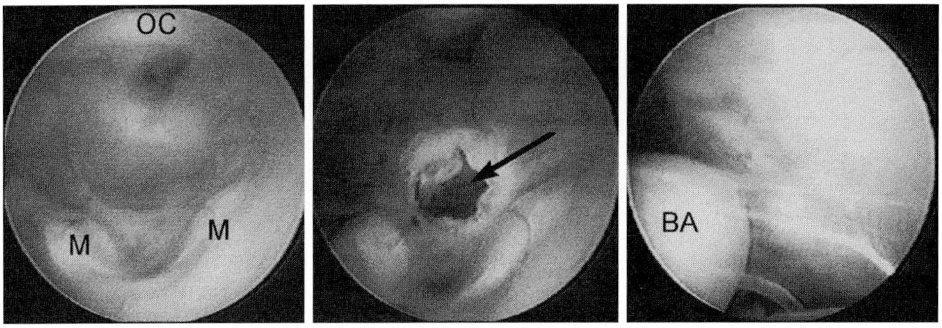 c

FIG. 1. Endoscopic appearance of third ventricular floor. **a** Before ventriculostomy. **b** After ventriculostomy. **c** The endoscope is advanced through the hole into the interpeduncular cistern. *M*, mamillary body; *OC*, optic chiasm; *Arrow*, site of ventriculostomy; *BA*, basilar artery

the basilar artery is visualized in front of both mamillary bodies. To perforate the third ventricular floor, the coagulating electrode is advanced via a working channel in the sheath. Monopolar electrocoagulation with the electrode can easily perforate the third ventricular floor under direct vision (Fig. 1). The telescope can be advanced through a thinned coagulated portion of the third ventricle floor.

A flow of CSF through the hole is usually seen after perforation. The hole is enlarged with the insertion of the telescope, and the basilar artery in the interpeduncular cistern is usually inspected. The telescope and its sheath are removed and the cortical incision is packed with a piece of gelfoam. The wound is closed, and an epidural pressure monitoring sensor can be inserted for postoperative intracranial pressure (ICP) monitoring.

Postoperative Management and Assessment of Outcome

Initially, ICP is monitored for 48 h until a trend is established. In patients who show high ICP for over 48 h postoperatively, lumbar drainage of CSF has been tried for 1 week. Brain MRI with T2 weighted axial and T2 weighted midsagittal thin slices is performed on the 10th postoperative day. A flow void in the floor of the third ventricle can usually be seen (Fig. 2). Cine MR would also be useful to confirm the CSF flow via the ventriculostomy site.

The assessment of outcome is based on a combination of (a) resolution of symptoms of raised ICP, (b) ICP measurements, and (c) a neuroimaging study, e.g., MRI with a CSF flow study or cine MR. There are two possible results:

1. success, i.e., the patient does not need a shunt and has improved clinical symptoms;
2. failure, i.e., there was no significant alteration in symptoms in the postoperative period and the patient required placement of an extracranial shunt postoperatively.

Results

Author's Cases

Fifty-seven patients with noncommunicating hydrocephalus underwent endoscopic third ventriculostomy. Ten of the 57 cases had third ventriculostomy with ventriculoperitoneal

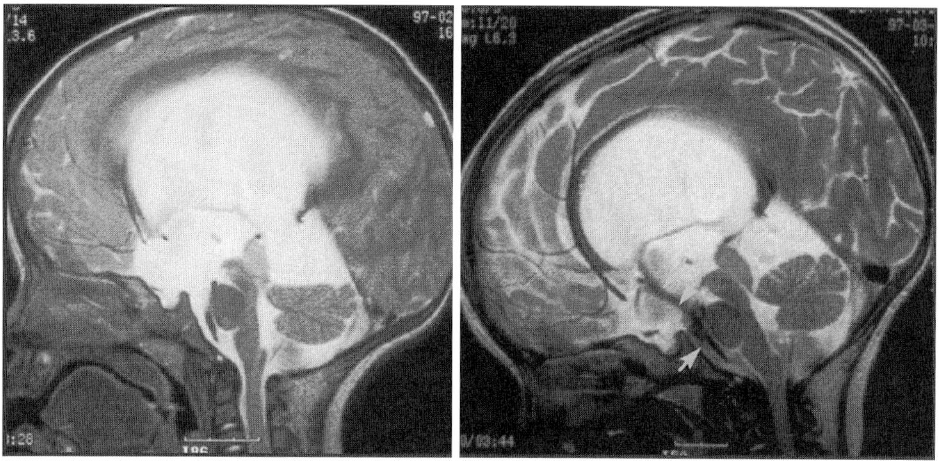

a b

FIG. 2. Brain MRI. **a** Before ventriculostomy. Aqueductal stenosis and dilated lateral ventricle are seen. **b** After ventriculostomy. Flow void is clearly seen between the third ventricle and the interpeduncular cistern (*arrow*)

TABLE 1. Results of endoscopic third ventriculostomy (group A)

Causes of hydrocephalus	Number of patients	Outcome	
		Success	Failure
Aqueductal stenosis	15	11	4
Aqueductal stenosis with tectal tumor	9	8	1
Aqueductal stenosis, s/p V-P shunt	6	6	
Aqueductal stenosis with arachnoid cyst	4	4	
Obstruction of fourth ventricle exit	2	2	
Pineal tumor	4	3	1
Thalamic tumor	1	1	
Posterior fossa tumor	6	6	
Total	47	41 (87%)	6 (13%)

shunt simultaneously because we thought that these patients might possibly have CSF absorption problems (group B). Forty-one out of 47 patients (group A) treated with endoscopic third ventriculostomy only were successful (87%). They did not need a shunting operation. Among the 41 successful cases, two patients showed delayed milestones. Endoscopic surgery failed in six cases who had to be treated with ventriculoperitoneal shunt (Table 1). Three of the six failed cases were patients with aqueductal stenosis under the age of 1 year.

The other failed cases were a 14-year-old boy who had aqueductal stenosis due to tectal tumor, and 12-year-old boy with a pineal tumor (Table 2). Endoscopy in those two patients were early in our experience. We judged failure of endoscopy after 48 h of ICP monitoring, but these cases might have been successful if we had tried lumbar CSF drainage for over 1 week. Two out of six failed cases were due to reobstruction of the fenestration site: a 5-month-old male with aqueductal stenosis after ventricular hemorrhage, and a 33-year-old male with obstructive hydrocephalus after meningitis.

TABLE 2. Unsuccessful endoscopic third ventriculostomy (failed group A)

Causes of hydrocephalus	Sex	Age	Treatment
Aqueductal stenosis	M	8/12	V-P shunt
Aqueductal stenosis	M	2/12	V-P shunt
Aqueductal stenosis, posthemorrhagic[a]	M	5/12	V-P shunt
Aqueductal stenosis, posthemorrhagic[a]	M	33	V-P shunt
Tectal tumor	M	14	V-P shunt
Pineal tumor	M	12	V-P shunt

[a] Obstruction of ventriculostomy site.

The other group (Group B) of our series consisted of the ten patients who had been treated with endoscopic third ventriculostomy and ventriculoperitoneal shunt simultaneously. Six patients had ventriculoperitoneal shunt owing to aqueductal stenosis previously at other hospitals, and they had presented with shunt malfunction. These patients were treated with third ventriculostomy with shunt revision. The other four cases presented with hydrocephalus with posterior fossa tumor under the age of 1 year. These ten patients were thought to need prompt relief of high intracranial pressure or they would have CSF absorption problems. Sixteen patients who had been treated with endoscopic third ventriculostomy and ventriculoperitoneal shunt have not had any shunt revisions for the last 4 years. There has been no operative mortality in our series of 57 patients.

We did have some postoperative complications: two transient diabetes insipidus, one delayed intraventricular hemorrhage (IVH), and one epidural hematoma. The IVH resolved spontaneously, and the epidural hematoma was evacuated and the patient did well.

Other Cases

Hoffman [13] reported his own experience of stereotactic third ventriculostomy, and reviewed 797 cases treated with third ventriculostomy from the literature. A total of 569 patients were treated with open craniotomy, and 228 cases with a percutaneous technique, mostly the stereotactic method. The over all success rate was about 53%. Operative mortality was 10.3% in the open method and 3.5% with the percutaneous technique.

Jones et al. [15] reported that eight of 14 patients with noncommunicating hydrocephalus were successfully treated using endoscopic third ventriculostomy (58%). Four cases out of 14 improved (29%), but one needed a shunting operation later. Three cases with noncommunicating hydrocephalus due to CNS tumors were treated with endoscopic surgery. Two cases were successful, and one was unsuccessful, with bradycardia being a limiting factor when the floor was approached.

Saint-Rose [24] reviewed two identical series of patients with aqueductal stenosis. Thirty-eight patients were treated by insertion of a ventriculoperitoneal shunt, and 30 had a third ventriculostomy. In a group of patients treated by third ventriculostomy, the ventricle remained enlarged despite clinical normalization in 60% of the patients. Fifty-eight percent of the shunted group developed slit-like ventricles on the CT scan during the same follow-up period. From a neurological, endocrinological, social, and behavioral point of view, there were no statistical differences between the two groups.

Two out of 20 of our endoscopic third ventriculostomy series showed marked reduction of ventricular size.

Discussion

Ventriculoscopy was first performed in 1910 by V.L. l'Espinasse, a surgeon from Chicago. He used a rigid cystoscope to fulgurate the choroid plexus bilaterally in two infants [11]. One child died immediately and the other lived for 5 years. The event received little attention and passed almost unnoticed at the time. In 1922, Dandy used a rigid cystoscope in an attempt at choroid plexus fulguration in two patients. The instrument was primitive and the procedures were only "partially successful." Dandy [5] correctly predicted that ventriculoscopy would be replaced by newer indirect methods of imaging the intracranical contents.

In 1923, Mixter [20] performed the first endoscopic third ventriculostomy for aqueductal stenosis. The patient was a 9-month-old girl with advanced noncommunicating hydrocephalus. Mixter introduced a small urethroscope into the lateral ventricle and then through the dilated foramen of Monro. Under visual guidance, he pushed a flexible sound through the floor of the third ventricle and successfully connected the third ventricle with the basal subarachnoid space.

Although investigators continued to perform ventricular endoscopy, the procedure gradually fell out of favor [26]. Its primary use was to inspect the ventricles, or to extirpate or cauterize the choroid plexus [23, 29]. Therapy was often ineffective, and morbidity and mortality rates were very high. Later, improved neuroimaging techniques made it unnecessary to inspect the ventricular system directly. In addition, the development of the valve shunt by Nulsen and Spitz in 1951 revolutionized the management of hydrocephalus. However, shunts are troublesome devices, plagued by many complications including infection, obstruction, misplacement, overdrainage, and underdrainage, etc. [11].

Technical advances in optics, miniaturization, and the steerability of instruments have created renewed interest in neuroendoscopy [1, 2]. The modern fiberoptic endoscope appears to provide a simple and safe means for performing third ventriculostomy. It has the advantage over the stereotactic technique of requiring less sophisticated equipment, and allowing direct visualization of the ventriculostomy site.

The real problem with third ventriculostomy, however, is selecting appropriate candidates for the procedure [12, 14–17]. It is first necessary for all patients to have adequately dilated third and lateral ventricles. Jones et al. [15] suggested that a suitable size for the third ventricle for endoscopic surgery is about 1 cm bicoronal diameter. Most successes reported in the literature were in patients with acquired aqueductal stenosis [17]. In our series, aqueductal stenosis also showed good results, especially in children above 1 year of age. We performed endoscopic third ventriculostomy and ventriculoperitoneal shunt simultaneously in six patients with aqueductal stenosis who showed malfunction of a previously inserted shunt, and in four young children with posterior fossa tumor who were supposed to have problems in extraventricular CSF circulation due to previous infection or hemorrhage. We anticipate that they will become less dependent on the shunts, which are now communicating above the level of the tentorium. If one could assess accurately the reabsorptive capacity or patency of the subarachnoid space prior to operation, it would be helpful in the selection of appropriate candidates for this procedure.

The best results for third ventriculostomy are achieved with patients in whom the onset of aqueductal stenosis occurred after 1 year of age; approximately 80% of these patients are shunt-independent after the procedure [24]. This is similar to the results in our series.

The major risks of third ventriculostomy are hypothalamic dysfunction by extending the fenestration into the infundibular recess, and hemorrhage from damage to arteries, ependymal veins, or choroid plexus. We experienced transient diabetes insipidus in two patients after third ventriculostomy, and one delayed IVH.

Conclusion

A simple technique for performing endoscopic third ventriculostomy and the results are described. We conclude that this procedure is simple, safe, and effective in appropriately selected cases with noncommunicating hydrocephalus.

References

1. Auer LM, Holzer P, Ascher PW, Heppner F (1988) Endoscopic neurosurgery. Acta Neuchir 90:1–14
2. Auer LM, Deinsberger W, Niederkorn K, Gell G, Kleinert R, Schneider G, Holzer P, Bone G, Mokry M, Korner E (1989) Endoscopic surgery versus medical treatment for spontaneous intracerebral hematoma: a randomized study. J Neurosurg 70:530–535
3. Backlund E, Grepe A, Lunsford LD (1981) Stereotaxic reconstruction of the aqueduct of Sylvius. J Neurosurg 55:800–810
4. Brocklehurst G (1974) Transcallosal third ventriculochiasmatic cisternostomy: new approach to hydrocephalus. Surg Neurol 2:109–114
5. Dandy WE (1922) An operative procedure for hydrocephalus. Bull Johns Hopkins Hosp 33:189–190
6. Dandy WE (1945) Diagnosis and treatment of strictures of the aqueduct of Sylvius (causing hydrocephalus). Arch Surg 51:1–14
7. Elvidge AR (1966) Treatment of obstructive lesions of the aqueduct of Sylvius and the fourth ventricle by interventriculostomy. J Neurosurg 24:11–23
8. Fukushima T (1978) Endoscopic biopsy of intraventricular tumors with the use of a ventriculofiberscope. Neurosurgery 2:110–113
9. Griffith HB (1975) Technique of fontanelle and presutural ventriculoscopy and endoscopic ventricular surgery in infants. Childs Brain 1:359–363
10. Guiot G (1973) Ventriculo-cisternostomy for stenosis of the aqueduct of Sylvius. Acta Neurochir (Wien) 28:275–289
11. Heilman CB, Cohen AR (1991) Endoscopic ventricular fenestration using a "saline torch". J Neurosurg 74:224–229
12. Hirsch JF (1982) Percutaneous ventriculocisternostomies in noncommunicating hydrocephalus. Monogr Neurol Sci 8:170–178
13. Hoffman HJ (1976) The advantages of percutaneous third ventriculostomy over other forms of surgical treatment for infantile obstructive hydrocephalus. In: Morley TP (ed) Current controversies in neurosurgery. WB Saunders, Philadelphia, pp 691–703
14. Hoffman HJ, Harwood-Nash D, Gilday DL (1980) Percutaneous third ventriculoscopy in the management of noncommunicating hydrocephalus. Neurosurgery 7:313–321
15. Jones RFC, Stening WA, Bradon M (1990) Endoscopic third ventriculostomy. Neurosurgery 26:86–92
16. Kelly P, Goerss S, Kall B, Kispert D (1986) Computed tomography based stereotactic third ventriculostomy: technical note. Neurosurgery 18:791–794
17. Manwaring KH, Rekate H, Kaplan A (1989) Hydrocephalus management by endoscopy: Ann Neurol 26:488 (abstract)
18. McNickle HF (1947) The surgical treatment of hydrocephalus: a simple method of performing third ventriculostomy. Br J Surg 34:302–307
19. Miler CF, White RJ, Roski RA (1979) Spontaneous ventriculocisternostomy. Surg Neurol 11:63–66
20. Mixter WJ (1923) Ventriculoscopy and puncture of the floor of the third ventricle. Boston Med Surg J 188:277–278
21. Patterson RH, Bergland RM (1968) The selection of patients for third ventriculostomy based on experience with 33 operations. J Neurosurg 29:252–254
22. Perlman BB (1968) Percutaneous third ventriculostomy in the treatment of a hydrocephalic infant with aqueduct stenosis. Int Surg 49:443–448

23. Powell MP, Torrens MJ, Thomson JLG, Horgan JG (1983) Isodense colloid cysts of the third ventricle: a diagnostic and therapeutic problem resolved by ventriculoscopy. Neurosurgery 13:234–237
24. Sainte-Rose C (1992) Third ventriculostomy. Neuroendoscopy Marg Ann Liebert, New York, pp 47–62
25. Sayers HP, Kosnik EJ (1976) Percutaneous third ventriculostomy: experience and technique. Childs Brain 2:24–30
26. Scarff JE (1935) Third ventriculoscopy as the rational treatment of obstructive hydrocephalus. J Pediatr 6:870–871 (abstract)
27. Scarff JE (1966) Evaluation of treatment of hydrocephalus. Reports of third ventriculostomy and endoscopic cauterization of choroid plexuses compared with mechanical shunts. Arch Neurol 382–391
28. Scarff JE (1966) Third ventriculostomy by puncture of the lamina terminalis and the floor of the third ventricle. J Neurosurg 24:935–943
29. Scarff JE (1970) The treatment of nonobstructive (communicating) hydrocephalus by endoscopic cauterization of the choroid plexuses. J Neurosurg 33:1–18
30. Volkel JS, Voris HC (1966) Third ventriculostomy in obstructive hydrocephalus: long term arrest in 4 cases. J Neurosurg 24:568–569
31. Vries J (1978) An endoscopic technique for third ventriculostomy. Surg Neurol 9:165–168
32. Vries JK (1980) Endoscopy as an adjunct to shunting for hydrocephalus. Surg Neurol 13:69–72
33. Vries JK, Friedman WA (1980) Postoperative evaluation of third ventriculostomy patients using III in DTPA. Childs Brain 6:200–205

Chronic Hydrocephalus Associated with Spina Bifida

Concezio Di Rocco

Summary. Chronic hydrocephalus associated with spina bifida constitutes a challenging problem for the neurosurgeon. Indeed, in spite of the numerous investigations carried out on the subject, the physiopathogenesis of this type of hydrocephalus remains relatively obscure in relation to its multifactorial etiology.

In utero and in the neonatal period, the ventricular dilation seems, in fact, to depend mainly on abnormal fluid exchanges between the ventricles and cerebral parenchyma, whereas in later life obstructive phenomena appear to play a major role. Such a variable interplay of functional and obstructive factors accounts for the difficulties experienced in establishing the surgical indication in untreated patients with chronic hydrocephalus, and in planning the correct surgical management. In this respect, the study of CSF dynamics may provide very useful information.

Key words. Hydrocephalus, Spina bifida, Aqueductal stenosis, CSF infusion test, CSF pressure recording

Introduction

In spite of numerous clinical and experimental investigations, the physiopathogenesis of the hydrocephalus associated with myelomeningocele (MM) remains relatively obscure. In fact, unlike other forms of hydrocephalus, this particular type of ventricular dilation appears to be compatible with life in several patients who have had no surgical treatment. A significant percentage of these subjects may even show a surprisingly limited impairment in mental performance, although their cerebral ventricles may be impressively enlarged. The possibility that hydrocephalus associated with myelodysplasia might reach apparent stabilization with an apparently acceptable low degree of secondary cerebral damage explains why some authors were reluctant in the past to perform CSF shunting in myelodysplasic children, especially at the light of the higher risk of complications caused by their hydrocephalus as compared with other forms of ventricular dilation.

This phenomenon—that is, the possibility of hydrocephalus associated with spina bifida occurring with relatively mild clinical manifestations—also accounts for the relatively low incidence of ventricular dilation requiring surgical treatment in reports concerning

Institute of Neurosurgery, Catholic University Medical School, 8 Largo Gemelli, Rome 00168, Italy

children with myelomeningocele when the surgical indication was based merely on clinical grounds.

In contrast to these reports, more recent studies on subjects operated on as a result of the findings provided by ultrasonography, computed tomography (CT), and magnetic resonance imaging (MRI) indicate that almost 100% of patients with myelodysplasia will require a CSF shunt procedure soon after birth or in subsequent years [1, 2].

In fact, two main aspects of the hydrocephalus associated with spina bifida suggest particular caution in accepting that the progression of ventricular dilation in subjects who have not had surgery has really come to a stop, even in patients who seem to tolerate their ventricular enlargement quite well.

The first aspect, the more dramatic one, is the possibility of an abrupt deterioration in the patient's clinical condition, eventually leading to death. Late deaths in myelodysplasic patients have been anecdotally reported, and are nearly always attributed to the effect of the concomitant Chiari type II malformation or to incidental causes, usually pneumonia. However, the observation of unexpected deaths in myelodysplasic children whose CSF shunt device has been removed because of a presumed diagnosis of shunt-independent "arrested" hydrocephalus should actually lead us to reconsider the possibility of a specific role for hydrocephalus in determining such a dismal outcome.

The second aspect concerns the actual cost of the untreated hydrocephalus in reaching its chronic stage. Indeed, as well as the characteristic compensatory changes which take place in all types of hydrocephalus during the transitional period from the acute to the chronic phase, such as enlargement of the skull volume, reduction of the cerebral vascular bed, increase in the ventricular surface, and flattening and tearing of the ependymal layer resulting in an enhanced transependymal CSF absorption, the hydrocephalus associated with spina bifida tends to find an important compensatory mechanism in the dilation of the central canal of the spinal cord. Consequently, in myelodysplasic subjects, a "false" arrest of the hydrocephalus may occur quite insidiously and be suggested by atypical clinical signs, such as a worsening of motor performances, progressive scoliosis, and spinal and radicular pain [3].

Natural History of Hydrocephalus

A relatively small amount of information is available concerning the natural history of hydrocephalus, although we can utilize the clinical observations made in the 1960s on populations of hydrocephalic children, the majority of whom had hydrocephalus associated with spina bifida and did not receive appropriate treatment because of the economic difficulties resulting from the effects of World War II. A second, though indirect, source of information is experimental observations on hydrocephalic animals.

Experimental Observations

By excluding the studies carried out on particular species of animals with inborn defects resulting in hydrocephalus, the findings of which are difficult to transfer directly to humans, most observations on the natural history of hydrocephalus have been obtained by inducing a mechanical block into the CSF circulation. Depending on the efficacy of such a block, two main cascades of events may occur.

In cases of a *complete block*, the rapid secondary dilation of the cerebral ventricles associated with an abnormally increased CSF pressure usually leads to the early death of the animal. The experiments performed in 1973 by Obenchain and Stern [4] may be considered a paradigm of this type of situation. A block in CSF circulation was obtained by injecting dental silicone material into the IVth ventricle of 5 adult monkeys. The obstruction actually involved the IVth ventricle, the aqueduct, and the posterior part of the IIIrd ventricle. Only 2 out of the 5 animals survived the duration of the experiment: 24 h, with an intracranial pressure of 750 and 1000 mm H_2O, respectively. Three animals died at times which coincided with peaks of increased ICP, i.e., at 5.5 h (with an ICP of 450 mm H_2O), at 17 h (with an ICP of 1300 mm H_2O), and 23.5 h (with an ICP of 2160 mm H_2O).

During this acute phase of the hydrocephalus, the rise in ICP was nonlinear, and was characterized by peaks over a few minutes followed by rapid falls to new levels which were slightly higher than those recorded prior to the build-up of each peak. Two types of pressure waves could be observed: (a) *fairly symmetrical undulations* (1–2/min, with an amplitude ranging between 25 and 40 cm H_2O), which occurred when the baseline ICP pressure increased to between 200 and 100 cm H_2O. These waves became more frequent and longer in duration with the progressive increase in mean ICP levels. They were associated with periodic respiration (hyperpnea with peaks of ICP pressure; hypopnea when the CSF pressure decreased after the peaks); (b) *monophasic increases in pressure* occurring at higher pressure levels, and lasting 4–5 min. These waves also tended to become more frequent and longer, up to 10 min, when the ICP further increased. They were associated with hyperventilation and, in the animals which did not survive, with apnea and medullary failure.

These two main patterns of ICP waves occurring in obstructive hydrocephalus in cases of a complete block in CSF circulation obviously correspond to the B waves and A waves recorded in humans with severely increased intracranial pressure [5]. Similar behaviour of the ICP can be observed in children harboring a posterior fossa occupying a space lesion associated with an acute ventricular dilation.

When the block into the CSF circulation *is not complete*, the secondary physiopathological changes tend to follow a biphasic pattern, as the animals can survive the acute phase and enter a chronic phase. In 1970, Milhorat et al. [6] used an inflatable balloon to occlude the caudal aqueduct in monkeys, and was able to demonstrate that gross ventricular dilation occurred within 1 h, and became well advanced within 3 h. The associated clinical manifestations included loss of normal alertness, progressive lethargy, and cerebellar signs. However, these clinical manifestations tended to become progressively less evident after 48–72 h, when the progression of the ventricular dilation seemed to continue at an obviously slower rate. During the chronic phase, the clinical manifestations also appeared to subside.

Similar observations were obtained by Hochwald et al. [7] in cats with obstructive hydrocephalus induced by injecting kaoolin into the cisterna magna; as many as 40% of the animals were severely ill during the acute phase of the experiment (the first 5–7 days after the cisternal injection), during which the ICP was high (mean ICP pressure 25.7 cm H_2O). About 50% of these animals died, and those which survived required hand-feeding as they were not able to reach their food. The cats which survived the acute phase after at least 1 month of hydrocephalus (mean 56.1 days) remained free of any gross neurological deficits. In these animals, the intraventricular CSF pressure was relatively low (mean 3.7 cm H_2O) and the CSF absorption ability exceeded the CSF formation rate. There are several functional and anatomical phenomena which account for the "compensation" of acute hydrocephalus: the abnormally elevated ICP is dissipated by an increase in CSF absorption in front of a "normal" CSF production, and the increased volume of intraventricular CSF is accommodated for by an increase in ventricular (and cranial) volume as well as by a decrease of the volume of the cerebral vascular bed, and, in the late phases, of the cerebral parenchyma.

In 1963, Bering and Sato [8] were able to demonstrate that CSF was absorbed within the ventricles in normal animals, and that such absorption occurred with a reduced resistance in the ventricles of chronic hydrocephalic dogs. The reduction in resistance to absorption was observed with time, as the ventricular volume increased and ependyma became flattened.

A phenomenon invariably noticed in periventricular structures in cases of chronic hydrocephalus is the spongy appearance of the subependymal white matter due to an increase in extracellular space. The subependymal fluid accumulation is more obvious in areas where the overlying ependyma is damaged or even lost, with the possibility, demonstrated by Ogata et al. [9], of the capillaries being directly exposed to the fluid within the ventricular cavity because of an apparent continuation of the subependymal extracellular space with the ventricles.

Three main hypotheses have been propounded to interprete the significance of the increased water content in the periventricular white matter in obstructive chronic hydrocephalus [10]: (1) edema resulting from an abnormal permeability of the ependyma induced by the increase in intraventricular pressure, which results in tearing and stretching of the structure; (2) the effect of the excess fluid produced within the ventricles because of the outflow obstruction; (3) the stasis of fluid produced within the cerebral tissue adjacent to the ventricles.

The first hypothesis may easily be discarded since edema implies an increased volume, whereas the white matter in chronic hydrocephalus is reduced. On the other hand, the second and third interpretations still remain open to discussion and justify further questions, namely about the importance of a possible transventricular absorption of CSF.

Transventricular bulk flow undoubtedly does occur in hydrocephalus: the phenomenon corresponds to fluid flow along routes of minor structural resistance—that is reflux of choroidal fluid into the periventricular tissues—and to a reduced gradient for bulk flow from the interstitial cerebral spaces into the cerebral ventricles.

The fate of the fluid confined to the extracellular space, in other words the "hydrocephalic edema" defined by Milhorat [11], is not well known, even though experimental evidence has been provided suggesting that it is absorbed, at least in part, across the fenestrated capillaries which line the ventricles [12, 13]. Such absorption could contribute to a slowing or arrest of the hydrocephalus. However, with progressive or persistent edema of the periventricular tissue, there is a significant reduction in local cerebral blood flow [14, 15], which could account for the functional disturbances observed in chronic hydrocephalus.

Clinical Observations

Most of the information concerning the neurological and mental development of untreated hydrocephalic subjects is derived from studies published in the 1960s. The economic difficulties faced in Europe following World War II, together with the insufficiency of surgical techniques at that time, resulted in an unacceptably high incidence of complications, and contributed toward a prejudiced attitude against surgery, especially in cases of severe ventricular dilation or in patients with associated neurological deficits, such as myelodysplasic children.

In 1962, Laurence and Coates [16] performed an extensive investigation on 239 cases of hydrocephalus under the age of 13 years. These cases were seen by Dr. McKissock at the Hospital for Sick Children, London, and at the Atkinson Morley Hospital between January 1938 and December 1957. Most of these children (182 out of 239) had not been operated on, particularly subjects with spina bifida cystica who were regarded as hopeless.

The authors stressed that the series could not be regarded as representative of the conditions in the community as a whole, as the most severe cases had probably not reached the hospital because of early death or because they had been considered beyond help. Indeed, in only 34 children (18.6%) in this series was the hydrocephalus associated with spina bifida, although the malformation, according to the authors, was the most common cause of hydrocephalus in the community.

At the time of the first observation, 31% of the patients were under 3 months of age, 67% were under 1 year, and only 8% were over 4 years. When the patients were reexamined at the end of 1958, 81 (44.5)% were found to be alive and well, as the hydrocephalus had arrested spontaneously. A further 3 subjects (1.1%) were presumed to be alive, even though they were no longer in the records. In 9 children (4.9%), all under 5 years of age, the ventricular dilation was still progressive.

Eighty-nine patients (48.9%) had died: two-thirds of them before the age of 18 months, 6 between 18 and 24 months, and 24 after the age of 2 years. Causes directly related to the hydrocephalus accounted for 46 deaths in the form of cardiorespiratory failure. Such events also occurred in 7 children in whom the hydrocephalus was regarded as having become arrested. A normal intelligence was present in about 17% of the survivors, and educational subnormality in 28 cases (15.3%). Twenty-two (12%) of the children were uneducable.

Taking into account the preliminary results of Pudenz et al. [17] and Spitz [18], who reported about a 70% chance of arresting hydrocephalus with CSF shunting procedures, Laurence and Coates [16] anticipated that with "more satisfactory operations now available, results better than 46% survival and 17% total survival with an intelligence quotient above 85 should be achieved."

It is worth noting that in 1967, 5 years after their first report, Laurence and Coates [19] published a second analysis of the 81 survivors from their series: the survival rate had dropped to 45%, as another 11 children had died.

The authors stressed that these subsequent deaths "highlight the precarious position of some patients with (arrested) hydrocephalus . . . those not retarded may have a recrudescence of a previously arrested hydrocephalus or they may suffer a very sudden disastrous attack of intracranial hypertension, from which they may not recover. Both conditions can be precipitated by some infection, but may occur without any apparent cause."

Since the observations of Schick and Matson [20], sufficient experience has been accumulated to indicate that the hydrocephalus associated with spina bifida is probably the one which has the best chance to reach an arrest. The difference is striking compared with other types of hydrocephalus which are overt at birth, but in which spontaneous arrest is a highly improbable event [10].

Nevertheless, there is also clinical evidence that myelodysplasic children with hydrocephalus may abruptly deteriorate and eventually die. In 1991, Rekate [21] reported on two teenagers with MM whose CSF shunting device had not been tested preoperatively, and who suddenly died during surgery for spinal stabilization. In one of these patients the shunt was found to be nonfunctioning and the brain showed evidence of intracranial hypertension with herniation. At Case Western Reserve University in Cleveland, trials of shunt occlusion were performed on 51 children with noncommunicating and communicating hydrocephalus [22]. However, out of 16 children with spina bifida who seemed to tolerate the occlusion, 4 suffered respiratory arrest 12 h to 5 years after the occlusion, none of them with warning signs of intracranial hypertension prior to the episode of acute deterioration. Two of these patients died, and two survived after resuscitation but with severe neurological downgrading. It is worth noting that unexpected deaths presumed to be due to sudden progression of the hydrocephalus have also been reported by Miyazawa et al. [23] in HTX rats with congenital hydrocephalus which had reached an apparent spontaneous arrest.

Hydrocephalus Associated with MM

A Physiopathogenetic Hypothesis

When considering the natural history of untreated hydrocephalus associated with MM, we should first consider that it remains, even in its chronic phases, a dynamic and ever-evolving disease.

Nowadays we have accumulated enough experience to know that the ventricular dilation occurs early in life, apparently independently of an obstruction in CSF circulation. This fetal hydrocephalus has specific morphological characteristics, e.g., the disproportional dilation of the occipital horns and atria in comparison with the anterior and temporal horns of the lateral cerebral ventricle. However, in spite of its precocity and the supposed weak resistance offered by the parenchyma and cerebral coverings at that age, the ventricular dilation tends to remain relatively stable, the head circumference relatively normal, or, in some case, even smaller than the normal limits. The cerebral convexity does not appear displaced against the inner surface of the skull, and the volume of the cisterns and the sulci is not reduced, in fact it is obviously enlarged.

There is experimental evidence [24] that a unique teratogenic agent—for example, trypan blue—utilized to induce a neural tube defect may also play a crucial role in altering the normal distribution of glycosaminoglycans, which in the fetus participate in water exchanges between the cerebral ventricles and the cerebral parenchyma [25].

In several instances during fetal life, the hydrocephalus associated with spina bifida may rely on the spinal defect itself to reduce the intrathecal excess of fluid.

The neonatal period represents a crucial time for the subsequent evolution of the hydrocephalus. As well as a role for surgical correction of the spinal defect to eliminate a possible compensatory mechanism, cerebrospinal inflammatory phenomena, and/or the development of the cerebellar structure within a hypoplasic posterior cranial fossa will more or less rapidly add a mechanical obstructive factor to the initially exclusively functional hydrocephalus.

Two main areas are particularly exposed to the secondary mechanical block: the cisterna magna and the upper spinal subarachnoid space and the aqueduct. The cisterna magna and the subarachnoid spaces at the cranial cervical junction may become progressively more crowded with the growth of the cerebellar hemisphere and the development of a medullary spur as well as a vermian peg on the midline. A further obstacle to CSF circulation is added by the variation in the diameter of the foramen magnum and by inflammatory connectival reactions of the fibrovascular tissue containing the choroid plexus, which also tends to be dislocated inferiorly, as can easily be observed from seriated CT-scan observations [26]. Further ventricular dilation, the effect of undampened supratentorial CSF pressure oscillations, and perhaps the effect of gravity when the child reaches a standing position, may all be factors contributing to the anatomical impact of the cerebellar and hindbrain structures at the cervico-cranial junction.

The aqueduct of Sylvius represents the second critical point. At this level, the mechanical compression exerted from the progressively enlarging lateral ventricles by distortion and abnormal angulation of the brainstem may result in a functional-mechanical obstacle, which in some cases may even transform the originally communicating hydrocephalus into a hydrocephalus where the aqueductal stenosis plays the predominant causative role.

Thus, the variable interplay of congenital abnormal regulatory fluid exchange mechanisms and the acquired impairment in CSF circulation may account for the different outcomes observed in hydrocephalic myelodysplasic patients, which range from the apparent arrest of the ventricular dilation to the abrupt occurrence of intracranial hypertension.

Given the unpredictable evolution of the hydrocephalus associated with MM, which typically shows phases of rapid progression which alternate with phases of apparent stabilization, the diagnosis of shunt-dependent or shunt-independent arrest is difficult to obtain, even nowadays when sophisticated methodology of morphological and functional analysis are available. Even more difficult may be predicting the prognosis.

As for other types of presumed arrested hydrocephalus, the clinical evaluation is of paramount importance. Intermittent headaches, increasing ataxia, ocular signs, changes in visual function, and worsening in seizure disorders are the frequent, although aspecific, neurological manifestations.

In 1991, Rekate [21] pointed to staring spells, which are similar to *absence attacks*, during which the child will stop talking in the middle of a sentence and stare into space for a few seconds or up to a minute, as specific clinical manifestations of the progression of chronic hydrocephalus in myelodysplasic children.

A decline in school performance and attention span may also be an important clinical sign which should be recognized by all caretakers. Neuropsychological testing may be particularly useful, although the learning disabilities of these patients may make interpretation of the results more difficult than usual.

The morphological studies have an ever increasing importance. Owing to the great variability of the morphological characteristics of this type of hydrocephalus, seriated examinations and accurate comparisons of examinations performed at different times are necessary in order to obtain a reliable evaluation. In 1979, Half et al. [27] first pointed out that chronic malfunctioning of CSF shunts could lead to hydromyelia and clinically progressive spinal deficit, i.e., the occurrence of scoliosis or the worsening of preexisting spinal deformities. More recently, the association between hydromyelia and hydrocephalus in myelodysplasia has been unequivocally demonstrated by the occurrence of hydromyelia and spinal deficits in children with MM in whom an attempt to arrest the hydrocephalus had been carried out by bandaging the head [28], as suggested by Epstein et al. in 1973 [29]. With the advent of MRI, the association of hydrocephalus and hydromyelia has become a fairly common finding in patients with MM. In some of these patients, analysis of the clinical course clearly demonstrates that the dilation of the central canal acts as a compensatory mechanism to accomodate the intrathecal excess of CSF fluid.

The study of CSF dynamics offers data of paramount importance for establishing the arrest of hydrocephalus in myelodysplasic patients as well as in other types of hydrocephalus. There are several ways to evaluate such dynamics, ranging from noninvasive investigations, e.g., the Diamox test, or the evaluation of CSF flow patterns using MRI, to invasive methodologies based on direct recordings of intrathecal CSF pressure [30–34]. In our experience, the constant subarachnoid infusion—manometric test and the prolonged recording of intracranial pressure have been shown to be very reliable methods [32, 35].

In myelodysplasic patients, variable patterns of pressure–volume curves can be observed during the infusion test: (1) intracranial pressures which remain within the normal limits correspond to true arrested hydrocephalus; (2) intracranial pressures which increase constantly during the examination until the discontinuation of the infusion are evidence of a false arrested hydrocephalus, in which the aqueductal stenosis plays an important role; (3) biphasic curves, characterized by an immediate rapid increase in intracranial pressure followed by a late return toward normal values, will suggest a false arrested hydrocephalus, with a predominantly communicating nature.

The biphasic response is not typical of chronic hydrocephalus associated with MM, as it can also be observed in some types of constrictive hydrocephalus, e.g., in some cases of craniosynostosis. We believe that the rapid increase in pressure following the start of the infusion corresponds to an induced decompensation of the baseline precarium equilibrium between CSF production and absorption, which accounts for the apparent arrest of hydrocephalus in several children with MM. In this connection, it is worth noting that as well as ventricular dilation and/or hydromyelia, children who seem to do reasonably well nearly always present an accumulation of fluid within the peripheral CSF spaces, which consequently cannot dilate further to accommodate for the extra fluid administered intrathecally during the intrathecal infusion. The late phase of reequilibrium probably represents the effectivess of the compensatory mechanisms for CSF absorption, which may still be called into action, although at higher pressure levels. The efficacy of these mechanisms explains why, in most cases, patients with MM and chronic hydrocephalus do not show episodes of obvious increases in intracranial pressure, although their CSF dynamics is impaired.

Long-term intracranial pressure recordings may reveal normal values during relaxed wakefulness in patients who show large increases in the mean pulse intraventricular CSF pressure during physiological sleeep, a finding which is characteristic of the so-called "normal pressure hydrocephalus" in adult patients [34].

In other words, the abnormally large and persisting phasic increases in intracranial pressure probably translate into the precarious equilibrium which may characterize patients with MM and chronic hydrocephalus [32]. In fact, the abnormal pressure elevations correspond to a limited ability to compensate for abrupt increases in intracranial volume, and are secondary to the dilation of the cerebral vascular bed associated with the increased blood flow which occurs during the REM phase of sleep.

Perspectives

Although several children with MM, both shunted and unshunted, may apparently reach an arrest of hydrocephalus, the physiopathogenetic characteristics of the hydrocephalus associated with spina bifida requires close follow-up, with periodic neurological and neuropsychological evaluations. In some patients, a misdiagnosis of arrested hydrocephalus may prevent remediable conditions being treated [22, 33, 36]. In some circumstances, a decompensation can be noticed, often necessitating urgent surgical therapy months or even years after an apparently uneventful clinical course. However, reversal of the arrest should not be considered an exceptional event, as it has been reported in about one-quarter of cases, even when normal intracranial pressure recordings have initially been demonstrated [37]. Progression of the ventricular dilation, even though mild, deterioration in intellectual performance, and the occurrence of neurological symptoms and signs such as recurrent headaches, decrease in visual acuity, staring spells, and increasing motor and sensorial deficits of the inferior limits should lead to a prompt reevaluation of the hydrocephalus. Most of the caution which exists about deciding to insert a CSF shunt device in myelodysplasic children with chronic hydrocephalus, or to revise a CSF shunt which is presumed not to be working, has arisen from the known high risk of complications related to the insertion of a CSF shunting device.

A recent reappraisal of CSF shunting procedures without tubes, namely third-ventriculostomy, may provide at least a partial answer to this problem. It is worth noting that the procedure seems to be less effective in the newborn period than in later life [38, 39], a finding which might further confirm the predominant role of intracranial fluid imbalance in

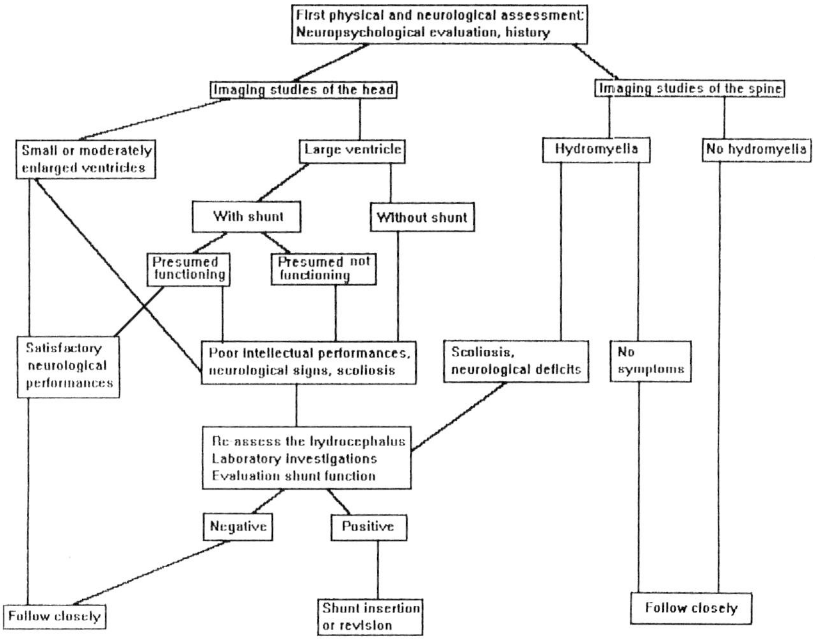

FIG. 1. Algorithm for chronic hydrocephalus associated with spina bifida

the early phases of ventricular hydrocephalus, and of obstructive factors in the late chronic phases.

Conclusions

Although the ventricular dilation associated with spina bifida seems to have a reasonable chance of reaching a state of chronic compensation ("arrest"), its possible evolution towards an obstructive hydrocephalus means that myelodysplasic patients are at risk of sudden deterioration for their entire life. In some patients where chronic hydrocephalus is presumed to be arrested, subtle neurological manifestations may actually correspond to the slow progression of the ventricular dilation, and thus suggest the need for further examination (Fig. 1). Neuroimaging studies, repeated neurological and neuropsychological examinations, and, in selected cases, the study of CSF dynamics, using indirect or direct evaluation of CSF flow pressure, should be considered in any case of doubt concerning the real arrest of the ventricular dilation.

References

1. McLone DG, Naidich TP (1989) Myelomeningocele: outcome and late complications. In: McLaurin RL, Epstein F (eds) Pediatric neurosurgery: surgery of the developing nervous system, 2nd edn. Saunders, Philadelphia, pp 53–70
2. Steinbock P, Irvine B, Cochrane DD, Irwin BJ (1992) Long-term outcome and complications of children born with myelomeningocele. Child's Nerv Syst 8:92

3. Caldarelli M, Di Rocco C, Colosimo C Jr, Fariello G, Di Gennaro M (1995) Surgical treatment of late neurological deterioration in children with myelodysplasia. Acta Neurochir 137:199
4. Obenchain TG, Stern WE (1973) Continuous pressure monitoring in experimental obstructive hydrocephalus. I. The dynamics of acute ventricular obstruction. Arch Neurol 29:287
5. Lundberg NG (1960) Continuous recording and control of ventricular pressure in neurosurgical practice. Acta Psychiatr Scand 36(Suppl 149):168
6. Milhorat TH, Clark RG, Hammock MK, McGrath PP (1970) Structural, ultrastructural and permeability changes in the ependyma and surrounding brain favoring equilibration in progressive hydrocephalus. Arch Neurol 22:397
7. Hochwald GM, Lux WE, Sahar A, Ransohoff J (1972) Experimental hydrocephalus. Changes in cerebrospinal fluid dynamics as a function of time. Arch Neurol 26:120
8. Bering EA, Sato O (1963) Hydrocephalus: changes in formation and absorption of cerebrospinal fluid within the cerebral ventricles: J Neurosurg 20:1050
9. Ogata J, Hochwald GM, Cravioto H, Ransohoff J (1972) Light and electron microscopic studies of experimental hydrocephalus. Acta Neuropathol (Berlin) 21:213
10. Di Rocco C (1987) The treatment of infantile hydrocephalus, vol 1. CRC Press, Boca Raton, pp 17–69
11. Milhorat TH (1987) Cerebrospinal fluid and the brain edemas. Neuroscience Society of New York, New York, p 145
12. Levin VA, Milhorat TH, Ferstermacher JD, Hammock MK, Rall DP (1971) Physiological studies on the development of obstructive hydrocephalus in the monkey. Neurology 21:238
13. McLone DG (1972) Development of brain extracellular space in hydrocephalic (Hy-3) mice. J Neurol Neurosurg Psychiatr 36:155
14. Rosenberg GA, Saland L, Kyner WT (1983) Pathophysiology of periventricular tissue changes with raised CSF pressure in cats. J Neurosurg 59:606
15. Endo S, Oka N, Nokade J, Harada J, Nagahori T, Tokaku A (1996) Changes of the cerebrovascular bed in experimental hydrocephalus. Curr Trends Hyd (Tokyo) 6:23
16. Laurence KM, Coates S (1962) The natural history of hydrocephalus. Arch Dis Child 37:345
17. Pudenz RH, Russell FE, Hurd AH, Shelden CH (1957) Ventriculo-auricolostomy: a technique for shunting cerebrospinal fluid into the right auricle (preliminary report). J Neurosurg 14: 171
18. Spitz EB (1959) Neurosurgery in the prevention of exogen mental retardation. Pediatr Clin N Am 6:1215
19. Laurence KM, Coates S (1967) Spontaneously arrested hydrocephalus. Results of the reexamination of 82 survivors from a series of 182 unoperated cases. Dev Med Child Neurol 9(Suppl 13):4
20. Schick RW, Matson DD (1961) What is arrested hydrocephalus? J Pediatr 58:791
21. Rekate HL (1991) Comprehensive management of spina bifida. CRC Press, Boca Raton, pp 93–111
22. Rekate HL, Nelsen FE, Mack HL, Morrison G (1982) Establishing the diagnosis of shunt independence. Monogr Neurol Sci 8:223
23. Miyazawa T, Sato K, Ikeda Y, Nakamura N, Matsumoto K (1997) A rat model of spontaneously arrested hydrocephalus. A behavioured study. Child's Nerv Syst 13:189
24. Di Rocco C, Rende M (1987) Neural defects. Some remarks on the possible role of glycosaminoglycans in the genesis of the dysraphic state, the anomaly in the configuration of the posterior cranial fossa, and hydrocephalus. Child's Nerv Syst 3:334
25. Torack RM, Grave M (1980) Subependymal glycosaminoglycan network in adult and developing rat brain. Histochemistry 68:55
26. Ruge JR, Masciopinto J, Storr BB, McLone DG (1992) Anatomical progression of the Chiari II malformation. Child's Nerv Syst 8:86–91
27. Hall P, Lindscth R, Campbell R, Kalisbeck JE, Desonsa A (1975) Scoliosis and hydrocephalus in myelocele patients. The effects of ventricular shunting. J Neurosurg 50:174
28. Baltshauser E, Cavanagh N (1976) Hydrocephalus treated by compressive head wrapping. Arch Dis Child 51:399
29. Epstein F, Hochwald GM, Ransohoff J (1973) Neonatal hydrocephalus treated by compressive head wrapping. Lancet 1:636

30. Miyake H, Ohata T, Kajimoto Y, Osaka K, Yamashita M (1996) Shunt system and shunt problems. The history of study in Osaka Medical College. Curr Trends Hyd (Tokyo) 6:32
31. Mase M, Yamada K, Banus T, Ohara S, Miyachi T, Nagai H (1996) CSF flow velocity in aqueduct and intracranial compliance in normal pressure hydrocephalus after subarachnoid hemorrhage. Curr Trends Hyd (Tokyo) 6:42
32. Di Rocco C, McLone DG, Shimoji T, Raimondi AJ (1975) Continuous intraventricular cerebrospinal fluid pressure recording in hydrocephalic children during wakefulness and sleep. J Neurosurg 42:683
33. Caldarelli M, Di Rocco C, Rossi GF (1979) Lumbar subarachnoid infusion test in pediatric neurosurgery. Dev Med Child Neurol 21:71
34. Di Rocco C, Maira G, Rossi GF, Vignati A (1976) Cerebrospinal fluid pressure studies in normal pressure hydrocephalus and cerebral atrophy. Eur Neurol 14:119–128
35. Di Rocco C (1982) Shunt dependency in myelomeningocele. Monogr Neurol Sci 8:117
36. Rekate HL (1988) Management of hydrocephalus and the erroneous concept of shunt independence in spina bifida patients. BNI Q 4:17
37. Whittle IR, Johnston IH, Besser M (1985) Intracranial pressure changes in arrested hydrocephalus. J Neurosurg 62:77
38. Teo C, Jones R (1996) Management of hydrocephalus by endoscopic third ventriculostomy in patients with myelomeningocele. Pediatr Neurosurg 25:57–63
39. Grant JA, McLone DG (1997) Third ventriculostomy: a review. Surg Neurol 47:210–212

Developmental Outcome in Spinal and Cranial Dysraphism

Shuzo Okuno, Tohru Hoshida, Tetsuya Morimoto, and Toshisuke Sakaki

Summary. We retrospectively investigated the factors affecting the independent social outcome of 23 patients with spinal or cranial dysraphism surgically treated in our department over 25 years. All patients were diagnosed at birth, and their social adaptability was assessed from the physical and mental viewpoints. Of the 12 spinal patients, two died due to gross congenital heart diseases. The follow-up periods ranged from 3 to 27 years (mean 10.9 years) for 10 survivors with spinal lesion, and from 2 to 28 years (mean 12.6 years) for 11 patients with cranial lesion. Six of the 12 spinal and 6 of the 11 cranial dysraphism patients were engaged in socially independent living. The neurologic level of L3 or above is suggested to be the sole factor affecting the prognosis in patients with spinal dysraphism. Hydrocephalus, if any, had no effect on the prognosis. In cranial dysraphism, the histological type and the existence of associated gross anomalies were thought to be of prognostic significance. The clinical evidence of primary, secondary, and no hydrocephalus also caused a significantly different outcome.

Key words. Spinal dysraphism, Cranial dysraphism, Hydrocephalus, Myelocele, Cephalocele

Introduction

Dysraphism in the central nervous system may occur alone or in association with other neurological conditions. Even if the reconstructive surgery succeeded in arresting the progression of symptoms and/or solving the cosmetic problems, the validity of aggressive treatment could not necessarily be justified. Occasionally, patients treated with early repair would suffer immensely from neurological, mental, and physical sequelae throughout their life [1, 7, 9]. The developmental outcome of dysraphism reported in large series has not been encouraging [2, 3, 5, 8, 10]. Some authors advocated the routine use of selection programs for infants with spinal dysraphism, and reported that the favorable prognosis in selected patients would be expected by early aggressive treatment [6, 9]. Cranial dysraphism has not been investigated in major series as a separate entity, and the selection of aggressive treatment has not been established. Although the ethical limitations indigenous to each country would influence decision making in the treatment of dysraphism, it is important to predict the social adaptability in the future of the affected infants. To serve this purpose, we have retrospectively eval-

Department of Neurosurgery, Nara Medical University, 840 Shijo-cho, Kashihara, Nara 634, Japan

uated the factors affecting the independent social outcome in 23 randomly selected and surgically treated patients (12 spinal and 11 cranial).

Materials and Methods

Patient Population

Between 1970 and 1995, 12 spinal and 11 cranial dysraphic patients were treated surgically at Nara Medical University (Tables 1 and 2). The spinal dysraphic patients were 5 males and 7 females. Two of them had meningomyelocele and died at 43 and 68 days after birth, due to severe congenital heart diseases. The 10 survivors ranged in age from 3 to 27 years (mean 10.9 years). There were 2 meningoceles, 8 meningomyeloceles (2 dead), and 2 lipomeningomyeloceles. Regarding the neurological level, 9 were below L3, and 3 were L3 or above. In two patients (cases 2 and 7) having L4 neurological level at birth, the activity of the lower limbs deteriorated later to involve L3 level. Hydrocephalus was present in 8 patients; 4 were primary at birth and 4 developed secondary to the surgical closure. Seven patients had some associated anomalies: serious congenital heart diseases in two, Arnold–Chiari malformation in two, and partial dysgenesis of the corpus callosum, exstrophy of the cloaca, and Chiari type 1 malformation complicated with microphthalmos in one each. The patients with cranial dysraphism were 7 males and 4 females with a mean age of 12.6 years (range 2–28 years). Seven had meningocele, 3 meningoencephalocele, and 1 meningoencephalocyctocele. Two of the 7 meningocele patients probably had an atretic type of cephalocele. Four were located in the parietal, 6 in the occipital, and 1 in the basisphenoidal region. The size of the sac ranged from 1 to 6 cm (mean 3.0 cm) in maximum diameter. Hydrocephalus was present in 3 at birth and in 4 following surgical reconstruction. Other associated anomalies were seen in 6 of the 11 patients: agenesis of the corpus callosum in two, and Arnold–Chiari malformation, porencephaly, holoprosencephaly, and cleft palate in one each. One patient had high cervical (C1-3) myeloschisis, which could not definitely be distinguished from Chiari type 3 malformation.

The patients' physical and mental conditions were separately analyzed and assigned as either "dependent" or "independent" after considering the clinical and radiological findings.

Clinical Presentation

The 10 survivors with spinal dysraphism had various degrees of motor weakness in their lower limbs. In 6 patients, paralysis was negligible and all could engage in a socially independent life without aids. Three suffered moderately, and were allowed to locomote with the assistance of braces and considerable medical support, and all were assigned as physically dependent. One had severe paraplegia, his locomotion was possible only with wheelchair, and her life entirely depended on constant medical support. In two patients, the neurological level deteriorated from L4 at birth to L3. In one of them, this event changed his quality of life from "independent" to "dependent." The surgical treatment might have caused this deterioration, but the actual reason is not clear. On the other hand, mentally disabilities were seen in 2 of the 10 spinal survivors; both of them were complicated with Arnold–Chiari malformation. The other 8 had enough intelligence to live independently with an IQ of more than 80. Of the 11 patients with cranial dysraphism, 6 had no motor weakness, and two had insignificant hemiparesis. The remaining 3 patients had critical hemiparesis or tetraparesis, and constant medical support was essential for living. Five of the 11 patients had mental retardation, with an IQ of less than 80. All of them had some associated anomalies, but no fatalities occurred in this group.

Table 1. Summary of 12 cases with myeloceles

Case	Age (years)/sex	Histology	Neurological level	Hydrocephalus	Other anomaly	Physical disability	Mental disability	Social outcome
1	27/F	MMC	S1	Primary	DCC	Mild	No	I
2	22/F	MMC	L3	Primary	Arnold–Chiari	Moderate	Yes	D
3	18/F	MC	S1	No	No	Mild	No	I
4	43 days/M	MC	S2	No	Severe heart disease	n/a	n/a	Dead
5	10/F	MMC	L5	Primary	Chiari type 1	Mild	No	I
6	9/F	LMMC	L3	No	Exstrophy of the cloaca	Severe	No	D
7	7/M	MMC	L3	Secondary	No	Moderate	No	D
8	5/M	LMMC	L5	Secondary	No	Mild	No	I
9	4/M	MMC	S1	Secondary	No	Mild	No	I
10	4/M	MMC	L1	Secondary	Arnold–Chiari, polydactyly	Moderate	Yes	D
11	3/F	MMC	S1	No	No	Mild	No	I
12	68 days/F	MMC	L3	Primary	Severe heart disease	n/a	n/a	Dead

M, meningocele; MMC, meningomyelocele; LMMC, lipomeningomyelocele; DCC, dysgenesis of the corpus callosum; n/a, not applicable; I, independent; D, dependent.

Table 2. Summary of 11 cases with cephaloceles

Case	Age (years)/sex	Histology	Site	Size (cm)	Hydrocephalus	Other anomaly	Physical disability	Mental disability	Social outcome
1	28/M	ME	P	3	Primary	Porencephaly, ACC	Mild	Yes	D
2	24/M	M	P	2	Primary	Holoprosencephaly	Severe	Yes	D
3	14/M	MEC	O	5	Secondary	C1-3 myeloschisis	Severe	Yes	D
4	13/M	M	P	2	No	No	No	No	I
5	13/F	M	O	3	No	No	No	No	I
6	10/F	M	BS	3	Secondary	Cleft palate	Mild	No	I
7	10/F	ME	O	5	Secondary	Arnold–Chiari	Moderate	Yes	D
8	9/M	M	O	1	No	No	No	No	I
9	8/F	ME	O	2	Primary	ACC	No	Yes	D
10	7/M	M	P	1	No	No	No	No	I
11	2/M	M	O	6	Secondary	No	No	No	I

M, meningocele; ME, meningoencephalocele; MEC, meningoencephalocystocele; P, parietal; O, occipital; BS, basisphenoidal; ACC, agenesis of the corpus callosum; I, independent; D, dependent.

Surgical Treatment

Simple dysraphism without major congenital anomalies is always treated surgically at our institution, regardless of the size, location, and histologic type of lesion. The surgical indication for highly complicated dysraphism should be determined according to whether the associated anomalies could have a gross effect on the future life of the patients or not. Although the physical disabilities, including the motor activity, could be guessed from routine radiological and neurological examinations, it is difficult to distinguish mentally disabled babies from normal ones during the neonatal period. Consequently, it becomes necessary to inform the parents fully about the future quality of life of their children, so that they can accept the sequelae of surgery. Two cases with spinal dysraphism and severe congenital heart diseases were considered unsuitable for any surgical treatment, but were operated on at the parents' request. The primary goal of surgery was to return the herniated neuronal elements, if any, to the spinal canal or the cranial cavity, which were fully covered by dura matter or patch graft to close the wound anatomically in layers with healthy muscle and skin. We performed surgery within the first 7 days of life on the majority of patients with spinal dysraphism. In cranial lesions, surgery was not urgent except for cases of CSF leakage, and was performed at a time when the parents had been fully informed and the risk of surgery was diminished.

For the surgical treatment of hydrocephalus, shunting procedures have been used. Routinely, we employed ventriculo-peritoneal shunts. The number of procedures in patients with hydrocephalus ranged from 1 to 7 in spinal dysraphism (mean 2.6) and from 2 to 4 in cranial dysraphism (mean 3.3). The shunt procedure was done early when necessary.

Developmental Outcome

For social independence, it is necessary to specify the requirements for "independent" in both physical and mental conditions. Physically, patients with "no" or "mild" disabilities were recognized to be "independent." In mental disabilities, "no" indicated patients with an IQ of more than 80.

In spinal dysraphism, 6 of the 10 survivors lived independently. All of them had minimal motor weakness but no gross mental retardation. Another two patients had almost normal intelligence, but were classified as "dependent" because of exstrophy of the cloaca in one and deterioration of neurological level from L4 to L3 in the other. The remaining 2 patients were severely disabled both physically and mentally. Regarding the cranial lesions, no medical support was or would be required in 6 of 11 patients: 5 had no apparent paralysis and were in a normal mental condition, and 1 had basisphenoidal meningocele associated with cleft palate but was intellectually normal. All of the 5 dependent patients had severe mental retardation, and motor activity was classed as normal in 1 and severely disabled in 4.

Results

First, the correlation of various factors with the social outcome in patients with spinal dysraphism is presented. The type of histology and the timing of surgery did not affect the outcome. A neurological level of L3 or above had a significant effect on the outcome (Table 3). From a practical point of view, the involvement of L3 neurological level is manifested by almost complete paralysis of the hip and knee joints. The presence and type of hydrocephalus had no prognostic value either. The presence of other anomalies, as seen in 7 of our series (5 of the 6 dependent patients and 2 dead), was not related to the outcome. Two patients lived independently despite having other anomalies, because of their minimal neurological man-

TABLE 3. Outcome and Neurological level of the 10 survivors with myeloceles

	L3 or above	Below L3
Independent	0	6
Dependent	4	0

For the correlation between neurological level and outcome, $P < 0.01$ (Fisher's exact test).

TABLE 4. Outcome and the histologic type of cephalocele

	M	ME	MEC
Independent	6	0	0
Dependent	1	3	1

M, meningocele; ME, meningoencephalocele; MEC, meningoencephalocystocele.
For the correlation between histological type and outcome, $P = 0.015$ (M: ME + MEC, Fisher's exact test).

TABLE 5. Outcome with hydrocephalus

	Hydrocephalus		
	Primary	Secondary	No
Independent	0	2	4
Dependent	3	2	0

For the correlation between independent and dependent patients in the three groups, $P < 0.05$ (χ^2 test).

ifestations; one had partial dysgenesis of the corpus callosum (case 1) and the second had Chiari type 1 malformation (case 5). In 11 patients with cranial dysraphism, the histology of the lesion was statistically significant for the prognosis (Table 4). All the 4 patients with obvious neuronal elements in the sac had a poor outcome. All the 7 meningocele patients, except one who had an associated holoprosencephaly at birth, had a good prognosis. The site of the cephalocele was not significant. The size of the cephalocele was measured in 9 of the 11 patients and had no prognostically significant effect, although it seemed that the larger lesions had a poorer outcome. The differences of symptoms with primary, secondary, or no hydrocephalus had a statistical significance on the outcome (Table 5). The existence of other anomalies had a significant impact on the outcome. In 5 of 6 complicated patients, the associated anomalies were thought to have a "gross" effect on the prognosis (Table 6). Only one patient had cleft palate and was not regarded as having "gross" anomalies. The timing of surgery had no influence on the prognosis.

TABLE 6. Outcome with other associated anomalies

	Yes	No
Independent	1	5
Dependent	5	0

For the correlation between other associated anomalies and outcome, $P = 0.015$ (Fisher's exact test).

Discussion

Spinal/cranial dysraphism is frequently associated with various physical and neurological anomalies. The surgical indication for patients with simple dysraphism may be straightforward, but for complex dysraphic patients, controversial arguments about the surgical treatment have been made, partly because of the ethical problems indigenous to various countries (6, 9). For spinal lesion, Lorber's adverse criteria have been used to exclude patients unsuitable for surgical treatment in some countries. However, this is not always true for other countries and all parents. Informed consent is essential, but the social adaptability of the patients should be the most important issue. Employment, pecuniary matters, and marriage will always be important in the patient's life [1, 7, 9]. The burden on the community must be taken into account. In our institution, the policy of whether aggressive treatment should be undertaken is not uniformly prescribed, and the decision about surgery has to be made individually. Our results from surgical treatment of spinal and cranial dysraphism were not satisfactory, and almost resembled the outcome of a large series of randomly selected cases [2–5].

We do not recommend surgical treatment for patients with critical mental retardation, although this cannot be satisfactorily proven at birth. Two of the patients with spinal lesion had mental disability, and both also had Arnold–Chiari malformation. Partial dysgenesis of the corpus callosum and Chiari type 1 malformation appeared to have no effect on the mental condition. In 5 mentally retarded patients with cranial dysraphism, 4 had meningoencephalocele or meningoencephalocystocele, and in all 5 patients these were complicated by both primary hydrocephalus and gross anomalies of the central nervous system. This indicated that the patients with cephalocele containing some brain tissue would have very complicated neuropsychological sequelae. Agenesis of the corpus callosum, as seen in 2 patients, affected the prognosis. The critical degree of dysgenesis of the corpus callosum is not known. It may be important to state that "gross" neurological anomalies were a negative indicator for aggressive treatment.

In spinal dysraphism, the involved level was the sole factor affecting the independent social outcome. The involvement of L3 level is crucial, and distinguishes locomotion requiring considerable support from that without support. From this standpoint, Lorber's criteria seem reasonable. Reconstructive surgery for patients with L4 neurological level should be conducted very carefully, because involvement of L3 would result in a critical deterioration in the quality of life. As to cranial dysraphism, 2 of the 3 patients with critical motor weakness had a huge cephalocele containing massive brain tissue. In one, holoprosencephaly was thought to cause the motor weakness. We believe that the motor function in patients with spinal and cranial dysraphism can, to some degree, be evaluated from a routine neurological check-up and anatomical examination by magnetic resonance imaging.

Some reports stated that the presence of hydrocephalus would worsen the prognosis of the spinal dysraphic patients [6, 8]. In our study, no significant effect was seen on the prognosis, and the shunt procedure was effective for the treatment of primary and secondary hydrocephalus. On the other hand, the presence of hydrocephalus in patients with cranial dysraphism was of some prognostic significance, and comparable to the results given in the previous reports [2, 4]. The degree of hydrocephalus and its responsiveness to the shunt procedure were not different between primary and secondary hydrocephalus. This indicates that primary hydrocephalus may represent only one of the anomalies in highly complex dysraphism, and the irreversible brain damage have existed at birth.

We concluded that, in spinal dysraphism, the level of neurological insults is the sole and most important indicator for social independence, although the associated neurological and physical anomalies should be considered when aggressive therapy is indicated. In cranial dysraphism, surgery for encephalocele or encephalocystocele patients may be performed selectively because of the common association with other gross anomalies in the central nervous system.

References

1. Begeer IH, Staal-Schreinemachers AL (1996) The benefits of team treatment and control of adult patients with spinal dysraphism. Eur J Pediatr Surg 6, Suppl 1:15–16
2. Brown MS, Sheridan-Pereira M (1992) Outlook for the child with a cephalocele. Pediatrics 90:914–919
3. Czech T, Reinprecht A, Matula C, Svoboda H, Vorkapic P (1995) Cephaloceles-experience with 42 patients. Acta Neurochir (Wien) 134:125–129
4. Date I, Yagyu Y, Asari S, Ohmoto T (1993) Long-term outcome in surgically treated encephalocele. Surg Neurol 40:125–130
5. Date I, Yagyu Y, Asari S, Ohmoto T (1993) Long-term outcome in surgically treated spina bifida cystica. Surg Neurol 40:471–475
6. Gross RH, Cox A, Tatyrek R, Pollay M, Barnes WA (1983) Early management and decision making for the treatment of myelomeningocele. Pediatrics 72:450–458
7. Kalucy M, Bower C, Stanley F (1996) School-aged children with spina bifida in Western Australia—parental perspectives on functional outcome. Dev Med Child Neurol 38:325–334
8. Lorber J (1971) Results of treatment of myelomeningocele. An analysis of 524 unselected cases, with special reference to possible selection for treatment. Dev Med Child Neurol 13:279–303
9. Lorber J, Salfield SAW (1981) Results of selective treatment of spina bifida cystica. Arch Dis Child 56:822–830
10. Martinez-Lage JF, Poza M, Sola J, Soler CL, Montalvo CG, Domingo R, Puche A, Ramon FH, Azorin P, Lasso R (1996) The child with a cephalocele: etiology, neuroimaging, and outcome. Child's Nerv Syst 12:540–550

Possibility of Ventriculoperitoneal Shunt (VPS) Removal in Hydrocephalic Patients with Meningomyelocele (MMC)

Yoshio Takahashi and Kohshi Tatewaki

Introduction

Although shunt operations are definitely effective in the management of hydrocephalus, the flow of cerebrospinal fluid becomes dependent on the shunt, and there is the disadvantage that the shunt cannot be removed even though reconstruction of the cerebrum itself has been achieved.

Therefore, children who have undergone shunt surgery are always anxious about shunt malfunction occurring, and the presence of the shunt itself is a handicap in countries such as Japan where discrimination exists.

Therefore, removal of the ventriculoperitoneal shunt is strongly desired by such children and their families after the clinical situation has stabilized. This is the great dream of these children and their families.

We attempted shunt removal in children with MMC and report the clinical outcome here. We also report the usefulness of a programmable valve in shunt removal.

Subjects and Methods

The subjects were 28 patients who had undergone shunt surgery for MMC associated with hydrocephalus, in whom removal was attempted when shunt malfunction occurred or when the shunt became too short during growth. Imaging of the shuntgraphy was performed in all subjects, and the shuntgraphy helped to decide if the shunt could be removed or not. The Medos programmable valve was used in 17 of the 28 subjects from the time of the initial shunt operation.

Shunt removal was attempted in 11 children in whom the programmable valve was not used in the initial shunt operation, and removal was possible in three (27%) of these. In five of the remaining eight patients, shunt removal was judged to be impossible based on the shuntgraphy imaging and operative findings, and reconstruction was performed. In three patients, shunt reconstruction was performed within 5 days after the operation because symptoms occurred and ventricular enlargement appeared after shunt removal.

Department of Pediatric Neurosurgery, Hokkaido Children's Hospital and Medical Center, 1-10-1 Zenibeko, Otaru, Hokkaido 047-02, Japan

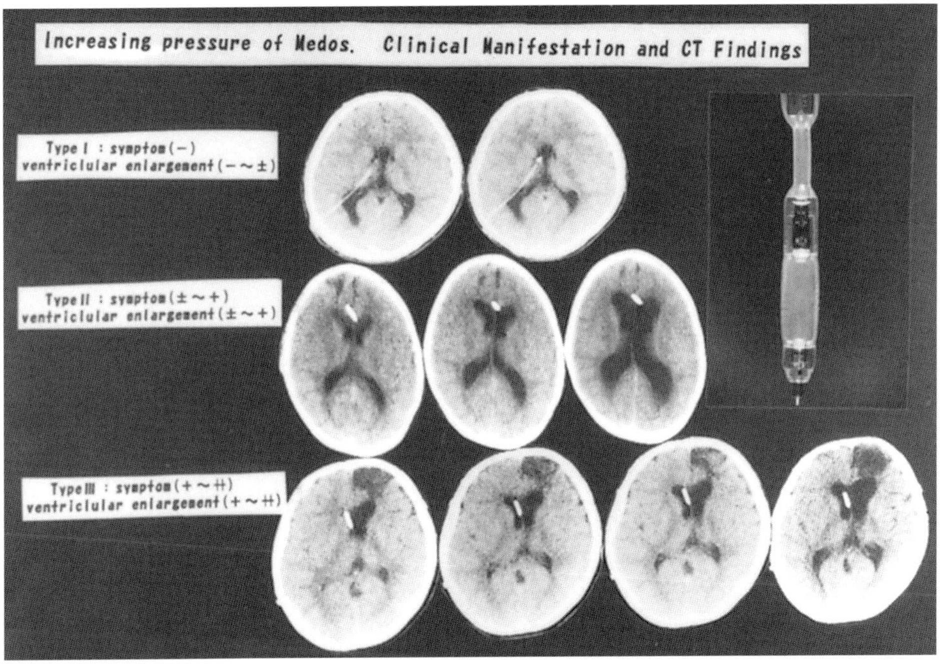

FIG. 1. Changes in computed tomography (CT) findings and symptoms after increasing setting pressure in Medos programmable valve

Shunt removal was attempted in 17 patients in whom the initial shunt pressure had gradually been increased using the programmable valve, and removal was possible in nine patients (53%).

Figure 1 shows changes in the computed tomography (CT) findings and symptoms after the pressure setting was increased in patients with a Medos programmable valve who had hydrocephalus without MMC. Changes after the pressure increase were divided into three types. In type I, no ventricular enlargement was observed on CT, and no symptoms appeared after the pressure increase. In type II, ventricular enlargement was observed on CT, but symptoms were mild. In type III, both ventricular enlargement on CT and prominent symptoms developed.

Almost the same course was observed in MMC patients with hydrocephalus who underwent shunt surgery. Shunt removal was impossible in eight of the 17 patients in whom it was attempted. Six of these eight patients showed prominent symptoms after the pressure was increased. Ventricular enlargement was also present, and they were classified as the type III pattern. The pressure was lowered when shunt reconstruction was performed. In two patients showing the type II pattern with ventricular enlargement but mild symptoms, removal was attempted but the shunt had to be reconstructed due to symptoms worsening and progressive ventricular enlargement at 2–3 weeks after removal.

Two of the nine patients showed the type I pattern, with a pressure increase but no symptoms and no ventricular enlargement, and their shunts were removed (Fig. 2). The type II pattern, with mild symptoms and slight ventricular enlargement, was observed in four of the nine patients. In these patients, the pressure was gradually increased over a period of 1–2

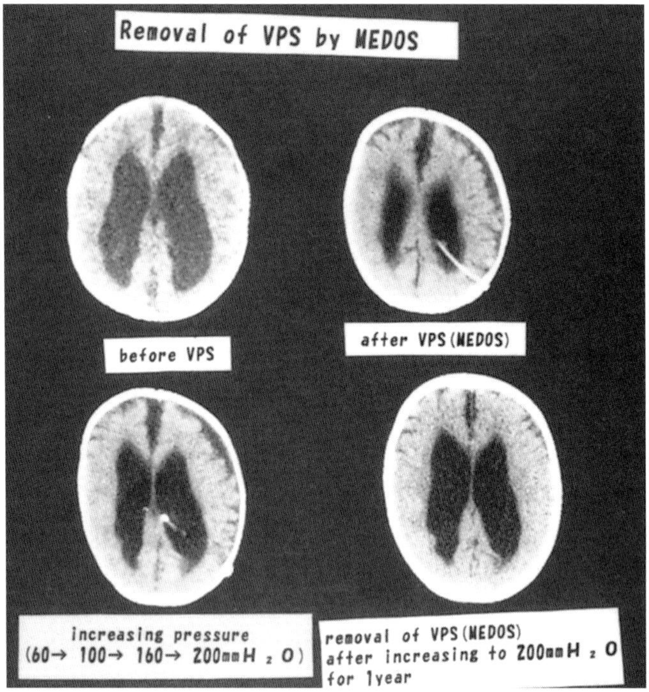

FIG. 2. Serial CT findings in removal of ventriculoperitoneal shunt (VPS) by programmable valve

years, and the shunt was finally removed (Fig. 3). In two of the nine patients, reconstruction was performed using a specially ordered Sophy valve, which permitted a pressure setting above 200 mm H_2O because of the symptoms and ventricular enlargement caused by pressure elevation. The pressure was subsequently increased over about 1 year, and then the shunt could be removed (Fig. 4). In one of the nine patients, the increase in pressure caused inactivity and ventricular enlargement, and the shunt was removed about 2 weeks after neuroendoscopic 3rd ventriculostomy (Fig. 5).

In patients with successful shunt removal, no worsening of clinical symptoms appeared over a follow-up period of 1–2 years.

Based on our experience, it appears that shunt removal was possible in six patients because of the efficacy of the programmable valves. Removal was also successful in two patients with no symptoms following an increase of pressure, and in one patient who had neuroendoscopy.

Discussion

One of the dreams after cerebral reconstruction by shunt surgery for hydrocephalus is releasing the child from dependency on the shunt. The probability of shunt removal was only about 30% before the introduction of programmable valves. Basically, the same was true for MMC shunts.

However, the present study showed that the use of programmable valves for patients in whom shunt removal was previously impossible allows a gradual increase of pressure at the

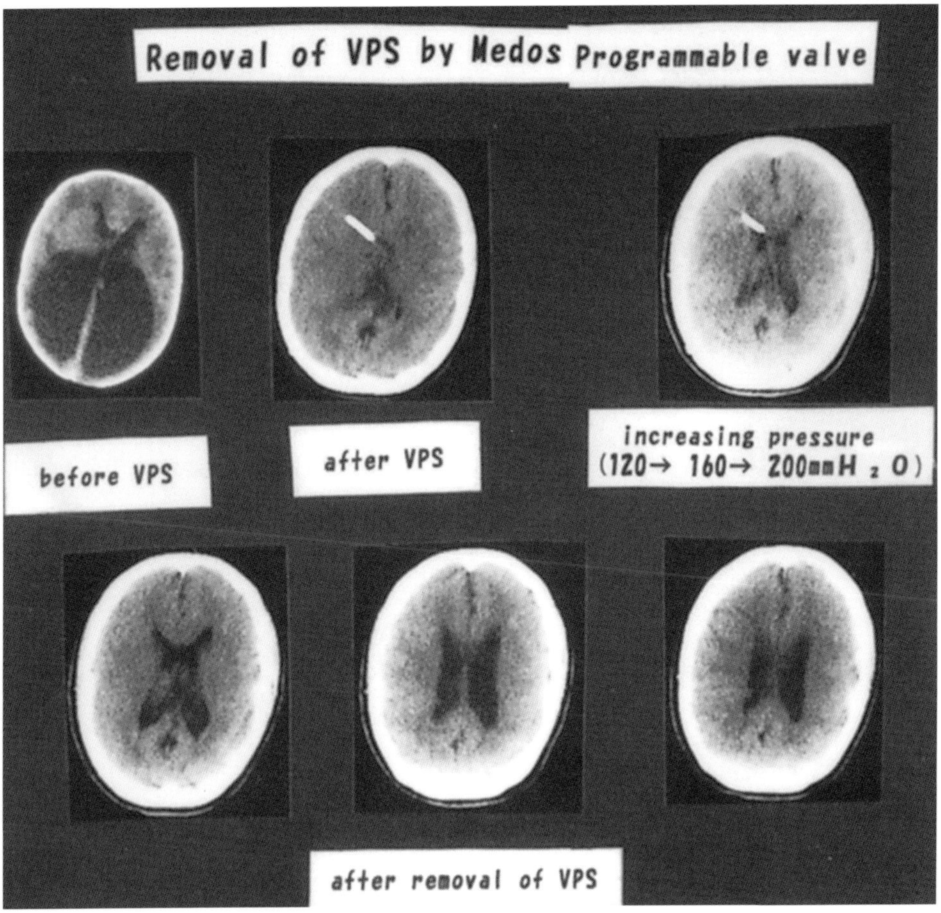

FIG. 3. Serial CT findings in removal of VPS after long-time high-pressure setting

stage of cerebral reconstruction, activates normal circulation of the cerebrospinal fluid, and increases the possibility of shunt removal.

The present study showed that shunt removal is possible in half of the patients with MMC shunts if a programmable valve is used. Aqueduct stenosis is often present in children with MMC and hydrocephalus. In such patients, pressure is increased with a programmable valve, the ventricles become enlarged, and neuroendoscopic 3rd ventriculostomy can be performed. Accordingly, the number of patients in whom shunt removal is possible can be further increased.

Among the various programmable valves available, the Medos valve is designed so that the maximum pressure is 200 mm H_2O, but the specially ordered Sophy valve has a higher pressure setting (above 200 mm H_2O) which should allow more cases of successful shunt removal.

Early shunt surgery is effective in achieving good therapeutic results in children with MMC and hydrocephalus, and also improves their quality of life. Shunt surgery should be attempted at the stage when it is possible to reconstruct the brain and promote development of the immature brain as a means of minimizing the handicap caused by shunting. It should be

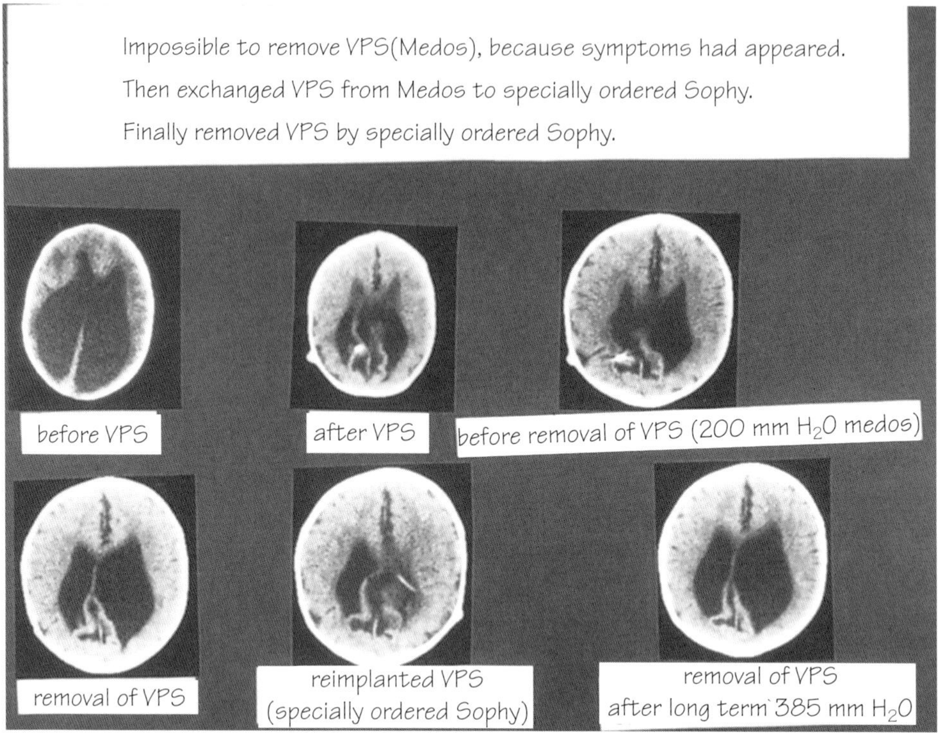

FIG. 4. Serial CT findings in removal of VPS, a case in which Medos was ineffective but specially ordered Sophy was effective

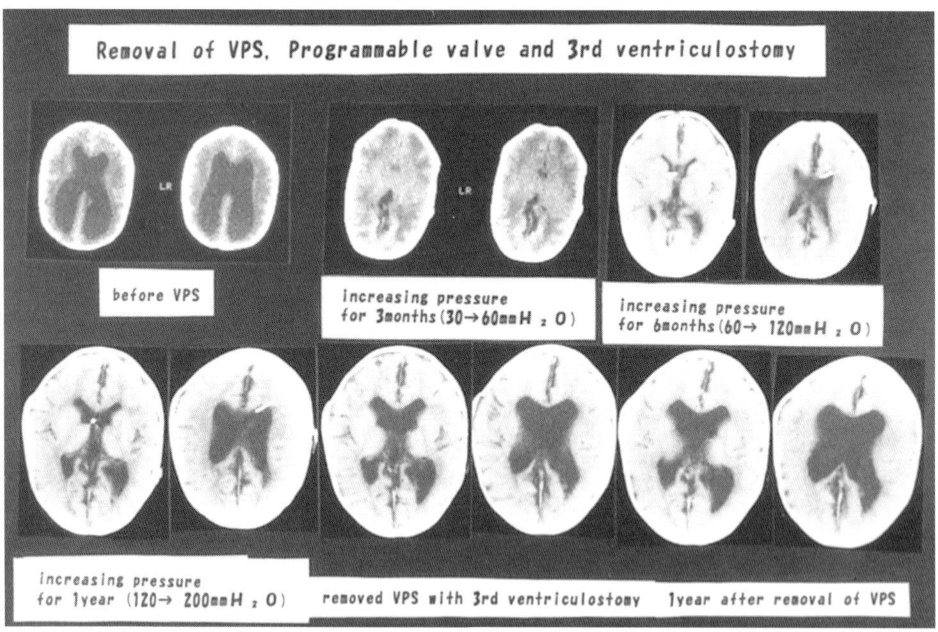

FIG. 5. Serial CT findings in removal of VPS (programmable valve and 3rd ventriculostomy)

emphasized that the probability of shunt removal is increased by using a programmable valve.

Programmable valves which can be used from the neonatal period are effective in ending dependence on the shunt and increasing the possibility of shunt removal. Shunts can be removed in about 50% of patients if the pressure is changed appropriately in accordance with age and cerebral development, and if their symptoms do not become worse. Thus, precise management in pediatric hydrocephalus is very important for the child's future.

Conclusions

1. Shunt removal and release of dependency on the shunt are possible in about 30% of children with MMC and hydrocephalus.
2. In about 30% of children whose shunts were thought not to be removable, removal became possible by gradually increasing the pressure with a programmable valve, thus changing their shunt-dependent cerebrospinal fluid circulation to a regular pattern. This means that shunt removal becomes possible in about 50% of patients with MMC if a programmable valve is used.
3. Since there is a high incidence of aqueduct stenosis in children with MMC and hydrocephalus, the frequency of shunt removal can probably be increased by ventricular enlargement via pressure increase using a programmable valve and subsequent neuroendoscopic 3rd ventriculostomy.

Neuroendoscopic Management of Shunt Complications

Michael Vloeberghs, Conor Mallucci, and Jonathan Punt

Summary. Because of our intense dissatisfaction with shunts and their secondary morbidity, endoscopic third ventriculostomy (ETV) as a primary treatment for hydrocephalus has been offered to 47 patients with shunt blockage, in whom 51 procedures were done. We report an overall success rate of ETV in patients with shunt blockage of 73%. Our conclusion is that ETV should be offered as first-line treatment of shunt blockage instead of shunt revision.

Key words. Neuroendoscopy, Third ventricle, Hydrocephalus, Shunt complications

Introduction

As paediatric neurosurgeons, a large part of our practice is the management of hydrocephalus. Despite advancements in materials, implantation techniques, and shunt design, we are still confronted with an appalling shunt failure rate (Tables 1 and 2).

Endoscopic third ventriculostomy (ETV) is an old procedure, which is now going through a renaissance because of renewed interest and recent advances in technology. Many questions regarding the indications and the correct technical execution of this procedure remain unanswered. However, this procedure is a major advance in the management of hydrocephalus, and gives the patient the opportunity to live a shunt-independent life.

In the global health care crisis and the sometimes extreme budgetary restrictions in which we work, ETV has important economic implications. Because of its "one off" character, the need for future interventions is greatly reduced.

Methods

The data presented are extracted from our permanently updated prospective database, which includes more than 150 neuroendoscopic procedures from August 1994 to August 1997. One hundred and three ETVs have been performed for the management of hydrocephalus, both as a primary treatment and as a treatment of shunt blockage. Fifty-one ETVs have been done in 47 patients with blocked shunts. Of these, 37 patients had been treated for hydrocephalus in our institution, and 10 patients were referred to our services for endoscopic treatment. The

Paediatric Neurosurgery, Queens Medical Centre, University Hospital, Nottingham NG7 2UH, UK

TABLE 1. History of the hydrocephalus

Age at first shunt: median 3 months (1 week to 240 months)
Number of shunt procedures: median 2 (1–18)
Number of shunt-related infectious episodes: 30 in 16 patients

TABLE 2. Fate of the original shunt

Left in place	25
Removed	11
Ligated	10
Liberated	2

All CSF diversions are ventriculo-peritoneal shunts.

median age is 118 months (9.8 years), ranging between 6 and 339 months (0.5–28.25 years), with a median follow-up of 13 months.

The history is obtained through a review of the national standardized notes, and a review of the imaging, clinical examination, and outpatient follow-up. The success of an ETV must be defined in two ways, i.e., clinical and technical success. An ETV can be technically successful but fail to relieve clinical symptoms, and so is to be considered as a failure of the technique. Clinical success of the procedure is defined as the absence of clinical symptoms, i.e., the absence of pressure signs, and control or stabilization of the head circumference where applicable. The clinical criterion is the most important. The technical outcome is defined as a successful operation with flux of CSF through the floor of the third ventricle at operation and on the postoperative magnetic resonance imaging (MRI). As mentioned above, this does not necessarily imply clinical success of the ETV. The presence of a flow jet through the floor of the third ventricle and redistribution of CSF around the brain is a measure of the technical success of the ETV on postoperative MRI. The postoperative imaging should be evaluated with regards to the clinical outcome. We have noted that after ETV the size of the ventricular system may remain static or decrease only slightly, and so we find ventricular size of only marginal importance as a measure of the success of the procedure.

Outcome

ETV was technically possible in 47 patients, and proved impossible or unsatisfactory in 4 patients. In 2 patients in whom ETV was not technically possible, the shunt catheter was freed from the ingrown scar tissue and the shunt resumed its function.

ETV alone relieved the symptoms of shunt blockage in 37 patients. Fourteen patients required an alternative procedure, of which 10 went on to have a shunt revision and 4 patients required the endoscopy to be redone (Table 3). Reseal of the ventriculostomy was seen in 2 patients who required an endoscopy to be redone. The ETV needed to be redone because of the presence of prominent membranes below the third ventricle floor, which caused failure of the first ETV. The remaining 2 patients required their endoscopy to be redone because Lilliequist's membrane had not been divided at the first endoscopy and pressure symptoms

TABLE 3. Time elapsed from ETV to alternative procedure (14 patients with failed ETV)

Shunt revision: median 1 week
Redone endoscopy: 4 patients
Success of redone ETV: 2 patients (15 months and 23 months after prior ETV)
Failure: 2 patients (1 month and 21 months after prior ETV)

TABLE 4. Etiology of the hydrocephalus

Aqueduct stenosis/dandy walker	13
Posthaemorrhagic	12
Postmeningitic	7
Dysraphic	7
Tumors	6
Other	2
Total	47

TABLE 5. Success of ETVin 47 patients by etiology

Tumour-related hydrocephalus	6/6	(100%)
Dysraphic	6/7	(88%)
Aqueduct stenosis/dandy walker	9/13	(69%)
Postmeningitic	4/7	(62%)
Posthaemorrhagic	6/12	(50%)
Other	1/2	(50%)

Overall success 73%.
50% of the ETVs performed for shunt blockages were done as an emergency because of the poor clinical status of the patient.

recurred. In both patients the floor of the third ventricle was open but Lilliequist's membrane was intact.

Results

The success rate of ETV is 73%, depending on the primary etiology of the hydrocephalus. Clearly obstructive hydrocephalus of whichever origin has the highest success rate, but in ETV for shunt blockage the success rate does not drop below 50% (Tables 4 and 5) [3, 5, 7]. On average the results of ETV show a 73% success. There are a limited number of complications (7 in 51 procedures), which are often of little consequence to the patient (Table 6).

The proper technique for third ventriculostomy is not established in the literature, and often little importance is given to the presence of Lilliequist's or other prepontine membranes [1, 4, 5, 7–9]. These membranes do have a pathological role and must be divided during the operation [1]. For the same reason the subarachnoid space below the third ventricle and in the optochiasmatic cisterns needs to be inspected. The presence of scarring of the sub-

TABLE 6. Complications of ETV for shunt malfunction

Infection	2 (1 superficial, 1 ventriculitits)
Paresis/palsy	2 (temporary IIIrd, permanent VIth)
Seizure	2
Haemorrhage	1 (the haemorrhage did not affect the procedure)
Total	7/51 procedures

arachnoid space or the impossibility of dividing an arachnoid membrane below the third ventricle is one cause of technical failure [2, 4, 6, 8, 9].

Many patients presented with a complicated shunt history, with multiple revisions or infectious episodes. The etiology of the hydrocephalus has a prognostic value for the success of the ETV, but it cannot predict which patient will benefit from ETV and which patient will fail (Table 5) [5].

So far no conclusive pattern has emerged which could allow us to predict the outcome for ETV in a particular patient. One possibility could be to do invasive isotope studies of the cerebro-spinal fluid circuit. Such studies would be very difficult in our patient population because of the often poor clinical status on admission and the urgency of the situation. For this reason we offer ETV indiscriminately to patients with shunt blockage, but counsel parents and patients by showing our statistics and offering a very basic overview of our success rate [3].

Conclusion

Endoscopic third ventriculostomy has become the cornerstone in the management of hydrocephalus in our department, both as a primary treatment and as a treatment for shunt blockage.

Because of the overwhelming success rate (73%) and low morbidity, we have come to the conclusion that ETV should be the first choice for the treatment of hydrocephalus of whichever origin. The success of ETV depends on the etiology of the hydrocephalus, the experience of the surgeon, and the proper execution of the technique.

Classic obstructive hydrocephalus has the highest success rate when compared with posthaemorrhagic and postmeningitic hydrocephalus. Because the effect of ETV on the relief of symptoms for the individual patient remains unpredictable at the moment, we consider this treatment as the first choice for the relief of hydrocephalus independent of age or the origin of the hydrocephalus.

References

1. Buxton N, Vloeberghs M, Punt J (1977) Lilliequist's membrane: a re-examination of its importance. Surg Radiol Anat J Clin Anat 19:14
2. Ellenbogen RG, Moores LE (1997) Endoscopic management of a pineal and suprasellar germinoma with associated hydrocephalus: technical case report. Minim Invasive Neurosurg 40:13–5
3. Ferrer E, Santamarta D, Garcia-Fructuoso G, Caral L, Rumià J (1997) Neuroendoscopic management of pineal region tumours. Acta Neurochir (Wien) 139:12–20

4. Grant JA, McLone DG (1997) Third ventriculostomy: a review. Surg Neurol 47:210; Jones RF, Kwok BC, Stening WA, Vonau (1996) Third ventriculostomy for hydrocephalus associated with spinal dysraphism: indications and contraindications. Eur J Pediatr Surg 6:5
5. Mallucci C, Vloeberghs M, Punt J (1997) Neuroendoscopic third ventriculostomy: the first-line treatment for blocked ventriculo-peritoneal shunts? Child's Nerv Syst 13:498
6. Teo C, Jones R (1996) Management of hydrocephalus by endoscopic third ventriculostomy in patients with myelomeningocele. Pediatr Neurosurg 25:57–63
7. Vinas FC, Dujovny N, Dujovny M (1996) Microanatomical basis for the third ventriculostomy. Minim Invasive Neurosurg 39:116–121
8. Vloeberghs M, Vangeneugden J, D'Haens J (1995) Third ventriculostomy using the "air bubble" technique. Acta Neurol Belg 95:119
9. Wilcock DJ, Jaspan T, Worthington BS, Punt J (1997) Neuro-endoscopic third ventriculostomy: evaluation with magnetic resonance imaging. Clin Radiol 52:50–54

Abstract

Clinical Significance of the Ventricular Size in Hydrocephalic Children

Shouhei Kitano and Hiroaki Sakamoto

Cerebrospinal fluid shunt for hydrocephalic children often induces slit-like ventricles, which may indicate reduced intracranial compliance. We tried to seek the most suitable size for the lateral ventricles in hydrocephalic children. Thirty-seven shunted hydrocephalic children (congenital hydrocephalus 15, myelomeningocele 12, other associated pathologies 10) who required emergent shunt revisions for obstructed shunt were analyzed retrospectively. The slit-like group ($n = 13$) consisted of cases in which the size of the lateral ventricles was less than 0.35 on Evan's index at the time of shunt obstruction, and the dilated group ($n = 24$) consisted of cases in which the size of the lateral ventricles was more than 0.36. Mean age in the slit-like group (from 2 to 17 years, with a mean of 7 years) was significantly greater than that in the dilated group (from 3 months to 9 years, with a mean of 3 years). In the slit-like group, the patients were hospitalized 0–5 days (mean 1.5 days) after onset, and 8 patients (62%) developed lethargy at the time of hospitalization. In the dilated group ($n = 24$), the patients were hospitalized 1–18 days (means 4.6 days) after onset, and only 4 patients (17%) showed lethargy. On the latest CT before shunt obstruction, all 13 patients in the slit-like group had an Evan's index of less than 0.33. In the dilated group. only 3 patients had small lateral ventricles of less than 0.33 on Evan's index. Because small ventricles may indicate significantly reduced intracranial compliance against shunt obstruction, it is recommended that the size of the lateral ventricles after shunting should be maintained at more than 0.33 on Evan's index in older children with hydrocephalus.

Department of Pediatric Neurosurgery, Osaka City General Hospital, 2-13-2 Miyakojima-hondori, Miyakojima-ku, Osaka 534, Japan

Abstract

Dual-Switch Valve: A New Concept in the Treatment of Hydrocephalus Avoiding Inappropriate Drainage

Hans Axel Trost[1], Christian Sprung[2], Christoph Miethke[3], Detlef Ernst Rosenow[4], and Wolfgang R. Lanksch[2]

Presently available hydrocephalus valves have two major drawbacks: they have a tendency to clog and/or they do not take into account the posture of the patient, resulting in unphysiological overdrainage in the upright position. School-age children and young adults bearing a low resistance shunt since their first years of life are prone to overdrainage-related problems such as subdural effusions, skull deformities, and slit ventricle syndrome. Changing these low-resistance shunts into medium- or high-resistance shunts may be one solution, but another way is the use of a siphon preventing device such as the ASD™ or the Delta™ valve, although these devices are prone to late malfunction due to shrinkage of the surrounding tissues. The development of a new hydrostatic controlled valve gives rise to a more optimistic view of shunt therapy.

The dual-switch™ valve has been implanted in more than 50 patients. Clinical performance is very satisfying. Ventricular size was reduced slowly and gently, with good clinical performance and—where applicable—normalized intracranial pressure values. There were no infectious problems, and no overdrainage-related complications were noted.

The very slow and slight reduction in ventricular size, as proved by CCT, is remarkable. This, together with the complete lack of overdrainage-related complications such as slit ventricles or subdural effusions, is thought to be the result of the more physiological drainage of CSF by the hydrostatic hydrocephalus valve. Clinical performance and patient acceptance of the dual-switch™ valve was encouraging.

---

[1] Department of Neurosurgery, Krankenhaus Bogenhausen, Technical University, München, Germany
[2] Department of Neurosurgery, Virchow-Klinikum, Humboldt-University, Berlin, Germany
[3] Christoph Miethke KG, Berlin, Germany
[4] Neurosurgical Clinic, University of Essen, Germany

Moderator's Comments on Sessions—Hydrocephalus

Tomio Tsuchida

In this session the treatment of hydrocephalus was discussed. Dr. Shouhei Kitano (Osaka City General Hospital, Japan) analyzed 37 cases of shunted hydrocephalic children (who required emergent shunt revisions for shunt obstruction) and tried to establish the most suitable size of lateral ventricle. He classified these cases into two groups, namely the slit-like group (n = 13), whose lateral ventricle was less than 0.35 on Evan's index at shunt revision, and the dilated group (n = 24), whose lateral ventricle was more than 0.36. Most patients belonging to the first group developed lethargy, and those in the second group did not. Small ventricles may indicate significantly reduced intracranial compliance against shunt obstruction. It was recommended that the size of the lateral ventricles after shunting should be maintained at more than 0.33 on Evan's index.

Dr. Yoshio Takahashi (Hokkaido Children's Hospital, Japan) analyzed 26 cases of shunt removal among 66 hydrocephalic children with MMC. Shunt removal was successful in 3/11 cases (27%) before the employment of programmable valves. When intracranial pressure had been gradually increased with programmable valves, shunt removal was performed successfully in 7/15 cases (45%). Takahashi reported that a high incidence of aqueductal stenosis had been found in these groups, and therefore the frequency of shunt removal would probably increase by performing neuroendoscopic 3rd ventriculostomy.

Dr. Hans Axel Trost (Technical University, Germany) proposed a new concept in the treatment of hydrocephalus which avoids inappropriate drainage, and showed his dual-switch valve. When this new hydrostatically controlled valve was used in 50 patients, ventricle size reduced slowly and steadily, while good clinical performance was maintained.

Dr. Michael Vloeberghs (University of Nottingham, UK) reported his experience of the treatment of hydrocephalic children using an endoscopic operation. From his own experience and from the literature on shunts, he found that in the past 25–40% failed within the first year of implantation. He has performed 40 neuroendoscopic third ventriculostomies. The overall success rate is 71%, and therefore he believes that neuroendoscopic third ventriculostomy should always be preferred as the first choice of treatment.

As described above, endoscopic surgery and/or a programmable shunt system (or a new model of such a system) were felt to be very useful for the treatment of hydrocephalus. When a suitable ventricular size can be maintained using these methods, they will be preferable for hydrocephalic children.

Tokyo Metropolitan Rehabilitation Center 3-17-2 Toyama, Shinjuku-ku, Tokyo 162-0052, Japan

Slit Ventricle Syndrome in Children: Clinical Presentation and Treatment

Joong-Uhn Choi and Dong-Seok Kim

Summary. The term "slit ventricle syndrome" (SVS) refers to an episodic occurrence of headache, vomiting, and possibly some degree of consciousness impairment in shunted hydrocephalic children in whom slit-like ventricles are seen on computed tomography (CT) scan or magnetic resonance imaging (MRI). We present six cases of SVS which we have seen at our institute in last 10 years.

From 1986 to 1996, 821 patients underwent shunt surgery for hydrocephalus. The etiology of the hydrocephalus included brain tumor (140 patients), posthemorrhagic hydrocephalus (62 patients), idiopathic normotensive hydrocephalus (64 patients), postmeningitic hydrocephalus (58 patients), posttraumatic hydrocephalus (54 patients), congenital hydrocephalus (48 patients), neurocysticercosis (31 patients), and unknown (364 patients). During the mean follow-up period of 68 months, shunt revision was performed on 232 cases, yielding a revision rate of 1.28 per patient. The incidence of SVS was 0.7% (6 cases).

Most of the patients had been operated on in infancy. The time from the first operation to the development of slit ventricle syndrome ranged from 4 to 8 years; the mean was 6 years. Shuntograms showed patent shunts in all patients. Two patients with less severe clinical symptoms improved with conservative treatment. Intracranial pressure (ICP) was not measured in these patients because of a good hospital course. One patient showed high ICP and needed only revision with the same pressure valve as in the previous shunt. Low ICP was noted in three patients. Pressure augmentation using an antisiphon device or an upgrading valve system were necessary in these patients.

The authors stress that determining the type of SVS is the first step in treatment, and that the best treatment is a strategy aimed at resolving the specific type of SVS responsible for the symptoms.

Key words. Slit ventricle syndrome, ICP monitoring, Overdrainage, Shuntogram, Shunt malfunction

Introduction

Complications of shunting due to overdrainage are poorly defined and understood, and therefore the treatment has been the subject of confusing literature. Slit ventricle syndrome (SVS) is one form of overdrainage problem in shunted children, and is defined as a symptom

Department of Neurosurgery, Brain Research Institute, Yonsei University College of Medicine, Severance Hospital, C.P.O. Box 8044, Seoul, Korea

complex suggestive of increased intracranial pressure with a slit-like appearance of the ventricular system on a computed tomography (CT) scan or magnetic resonance imaging (MRI).

The incidence of SVS is not well documented because of the variable way it has been defined, but it is probably 3–5%. The clinical characteristic of SVS differ so widely as to suggest that different clinical conditions are being described.

Materials and Methods

From 1986 to 1996, 861 patients underwent shunt surgery for hydrocephalus. The etiology of the hydrocephalus included brain tumor (140 patients), posthemorrhagic hydrocephalus (62 patients), idiopathic normotensive hydrocephalus (64 patients), postmeningitic hydrocephalus (58 patients), posttraumatic hydrocephalus (54 patients), congenital hydrocephalus (48 patients), neurocysticercosis (31 patients), and unknown (364 patients). During the mean follow-up period of 68 months, shunt revisions were performed in 232 cases. Among these 232 revisions, 43 (19%) were the elective lengthening of the distal catheter. Proximal obstruction (42.7%) was more frequent than distal obstruction (35.3%). There were 6 cases (0.7%) of SVS in our series. The treatments carried out were insertion of an antisiphon device in 3 patients, conservative treatment in 2 patients, and revision of the same pressure valve in 1 patient. All patients were followed for over 2 years by brain CT or MRI. The hospital records, the results of shuntograms and intracranial pressure (ICP) monitoring, and radiographic studies of these patients were reviewed.

Results

The symptoms of SVS consisted of intermittent episodes of headache, vomiting, and lethargy, and occasionally some neurological signs such as upward gaze paresis and ataxia. No one progressed to an unconscious state. All patients showed sluggish or absent refill of the pumping device and collapsed ventricle on brain CT or MRI.

All of them had been operated on in infancy (the age at the time of the initial shunting ranged from 5 months to 14 months). The time from the initial shunting operation to the development of slit ventricle syndrome ranged from 4 to 8 years; the mean duration was 6 years. Shuntograms showed patent shunt function in all patients. The pressure types of the initially inserted shunt valves were low in 4 patients and medium in 2 patients (Table 1).

ICP monitoring was performed in 4 patients. One patient showed high ICP and needed only revision with the same pressure valve as in the previous shunt system; this patient then improved. We thought that his clinical symptoms could result from partial obstruction of the

TABLE 1. Summary of patients with slit ventricle syndrome

Case	Age		Valve pressure	Shuntogram	ICP monitoring	Treatment
	Initial	SVS				
1	6 months	4 years	Low	Patent	Low	Valve upgrading
2	8 months	5 years	Low	Patent	Low	Valve upgrading
3	5 months	5 years	Low	Patent	Low	Valve upgrading
4	9 months	7 years	Medium	Patent	High	Revision with same pressure
5	12 months	6 years	Low	Patent	Not checked	Conservative
6	14 months	8 years	Medium	Patent	Not checked	Conservative

proximal shunt catheter in the slit ventricle even if the shuntogram was interpreted as normal. Low ICP was noted in 3 patients. Pressure augmentation using an antisiphon device or an upgrading valve system were necessary in these patients. Two patients with less severe clinical symptoms improved with conservative treatment. The ICP in these patients was not checked because of a good hospital course. We thought that the symptoms of SVS in these patients could be differentiated from those of migraine in the same patients.

Discussion

Clinical Manifestation and Incidence

"Slit ventricle syndrome" was first described by Becker and Nulsen [1], who in the early 1960s pointed out the possibility of inadequate drainage secondary to small ventricles in shunted hydrocephalic subjects. This syndrome is still a rather poorly understood clinical entity in spite of its wide acceptance in the medical literature and in numerous reports. The syndrome consists of recurrent episodes of headache, malaise, vomiting, and varying degrees of impairment of consciousness. However, the complete SVS syndrome is not based entirely on clinical symptoms and neurological signs. These must be accompanied by a sluggish or absent refill of the pumping device, and radiological evidence of a slit-like ventricle on the side of the shunt. The demonstration of slit-like lateral ventricles with CT scan or MRI is a mandatory, though not sufficient, finding for a diagnosis of SVS. The diminished size of the lateral ventricles is a relatively common observation in hydrocephalic children harboring shunt devices; this was seen in as many as 50–60% of the cases in some series reported in the literature [29, 30]. Most of the patients with slit-like ventricles do not develop any kind of clinical manifestation during life. On the other hand, the symptomatology regarded as typical of SVS is also found in patients with normal or even large cerebral lateral ventricles [10, 21, 26].

The time interval from the original shunt and the age of the patient are also helpful when making a diagnosis. SVS typically arises after several months or years of adequate functioning of the CSF shunt device [4, 21, 24]. All patients in this paper had a different latent period. These ranged from 4 to 8 years after shunting to the onset of SVS symptoms. Such a long time-interval has led some authors to classify the syndrome as one of the complications of chronic CSF overdrainage [11, 22, 24]. However, the headache associated with SVS differs from that accompanying intracranial hypotension: it is not related to posture and it is not relieved by recumbence. The headache due to chronic intracranial hypotension is not generally accompanied by malaise, vomiting, or signs of neurological dysfunction. The intermittent character of the symptoms is also significant in distinguishing SVS from the symptoms of intracranial hypotension.

The diagnosis of SVS should be avoided, and substituted by a correct diagnosis of disturbances unrelated to CSF shunting therapy, etc., or childhood migraine. Headache, vomiting, and altered sensorium can be seen in childhood migraine as well as in patients with SVS. A majority of children with migraine have a family history of migraine, and responds to propranolol or verapamil therapy [16].

The actual incidence of SVS is not known. In the literature, the reported frequency of the syndrome varies surprisingly widely in different articles (Table 2), with values ranging from 1% to 24%, and even up to 37% [2, 4, 6, 17, 21, 24].

The incidence of SVS does not seem to be related to the etiology of the hydrocephalus: in most reports it appears to be associated with all the various types of hydrocephalus, such as malformative, posthemorrhagic, postinfective, and posttraumatic [4, 13, 15, 21, 24]. Some

TABLE 2. Incidence of slit ventricle syndrome

Reference	Period (years)	No. of patients	No. of SVS cases	%
Benzel et al. [2]	5	92	22	24
Choux and Genitori [4]	18	?	28	0.9
DiRocco [6]	17	625	6	0.9
Keucher and Mealey [17]	12	228	3	1.3
McLaurin and Olivi [21]	7	?	15	3.5
Oi and Matsumoto [23]	?	164	5	3
Choi and Kim	10	821	6	0.7

TABLE 3. Opening valve pressure in slit ventricle syndrome

Reference	Opening pressure (No. of patients)				Total number of patients
	Low	Medium	High	Unknown	
Benzel et al. [2]	20	2			22
Choux and Genitori [4]	6	21		1	28
DiRocco [6]		6			6
Hyde-Rowan et al. [15]	6				6
Choi and Kim	4	2			6

series show a higher risk of this kind of complication in patients with posthemorrhagic or postinfective hydrocephalus [2, 4], but we could not find any etiologic factors related to the incidence of SVS.

Other factors, such as the number of previous CSF shunting surgical procedures or the characteristics of the valve system used for treating the hydrocephalus, do not show any demonstrable correlation with the occurrence of the syndrome (Table 3). Our series strongly suggested that low-pressure valves would be responsible for the occurrence of SVS. Even though other authors have also found a higher incidence in patients originally treated with low-pressure valves [2, 14, 15], some have observed the complication in subjects operated on with medium-pressure or even high-pressure valves [4, 6, 30].

The age distribution of SVS presents a peak in incidence in the first decade of life, with most authors indicating a preferential age of diagnosis between 4 and 7 years [2, 4, 6, 21, 24]. The syndrome is definitely rare after the second decade of life. All of the patients in our series had been operated on in infancy. Their ages at the onset of SVS symptoms was below 10 years.

Pathogenesis

The results of laboratory investigations, such as tests for evaluating shunt function and ICP recordings, appear to vary considerably. However, SVS is basically due to an overdrainage of CSF leading to collapse of the cerebral ventricles. It is recognized that in the normal individual a negative intraventricular pressure, approximately −70 mm H_2O, exists in the upright posture. In the shunted person this negative pressure is increased several-fold as a consequence of a siphon effect by the hydrostatic column of the shunt catheter.

Serlo et al. [29, 30] stated that blockage of the ventricular catheter causes cerebral edema and subarachnoid accumulation of CSF, which is usually accompanied by signs of increased intracranial pressure. There appears to be no evidence to support this explanation. Some authors affirm that the symptomatology of the syndrome depends on transitory phases of increased intracranial pressure [5, 8, 12, 18]. These phases of intracranial hypertension are thought to occur because of ventricular catheter trapping between the abutting ventricular walls, which causes transient obstructions of the catheter itself. Transitory enlargement of the cerebral ventricle during the acute phase of the syndrome is thought to be indirect evidence of a transitory malfunction of the shunt system [10]. However, the hypothesis of transitory occlusion of the ventricular catheter causing an intermittent shunt malfunction has never been demonstrated directly [9, 12, 14, 19, 26, 30]. When tested with a radionuclide shuntogram, the CSF shunts in subjects with SVS interpreted as an intermittent CSF shunt malfunction have never been found to be patent [8].

In facts, the reports describing the condition of the shunt device for the pathogenetic interpretation of the syndrome differ considerably: the shunt has been found to be patent [10, 26], occluded either at the proximal [11, 15] or at the distal [7] end, or only partially occluded [19]. Such variability has led to a demand for a change in the pathogenetic interpretation of the syndrome in subsequent reports, and has justified attempts to classify patients in various groups according to the functioning of the CSF shunt devices. Epstein et al. [10] have proposed that children with SVS and intermittent shunt malfunction, who can be treated by simple revision of shunt, should be differentiated from children with increased ICP and patent shunt, who would need cranial expansion. Recently Rekate [28] classified SVS into five distinct syndromes by ICP monitoring: (1) intermittent low-pressure headache, (2) intermittent proximal obstruction, (3) shunt failure with a small ventricle (normal volume hydrocephalus), (4) intracranial hypertension with working shunts (hydrocephalic pseudotumor), (5) headache unrelated to shunt function. (1)–(3) can be treated with shunt revision or upgrading, and (4) with cranial expansion.

We performed ICP monitoring for a period of 24 h in 4 patients. One patient showed high ICP and 3 patients low ICP. We found that the proximal shunt catheter of patient with high ICP was partially obstructed in spite of a normal shuntogram. He was well after only shunt revision, changing the proximal catheter, and the same pressure valve as in the previous shunt. The clinical symptoms of the 3 patients with low ICP resulted from overdrainage of CSF and intermittent obstruction of the proximal shunt catheter. Pressure argumentation was the treatment of choice in these cases.

The concept of rigid ventricular walls as the pathogenetic mechanism accounting for persistence of slit-like cerebral ventricles leading to increased intraventricular pressures has been widely accepted [23, 30]. Oi and Matsumoto [23] noted dilatation of cortical veins and Virchow–Robin spaces, destruction and disorganization of the ependyma, gliosis in the subependymal area, and decreased CSF edema in the subependymal white matter in morphological studies of a postshunt slit ventricle in dogs. Rekate [28] detected high brain elastance in the case of SVS characterized by high intraventricular pulse pressures not associated with intracranial hypertension. They pointed out that the reduced ability of the cerebral ventricle to expand would take into account the possibility of a high brain turgor, mainly related to compression by the intracranial venous pressure.

Investigation and the Treatment Options of Slit Ventricle Syndrome

The treatment of SVS has also been the subject of varying recommendations. Probably the first report in the literature dealing with slit-like ventricles was that of Yein and Ehni [31]. They described insertion of a red rubber catheter around the ventricular catheter, via a transcallosal approach, in order to prevent blockage of the ventricular catheter by the collapsed ventricle.

In 1973, Portnoy et al. [25] described the antisiphon device (ASD) which prevents the flow of CSF through the shunt whenever a negative pressure of 100–200 mm H_2O is exerted at the outlet of the device. Epstein et al. [9] advocated a subtemporal craniectomy to decompress the intracranial contents, to permit dilatation of the ventricles, and to provide a means of assessing intracranial pressure by palpation. This procedure was also recommended by Holness et al. [14]. It is significant, however, that 10 of the 22 patients had postcraniectomy shunt revisions, and in 8 of them the revisions were for ventricular end obstruction.

The CT scan or MRI is the paramount neurodiagnostic examination. It is essential that the study be performed during a symptomatic period and compared with a baseline scan made during an asymptomatic period. Any increase in previous slit ventricles may be only an objective sign of intermittent shunt obstruction. If the ventricles' size is unchanged, a radionuclide study (shuntogram) for the evaluation of shunt patency is performed: partially occluded catheters will usually demonstrate a prolonged clearance time. These catheters may be unable to increase the rate of CSF drainage in response to an increase in intracranial volume, and result in high ICP. ICP monitoring is reserved for those children with normal shunt patency and slit ventricle in radiological studies. If ICP is low, upgrading of the CSF shunt resistance and incorporation of an antisiphon device into the existing CSF shunt system is the treatment of choice. This option is based on the hypothesis that the cause of SVS is an intermittent obstruction of the ventricular catheter trapped between the abutting ventricular walls. The rationale of these operations is that they favor an increase in the volume of the ventricle harboring the shunt catheter by augmenting its inner pressure, thus freeing the catheter and reducing the risk of further obstruction (Fig. 1). In fact, some degree of enlargement of the cerebral ventricle following the placement of a higher opening pressure valve or an antisiphon device has been described in a few reports [12, 15]. However, the effectiveness of the ASD has not been well understood in the majority of cases, because a disappearance of symptoms has not been accompanied by obvious modifications in the volume of the cerebral ventricles [2, 21, 30].

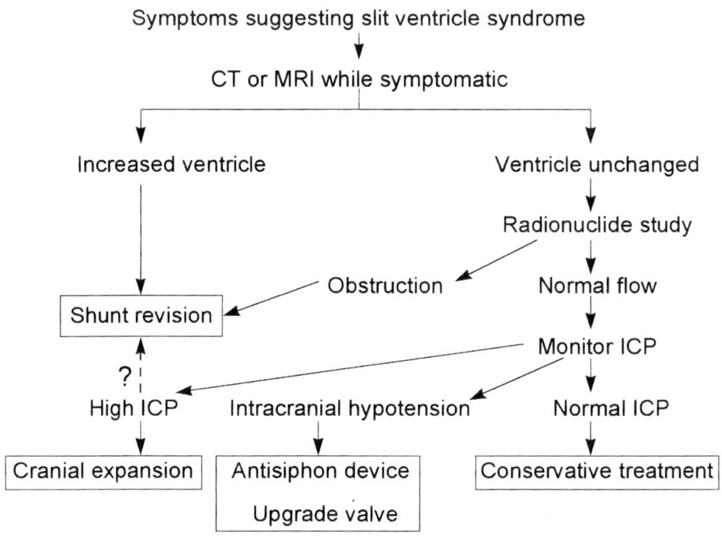

FIG. 1. Algorithm for the treatment of slit ventricle syndrome

ICP monitoring is necessary for at least 24h either through a subarachnoid screw, or directly into the shunt reservoir, usually with a portable monitor that permits ambulation and simultaneous pressure recording with postural alterations. In children with paroxysms of increases in ICP and normal shunt function, cranial expansion is the preferred treatment. Subtemporal craniectomy was introduced with the main goal of "freeing" the trapped ventricular catheter by allowing the ventricular wall to expand towards the area of diminished resistance. The first positive results obtained with this type of operation have been attributed to some degree of postoperative ventricular enlargement [15]. However, other authors have noted the decreased volume of the ventricular system following subtemporal craniectomy, with the reduction being more prominent on the side of the ventricle harboring the draining catheter [3,20]. They postulate that a decrease in the ventricular pulse pressure by this type of operation is the main factor in the disappearance of the clinical symptomatology. Other authors carried out a craniotomy with morcellation of the posterior calvarium from the coronal suture to the inion, as well as laterally to the squamosal suture [10]. They pointed out that posterior calvariotomy would provide more extensive expansion of intracranial volume than subtemporal craniectomy. This type of operation aims at increasing cranio-cerebral compliance. In one of our patients who showed high ICP, a shuntogram was interpreted as normal, but we found a partial obstruction of the proximal catheter at the time of revision. This patients was improved by simply changing the proximal catheter. In our small series we have no experience of cranial expansion. In cases of SVS with high ICP, the patency of the shunt system would have to be investigated carefully before deciding on calvarial expansion.

Other important point in SVS is that the initial shunt operation should be designed for the restoration of the CSF circulation or correction of the impaired CSF absorption, as well as trying to decrease the risk of shunt malfunction by favoring the diversion of CSF to an extraventricular level (lumboperitoneal shunt, endoscopic third ventriculostomy) [27]. All these operations have been so rarely used in patients with SVS that a reliable evaluation of their efficacy is not yet possible. We hesitate to perform lumboperitoneal shunt in infants with an unstable and growing spine. However, we believe that endoscopic third ventriculostomy, or a combination of endoscopic procedure and shunt, is a simple and effective method to avoid shunt dependency and the overdrainage of CSF in hydrocephalus of an infant with the presence of a dilated the third ventricle, and to decrease the risk of shunt malfunction.

Conclusions

Slit ventricle syndrome is not a pathological entity, and is distinguishable from low-pressure headaches and from irreversible shunt obstruction. The pathogenesis of SVS is not entirely clear, but various suggestions have been proposed such as an intermittent shunt obstruction due to collapsed ventricles, etc. Determining the type of SVS by investigation is important before selecting the treatment. The placement of an antisiphon or upgrading the valve resistance was effective in relieving the symptoms of SVS in most patients in our series.

Reference

1. Becker DP, Nulsen FE (1968) Control of hydrocephalus by valve-regulated venous shunt: avoidance of complications in prolonged shunt maintenance. J Neurosurg 28:215–226
2. Benzel EC, Reeves JD, Kesterton L, Hadden TA (1992) Slit ventricle syndrome in children: clinical presentation and treatment. Acta Neurochir (Wien) 117:7–14

3. Cardoso ER, Del Bigio MR, Schroeder G (1989) Age-dependent changes of cerebral ventricular size. I. Review of intracranial fluid collections. Acta Neurochir (Wien) 97:40–46
4. Choux M, Genitori L (1990) Slit ventricle syndrome. Presented at the International Symposium on Hydrocephalus, Kobe, 1990
5. Collmann H, Mauersberger W, Mohr G (1980) Clinical observations and CSF absorption studies in the slit ventricle syndrome. Adv Neurosurg 8:183–185
6. DiRocco C (1994) Is the slit ventricle syndrome always a slit ventricle syndrome? Child's Nerv Syst 10:49–58
7. Engel M, Carmel PW, Cantorian AM (1979) Increased ventriculomyelomegaly in children with shunts: "normal volume" hydrocephalus. Neurosurgery 5:549–552
8. Epstein FJ (1983) Increased intraventricular pressure in hydrocephalic children with functioning shunts: a complication of shunt dependency. Concepts Pediatr Neurosurg 4:119–130
9. Epstein FJ, Fleischer AS, Hochwald GM, Ransohoff J (1974) Subtemporal craniectomy from recurrent shunt obstruction secondary to small ventricles. J Neurosurg 41:29–31
10. Epstein FJ, Lapras C, Wisoff JHI (1988) Slit ventricle syndrome: etiology and treatment. Pediatr Neurosurg 14:5–10
11. Faulhauer K, Schmitz P (1978) Overdrainage phenomena in shunt-treated hydrocephalus. Acta Neurochir (Wien) 45:89–101
12. Gruber R, Jenny P, Herzog B (1984) Experiences with the anti-siphon device (ASD) in shunt therapy of pediatric hydrocephalus. J Neurosurg 61:156–162
13. Hirayama A (1981) Slit ventricle—a reluctant goal of ventriculo-peritoneal shunt. In: Choux M (ed) Shunts and problems in shunts. Karger, Basel, pp 108–111
14. Holness RO, Hoffman HJ, Hendrick EB (1979) Subtemporal decompression for slit ventricle syndrome after shunting in hydrocephalic children. Child's Brain 5:137–144
15. Hyde-Rowan MD, Rekate HL, Nulsen FE (1982) Reexpansion of previously collapsed ventricles: the slit ventricle syndrome. J Neurosurg 56:536–539
16. James HE, Nowak TP (1991–92) Clinical course and diagnosis of migraine headache in hydrocephalic children (discussion). Pediatr Neurosurg 17:310–316
17. Keucher TR, Mealey J (1979) Long-term results after ventriculo-atrial and ventriculo-peritoneal shunting for infantile hydrocephalus. J Neurosurg 50:179–186
18. Kickens R, Mortier W, Pothmann R, Bock WJ, Seibert A (1982) The slit ventricle syndrome after shunting in hydrocephalic children. Neuropediatrics 13:190–194
19. Korfali E, Aksoy K, Saf-i I (1988) Slit ventricle syndrome presenting with paroxysmal hypersomnia in an adult case report. Neurosurgery 22:594–595
20. Linder M, Diehe J, Sklar FH (1983) Subtemporal decompression for shunt-dependent ventricles: mechanism of action. Surg Neurol 19:520–523
21. McLaurin R, Olivi A (1987) Slit ventricle syndrome: review of 15 cases. Pediatr Neurosci 13:118–124
22. Murros K, Fogetholm R (1983) Spontaneous intracranial hypotension with slit ventricles. J Neurol Neurosurg Psychiatr 46:1146–1151
23. Oi S, Matsumoto S (1986) Morphological findings of post-shunt slit-ventricle in experimental canine hydrocephalus. Aspects of causative factors of isolated ventricles and slit-ventricle syndrome. Child's Nerv Syst 2:179–184
24. Oi S, Matsumoto S (1987) Infantile hydrocephalus and the slit-ventricle syndrome in early infancy. Child's Nerv Syst 3:145–150
25. Portnoy HD, Schulte RR, Fox JL, Croissant PD, Tripp L (1973) Anti-siphon and reversible occlusion valves for shunting in hydrocephalus and preventing post-shunt subdural hematomas. J Neurosurg 38:729–738
26. Rapaport A, Siderer M, Sarova I (1989) Slit-ventricle and intracranial pressure. Neurosurgery 25:667–670
27. Reddy K, Fewer HD, West M, Hill NC (1988) Slit ventricle syndrome with aqueduct stenosis: third ventriculostomy as definitive treatment. Neurosurgery 23:756–759
28. Rekate HL (1993) Classification of slit-ventricle syndromes using intracranial pressure monitoring. Pediatr Neurosurg 19:15–20

29. Serlo W, Heikkinen E, Sankkonen AL, Wendt L von (1985) Classification and management of the slit ventricle syndrome. Child's Nerv Syst 1:194–199
30. Serlo W, Saukkonen AL, Heikkinen E, Wendt L von (1989) The incidence and management of the slit-ventricle syndrome. Acta Neurochir (Wien) 99:113–116
31. Yein FS, Ehni G (1969) Pericallosal sump ventriculostomy for shunt-dependent hydrocephalic patient with small ventricle. J Neurosurg 31:570–573

Abstract

Treatment of Hydrocephalus Associated with Spina Bifida

MASSIMO CALDARELLI

The advent of echoencephalography, CT, and MRI has unequivocally demonstrated the almost constant association between myelomeningocele (MM) and hydrocephalus. Consequently, most authors agree nowadays on shunting myelodysplasic children even before the clinical findings demonstrate the progression of the underlying hydrocephalus. However, even though the need for early shunting for myelodysplasic children is no longer discussed, controversy still exists as to the timing and modalities of treatment. In newborns, opinions vary on the sequence to be followed between MM repair and CSF shunting. Although few authors have reported a higher incidence of infectious complications in children operated on simultaneously, there is some evidence that excessively early CSF shunting may bear an increased risk of infection. Indeed, in our experience there is a correlation between the incidence of mechanical and/or infectious complications and increased protein content in the CSF at operation when it is performed soon after birth. This correlation was even more significant in cases with possible CSF contamination, even in the absence of clear signs of CSF infection.

All the series in the literature emphasize the high risk of complications when treating hydrocephalus associated with MM in infants or young children, whereas this risk seems to decrease in toddlers and adolescents, both because of the improvement in their general condition and, above all, because of the development of some kind of compensatory mechanisms for CSF absorption. The latter hypothesis is supported by the elevated success rate of 3rd-ventriculostomy in myelodysplasic children and adolescents, compared with the failure of the same procedure when performed on infants.

Department of Neurosurgery, Catholic University Medical School, Rome, Italy

Abstract

Shunt Complications in School-Age and Adolescent Patients with Spina Bifida

Fernando Rueda-Franco

During the last 25 years, advances in neonatal care, neuroimaging, neurosurgical techniques, antibiotics, etc., have permitted the long-term survival of patients with spina bifida and hydrocephalus. Shunt failure and infections remain the most frequent complications in the treatment of hydrocephalus of any etiology. Infection is the single most serious problem after a shunt implantation or revision, with rates of between 0.7% and 25%, and *S. epidermidis* is the most frequent germ involved. Choux et al., in 1992, proposed a strict protocol for shunt implantation in order to reach a 0% infection rate, something that many authors still consider "an impossible dream." In school-age and adolescence, complications related to the hardware are overdrainage, disconnection, obstruction, migration with externalization e.g., annal, vaginal, or even through the umbilicus, and rarely an allergy to the silicon. Other complications are the development of abdominal cysts, almost always associated with infections, and epilepsy and vein thrombosis in patients with ventriculoatrial shunts. The so-called slit ventricle syndrome (SVS) is a controversial and often frustrating clinical problem, with an estimated frequency in children of 0.9–3.3%. SVS is actually a mixed group of disorders, all causing symptoms of headache, vomiting, and lethargy in the presence of slit ventricles with normal, hypertensive, or hypotensive intracranial pressure. There are many theories about the pathogenic mechanism, as well as many approaches to the treatment of SVS, so there is not a complete answer to this problem as yet. The revisited third ventriculostomy using neuroendoscopic techniques also has complications which, according to Teo (1997), are of two distinct categories: intraoperative and clinically significant. In Teo's series of 340 cases, the former occurred in 11% and the latter in 6% of patients. The prevention of shunt complications should include: (1) selection of the patient; (2) refined surgical techniques; (3) use of the most suitable system or noninvasive treatment; (4) strict follow-up of the patient, which can include the use of software facilities (Hladky 1997) or telephone triage (Rekate 1997).

Division of Pediatric Neurosurgery, Instituto Nacional de Pediatría, Mexico City, Mexico

Abstract

Long-Term Management of Shunt Problems for Spina Bifida in School-Age and Adolescent Patients

Maurice Choux

More than 80% of patients with myelomeningocele are shunted. Late complications are mostly the same as for hydrocephalic patients of different etiologies, but some differences may be detected. In our series of cases, manifestations of hyperdrainage, as slit ventricle syndrome or subdural collection, are more rare than in posthemorrhagic or postinfection hydrocephalus. Mechanical complications such as disconnection or rupture of the material are more frequent in patients suffering frequent traumas. In several patients where a rupture of the material has been detected without any symptoms of increased intracranial pressure, it was possible to remove all the material safely. In our experience (31 cases in our series), is only possible in patients with myelomeningocele.

An other complication is related to extensive calcification of the catheter, especially at the cervical and thoracic level. It is not easy to understand why such a complication occurs in some patients and not in others. When a revision is needed, the removal of different calcified pieces of the peritoneal shunt is not always easy.

An other problem which may occur in shunted patients with a myelomeningocele is the management of multiloculated ventricles when a shunt infection was present initially. These cavities may become symptomatic secondary complications. Endoscopic procedures may be very useful in these cases. In case of secondary manifestations of Chiari II malformation, a shunt revision could be the first management step.

Department of Pediatric Neurosurgery, Hôpital des Enfants, La Timone, Marseille, France

Moderator's Comments on Sessions—Hydrocephalus

Koreaki Mori

Patients with myelomeningocele (MMC) frequently have hydrocephalus. Hydrocephalus associated with MMC is different from other forms of congenital hydrocephalus, both clinically and pathophysiologically. Such hydrocephalus may become shunt-independent a few years after a shunting operation; i.e., the patient is found to be doing well in spite of a malfunctioning shunt (shunt-independent arrested hydrocephalus).

Hydrocephalus may not be evident at birth in some patients with MMC, but some may present marked hydrocephalus at birth. The timing of CSF shunting still remains controversial. Some pediatric neurosurgeons insert a shunt simultaneously at the time of the repair of the MMC. Others treat hydrocephalus in toddlers or adolescents whose general condition has improved, because of the high risk of infection when treating hydrocephalus with MMC in neonates or infants.

When hydrocephalus in patients with MMC is treated depends on the severity of the hydrocephalus. Even if the head is kept lower than the spine after repair of MMC in order to reduce CSF pressure exerted on the operative wound, CSF leakage from the wound may occur in patients with marked hydrocephalus. In such cases, CSF shunting should be performed simultaneously at the time of repair of MMC or soon after wards. Delayed treatment for hydrocephalus may also cause irreversible brain damage.

Shunt malfunction and infections are the most frequent complications in the treatment of hydrocephalus of any age or etiology. Among shunt complications, infection is the most serious problem, with rates raging from 0.7 to 25%.

Late complications relatelated to the shunt system are overdrainage and mechanical complications. Shunt infection may result in an abdominal CSF cyst. As well as shunt obstruction, disconnection, migration, and protrusion of the abdominal catheter through the vagina, umbilicus, etc. may occur as mechanical complications.

The so-called slit ventricle syndrome (SVS) is one of the late complications of shunting for hydrocephalus in children, with an estimated incidence of 0.9–3.3%. SVS consists of different disorders. Patients with SVS present with headache, vomiting, and lethargy, with hypertensive, normal, or hypotensive intracranial pressure. Since many pathogenetic mechanisms and many approaches to treatment have been advocated, SVS is still a controversial clinical problem. Most patients with SVS were shunted in infancy, and SVS may developed 4–8 years later. When we manage patients with SVS, we have to determine which type of SVS is present.

Department of Neurosurgery, Kochi Medical School, Kochi, Japan

To prevent late shunt complications, the following should be considered: (1) selection of the patient; (2) a refined surgical technique; (3) use of the most suitable shunt system; (4) strict long-term follow-up.

Most patients with MMC are shunted for hydrocephalus. The shunted patients may develop not only early, but also late complications of the shunt, as in patients with hydrocephalus of different etiologies.

Overdrainage of the shunt may result in slit ventricle syndrome or subdural fluid collection. Fortunately, these complications are rare in hydrocephalus associated with MMC compared with hydrocephalus of other etiologies.

Mechanical complications such as disconnection or rupture of the shunt system are more frequent in patients with MMC because they suffer from frequent traumas. In some patients, the shunt becomes obliterated without any symptoms or signs of increased intracranial pressure. In these patients, the shunt may be removed.

One late shunt complication, an extensive calcification of the catheter, has been reported in some patients. When shunt revision is needed, the removal of the catheter may be difficult in these patients.

Multiloculated ventricles are another problem in shunted patients with MMC where shunt infection was present at the time of shunt insertion. This complication may become symptomatic. For the treatment of loculation within the ventricle, endoscopic procedures may be useful.

Patients with MMC may develop late manifestation of Chiari II malformation. For late-onset symptomatic Chiari II malformation, a shunt revision should be the first treatment. If the shunt is functioning, decompression procedures should be considered.

Abstract

The "Ideal" Management of Children with Spina Bifida in the Future

Fred J. Epstein

In addressing the subject, I am sure that there are many more questions than answers in terms of what will be "state of the art" treatment twenty or thirty years from now. Perhaps to understand more completely where we will be in the future, it is appropriate to briefly consider where we have come from, in the evolution of treatment over the past twenty or thirty years.

Twenty-five years ago, there was no practical way to detect afflicted children during pregnancy. Certainly, prenatal detection has at least made it technically possible to consider whether intrauterine surgery, in the future, may have some role in terms of limitation of postnatal disability.

Twenty-five years ago, the "Lorber" criterion was widely accepted as being indicative of a poor prognosis in children with spina bifida and was utilized in many major centers as an indication for withholding treatment. I believe that this philosophy has been relegated to "history" but it is important to remember that universal pessimism was associated with the birth of a child fulfilling these "crude" criteria.

Twenty-five or thirty years ago, hydrocephalus had an entirely different prognosis, particularly prior to the introduction of CAT scanning in 1974. For this reason, hydrocephalus associated with meningomyelocele, in and of itself, was a formidable long-term therapeutic problem associated with multiple complications and often an abbreviated life span.

The most common cause of fatality in these patients was directly related to urological problems associated with a neurogenic bladder. There was little understanding of the necessity of the supervision of a pediatric urologist with particular expertise in caring for the neurogenic bladder. Intermittent catheterization had not been introduced and the spectrum of therapeutic options from a urological perspective was limited.

Twenty-five years ago, we did not understand the role of "tethered cord" in evolving disability in this patient population. We were taught by our predecessors that children with a relatively "low" level often ended up in wheelchairs in their adolescence as a result of weight gain and the fact that wheelchair propulsion was physically less demanding than utilizing braces and crutches. It was only many years later that we recognized that this was a completely erroneous concept and that many of these children, in fact, had a tethered spinal cord and that properly timed surgery prevented the evolution of the disabilities that often resulted in total functional dependence.

Department of Neurosurgery, Institute for Neurology and Neurosurgery, Beth Israel Medical Center, New York, NY USA

In summary, then, it is very clear that the contemporary state of the art would have been considered "fantasy" just two or three decades ago. Inasmuch as we have come so far in such a relatively short period of time, it is almost impossible to predict the future (but I will try!).

Clearly, with prenatal detection, the issue of intrauterine surgery will be "revisited" in the future. Is it possible that prenatal closure of the meningomyelocele will prevent the neural toxicity of amniotic fluid from contributing the severity of postnatal deficit? Is it possible that treating hydrocephalus prior to birth will likewise alter prognosis for the better? Certainly, intrauterine surgery will be seriously examined in the coming decades.

Much work is being directed towards nerve transfer to restore function to weak or paralyzed limbs. I believe that, in the future, work that I carried out some years ago will be reassessed and perhaps techniques will be developed for utilizing proximal peripheral nerves to "jump the gap" of the placode and connect up directly to intact nerves peripheral to the neural plate to restore some element of function to the bladder or the lower extremities.

Certainly, clinical research that has been carried out in terms of "bladder stimulation" is promising with regard to restoring continence of bowel and bladder. I am confident that this will evolve rapidly and that sacral root stimulation will become one of the accepted therapeutic procedures in this endeavor.

Finally, we will become more sensitive to the needs of the "aging" spina bifida population. Insidious and unusual manifestations of neurological deterioration from inadequately treated tethered cord, Arnold-Chiari malformation, neurogenic bladder, and hydrocephalus will be recognized and treated effectively.

Perhaps most importantly, the attitude of physicians and society will change significantly and become more uniformly optimistic. While there is no question that a multiplicity of procedures will evolve in the coming decade, it is equally important that the willingness of society in general to support both the costs and the growing population of children with residual disability be very strong. There is no question that it is easy to speak in generalities and to espouse optimism, but this must be grounded in "geographical reality". All of the future treatments will be expensive and require much expertise and will remain the "luxury" of an affluent society. It should, therefore, be clear that these comments are only referable to the ideal world and will be unavailable in many countries in which treatment by economic necessity will remain "expectant".

Neurosurgical Perspective in Ideal Treatment and Therapy for Children with Spina Bifida

Tadanori Tomita

Introduction

A neurosurgeon is the first clinical specialist to evaluate and treat a child with spina bifida shortly after birth. Neurosurgery plays an integral part in the care of children with spina bifida in a multidisciplinary clinic, which also includes pediatric specialists in such fields as orthopedics, urology, and rehabilitation medicine. Neurosurgical roles include not only the initial repair of the myelomeningocele and treatment of hydrocephalus, but also treatment of CSF diversion shunt, Chiari II malformation, tethered cord, and hydromyelia. In order to identify these late-onset complications, patients are best assessed by a multidisciplinary team.

Initial Therapy

The initial therapy for children with spina bifida is the repair of the open neural tube defect. This procedure includes a reconstruction of the neural tube, untethering of the spinal cord, which includes dissection of the skin surrounding the neural placode and the section of thick filum terminalis, and the creation of the dura sac, which needs to be closed in a watertight fashion.

Hydrocephalus

Hydrocephalus is present in approximately 90%–95% of children with spina bifida. Most cases of hydrocephalus associated with spina bifida are multifactorial, and various pathological anatomical changes are well documented. One is a dilated lateral ventricle similar to that seen in colpocephaly of the fetal ventricular system. The choroid plexus tissues in the lateral ventricles can be voluminous. In the 3rd ventricle, the massa intermedia is sometimes unusually developed. At the aqueduct of Sylvius, the beaking tectal plate is sometimes thick, which may result in aqueductal stenosis. The 4th ventricle can be elongated, and the 4th ventricle tends to be present in the upper cervical cord because of Chiari II malformation. In the subarachnoid space, there might be severe arachnoiditis at the tentorial notch, which keeps the CSF

Divison of Pediatric Neurosurgery, Children's Memorial Hospital and Northwestern University Medical School, 2300 Children's Plaza, Chicago, IL 60614, USA

from circulating into the supratentorial subarachnoid space. All these pathological processes can cause both obstructive and communicating types of hydrocephalus.

Neonates with hydrocephalus often present with an enlarging head circumference, full anterior fontanelle, lethargy, bradycardia, and emesis. At the present time, a ventriculoperitoneal (VP) shunt is the most commonly used CSF diversion. In the past, a ventriculoatrial shunt was used, but this is not recommended, at least not as the first choice of CSF diversion, owing to the high incidence of shunt nephritis, cor pulmonare, and superior vena cava occlusion. The pleural space is ideal for CSF diversion, but ventriculopleural shunt may not be suitable when the patient is younger than 6 years of age owing to the limited pleural space in small children and also because of the possibility of kyphoscoliosis in children with spina bifida.

Shunt Malfunction

The most frequent shunt complication in children with spina bifida is a shunt malfunction. Owing to the voluminous choroid plexus and the colpocephalic shape of the ventricule, together with the frequent development of a slit ventricle due to shunt placement in the neonatal period, proximal shunt obstruction is a common occurrence. Distal obstructions are relatively uncommon. Distal slit valve obstruction, shunt disconnection, or the development of a CSF pseudocyst can account for distal obstruction of a VP shunt. Occasionally a functional shunt malfunction develops after the application of a body cast or a high degree of constipation, both of which are common in children with spina bifida, because increased abdominal pressure eliminates the pressure differential between head and abdomen. Another problem with shunts in children with spina bifida is contralateral ventricle enlargement after a shunt placement due to a poor connection between the bilateral ventricles. This can occur in 15% of children with spina bifida requiring bilateral placement of the VP shunt and may require septostomy using ventriculoscopic guidance. Numerous shunt valves have been manufactured and used, but to date there is no perfect shunt.

A common question from parents of children with spina bifida is whether a shunt would be permanent. Current advancements in ventriculoscopic techniques enables us to perform third ventriculostomy, which could eliminate the need for an internal shunt. However, owing to a massive massa intermedian together with the short distance between the mamillary body and the infundibular recess in the floor of the 3rd ventricle, technical difficulties have arisen during 3rd ventriculostomy for hydrocephalus among children with spina bifida. Even though 3rd ventriculostomy is carried out, the success rate of the patency remains quite poor in myelomeningocele children, particularly those younger than 2 years of age. These poor results may be due to the lack of subarachnoid space secondary to adhesive arachnoiditis. Also, the patient's hydrocephalus may recur several months after successful ventriculostomy. These late failures are most likely due to closure of the 3rd ventriculostomy or the development of arachnoiditis in the subarachnoid space beyond the 3rd ventriculostomy.

The signs of a shunt malfunction in children with spina bifida are most often frontal headaches, emesis, and lethargy. Brachycardia and hypertension, so-called Cushing's phenomenon, are often present. When the patient experiences a suboccipital pain with or without opisthotonos, one should be aware that acute respiratory arrest may ensue. The explanation of this complication is that the lack of the tentorium allows direct compression upon the cerebellum by the mesial temporal and occipital lobe due to acute shunt malfunction. This acute compression upon the cerebellum directly causes the compression of the medulla oblongata at the foramen magnum and paralyzes the medullary respiratory center. Occasionally the patient may present with an aggravation of Chiari II malformation (i.e., increasing stridor), or low back pain due to aggravation of the existing hydromyelia. Some patients may present without any acute symptoms but with decreasing school performances.

Other Problems

Other than shunt malfunctions, neurological deterioration in children with spina bifida could be due to Chiari II malformation, tethered cord, hydromyelia, or repair-site dermoid. Nonetheless, if the patient presents with neurological deterioration, one should remember that a shunt malfunction must be suspected and checked first. Once shunt malfunction has been ruled out, one should perform appropriate diagnostic tests and therapy for other anatomical pathologies related to spina bifida.

Chiari II malformation is present in all children with myelomeningocele. In young children, particularly newborns, respiratory stridor, vocal cord palsy, or central apnea are the most serious complications of Chiari II malformation. A posterior fossa decompression, or more appropriately upper cervical decompression, for Chiari II malformation may provide some relief from the symptoms, but the vast majority fail to repond to surgical decompression. Perhaps this is because the symptoms are not caused by simple mechanical brain stem compression, but rather by an incomplete formation of the brain stem nuclei. If the patient is normal at birth but deteriorates with stridor or opisthotonic posturing during infancy, decompressing the Chiari II malformation should be considered. However, again, one should rule out a shunt malfunction before undertaking the decompression.

A tethered cord is present in 100% of myelomeningocele cases, but the majority are asymptomatic. The symptoms related to a tethered cord are spasticity, scoliosis, spastic bladder, low back pain, and frequent urinary tract infections. The tethered cord is due to arachnoid adhesion of the spinal cord to the dural surface. Numerous techniques have been applied to prevent this tethering. The problem of preventing tethering and at the same time repairing the spina bifida is quite difficult because of lack of dura space in neonates. However, when a patient presents with the signs of tethered cord, one should actively untether it.

Hydromyelia is present in 50% of patients with spina bifida. However, only 20% of patients require treatment for severe hydromyelia. Usually patients with hydromyelia present with back pain, scoliosis, spasticity, or hypotonia. When hydromyelia is diagnosed, a shunt malfunction needs to be ruled out. Symptomatic hydromyelia often responds to a shunt revision. If the hydromyelia is persistent, it can be controlled with a syringopleural shunt. Unfortunately, a syringotomy or a stent placement to the spinal subarachnoid space for hydromyelia associated with spina bifida are often unsuccessful because of existing spinal arachnoiditis.

Conclusions

Neonatal and infantile hydrocephalus are best treated with a VP shunt. The ideal placement of a shunt is achieved with the aid of a ventriculoscope. At the present time, an ideal shunt system has yet to be found. While often unsuccessful during infancy, a 3rd ventriculostomy in older children may be a useful alternative way to treat hydrocephalus, hopefully eliminating the need for a shunt. Clinicians should be aware of shunt malfunction as the primary cause of neurological deterioration in children with spina bifida. Symptoms due to shunt malfunction may mimic those of a tethered cord, hydromyelia, or Chiari II malformation. One should rule out a shunt malfunction before treating other possible causes of neurological deterioration.

Experimental Analysis: The Causes of Neural Tube Defects and Chiari II Type Malformation, and the Important Role of Normal Neurulation in Their Prevention

Takayuki Inagaki[1], Gary C. Schoenwolf[2], Yasuo Yamanouchi[1], and Keiji Kawamoto[1]

Introduction

The early development of the embryo, during the 4th week of human gestation, has important consequences for the later development of the entire nervous system. The primitive neural tube is the forerunner of the entire central nervous system, the brain, and the spinal cord. Unfortunately, in about 1 in every 1600 babies, i.e., more than 2500 babies per year in the United States alone, neurulation occurs abnormally, resulting in serious, life-threatening birth defects called anencephaly and spina bifida that result in paralysis.

We use both normal animal models to study the formation of the neural tube, and genetic mutations and environmental insults to study the formation and prevention of neural tube defects. We present our experimental data to demonstrate the following conclusions: (1) the failure of neural tube closure at the critical time is a major cause of neural tube defects; (2) some types of closed neural tube defects may be due to the same cause as that involved in open neural tube defects, but acting at different stages of embryonic development; (3) leakage of cerebro-spinal fluid through the opening in the caudal spine may be a major cause of the brain abnormalities which can be seen in a patient with myelomeningocele; (4) Hensen's node plays an important role in early neurulation events.

Part 1

Since Von Recklinghausen [1] proposed a theory of the cause of myelomeningocele, many investigators have tried to find the cause of open neural tube defects. Von Recklinghausen proposed that failure of the embryonic neural plate to close, forming the neural tube, at about 26–28 days of gestation led to myelomeningocele. Patten [2] observed overgrowth of the dorsal caudal neural plate in chick and human embryos, and suggested that this was the primary event preventing neural tube closure. Most investigators agree that myelomeningocele and anencephaly result from failure of initial closure rather than from reopening of the once-closed neural tube [3–6]. On the other hand, Gardner [7] and Oi et al. [8, 9] proposed that reopening of the once-closed spinal cord may be a cause of the dysraphic state. A hypothesis for embryo pathogenesis of myeloschisis is described on the basis of experimental studies

[1]Department of Neurosurgery, Kansai Medical University, 10-15 Fumizono-cho, Moriguchi, Osaka 570, Japan, and [2]Department of Neurobiology and Anatomy, University of Utah School of Medicine, Salt Lake City, Utah 84132, USA

analyzing the stage-specificity and histological characteristics of the open neural tube [10, 11]. There is a relationship between the timing of treatment, for example with Concanavalin-A and Vitamin-A, and the type of neural tube defect. Early treatment results in exencephaly or an extensive opening. Relatively delayed treatment results in a small opening at the more caudal spinal level. The critical timing for developing neural tube defects may be at the period of neural tube fusion and/or adhesion.

Part 2

McLone et al. [12] concluded that some of the various forms of spina bifida may be related to (1) abnormal development of the neural tube, (2) separation of the superficial ectoderm, or (3) migration of the mesoderm toward the cleavage space between the superficial ectoderm and the neuroectoderm. The results of Concanavalin-A-induced abnormal spinal cords in chicks [11] showed that the patterns of abnormal development of the neural tube varied at the closed and opened levels of the neuraxis at the time of treatment. Thus the resulting opened neural tubes were, (1) with or without a superficial ectodermal covering, (2) consisting of disorganized neuroectodermal cells rather than overgrowth of the neuroectoderm, or (3) covered by mesenchymal cells which intervened between the neuroectoderm and overlying superficial ectoderm. The disjunction between the surface ectoderm and neural ectoderm was seen as a common feature in this study, and may be followed by mesenchymal accessing to the central portion of the neuroectoderm, in a similar way to clinical lipomyelomeningocele cases. This leads to the possible interpretation that the same causes may create various types of open and/or closed neural tube defects depending on the timing, and that different timing will have different effects on the embryo.

Part 3

The fact that Type II Chiari malformations are associated with myelomeningocele is well established [13, 14]. Theories about the cause of Chiari II malformation have been debated since Chiari proposed that the herniation of the posterior fossa contents was the result of supratentorial hydrocephalus [15]. There are now many theories, such as the hydrocephalus/hydrodynamic theory [16–20], the traction theory [21, 22], the dysgenesis of the hindbrain/development arrest theories [23–26], and the overgrowth/small posterior fossa theories [27–31].

From our own experimental study [32], we concluded that surgical reopening of the once-closed neural tube is the cause of abnormal development in the ventricular system. This abnormality is thought to be the early phase of the maldevelopment of the cerebrum and cerebellum seen in the Spd/Spd mutant and vitamin-A-induced mice embryos on gestation days 12–14. This leads to the conclusion that the failure of distention of the primitive ventricle may be a cause of Chiari II malformation.

Part 4

Hensen's node, considered to be the avian and mammalian equivalent of the amphibian organizer, has been the subject of intensive study in recent years. Several investigators have shown that Hensen's node has two abilities: the potential to self-differentiate, and the power to act as an organizer [33–45]. We also conducted a series of experiments consisting of transplantation of Hensen's nodes to examine axis development in avian embryos [46]. In these experiments, only the central one-third to one-half of the width of the node was transplanted to host blastoderms, and yet ectopic embryos, complete with an induced neuraxis, were formed. From these results, we deduced the strong ability of Hensen's node to self-differentiate. The results also suggest that once morphogenetic movements are under way, neuraxial structures can form and characteristic rostrocaudal patterning of the neuraxis can occur without sustained influence from Hensen's node. More recently, Dias and Walker [47] have proposed a theory of complex dysraphic malformations described by abnormal migration of multipotential primitive-streak cells prior to neurulation.

Conclusion

Traditionally, neural tube defects have been explained by errors in closure of the neural tube, or post-neurulation rupture, as described above. We have described the results of our own experiments. The results of our own investigations and those of other researchers have shown that the cause of spina bifida may be multifactorial. To prevent spina bifida, further investigations are needed.

References

1. von Recklinghausen FD (1886) Untersuchungen über die Spina Bifida. Virchow's Arch 105:243–330
2. Patten BM (1952) Overgrowth of the neural tube in young human embryos. Anat Rec 113:381–393
3. Dekaban AS, Bartelmez GW (1964) Complete dysraphism in 14 somites in human embryos. Am J Anat 115:27–42
4. Emery JL, Lendon RG (1973) The local cord lesion in neurospinal dysraphism (meningomyelocele). J Pathol 110:83–96
5. Ferm VH (1966) Severe developmental malformations: malformations induced by urethane and hydrozyurea in the hamster. Arch Pathol 81:174–177
6. Lemire RJ, Loeser JD, Leech RW, Allvord EC Jr (1975) Normal and abnoraml development of the human nervous system. Harper and Row, Hagerstown, pp 144–165
7. Gardner WJ (1977) Etiology and pathgenesis of the development of myelomeningocele. In: McLaurin RL (ed) Myelomeningocele. Grune and Stratton, New York, pp 3–30
8. Oi S, Kokunai T, Okuda Y, Sasaki M, Matsumoto S (1990) Identical embryopathogenesis for exencephaly and myeloschisis: an experimental study. J Neurosurg 72:450–457
9. Oi S, Saya H, Matsumoto S (1988) A hypothesis for myeloschisis: overgrowth and reopening. An experimental study. J Neurosurg 68:947–954
10. Nakahara S, Tanaka H, Nakazawa K, Matsumoto M, Inagaki T, McLone DG, Knepper PA (1992) Vitamin-A-induced neural tube defect with Chiari II malformation in mice (in Japanese). Shoni No Noshinkei 17:135–142
11. Inagaki T, Wang Kyu-Chang, Higbee GH, McLone DG, Knepper PA (1996) Concanabalin-A-induced open neural tube defects in chick embryos. Neurol Med-Chir 36:691–697
12. McLone DG, Suwa J, Collins JA, Poznanski S, Knepper PA (1983) Neurulation: biochemical and morphological studies of primary and secondary neural tube defects. In: Humphreys R (ed) Concepts in pediatric neurosurgery, vol 4. Karger, Basel, pp 15–19
13. Hoffman HJ, Hendrich EB, Humphreys RP (1975) Manifestations and management of Arnold-Chiari malformation in patients with myelomeningocele. Childs Brain 1:255–259
14. Park TS, Hoffman HJ, Hendrick EB, Humhreys RP (1983) Experience with surgical decompression of the Arnold-Chiari malformation in young infants with myelomeningocele. Neurosurgery 13:147–152
15. Chiari H (1896) Über Veränderungen des Kleinhirns, des Pons und der Medulla oblongata infolge von Kongenitaler Hzdrocephalie des Grosshirns. Denkschr Akad Wiss Wien 63:71–116

16. Weed LH (1917) Development of the cerebrospinal fluid spaces in pig and man. Contrib Embryol 5:1–6
17. Gardner WJ (1959) Anatomic features common to the Arnold–Chiari and the Dandy–Walker malformations suggest a common origin. Cleve Clin 26:206–222
18. Gardner WJ (1965) Hydrodynamic mechanism of syringomyelia: its relationship to myelocele. J Neurol Neurosurg Psychiatr 28:247–259
19. Cameron AH, Osman Hill WC (1955) The Arnold–Chiari malformation in a sacred baboon (*Papio hamadryas*). J Pathol Bacteriol 70:552–554
20. Cameron AH (1957) Malformations of the neurospinal axis, urogenital tract and foregut in spina bifida attributable to disturbances of the blastopore. J Pathol Bacteriol 73:213–221
21. Penfield W, Cone W (1932) Spina bifida and cranium bifidum: results of plastic repair of meningocele and myelomeningocele by a new method. JAMA 98:454–461
22. Lichtenstein BW (1942) Distant neuroanatomic complications of spina bifida (spinal dysraphism). Hydrocephalus, Arnold–Chiari deformity, stenosis of the aqueduct of Sylvius, etc: pathogenesis and pathology. Arch Neurol Psychiatr 47:195–214
23. Cleland J (1883) Contribution to the study of spina bifida, encephalocele, and anencephalus. J Anat Physiol 17:257–292
24. Daniel PM, Strich SJ (1958) Some observations on the congenital deformity of the central nervous system known as the Arnold–Chiari malformation. J Neuropathol Exp Neurol 17: 255–266
25. Peach B (1964) Cystic prolongation of fourth ventricle: an anomaly associated with the Arnold–Chiari malformation. Arch Neurol 11:609–612
26. Peach B (1965) Arnold–Chiari malformation: anatomic features of 20 cases. Arch Neurol 12:613–621
27. Barry A, Patten BM, Stewart BH (1957) Possible factors in the development of the Arnold–Chiari malformation. J Neurosurg 14:285–301
28. Brocklehurst G (1971) The pathogenesis of spina bifida: a study of the relationship between observation, hypothesis, and surgical incentive. Dev Med Child Neurol 13:147–163
29. Padget DH (1972) Development of so-called dysraphism: with embryologic evidence of clinical Arnold–Chiari and Dandy–Walker malformations. Johns Hopkins Med J 130:127–165
30. Padget DH, Lindenberg R (1972) Inverse cerebellum morphogenetically related to Dandy–Walker and Arnold–Chiari syndromes: bizarre malformed brain with occipital encephalocele. Johns Hopkins Med J 131:228–246
31. Marin-Padilla M, Marin-Padilla TM (1981) Morphogenesis of experimentally induced Arnold–Chiari malformation. J Neurol Sci 50:29–55
32. Inagaki T, Schoenwolf GC, Walker ML (1997) Experimental model: changes in the posterior fossa with surgically induced spina bifida aperta in mouse. Pediatr Neurosurg 26:185–189
33. Waddington CH (1932) Experiments of the development of chick and duck embryos, cultivated in vitro. Philos Trans R Soc London, Ser B 221:179–230
34. Waddington CH (1933) Induction by the primitive streak and its derivatives in the chick. J Exp Biol 10:38–46
35. Waddington CH, Schmidt GA (1933) Induction by heteroplastic grafts of the primitive streak in birds. Arch Entwicklungsmech Org 128:522–563
36. Woodside GL (1937) The influence of host age on induction in the chick blastoderm. J Exp Zool 75:259–281
37. Grabowski CT (1957) The induction of secondary embryos in the early chick blastoderm by grafts of Hensen's node. Am J Anat 101:101–133
38. Grabowski CT (1962) Neural induction and notochord formation by mesoderm from the node area of the early chick blastoderm. J Exp Zool 150:233–245
39. Sher-Pu S, I-Lan N, Shu-Dung T (1963) Studies on the inductive action of the Hensen's node following its transplantation in ovo to the early chick blastoderm. Acta Bilo Wxp Sin 8:441–462
40. Sher-Pu S, I-Lan N, Shu-Dung T (1965) Experimental analysis on the reactive capacity of the epiblast of the chick blastoderm. Acta Anat Sin 8:1–10
41. Gallera J, Ivanov I (1964) La compétence neurogène du feuillexterne du blastoderme de poulet en fonction du facteur "temps." J Embryol Exp Morphol 12:693–711

42. Vakaet L (1984) Early development of birds. In: LeDouarin N, McLaren A (eds) Chimeras in developmental biology. Academic Press, London, pp 71–88
43. Dias MS, Schoenwolf GC (1990) Formation of ectopic neurepithelium in chick blastoderms: age-related capacities for induction and self-differentiation following transplantation of quail Hensen's nodes. Anat Rec 229:437–448
44. Garcia-Martinez V, Schoenwolf GC (1992) Positional control of mesoderm movement and fate during avian gastrulation and neurulation. Dev Dyn 193:249–256
45. Selleck MAJ, Stern CD (1992) Commitment of mesoderm cells in Hensen's node of the chick embryo to notochord and somite. Development 114:403–415
46. Inagaki T, Schoenwolf GC (1993) Axis development in avian embryos: the ability of Hensen's node to self-differentiate, as analyzed with heterochronic grafting experiments. Anat Embryol 188:1–11
47. Dias M, Walker M (1992) The embryogenesis of complex dysraphic malformation: a disorder of gastrulation? Pediatr Neurosurg 18:229–253

The Pathogenesis of Myeloschisis: Experimental Studies

K. Takahashi[1], H. Tanaka[1], S. Nakahara[2], H. Nakazaki[1], T. Terao[1], and T. Abe[1]

Summary. In order to clarify the pathogenesis of dysraphism, we performed experimental studies on: (1) neural tube defect (NTD) induced by Concanavalin-A (Con-A); (2) the proliferation of spinal neurons under the influence of amniotic fluid; (3) immunohistochemical analysis of myeloschisis in the Splotch-delayed mouse. We found that the effects of Concanavalin-A (Con-A) depended on the time of administration, and Con-A administration resulted in target-specific NTD. Cultures in amniotic fluid showed a dose-dependent proliferation of neural cells. Therefore, amniotic fluid may have some effect on neural cells. Glial fibrillary acidic protein (GFAP) was confirmed on the neural placode in Splotch-delayed mice. In contrast, GFAP was not detected in normal mice. Therefore, gliosis was in progress at the neural placode. These findings suggested that Con-A may bind to carbohydrates of the neuroepithelium during neurulation and induce NTD by disturbance of the cell-to-cell interaction. We speculate that the overgrowth is a secondary phenomenon caused by the amnion.

Key words. Neural tube defect, Neurulation, Lectins, Amnion, Splotch delayed mouse, GFAP

Introduction

Spina bifida is one of the most common congenital malformations of the central nervous system. The incidence is 1 per 1000 live births in Japan. Myeloschisis is especially representative of spina bifida, and almost all of the neural placode is irreversibly damaged.

The embryopathogenesis of dysraphism has been extensively studied, but no theory has been agreed upon. In order to analyze the pathogenesis of myeloschisis, we performed experimental studies on: (1) neural tube defects induced by amnion injected with Concanavalin-A in mouse embryos; (2) the proliferation of spinal neurons in a normal mouse fetus under the influence of amniotic fluid; (3) immunohistochemical analysis of myeloschisis in the Splotch-delayed mouse.

[1]Department of Neurosurgery, The Jikei University of Medicine, 3-25-8 Nishi-shinbashi, Minatoku, Tokyo 105, Japan
[2]Department of Neurosurgery, Meitokukai Sotoh Daiichi Hospital

Neural Tube Defects Induced by Amnion Injected with Concanavalin-A in Mouse Embryos

Materials and Method

Carbohydrates on a cell surface may serve as determinants of cell differentiation in cell-to-cell interactions and maturation. Nakahara [1] tested the possibility that exogenous lectin may be bound with glycoconjugates of neurulation and induce neural tube defects.

We injected 200 ng/0.2 ml of Concanavalin-A into the amniotic cavity on gestation days 8.2 and 8.4 (prior to anterior neuropore closure, which normally occurs on gestation day 8.5), and 9.0 and 9.2 (prior to posterior neuropore closure, which normally occurs on gestation day 9.5).

Observations and Results

Concanavalin-A administered prior to anterior neuropore closure resulted in cranioschisis without spinal neural tube defects, whereas Concanavalin-A administered prior to posterior neuropore closure resulted in spinal neural tube defects without cranioschisis (Table 1).

The results indicated that the effects of an exogenous lectin were dependent on the time of its administration, and Concanavalin-A administration resulted in target-specific neural tube defects. The dysraphism seen in this experiment may be caused by a disturbance in the recognition and interaction of neural cells and a failure of neural tube closure.

Proliferation of Spinal Neurons of a Normal Mouse Fetus Under the influence of Amniotic Fluid

Materials and Method

Myeloschisis presents as skin defects on the back or lumbar region, and cerebrospinal fluid leakage may be found here. These problems are traditionally called overgrowth. Some researchers have reported that this overgrowth is an important cause of dysraphism [2, 3]. However, we believe that the overgrowth is a secondary reaction to the open neural tube bathed in amniotic fluid.

The spinal cord of a normal mouse fetus on gestation day 12 was extracted and cultured. 0%, 10%, or 30% of amniotic fluid was added to the cultures and the growths of these cultures were compared.

TABLE 1. CNS anomalies induced by exogenous lectin

	Cranioschisis		Caudal NTD	
Gestation Day	*n*	%	*n*	%
8.2 ($N = 14$)	3	21.4	0	0
8.4 ($N = 17$)	2	11.8	0	0
9.0 ($N = 33$)	0	0	10	30.3
9.2 ($N = 18$)	0	0	1	5.6

NTD, neural tube defect.

Observations and Results

Over time, the cultures with amniotic fluid, showed a dose-dependent proliferation of cells (Fig. 1). This result suggested that amniotic fluid may have some effect upon neural cells.

Immunohistochemical Analysis of Myeloschisis in the Splotch-Delayed Mouse

Materials and Method

Splotch-delayed mice are known to have a 25% possibility of developing myeloschisis during gestation. Using Splotch-delayed mice in order to analyze the pathogenesis of the opened neural placode, we studied the immunohistochemical localization of glial fibrillary acidic protein (GFAP) in the neural placode and compared in with that of normal mice. Embryos

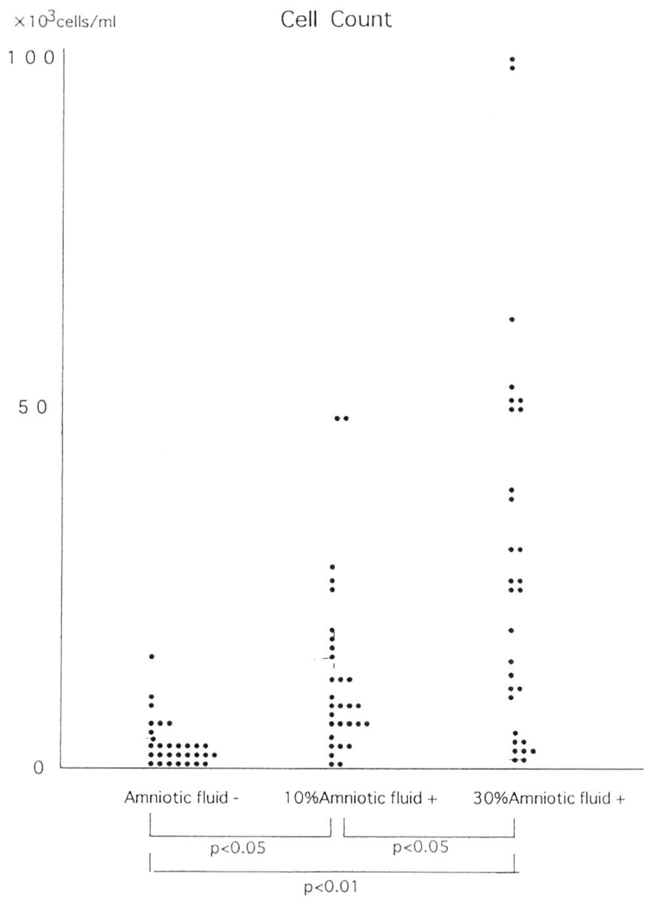

FIG. 1. Result of viable cell count

were removed from the uterus on gestation days 15, 16, or 18. Horizontal sections of the lumbosacral region were prepared as specimens. We used anti-GFAP rabbit serum for the first antibody.

Observations and Results

GFAP was not detected in the neural placode on the 15th fetal day. On the 16th fetal day, GFAP was confirmed in the cytosome of the neural placode on the dorsal surface of a Splotch-delayed mouse (Fig. 2A). GFAP was particularly evident where the amniotic fluid came into direct contact with the neural placode. By the 18th fetal day, GFAP-positive cells had increased and could be confirmed extending inwards (Fig. 2B). In contrast, GFAP was not detected at the same time periods in normal mice (Fig. 3).

These experiments using Splotch-delayed mice suggested that gliosis was in progress at the neural placode.

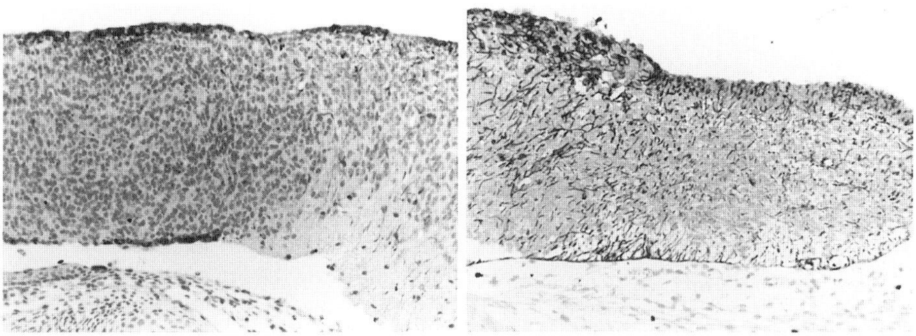

A B

Fig. 2. Staining for glial fibrillary acidic protein (GFAP) in a Splotch-delayed mouse with myeloschisis. ×100. GFAP is confirmed on the dorsal surface of the neural placode on the 16th fetal day (**A**), and GFAP expression has increased by the 18th day of gestation (**B**)

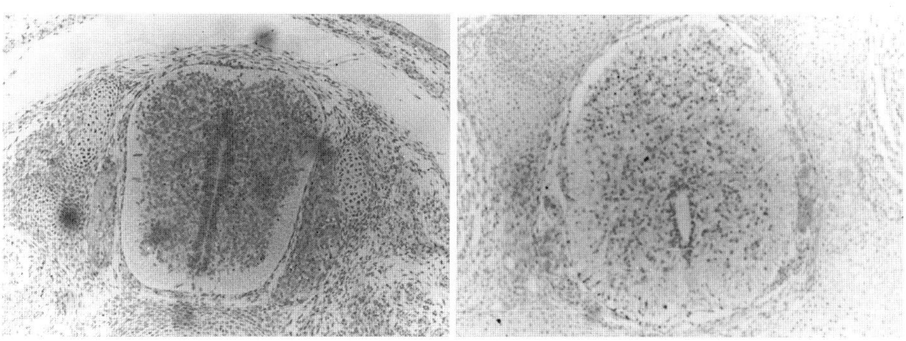

A B

Fig. 3. Staining for GFAP in a normal mouse. ×100. GFAP was not detected on the 16th (**A**) or 18th (**B**) fetal day

Discussion

Several theories have been suggested for the embryopathogenesis of myeloschisis. Weed [4] proposed a hypothesis of rupture of the closed neural tube. Gardner [5] proposed that overdistension and rupture of the neural tube could occur as a result of elevated cerebrospinal fluid pressure. This theory was based on the background work of Weed. On the other hand, Von Recklinghausen [6] proposed that the embryonic neural tube fails to close (simple nonclosure theory). Jones et al. [7] proposed a mesodermal origin for axis dysraphic disorder, which is also regarded as an early effect of fetal environmental factors before the neural tube closes (chordoaxial mesodermal origin theory). McLone and Knepper [8] suggested that a certain teratogen interferes with the synthesis of complex carbohydrates that play a role in the closure of the neural tube. From the result that neural tube defects were induced by exogenous lectin, we believe that myeloschisis is caused by a disturbance of the recognition and interaction of neural cells, followed by failure of neural tube closure.

Some researchers have observed morphological findings in the neural placode known as overgrowth. Patten found evidence of overgrowth of the neural tube in young human embryos, and emphasized the possibility that local overgrowth of the neural plate in the early stages of its development might be a factor in the genesis of myeloschisis and spina bifida (overgrowth and nonclosure theory) [2]. Oi et al. [3] proposed experimental studies to analyse the stage-specificity using chick embryos. They suggested that myeloschisis could be produced by some mechanism of reopening the once closed neural tube, and overgrowth of the neural plate was an attempt at reopening. However, from the results of immunohistochemical analysis and culture, we consider that one cause of our histological findings on the overgrowth of the neural placode is a secondary reaction of the opened neural placode in amniotic fluid. Patients with myeloschisis have severe neurological defects, such as paraplegia. Severe irriversible neurological defects may be caused by the progression of gliosis.

Conclusion

We have reported on three studies of the pathogenesis of myeloschisis.

Myeloschisis is considered to be caused by a failure to recognize the interaction of neural cells during neural tube closure. It is suggested that the histological changes represented by gliosis at the myeloschisis is a secondary response induced by amniotic fluid coming into contact with the opened neural placode.

References

1. Nakahara S (1992) Exogenous lectins and neurulation defects. Off J Jpn Soc Pediatr Neurosurg 17:325–332
2. Patten BM (1946) Embryological stages in the development of spina bifida and myeloschisis. Anat Rec 94:487 (abstract)
3. Oi S, Saya H, Matsumoto S (1988) A hypothesis for myeloschisis: overgrowth and reopening; an experimental study. J Neurosurg 68:947–954
4. Weed LH (1917) The development of the cerebrospinal spaces in pig and man. Contrib Embryol 15:1–116
5. Gardner WJ (1965) Hydrodynamic mechanism of syringomyelia: its relationship to myelocele. J Neurol Neurosurg Psychiatr 28:247–259

6. Von Recklinghausen F (1886) Untersuchungen uber die Spina Bifida. Virchows Arch (A) 105:243–330, 373–455
7. Jones MC, Jones KL, Chernoff GF (1982) Possible mesodermal origin for axial dysraphic disorders. J Pediatr 101:845–849
8. McLone DG, Knepper PA (1986) Role of complex carbohydrates and neurulation. Pediatr Neurosci 12:2–9

Functional Roles of Basic Helix–Loop–Helix (bHLH) Transcription Factors in Proliferation and Differentiation of Neural Tube Cells

Kikuo Suda[1], Masakazu Miyajima[2], Hajime Arai[2], and Kiyoshi Sato[2]

Summary. Clinical studies demonstrate that folic acid supplementation in early pregnancy can prevent up to 70% of neural tube defects, whereas the remaining neural tube defects are resistant to folate. The molecular mechanism of neural tube defects still is unclear. We have isolated helix–loop–helix (HLH) transcription factor GE1, GE12 cDNA and demonstrated its expression in developing neural tube interneurons. To examine the function of class A bHLH transcription factors, including GE1, GE12, we intend to block their expression using antisense oligonucleotides. Simultaneous blocking of class A bHLH transcription factors in cultured neural tube cells results in the reduction of differentiating neurons. Blocking the expression of individual class A bHLH transcription factors has no detectable effect. These results demonstrate that class A bHLH transcription factors have a functional redundancy during neuronal development, and suggest that a single gene mutation does not cause neural tube defects.

Key words. bHLH, Neural tube, Neuronal differentiation

Introduction

Clinical studies demonstrate that folic acid supplementation in early pregnancy can prevent up to 70% of neural tube defects, whereas the remaining neural tube defects are resistant to folate [5, 11]. The molecular mechanism of neural tube defects still is unclear.

Helix–loop–helix (HLH) transcription factors are involved in the regulation of neurogenesis from insects to vertebrates [3, 8]. Basic HLH (bHLH) transcription factors are expressed either ubiquitously, class A, or have cell- and tissue-type-specific expression, class B [13]. Class A bHLH transcription factors interact with class B bHLH proteins [7, 12, 13] as well as with Id-like negative regulators [2, 16] and the HES family of HLH transcription factors [1].

Class A bHLH transcription factors GE1 and GE12 (chick) are expressed at relatively high levels in developing neuroepithelium during the early stages of neurogenesis. The expression of GE1 is highest in the distal region of the ventricular zone. Also, the highest expression of GE12 is in the distal region of the ventricular zone and the newly formed intermediate zone

[1] Department of Neurosurgery, Saiseikai General Hospital, 5-12-1 Nishikawaguchi, Kawaguchi-city, Saitama 332, Japan
[2] Department of Neurosurgery, Juntendo University School of Medicine, 2-1-1 Hongo, Bunkyo-ku, Tokyo 113, Japan

[15, 19]. The distal region of the ventricular zone is composed of cells in the DNA synthesis phase of the cell cycle and early stages of differentiation. Another class A bHLH transcription factor, E2A, gene is expressed in proliferative zones of the developing brain, and no E2A expression is detectable in nonproliferative regions of the brain spinal cord of rats [17]. The expression patterns of these different HLH transcription factors suggest the existence of a dynamic network of these proteins during neurogenesis.

Within this interacting network of different HLH transcription factors, class A bHLH genes are expressed while cells are in the transition from proliferation to differentiation. This expression pattern and the molecular interactions of class A proteins suggest that they have a critical role in the neurogenesis. Overlapping expression of class A bHLH transcription factors in developing neural tube enables us to hypothesize that a network of HLH transcription factors is involved in the regulation of the initial stages of neurogenesis. To test this hypothesis, we blocked expression of class A bHLH proteins using antisense oligonucleotides. In this chapter, we present data which demonstrate that class A bHLH transcription factors have functional redundancy, and that blocking their expression results in the death of differentiating interneurons.

Materials and Methods

Cloning

PCR amplification was used to isolate class A bHLH transcription factor GE1, GE12 cDNA from the developing nervous system of chick, as described elsewhere [15, 19]. The oligonucleotide primers 5′-GC(A,C,G,T)AA(C,T)AA(C,T)GC(A,C,G,T)(A,C)G(A,C,G,T)GA(A,G)(A,C)G and 5′-CYCT(A,C,G,T)AC(C,T)TG(C,T)TG(C,T)TC(A,C,G,T)A were used in the amplification reaction. Clones obtained by screening the library were used to confirm and extend the sequence obtained from the original PCR amplified cDNA.

Cell Culture

Neural tubes (from midmyelencephalon to thoracic level of chick embryo, stage 14–17 [6]) were isolated as described elsewhere (K. Suda et al., unpublished) and dissociated into single cells using 0.25% trypsin and 50 mM EDTA in calcium-magnesium-free Dulbecco medium (Gibco). Cells ($2–5 \times 10^4$ per well) were cultivated on poly-L-lysine and laminin (50 μg/ml) coated tissue culture 8-chamber slides in DME/F12 serum-free medium with N-2 supplement (Gibco) in the presence of EGF (20 ng/ml) and antibiotics.

Antisense Oligonucleotides

Antisense oligonucleotides specific for GE1 and GE2 as well as degenerate oligonucleotides recognizing both GE1 and GE2 were synthesized.

GE1a1—5′-CCAAGCGCATCGCCTGTCTG
GE1a2—5′-GTACTGCTTGTTCTTCCTCTA
GE12a1—5′-GCTTCGTCCAACCTGTCTTCC
GE12a2—5′-CAGCTCCTTCTTCTCCTCTTC
GEa1—5′-A(GC)GCCTCGTTGATGACACGGAC
GEa2—5′-T(CT)AGCAGTTT(GC)GTCTGTGGT
GEa3—5′-TTCAGGATGACCGAGACAGCC
Nonsense oligo—randomly synthesized 21-mer

Antisense oligonucleotides were added directly into culture media at a final concentration of 50 μM.

Immunohistochemistry

Double-staining of neuronal cultures was used to identify proliferating and differentiating into neuron cells.

5-Bromo-2′-deoxyuridine (BrdU; Boehringer, Mannheim, Germany) was added to the culture media at a concentration of 10 μM for 24 h soon after plating. After 48 h, the cells were rinsed with PBS and fixed by cold methanol at 4°C. DNA was denatured by incubation in 2N HCl for 30 min followed by washing twice with borate buffer and three times with PBS. BrdU incorporation was detected by mouse anti-BrdU monoclonal antibody (Boehringer, Mannheim). Slides were incubated with antibody, washed with 0.05% Triton X-100/PBS and incubated with secondary HRP-conjugated goat anti-mouse IgG (Sigma, St. Louis). After an additional wash, bound antibody was detected using 0.05% diaminobenzidine (DAB-4HCl). Neurofilament immunostaining was performed after treatment of slides with 0.1 M glycine-HCl to remove anti-BrdU and HRP-conjugated anti-mouse antibodies [14]. After washing with PBS, mouse monoclonal antibody against the 68 Kd neurofilament protein (Sigma, St. Louis) was added and incubated. HRP-conjugated goat anti-mouse IgG and 0.02% 4-chloro-1-naphthol were used to detect NF-L immunoreactivity.

^{3}H-thymidine Incorporation Assay

Dissociated cells were plated on poly-L-lysine and laminin coated 48-well plates and incubated in the presence of [6-^{3}H] thymidine (1 μCi/ml). After 24 h, the medium was removed, and cells were washed three times with PBS. Aliquots were saved for counting cell numbers. Cells were disrupted in 75 μl distilled water and transferred to 2.4-cm glass fiber filter discs. After drying, filters were immersed in cold 10% trichloroacetic acid followed by cold absolute ethanol. Radioactivity in dried filters was counted using a liquid scintillation counter (LS 7000; Beckman). Cells were counted using a hemocytometer and the *t*-test was used for statistical analyses of data.

Flow Cytometry

Cultured cells for 24 h were fixed in 70% ethanol/PBS and stained with propidium iodine (50 μg/mol). The DNA content of individual cells was measured using a flow cytometer Coulter Epics 5, and cell cycle analyses were performed using multicycle analysis software (Phoenix Flow Cytometry System).

Results

Altering the Expression of GEs Using Antisense Oligonucleotides

The expression pattern indicates that class A bHLH transcription factors GE1 and GE12 are expressed in either proliferating or differentiating cells or in both. To determine the function of GEs in these cells, a tissue culture system was developed where neuroblasts proliferate and differentiate in vitro. Antisense oligonucleotides were added to these cultures to block the expression of class A bHLH transcription factors. Expression of GE1 or GE12 (GE1a1, GE1a2, GE12a1, and GE12a2) was blocked individually using two different antisense oligonu-

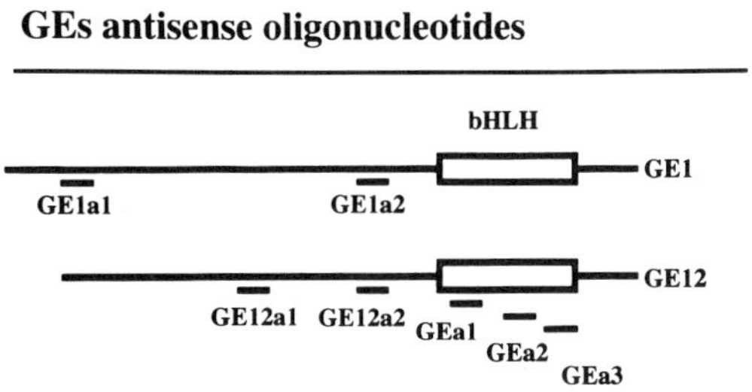

FIG. 1. Schematic representation of the localization of antisense oligonucleotide sequences on GE1 and GE12 mRNA. Antisense oligonucleotides GE1a1 and GE1a2 are specific for GE1 gene, GE12a1 and GE12a2 are specific for GE12 gene, GEa1, GEa2, and GEa3 are common for all known GEs

cleotides, and GE1 and GE12 were blocked simultaneously using degenerate antisense oligonucleotides (GEa1, GEa2, Gea3) corresponding to the HLH region (Fig. 1).

Proliferation and Differentiation of Neuroblasts

In the first experiment, proliferation and differentiation of neuroblasts were analyzed simultaneously. DNA synthesis was detected by 5-bromo-2′-deoxyuridine (BrdU) incorporation, and neurofilament L (NF-L) immunostaining was used as a neuronal marker. BrdU was present in cultures during the first 24 h, and cells were fixed and stained for neurofilament and BrdU immunoreactivity after 48 h. At this time, 40–50% of cells were NF-L positive and 70% of cells synthesized DNA (BrdU+). About 60% of NF-L-positive cells in control cultures were BrdU-positive, which indicates that neuroblasts continue proliferation and differentiation in vitro.

Antisense oligonucleotides are known to be unstable in cell culture. To optimize the treatment of neural tube cultures with antisense oligonucleotides, degenerative oligonucleotide GEa3 was added to the cell culture once (at the beginning of the experiment), twice (at the beginning and after 12 h), or five times (after every 6 h). In all treatments, the percentage of double-labeled cells is reduced compared with control oligonucleotide or PBS (Fig. 2). The addition of antisense oligonucleotides once, twice, or five times reduces the percentage of double-labeled cells by 6%, 13%, and 21%, respectively. Based on these data, all subsequent experiments were done with the addition of antisense oligonucleotides five times. All three degenerative antisense oligonucleotides which correspond to sequences in the HLH region of GE1 and GE12 genes caused about a 20% reduction of double-labeled cells, whereas control oligonucleotides had no effect. Also GE1- and GE12-specific antisense oligonucleotides had no detectable effect on the number of double-labeled cells (Fig. 3). Sense oligonucleotides were not used as controls in these experiments because of the possibility of forming triple helical structures with the gene, and thus affecting gene expression. The fact that antisense oligonucleotides complementary to the HLH region cause a reduction in double-labeled cells, while control as well as GE1- and GE12-specific oligonucleotides do not, suggests that the effect is specific, and is not caused by the high concentration of oligonucleotides.

These experiments demonstrate that either proliferation or differentiation of neuroblasts is affected when the expression of GE1 and GE12 are blocked simultaneously. However, blocking GE1 and GE12 individually has no detectable effect.

Furthermore, electrophoretic mobility shift assay (EMSA) was used to demonstrate the effectiveness of antisense oligonucleotides in blocking the synthesis of class A bHLH transcription factors in neural tube cultures, as described elsewhere [19]. The immunoglobulin enhancer kE2, which is a binding site for all known class A bHLH transcription factors [12],

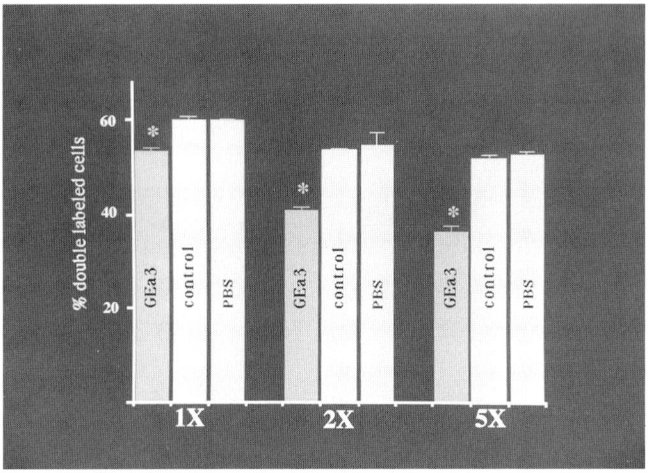

FIG. 2. Effect of repetitive addition of antisense oligonucleotide GEa3 to neural tube cell cultures on the number of DNA synthesizing and neuronally differentiating cells (double-labeled cells). DNA synthesis was analyzed using BrdU incorporation into DNA followed by immunocytochemical detection, and neuronal differentiation was detected using antibodies against neurofilament light (NF-L) subunit. Cells were fixed and immunostained after 48 h, and the number of BrdU- and NF-L-positive cells was counted in five randomly picked areas. Antisense oligonucleotides were added once (*1X*), twice (*2X*), and five times (*5X*). $^*P < 0.05$

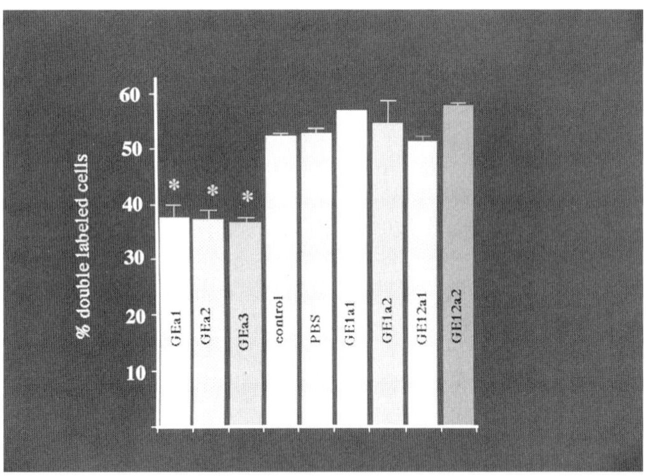

FIG. 3. Effect of different antisense oligonucleotides on the number of double-labeled cells. Fresh aliquots of antisense oligonucleotides were added to the culture media every 6 h, and the cells were fixed after 48 h. $^*P < 0.05$. All experiments were done at least in triplicate

was used. EMSA detects three DNA-protein complexes in control cultures. The amount of all three DNA-protein complexes is highly reduced in cultures treated with antisense oligonucleotides GEa1, GEa2, and GEa3, which are complementary to all GE RNAs. These analyses demonstrate indirectly that antisense oligonucleotides reduce the synthesis of bHLH proteins which form complexes with the kE2 binding site.

Does Reduction of GE Expression Affect Proliferation or Differentiation?

The experiments described above demonstrate about a 20% reduction in the number of cells that proliferate and differentiate to neurons in vitro when the expression of GEs is reduced. The following experiments are designed to determine which of these processes, proliferation or differentiation, is affected by altering the expression of class A bHLH transcription factors.

Cell Number and DNA Synthesis

DNA synthesis and the number of cells in neural tube cultures were analyzed after a 24-h treatment with antisense oligonucleotides (GEa1, GEa2, and GEa3) that reduce the expression of GEs. DNA synthesis is not affected, but there is about a 40–45% reduction in the number of cells after treatment (Fig. 4). Possible explanations for this reduced number of cells in culture is either the arrest of the cell cycle between the S phase and mitosis, or cell death. To clarify this problem, cell-cycle analyses were performed using flow cytometry.

Cell-Cycle Analyses

If there is a block in the cell cycle between the S and M phases, there will be an increase in the number of cells in the G2 phase of the cell cycle. In control cultures, 51% of the cells were

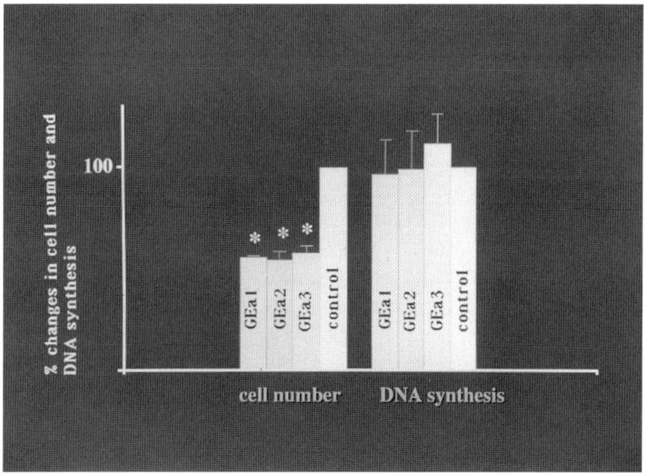

FIG. 4. Effect of antisense oligonucleotides on cell number and DNA synthesis of chick neural tube cells after 24 h in culture. Chick neural tube cultures were treated with antisense oligonucleotides GEa1, GEa2, and GEa3, and thymidine incorporation and cell number were analyzed in thrree independent experiments. Changes in cell number and DNA synthesis in the treated cultures are presented as percentages of the nonsense oligonucleotide control. $^{*}P < 0.05$

TABLE 1. Effect of antisense oligonucleotides GEa1 and GEa2 on the cell cycle

Oligonucleotide	% cells		
	G1	S	G2/M
Control oligonucleotide	51 ± 2	23.5 ± 2	25.5 ± 3
GEa1	52 ± 3	21 ± 1	27 ± 4
GEa2	52 ± 3	17 ± 3	31 ± 2

Chick neural tube cultures were treated with nonsense and antisense oligonucleotides GEa1 and GEa2 for 24h. The DNA content was determined by flow cytometry of propidium iodine-stained cells. There is no statistical difference (*t*-test, three experiments) in the portion of cells in different phases of the cell cycle between control- and antisense-treated chick neural tube cells.

in the G1, 24% in the S, and 25% in the G2 phase of the cell cycle (Table 1). There was no statistically significant change in the number of cells in different phases of the cell cycle following antisense oligonucleotide treatment. This result favors the second explanation, namely that cell death occurs after reducing the expression of class A bHLH transcription factors. Further, since DNA synthesis and the cell cycle are not affected, the cells which die have not synthesized DNA in culture during antisense oligonucleotide treatment.

Discussion

We have characterized the expression of class A bHLH transcription factors GE1 and GE12 in the developing neural tube. Both are expressed at high levels in the distal region of the ventricular zone, and blocking their expression causes cell death of differentiating neurons. Since the discovery of class A bHLH transcription factors, many details of their molecular interactions have been clarified, although their biological role remains unknown. In vertebrates, several members of class A bHLH transcription factors are expressed in the developing nervous system [15, 17].

To determine the biological role of class A bHLH transcription factors in neurogenesis, we used chick embryo neural tube cells. Two class A bHLH transcription factors are expressed in the developing neural tube of a chick. There is a high expression of GE1 [15] and GE12 [19] in the distal region of the ventricular zone, where cells are in the S phase of the cell cycle or at the beginning of differentiation. When cells migrate out from the ventricular zone, the expression of GE1 decreases and the expression of GE12 remains high in newly differentiating interneurons [19]. The expression pattern of GEs (GE1 and GE12) suggests that they function in proliferation or differentiation or in both processes in developing interneurons. We used antisense oligonucleotides complementary to all known GEs to reduce their expression in chick neural tube cells in vitro. The results of these experiments demonstrate that blocking GEs during first 24h in vitro causes a reduction in the number of cells at 24h, and the reduced number of double-labeled cells after 48h are presumably postmitotic interneurons.

In our culture conditions, the population of neural tube cells that synthesized DNA during the first 24h and became neurofilament-positive by 48h initiated differentiation relatively late in the 24-h period (K. Soda et al., unpublished). Since DNA synthesis is not affected by antisense oligonucleotides, the reduction in the number of double-labeled cells by 48h is again a result of the death of postmitotic neurons which proliferated and became exposed to antisense oligonucleotides in the initial stages of their differentiation. The expression pattern of GEs, as well as the reduction in the number of differentiating cells following antisense treatment, suggests that these factors are involved in the differentiation of interneurons. We hypothesize that blocking GEs in cells committed to differentiate into interneurons causes cell death. Another example where blocking differentiation causes cell death is when overexpression of simian virus (SV40) large T antigen in cerebellar Purkinje cells in transgenic mice blocks differentiation and results in massive cell death [4].

The second important conclusion from this study is that there is a redundancy in function of class A bHLH transcription factors during neurogenesis. Blocking a single class A bHLH transcription factor has no effect on development of neural tube cells, and simultaneous blocking of all known GEs causes cell death. The biological significance of redundancy is unknown, but it is a general phenomenon which exists in several gene systems [9, 10, 18]. Therefore we can suggest that a single gene mutation does not cause neural tube defects.

Following this study, we need to establish a neural plate explant culture from early chick embryo and examine whether or not neural tube defects occur by blocking their expressions of GEs using antisense oligonucleotides. We hope that these experiments will be useful in attempts to understand the molecular mechanism of neural tube defects.

Acknowledgments. We are deeply grateful to Howard O. Nornes and Toomas Neuman, in the Department of Anatomy and Neurobiology, Colorado State University, for helpful discussions and for reading the manuscript.

References

1. Akazawa C, Sasai Y, Nakanishi S, Kageyama R (1992) Molecular characterization of a rat negative regulator with a basic helix-loop-helix structure predominantly expressed in the developing nervous system. J Biol Chem 267:21879–21885
2. Benezra R, Davis RL, Lockshon D, Turner DL, Weintraub H (1990) The protein Id: A negative regulator of helix-loop-helix DNA binding proteins. Cell 61:49–59
3. Campos-Ortega JA, Jan YN (1991) Genetics and molecular bases of neurogenesis in *Drosophila melanogaster*. Annu Rev Neurosci 14:399–420
4. Feddersen RM, Ehlenfeldt R, Yunis WS, Clark HB, Orr HT (1992) Disrupted cerebellar cortical development and progressive degeneration of Purkinje cells in SV40 T antigen transgenic mice. Neuron 9:955–966
5. Greene NDE, Copp AJ (1997) Inositol prevents folate-resistant neural tube defects in the mouse. Nature Med 3:60–66
6. Hamburger V, Hamilton HL (1951) A series of normal stages in the development of the chick embryo. J Morphol 88:49–91
7. Hu JS, Olson E, Kingston RE (1992) A helix-loop-helix protein related to E2A and ITF2 that can modulate the DNA-binding ability of myogenic regulatory factors. Mol Cell Biol 12:1031–1042
8. Johnson JE, Birren SJ, Anderson DJ (1990) Two rat homologues of *Drosophila achaete-scute* specifically expressed in neuronal precursors. Nature 346:858–861
9. Joyner AL, Herrup K, Auerbach CA, Rossant J (1991) Subtle cerebellar phenotype in mice homozygous for a targeted deletion of the *En-2* homeobox. Science 251:1239–1243
10. Lufkin T, Dierich A, LeMeur M, Mark M, Chambon P (1991) Disruption of the Hox-1.6 homeobox gene results in defects in a region corresponding to its rostral of expression. Cell 66:1105–1119
11. MRC Vitamin Study Research Group (1991) Prevention of neural tube defect: result of the Medical Research Council Vitamin Study. Lancet 338:131–137

12. Murre C, McCaw PS, Baltimore D (1989) A new DNA binding and dimerization motif in immunoglobulin enhancer binding, daughterless, MyoD, and myc proteins. Cell 56:777–783
13. Murre C, McCaw PS, Vaessin H, Caudy M, Jan LY, Jan YN, Cabrera CV (1989) Interactions between heterologous helix–loop–helix proteins generate complexes that bind specifically to a common DNA sequence. Cell 58:537–544
14. Nakan PK (1968) Simultaneous localization of multiple tissue antigens using the peroxidase-labeled antibody method: a study on pituitary glands of the rat. J Histochem Cytochem 16:557–563
15. Neuman T, Keen A, Knapik E, Shain D, Ross M, Nornes HO, Zuber MX (1993) ME1 and GE1: basic helix–loop–helix transcription factors expressed at high levels in the developing nervous system and in morphogenetically active regions. Eur J Neurosci 5:311–318
16. Neuman T, Keen A, Kristjansson G-I, Gruss P, Nornes HO (1993) Neuronal expression of regulatory helix–loop–helix factor *Id2* gene in mouse. Dev Biol 160:186–195
17. Roberts VJ, Steenbergen R, Murre C (1993) Localization of E2A mRNA expression in developing and adult rat tissues. Proc Natl Acad Sci USA 90:7583–7587
18. Rudnicki MA, Braun T, Hinuma S, Jaenisch R (1992) Inactivation of MyoD in mice leads to up-regulation of the myogenic HLH gene Myf-5 and results in apparently normal muscle development. Cell 71:383–390
19. Suda K, Nornes HO, Neuman T (1994) Class A basic helix–loop–helix transcription factors in early stages of chick neural tube development: evidence for functional redundancy. Neurosci Lett 177:87–90

Pathogenesis of Cerebellar Deformity in Chiari Type I Malformation Caused by Mumps-Associated Hydrocephalus in Hamsters

Tomoyuki Takano

Summary. This study was undertaken to elucidate the pathogenesis of Chiari type I malformation using an experimental model of hydrocephalus produced by inoculating hamsters with mumps virus. Dilatation of the lateral ventricles was detected in all brains inoculated at 2, 10, or 25 days of age. The cerebellum in hamsters inoculated at 2 or 10 days of age showed elongation and flattening of the vermis, and protrusion or notching of the uvula. All layers, i.e., the molecular, Purkinje cell, and granular layers, and the white matter were preserved, but had narrowed. Purkinje cells remained normal. Hamsters inoculated at 25 days of age did not develop cerebellar deformity. Mumps virus antigen was detected in all ependymal cells and in some epithelial cells of the choroid plexus in all hamsters that had been inoculated at 2, 10, or 25 days of age. The results suggest that Chiari type I malformation is caused by two main factors occurring simultaneously: (1) increasing intracranial pressure, and (2) rapid histogenesis of the cerebellar cortex.

Key words. Chiari malformation, Mumps virus, Hydrocephalus

Introduction

Deformities characterized by cerebellar elongation and protrusion through the foramen magnum into the cervical spinal canal are known as the Chiari malformation. In the type I malformation, cone-shaped tonsils and medial aspects of the posterior lobe of the cerebellum, as well as an elongated caudal medulla, can be found in the upper cervical vertebral canal [1]. The pathogenesis of this malformation is still a matter of controversy [3].

In a series of experimental studies on the pathogenesis of congenital hydrocephalus caused by the inoculation of myxoviruses in hamsters, we reported that extensive damage to the ependymal cilia might have accounted for early ventricular dilatation, and that the subsequent aqueductal stenosis with glial proliferation was the main cause of the advanced hydrocephalus [15]. Moreover, we found that most hamsters thus inoculated later developed not only hydrocephalus, but also a cerebellar deformity [15, 16]. The cerebellar deformity in these hamsters was thought to be comparable to Chiari type I malformation. The present experiment was undertaken to elucidate the pathogenesis of Chiari type I malformation using the experimental model of hydrocephalus caused by inoculation of mumps virus in hamsters.

Department of Pediatrics, Shiga University of Medical Science, Seta-Tsukinowa, Ohtsu 520-21, Japan

Materials and Methods

The mumps virus used was isolated from the saliva of a patient with parotitis. Virus infectivity was expressed as the reciprocal of the dilution causing infection in 50% of cultures (TCD_{50}).

In the experimental group, a total of 39 Syrian hamsters, 2, 10, and 25 days old, were inoculated intracerebrally with 10 μl of $2TCD_{50}$ mumps virus through a 27-gauge needle. As controls, 14 animals of 2, 10, and 25 days of age were injected with the same amount of minimum essential medium in a similar manner. These animals were anesthetized with ether or pentobarbital, perfused with saline solution, and then killed either 8 or 14–18 days after each inoculation. Some of the excised brains were used for macroscopic examination. Others were fixed in phosphate-buffered 10% formalin and embedded in paraffin; serial 5-μm sagittal sections of cerebellum were then stained by the Bodian method. For immunohistochemical identification of the sites of mumps virus antigen, nine animals were killed 5 days after each mumps virus inoculation. Their brains were prepared by perfusion with 4% paraformaldehyde, 0.3% glutaraldehyde, and 0.2% picric acid in 0.1 M phosphate buffer. After immersion in 15% sucrose solution for more than 2 days at 4°C, the cerebellum of each brain was cut into 20-μm-thick serial sagittal sections on a cryostat. These sections were mounted on glass slides and incubated for 2 days at 4°C in rabbit anti-mumps virus hyperimmune serum (Denkaseiken, Tokyo, Japan), diluted 1:1200 in phosphate-buffered saline. These slides were then incubated serially at room temperature in 1:2000 biotinylated anti-rabbit IgG (Vector Lab, Burlingame, CA, USA) for 2 h, in avidin–biotin–peroxidase complex (Vector Lab) for 2 h, and in 0.05% diaminobenzidine solution containing 0.01% hydrogen peroxide for 5 min.

Results

Macroscopic Examination

All brains in the experimental group showed dilatation of the lateral ventricles on the 14th day after each inoculation of mumps virus. Dilatation of the lateral ventricles was more pronounced when mumps virus had been inoculated at an earlier age. The cerebellum in hamsters inoculated at 2 days of age did not show any macroscopic abnormalities on the 8th day. However, when these brains were examined on the 18th day after inoculation, the cerebellar vermis and caudal half of the hemisphere were flattened and displaced downward, and showed an elongated, atrophic, and sleeve-like structure (Fig. 1A).

When we compared the midsagittal section of the entire head and neck of a 16-day-old hamster that had been injected with mumps virus at 2 days of age with that of its age-matched control, it was apparent that the quadrigemina, thalamus, and cerebellum in the former were deformed and displaced caudally and/or ventrally (Fig. 1B,C). The cervical cord of the infected hamster was bent rectangularly at the caudal end of the medulla oblongata, which was covered by elongated folium of the vermis.

When mumps virus was inoculated at 10 days of age and the cerebellum was examined 18 days later, the caudal half of the vermis and one-third of the hemisphere were flattened and elongated, showing a notched appearance (Fig. 1E). These abnormal changes were less severe than those resulting from inoculation at 2 days of age. There was no macroscopic deformity of the cerebellum in hamsters inoculated 25 days after birth.

No control brains showed any macroscopic abnormalities (Fig. 1D).

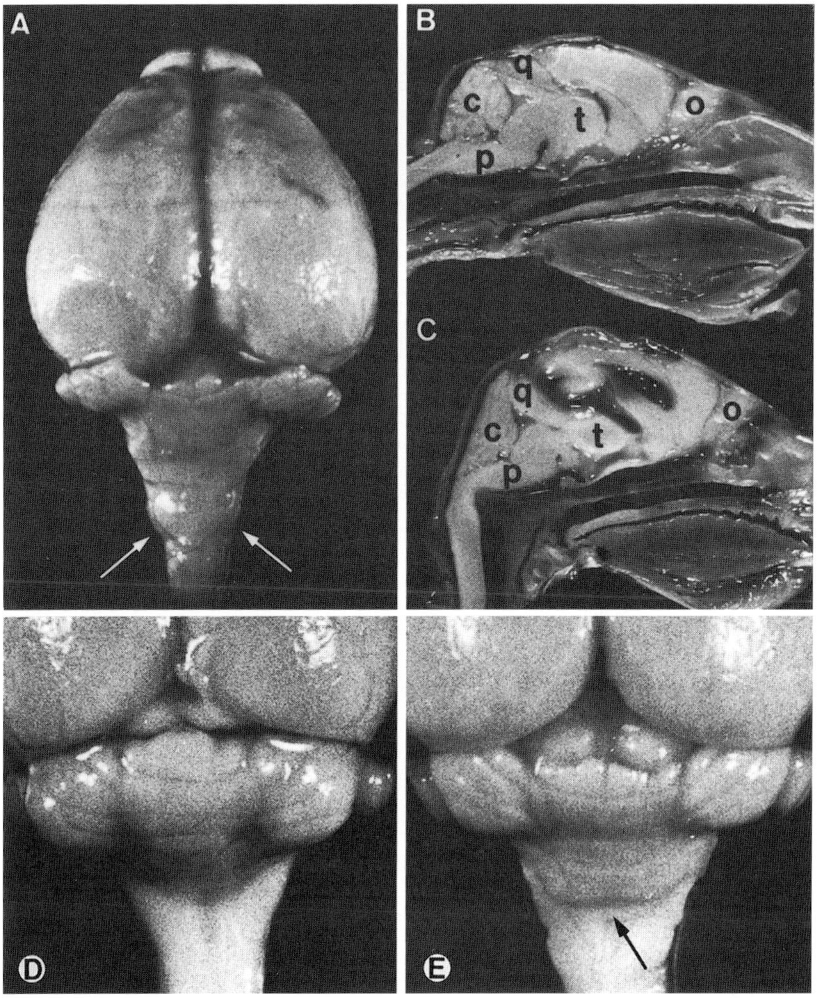

Fig. 1. **A** A dorsal view of a whole brain removed 18 days later from a hamster inoculated at 2 days after birth. **B,C** Midsagittal sections of the entire head and neck 14 days later in control (**B**) and infected (**C**) hamsters inoculated at 2 days after birth. Note the cone-shaped deformity of the posterior groove and hindbrain (**C**) (*o*, olfactory bulb; *t*, thalamus; *q*, quadrigemina; *p*, pons; *c*, cerebellum). **D,E** Dorsal views of the cerebellum in control (**D**) and infected (**E**) hamsters inoculated at 10 days after birth. Note the notched appearance on the flattened and elongated vermis (*arrow* on **E**)

Histological Examination

The midsagittal section of the cerebellar vermis of the 16-day-old control hamsters was composed of five different layers, i.e., from the outer to the inner layers, the vestigal external granular layer, the molecular layer, the Purkinje cell layer, the internal granular layer, and white matter. The brain inoculated at 2 days of age was examined on a midsagittal section of the cerebellar vermis, pons, and medulla oblongata 14 days later. Cone-shaped and flattened

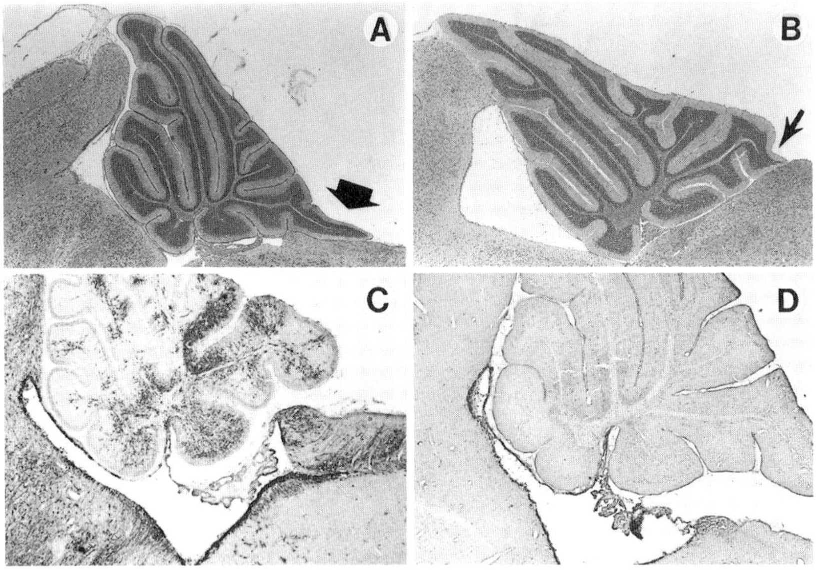

FIG. 2. **A**,**B** Midsagittal sections of the cerebellar vermis 14 days later in hamsters inoculated at 2 (**A**) and 10 (**B**) days after birth. Bodian stain. The elongation (*arrow* in **A**) and notching (*arrow* in **B**) of the uvula are characteristic. **A** ×12; **B** ×10. **C**,**D** Immunohistochemical detection of mumps virus antigen in the midsagittal section of the vermis examined 5 days after inoculation at 2 (**C**) and 10 (**D**) days of age. Strong immunoreactivity is found in the ependymal cells of the fourth ventricle (**C**,**D**), although mumps virus antigen is also detected in some granule cells in brains inoculated at 2 days of age (**C**). **C**,**D** ×30

folia of the vermis were elongated toward the caudal area (Fig. 2A). The uvula of the vermis, as well as an elongated caudal medulla, were found in the vertebral canal at the upper cervix. Each layer, i.e., the molecular, the Purkinje cell, and the granular layers, and the white matter were perserved and well differentiated, but were considerably narrowed. Purkinje cells remained normal.

When brains inoculated at 10 days of age were examined 14 days later, cone-shaped and elongated folia of the vermis were also found, but were less severely deformed than the corresponding structures in brains inoculated at 2 days of age. The caudal portion of the uvula showed a notched appearance that may have been produced by the upper cervical vertebrae (Fig. 2B). When hamsters were inoculated with mumps virus at 25 days of age and examined 14 days later, no elongation of the cerebellar vermis was found.

Immunohistochemical Examination

Mumps virus antigen was detected in all ependymal cells and in some epitherial cells of the choroid plexus of all hamsters inoculated with mumps virus at 2 (Fig. 2C), 10 (Fig. 2D), and 25 days of age. In brains inoculated at 2 days of age, mumps virus antigen was also detected in some granule cells in the cerebellar cortex (Fig. 2C).

Discussion

Margolis and Kilham [7] reported downward displacement and distortion of the cerebellum and hindbrain similar to the Arnold–Chiari malformation induced in suckling hamsters by inoculation of reovirus type I. Cerebellar deformities observed in their experiment were similar to those found in hydrocephalic hamsters in our experiment. In our previous report [15], we demonstrated that in experimental hydrocephalus induced by mumps virus inoculation in suckling hamsters, dilatation of the lateral ventricles appears during the acute phase of virus infection, preceding the appearance of aqueductal stenosis. Aqueductal stenosis is caused by periaqueductal glial proliferation, which occurs as a healing process after severe and extensive ependymal cell damage [15]. These results differ from those of Margolis and Kilham in that hydrocephalus is not a consequence of aqueductal stenosis. We suggested that the early ventricular dilatation before aqueductal stenosis in our experiment may have been related to functional and morphological disturbances of infected ependymal cells [17].

The present experiment demonstrated that the dilatation of the lateral ventricles was more pronounced when mumps virus had been inoculated at an earlier age. Generally, central nervous system susceptibility to viral infection is often age-dependent for any of a number of reasons [5, 10, 12]. Our colleagues examined the age-dependent susceptibility of the brain in mumps virus-induced hydrocephalus in hamsters, and evaluated the relationship between neuropathologic features and brain barriers using glial fibrillary acidic protein and zonula occludentes (ZO-1) immunohistochemistry [18]. In a group intracerebrally inoculated with mumps virus at 2 days of age, pathologic findings, including periventricular edema, ependymal cell loss, and ventricular dilatation, were more prominent and the distribution of mumps virus antigen was wider than in a group inoculated at 30 days of age. ZO-1-immunoreactive tight junctions in the hydrocephalic brains of the 2-day group were severely damaged in the choroid plexus and ependyma, and in white matter capillaries as early as 3 days after inoculation. These changes were not apparent in the hydrocephalic brains of the 30-day group. Prominent cortical dissemination of virus in the 2-day group was related to underdeveloped perivascular glial processes in brain parenchyma. Periventricular edema in the 2-day group was linked to ependymal and blood–brain barrier tight-junction permeability. These results suggest that tight junctions in the early postnatal period are more immature and fragile than in the adult stage. Based on these considerations, we concluded that brain susceptibility in mumps virus-induced hydrocephalus is intimately related to the maturity of brain barriers.

Hypotheses on the pathogenesis of the Chiari malformation may be classified into four groups [3]: (1) traction from below [6, 11]; (2) pressure from above [4, 8]; (3) a primary malformation of the hindbrain [2]; (4) a primary malformation of the basicranium [9]. Case reports and experimental studies have provided evidence both for and against these hypotheses, but there has been no consensus about the pathogenesis of the Chiari malformation.

The pathogenesis of hydrocephalus and cerebellar deformity in our experiment is quite different from "traction from below," since our hamsters did not have spina bifida. Characteristic appearances observed on the macroscopic midsagittal section of the head and neck showed that the cone-shaped deformity of the posterior groove did not result from "a primary malformation of the basicranium," but rather from the enlarged cerebral hemispheres. Although mumps virus antigen was found in some granule cells in the cerebellar cortex several days after virus inoculation, no apparent histological abnormalities had resulted. These findings show that the histogenesis of the cerebellum may have been unaffected by mumps virus inoculation. Thus, we consider "pressure from above" during active histogenesis to be the main cause of the cerebral deformity obtained in our experiment.

In the present experiment, hydrocephalus was caused in each hamster that had been inoculated with mumps virus at 2, 10, or 25 days after birth. Cerebellar deformities, however, were found only in those animals inoculated at 2 or 10 days of age; no cerebellar deformities were found in hamsters inoculated with virus at 25 days of age, although they showed moderate hydrocephalus. These results show that "pressure from above" per se is not enough to cause elongation, flattening, and protrusion of the cerebellum, and indicate that the particular histogenesis of the cerebellar cortex during early postnatal life also plays an important role in the development of such malformations.

In the cerebral cortex of newborn hamsters, neuron production and migration have almost been completed, whereas in the cerebellar cortex, all microneurons, i.e., granule, stellate, and basket cells, are produced in the external granular layer postnatally [13, 14]. The granule cells, which occupy more than 85% of the neurons in the cerebellar cortex, are produced between 3 and 18 days after birth in the hamster, indicative of accelerated growth during this period. It may therefore be concluded that the Chiari type I malformation is caused by two main factors occurring simultaneously: increasing intracranial pressure and rapid histogenesis of the cerebellar cortex.

References

1. Caviness VS (1976) The Chiari malformation of the posterior fossa and their relation to hydrocephalus. Dev Med Child Neurol 18:103–116
2. Daniel PM, Strich SJ (1958) Some observations on the congenital deformity of the central nervous system known as the Arnold-Chiari malformation. J Neuropathol Exp Neurol 17:255–266
3. Friede RL (1989) Forms of hindbrain crowding, including the Arnold-Chiari malformation. In: Reinhard L, Friede (ed) Developmental neuropathology, 2nd edn. Springer Berlin, Heidelberg, New York, Tokyo, pp 263–276
4. Gardner WJ, Goodall RJ (1950) The surgical treatment of Arnold-Chiari malformation in adults: an explanation of its mechanism and importance of encephalography in diagnosis. J Neurosurg 7:199–206
5. Griffin DE, Levine B, Tyor WR, Tucker PC, Hardwick JM (1994) Age-dependent susceptibility to fatal encephalitis: alphavirus infection of neurons. Arch Virol [Suppl] 9:31–39
6. Lichtenstein BW (1942) Distant neuroanatomic complications of spina bifida (spinal dysraphism). Hydrocephalus, Arnold-Chiari deformity, stenosis of the aqueduct of Sylvius, etc.: pathogenesis and pathology. Arch Neurol Psychiatr 47:195–214
7. Margolis G, Kilham L (1969) Experimental virus-induced hydrocephalus: relation to pathogenesis of the Arnold-Chiari malformation. J Neurosurg 31:1–9
8. Masters CL (1978) Pathogenesis of Arnold-Chiari malformation: the significance of hydrocephalus and aqueduct stenosis. J Neuropathol Exp Neurol 37:56–74
9. Müller F, O'Rahilly R (1980) The human chondrocranium at the end of the embryonic period proper, with particular reference to the nervous system. Am J Anat 159:33–58
10. Ogata A, Nagashima K, Hall WW, Ichikawa M, Kimura-Kuroda J, Yasui K (1991) Japanese encephalitis virus neurotropism is dependent on the degree of neuronal maturity. J Virol 65:880–886
11. Penfield W, Cone W (1932) Spina bifida and cranium bifidum: results of plastic repair of meningocele and myelomeningocele by a new method. JAMA 98:454–461
12. Sherman LA, Griffin DE (1990) Pathogenesis of encephalitis induced in newborn mice by virulent and avirulent strains of Sindbis virus. J Virol 64:2041–2046
13. Shimada M, Langman J (1969) Cell proliferation, migration and differentiation in the cerebral cortex of the golden hamster. J Comp Neurol 139:227–244
14. Shimada M, Langman J (1970) Repair of the external granular layer of the hamster cerebellum after prenatal and postnatal administration of methylazoxymethanol. Teratology 3:119–134
15. Takano T, Ohno M, Yamano T, Shimada M (1991) Experimental hydrocephalus in suckling hamster induced by myxovirus infection. I. Pathogenesis of hydrocephalus caused by mumps virus. Congenital Anomalies 31:115–128

16. Takano T, Ohno M, Yamano T, Shimada M (1991) Experimental hydrocepalus in suckling hamster induced by myxovirus infection. II. Pathogenesis of hydrocephalus caused by parainfluenza virus type 3. Congenital Anomalies 31:129–139
17. Takano T, Mekata Y, Yamano T, Shimada M (1993) Early ependymal changes in experimental hydrocephalus after mumps virus inoculation in hamsters. Acta Neuropathol 85:521–525
18. Uno M, Takano T, Yamano T, Shimada M (1997) Age-dependent susceptibility in mumps-associated hydrocephalus: neuropathologic features and brain barriers. Acta Neuropathol 94:207–215

Orthopedics

Gait Disturbance
Hip Pathology
Spine Pathology
Foot Pathology

A Social History of People with Physical Disabilities, Including Spina Bifida

James G. Gamble

Summary. The social history of people with physical disabilities shows that their status has been heavily influenced by emotions such as fascination and fear on the part of nondisabled people, and these emotions foster prejudices that act as powerful forces of discrimination and tell us a great deal about the sensibilities of the time. Currently, developments in health care financing in North America, coupled with the social implications of molecular genetics, threaten to erode many of the gains that disabled people have realized in this century. A socially active and politically empowered disability rights group is the vital protection that disabled people must have from medical cost cutting and a resurgence of eugenics based on molecular medicine.

Historically, people with disabilities have held an inferior social and economic status, presumably owing to the physical impairments imposed by the disability. However, nondisabled people frequently have uncomfortable feelings and even negative views of disabled persons, in part from fears and anxieties about their own vulnerability. Such anxieties come from the thought that all of us are vulnerable, generating a need to avoid identification with the disabled to assuage those anxieties. Negative feelings and beliefs on the part of nondisabled people act as powerful, prejudicial forces that foster discrimination and cause isolation, frustration, and even harm to the disabled.

In recent years, changes in public attitudes, coupled with the passage of federal legislation, has improved the prospects for people with disabilities, but modern society continues to be preoccupied with inabilities rather than with capabilities. The purpose of this paper is to present a social history of persons with physical disabilities, including spina bifida. This social history will show that the status of disabled people in society has been influenced by emotions such as fascination and fear, and that these emotions foster prejudice and discrimination against people with disabilities.

Physical Disability

Arbitrary judgments as to what constitutes a "normal person" are heavily influenced by the salient physical characteristics and distinct aesthetic viewpoint of the society or the person seeking the definition. What the ancient Romans would have considered normal is different

Division of Orthopaedic Surgery, Stanford University School of Medicine, Packard Children's Hospital at Stanford, 300 Pasteur Drive, Edwards Bldg. R-144, Stanford, CA 94304-5341, USA

from what the British in Victorian times would have considered normal. Terms used to describe those who differ from the norm, particularly the terms for the physically disabled, reflect the prevailing social attitudes and prejudices. For instance, to label a physically disabled person as unfit, deformed, misshapen, crippled, invalid, or handicapped—as has been common—reflects a prejudice that the disabled person is less than a complete human being, unsound, or even a freak of nature. Such a definition focuses attention on their physical status, and denies recognition of their individuality.

Another problem with arriving at a definition of disability is the necesssity of accounting for a broad spectrum of conditions and causes. Disabilities can result from birth defects, accidents, chemical toxicity, military action, and even the process of aging. There are hundreds of different disabilities with different appearances and different degrees of impairment, of which some are progressive and some are static. The medical condition and physical appearance of someone with cerebral palsy is different from that of someone with spina bifida, but the environmental problems, the stereotypes, and the prejudices they face have the same social result: exclusion and isolation. The common denominator uniting people with a variety of different disabilities is their experience with stigmatizing cultural values that have resulted in segregation, degradation, denial of opportunity, hostility, and even open aggression [8, 23, 30].

In the United States a legal definition of disability was put forth in the Americans with Disabilities Act of 1990 (Public Law 101-336). A physical impairment is defined as any physiological disorder or condition, cosmetic disfigurement, or anatomical loss affecting one or more body systems resulting from disease, genetic abnormality, or accident. The physical impairment is considered to produce a physical disability if it substantially limits one or more of the major life activities such as walking, lifting, learning, seeing, or hearing. A person with the physical disability is considered to be handicapped only in a specific set of environmental conditions. I will use the term "malformation" for a clearly visible anatomic impairment that is present at birth, and the term "physical disability" for any impairment of the musculoskeletal system that prevents a person from independently performing at least one of the major activities of daily living (thus requiring the help of other people or the use of assistive devices such as a wheelchairs, prosthetics, or orthotics).

Using these definitions, the Census Bureau estimates that there are 48 million disabled persons in the United States, 8 million of whom have obviously visible, severe physical impairments such as cerebral palsy, spina bifida, limb deficiencies, or major neurological damage, and another 5 million of whom have mobility problems and must rely on various devices to get around [7, 17]. Only 15% of disabled Americans were born with their disabilities, while the remainder acquired their disability at some time during their lives.

People with disabilities may be a minority, but at 48 million in American society, they do not constitute a small or insignificant minority. The prevalence of people with disabilities in the general population was not always this large. Prior to the 1940s when antibiotics became available, people with disabilities seldom died because of the disability; usually they died because of pneumonia, urinary tract disease, or some other infection. In ancient times, both environmental and social pressures worked to keep the prevalence of people with disabilities very low.

Prehistoric Times: An Impossible Burden

According to the fossil record, early humans were hunters and foragers. Since humans were slow, awkward, and relatively defenseless, they had to depend on other humans for survival. This meant that each person was vital to the continued existence of the group, which could ill afford anyone who did not contribute his or her share of the work. Furthermore, early humans were nomadic, following the herds of wild animals as they migrated. We have no way of knowing how primitive people felt about those with physical disabilities, but most likely, those who could not keep up with the group would have been left behind. The group had little choice, since an infant with a malformation or a member of the tribe who could no longer walk was a great liability and a threat to the survival of all [3, p. 3]. Consequently, an infant with a clubfoot or a hunter with a fractured femur probably would have been left to die—possibly even be killed—in the best interests of the group.

The Graeco-Roman World: Useless and Unfit to Live

For most people in the ancient world, life was harsh. The average life-span for men was 44 years and for women was 37 years [12, p. 11]. In classical antiquity, the social response to people with disabilities was influenced greatly by religious beliefs. Beauty and wholeness were considered a mark of divine favor, whereas ugliness and disability were signs of the Gods' displeasure. It was assumed that the structure of body reflected the substance of the soul.

The birth of a child with a condition like spina bifida was interpreted by the Greeks as a punishment inflicted upon the parents by the Gods. Given these circumstances, it would have been prudent for a family to eliminate a child as fast and as quietly as possible to avoid any social consequences of the birth. Religious beliefs as well as practical considerations worked against the raising of such a child, who would be a severe economic and social burden on the family. The Greeks and Romans had no compunction about abandoning any child who they thought was incapable of leading a full, active, and independent life.

Because of people's beliefs and fears, even adults with disabilities must have led lives of isolation and suffering on the margins of society, generally held in disdain by their families and by other members of the community. The anguish of people with disabilities may have been projected into the story of the Greek God Hephaestos, who was lame due to abnormal lower extremities, probably clubfeet. Hephaestos, the god of smiths and metalworkers, had the magical power to infuse life into inanimate materials and to forge armor of incomparable excellence. Hera bore him on her own, without having intercourse with Zeus, to spite Zeus for having brought forth Athena. Hera rejected her deformed son by hurling him into the sea, perhaps reflecting the emotional response of an average Greek mother to the birth of a disabled child.

The Roman attitude towards disability was shaped by extreme militarism coupled with a fascination with the exotic. Some disabled people who the Romans thought "exotic" had a special role during the Imperial period. Many royal families and members of the upper classes favored the company of people with malformations as a source of entertainment [12, p. 45]. Dwarfs, cretins, hunchbacks, and obese women were brought out at dinner parties and other festive occasions, often to undergo degrading and painful humiliation. People with disabilities were treated as objects of curiosity and amusement, in much the same way as exotic animals and other curiosities of nature were treated.

Judeo-Christian Tradition: An Immutable Act of God, A Source of Shame

The Judeo-Christian tradition, which historically overlapped the Greco-Roman period, held that humans were physically constructed in God's image. People with disabilities—who would not have been made in God's image—were presumed to be an expression of God's displeasure, which meant that either the disabled person or some close relative was a sinner [19, 25].

The medical profession was of little help to those with physical disabilities. Physicians reasoned that since God had sought to render a person malformed from birth, the profession had no business attempting to interfere with His decision. The primary function of the medieval hospital was to assist the patients in the worship of God. In fact, most of these establishments were filled with lepers, and in general, people went to hospitals to die. What little help that was available to people with disabilities came from the charity of the Church, where the occasional parish took to heart Christ's words of compassion and good will, but in general, people with physical disabilities were feared, ridiculed, excluded, or made the objects of persecution.

The parents of a child with spina bifida would have had to cope not only with feelings of sadness and inadequacy, but also with feelings of guilt and shame. They naturally would have looked for an explanation as to why something so terrible could have happened to them, and it would be preferable to have an explanation that could both alleviate some of the guilt and assume the blame. Such an explanation, that was popular in Europe throughout the Middle Ages, was that of the "changeling" [14]. A changeling was held to be a child of the demons which lived under the earth or in the water. Demons envied man for his beauty and for his immortal soul, both of which the demons lacked. It was thought that the demons could ennoble their stock by stealing a human child and later marrying it to one of their own, or if they could trick a human mother into suckling the changeling, it would eventually acquire beauty and a soul. Identification of a child with spina bifida as a changeling could shortcircuit the idea of parental sin, and would alleviate the parents guilt by focusing their anger on the child, who was considered an intruder.

During the fourteenth century, the church adopted and Christianized the idea of a changeling. It was held that the devil was the one who stole the child. Various saints were said to have been stolen from the cradle. Saints Stephen, Lawrence, and Bartholomew were said to have been swapped for a changeling, only to be rescued by the intervention of someone of great faith and purity. Even during the Reformation, the belief in changelings persisted. Martin Luther believed in the existence of changelings, and he recommended throwing these babies, most of whom had physical malformations, directly into the water. In the context of the Middle Ages, this was not considered an act of infanticide; it was exorcism.

Throughout the sixteenth century, Christian attitudes reflected the strong association of sexuality with embarrassment, shame, and guilt. The idea regained popularity that parents who did not behave properly were punished by God with the birth of a malformed child. In most cases, the sin was said to be one of a sexual nature, often sexual overindulgence, and the parents were expected to atone for the sin and suffer with the presence of the child.

A sixteenth-century illustrated document [1], *The Forme and Shape of a Monstrous Child, Born in Kent* (1568), describes a child that was born with a cleft lip, genu recurvatum, and spina bifida, that was considered to be God's punishment for immorality, since the mother, a woman named Marget Mere, was unmarried (Fig. 1). During these times, simply giving birth to a child with a physical abnormality was considered as incriminating evidence of unchastity, and could even serve to bring a woman to the stake. No wonder that the birth of a child with spina bifida would inspire such fear as to cause the parents to conceal and get rid of the child as soon as possible.

At the beginning of the seventeenth century, the increased number of people in poverty, including those with disabilities, began to make an impact on public consciousness. England endeavored to deal more favorably with the poor and the disabled by the codification of the Elizabethan poor laws, first adopted in 1601. These laws used a number of criteria to classify

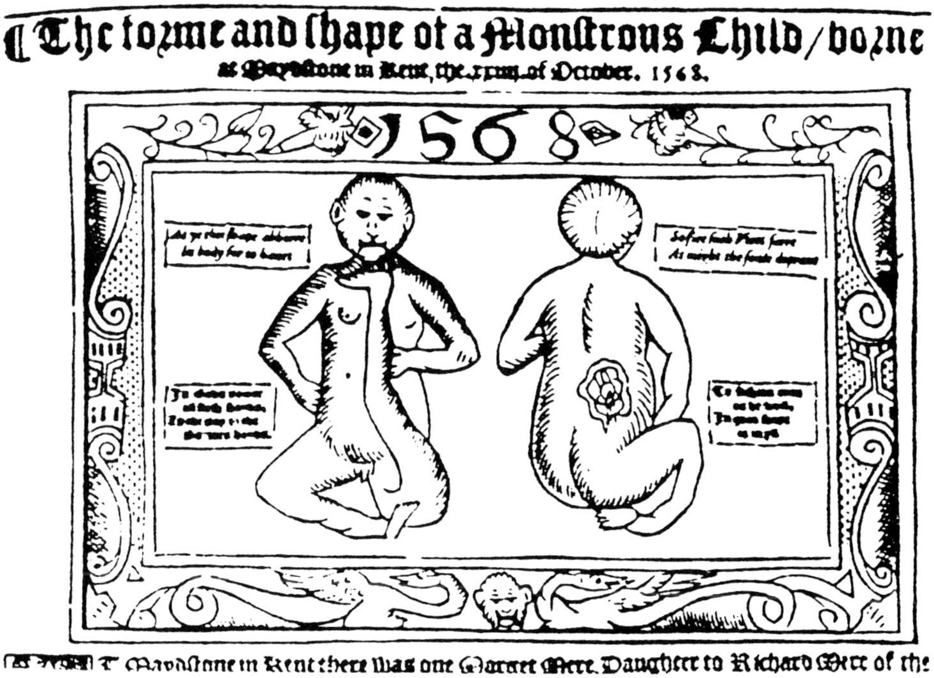

FIG. 1. Sixteenth-century document describing a case of multiple congenital anomalies, including spina bifida

people into deserving and nondeserving categories. Orphaned children, the blind, and the crippled were deemed deserving and received charity, whereas those who were judged nondeserving received no public assistance [34]. These laws helped to alleviate some of the overt neglect, but the public attitude remained hostile, and charity was handed out rather begrudgingly.

The Elizabethan poor laws were inherited almost intact by the American colonies, and they became the basis for early Colonial laws concerning the poor and the disabled. It was still the case that those who relied on public assistance were certain to be looked down on as a lower class of person, somehow personally responsible for their condition regardless of the source of the disability. Community values, based on Protestant mores, stressed the importance of independence, industry, and self-support. Indolence was seen as the principal source of poverty, not personal misfortune, and the association of disability with impurity and retribution remained strong [3]. Consequently, a disabled person would have been given little chance to achieve and to maintain self-sufficiency. People with physical disabilities were prevented from immigration. Any child with a congenital malformation was thought to have an immutable condition caused by an act of God, most likely as a result of the sins of the parents.

The Puritan ethic rejected homicide or infanticide as a way of dealing with the disabled. The only possible treatment could be absolution of the sin and redemption of the soul. The disabled were expected to remain at home and out of sight to be cared for by their families and to be prayed for on a regular basis.

By the beginning of the eighteenth century, institutions had been established in America and in Europe specifically to care for disabled people [36]. These institutions, while not providing great care by any standard, were an improvement over the policy of total social neglect. The establishment of these institutions indicated that society felt a responsibility for providing at least a minimal level of care to disabled people [10, p. 10]. Unfortunately, in most cases this minimum level of care simply translated into custodial care, basically a move out of an attic and into a warehouse.

The Eighteenth and Nineteenth Centuries: A Biological Deficit; a Chance to Cure

A new view of humanity emerged in Europe and America due to the ideas of the Enlightenment. Philosophers such as Voltaire (1694–1778), Rousseau (1712–1778), and Montesquieu (1689–1755) laid the foundations for an ethics based on reason, and not simply on faith and blind obedience to scripture. Scientists such as Isaac Newton (1642–1727), Robert Boyle (1627–1691), and Carl von Linné (1707–1778) showed that even nature was subject to understanding by human reason. There was a general feeling that people could take charge of their lives and destinies.

One of the prominent ideas of the Enlightenment was that humanity would make great progress once reason and knowledge became widespread. The promise of this idea was apparent in the field of medicine, where reason and informed observation improved the understanding of disease. Many of the world's greatest clinicians were alive during the eighteenth century. These men, along with the philosophers of the Enlightenment, shifted the center of interest from a preoccupation with the fate of the soul to a more secular concern with the improvement of life on earth. Within the optimistic intellectual environment of the Enlightenment, physicians such as Venel and Hunter began to think about disabilities in a new way that has come to be known as the medical model. According to this model, people with deformities and disabilities were looked upon as having a biological deficit derived from an illness or an injury to the body, as opposed to having an immutable condition as a result of divine punishment [22]. Furthermore, it was held that with proper treatment the individual could be cured, or at least trained to be functional enough to perform socially or vocationally.

With the medical model as their theoretical framework, physicians and educators established organizations and special schools that were dedicated to people with specific conditions such as blindness and deafness. In 1780, Venel was the first to treat crippled children in a systematic fashion, with attention to their social as well as their medical needs, in an institutional setting. The first institution for deaf children was founded in Hartford, Connecticut, in 1817, and by the late 1880s, many states had institutional–educational programs for children with physical and mental disabilities.

Towards the end of the nineteenth century, many professionals had lost confidence in their ability to perfect or even to improve most people with disabilities. Medicine once promised to wipe out disability by finding cures, but instead, doctors had only increased the disabled population by keeping these people alive longer. A few rare cases of individuals with spina bifida survived into adulthood, provided that the meningocele was covered and they had no hydrocephalus. However, it must have been a lonely and frightening existence. Most forms of medical treatment were dangerous. A case in point was reported in 1852 (Lancet, p. 56) from St. George's hospital in London of a 20-year-old man with a cyst, said to be about the size of two men's heads, extending from the lumbar to the sacral areas. Unfortunately, the physicians punctured the cyst and the patient died from infection.

It was at this time that the theories of social Darwinism began to make an appearance. These theories held that no intervention could cure people with disabilities because the laws of natural selection and the laws of genetics made them unfit for participation in life. Under the influence of these ideas, the social policy for people with disabilities began to shift back to the provision of crude custodial care in institutions. A malformation or a disability was now considered to be a genetic defect residing in the individual, making the person incompetent to function in society, unable to manage his life, and even socially dangerous and therefore in need of lifelong supervision.

It was also during this time that people with malformations and disabilities were exploited on a grand scale as human curiosities for entertainment and profit by various circuses and "freak shows" [2, 33]. In addition to watching the usual lion tamers and tightrope walkers, people would pay a fee to gawk at those with gross anatomical anomalies. This form of entertainment was popular in both Europe and the United States. Many well-appointed homes had a photo album filled not only with pictures of family members, but also with daguerreotypes of human oddities like General Tom Thumb, Henry "Zip" the Pin Head, and Chang and Eng, the so-called Siamese twins.

The First Half of the Twentieth Century: From Segregation to Social Concern

The early twentieth century was a time of contradiction for social policy towards the disabled. Philanthropic groups were organized in America and Europe to provide charity care for what was referred to as the "crippled child." On the other hand, prejudice and discrimination against disabled people was widespread. The idea still persisted that people with disabilities were unhealthy, defective, and morally unsound, best dealt with by residential care in an institution. Labels such as "subnormal," "idiotic," "handicapped," or "feeble-minded" were common [13]. An orthopedic textbook in 1911 stated that, "A Failure in the moral training of a cripple means the evolution of an individual detestable in character, a menace and burden to the community, who is only too apt to graduate into the mendicant and criminal classes" [11, p. 30].

Exclusion from society actually had a legal basis in Chicago, which passed the so-called "ugly law" in 1901, City Ordinance 36-34. This law stated that, "No person who is diseased, maimed, mutilated, or in any way deformed so as to be an unsightly or disgusting object or improper person to be allowed in or on the public ways or other public places in this city, shall therein or thereon expose himself to public view" [4]. It was only in 1974 that this law was repealed.

In a widely publicized case in 1915, Joseph Roberts of New York City refused surgery for his daughter who was born with spina bifida, and she eventually died. The case was extensively discussed in the newspapers, and in general, the father's decision was supported, even by noted pediatrician L. Emmett Holt. In 1919, a boy with cerebral palsy was expelled from public school in Wisconsin because the teachers and other children found him depressing and nauseating. A New York State study found that physically disabled children were neglected at home and rejected by the public schools [11, p. 29]. The majority of people with deformities or severe disabilities were simply placed in institutions, where they were massively neglected.

The ideas of social Darwinism and those of the new field of eugenics gained considerable academic and social respect in the early twentieth century. Helping the weak and the malformed to live, according to social Darwinism, contributed in the long run to weakening the whole human race. Eugenicists held that attention must be paid to hereditary hygiene or the human race would face degradation and eventually extinction. They wrote that the physical, mental, and behavioral qualities of the human race should be improved by suitable management and manipulation of heredity [18, p. ix]. People with disabilities should not be permitted to marry or have children in order to prevent the propagation of their imperfections.

The eugenics movement gained popularity with arguments claiming that people with disabilities were unproductive, and that their lives were of low quality or meaningless. The disabled were considered to be a burden to their families, and, more importantly, they were thought to drain scarce social and economic resources. The eugenicists and other professionals proposed the sterilization of all disabled people, including the deaf, the blind, and all those with developmental disabilities. European and American eugenicists did not advocate homicide or infanticide, but they did propose forced sterilization of all "socially unfit" people, and the definition of the unfit was broad and included children and adolescents with even minor malformations.

In 1917, Indiana enacted the first law in the United States to permit sterilization of "the unfit." The constitutionality of the law was upheld by the Supreme Court in 1927, "in order to prevent our being swamped with incompetence." [12, p. 180]. By the beginning of the First World War, 16 states had adopted sterilization statutes to be used against those who were considered socially unfit. The international eugenics movement reached its greatest extreme in Nazi Germany, where a law was passed in 1933 entitled "For the Prevention of Congenital Diseases Among the Rising Generations" and where an estimated 100000 people with disabilities were exterminated and more than 320000 others were sterilized [35]. It was not until 1941 that the sterilization laws were repealed in the United States, but by then, 36000 Americans had been forceably sterilized [12, p. 181].

The 40 years from 1920 to 1960 was a time when American public policy toward people with disabilities began to change from one of hostility, neglect, and indifference to one of charitable care, with the new provision of opportunities for rehabilitation [32]. Americans had remained immune to the plight of disabled soldiers, despite the great toll of the Civil War. The turning point of public opinion occurred towards the end of the First World War when large numbers of disabled soldiers, who were returning from the European conflict, could no longer be ignored. These maimed and disabled veterans had been the sons, brothers, and friends who had marched off to "save the world for democracy" only a few years earlier. Responding to public opinion, Congress passed the Vocational Education Act of 1917 (Public Law 64-347), also known as the Smith–Hughes Act, which created the Federal Board for Vocational Education to provide educational assistance to injured war veterans. This act was followed in 1918 by the Soldiers Rehabilitation Act (Public Law 65-178), also called the Smith–Sears Act, which provided for vocational retraining of veterans after their discharge from military service. Then in 1920, Congress passed the first legislation for civilian vocational training, the Industrial Rehabilitation Act (Public Law 66-236), the Smith–Fess Act. The extension of the legislation to the civilian sector was due, in part, to the recognition that America needed all the potentially available labor to support an expanding economy [28]. Although overt prejudice and discrimination against disabled people diminished in the years following the First World War, Western society continued to stigmatize those with physical deformities or those who used wheelchairs, leg braces, or other assistive devices.

The carnage of World War II greatly increased the numbers of men with disabilities. During World War I, only about 400 men survived with wounds that paralyzed them from the waist down, but during World War II, due to better evacuation and better medical care, more than

2000 paraplegics survived, as did thousands of amputees and others with major physical disabilities [33, p. 5]. The government responded by increasing veterans' services and increasing funding of basic research, which greatly improved the medical prospects for all people with disabilities. Unfortunately, the business community was less progressive, and remained under the influence of prejudice and stereotypes that prevented most disabled people from joining the work force and making significant contributions to society.

Then came the polio epidemic of the late 1940s and 1950s. Poliomyelitis was a disease that cross-cut all socio-economic groups and riveted public attention on the plight of the newly disabled, who could easily be you or your neighbor. In response to the increased public concern about illness and disability, the number, size, and power of charity organizations increased, not only to combat polio, but also to fight other acquired and congenital diseases as well. Groups were established such as the March of Dimes, the Easter Seal Society, and the Muscular Dystrophy Society, with the goals of improving disability services and funding research to find a cure for the disability in question. These groups also played an important role in changing public attitudes toward disabled people by mounting public relations campaigns such as the National Poster Child.

Scientific and medical knowledge expanded greatly during the 1950s. Government-funded educational programs increased the numbers and sophistication of medical and rehabilitation professionals, who provided new research findings which offered hope and ever-improving care to the disabled. Social attitudes began to reflect the view that people with disabilities were unfortunate humans who deserved at least a minimum level of care. Physicians continued to provide services within a medical model that defined the role of disabled persons as dependent and nonparticipatory in decisions about everything from their medical care and education to their transportation and employment [10, p. 13]. Independent access to public facilities and transportation continued to be extremely difficult, if not impossible, for people with disabilities.

The 1960s and 1970s: Civil Rights and the Birth of Independent Living

The 1960s were a time of social turmoil and a time of civil rights reform. Public policy began to change for people with disabilities as well as for other minorities, but unlike most of the other civil rights movements, the disability rights movement was a behind-the-scenes action carried out by advocates, and legislative protection for disabled people occurred in the absence of an active political movement. Disability policy and reform grew out of the efforts of advocates for the disabled who expressed their concern and indignation to a sympathetic Congress during this progressive social era [13, p. 15]. Advocates stressed that disabled people are seldom evaluated on the basis of their knowledge, abilities, or skills. Their disability will color all their activities and potentialities in the eyes of the nondisabled, and they will be considered incapable, weak, and inferior [31, p. 111]. Based on arguments like this, Congress recognized that people with disabilities were being oppressed by attitudes and images, and passed a body of legislation that extended civil rights statutes to the disabled.

Also during this era, residential institutions that had been holding people with disabilities for hundreds of years came under attack for what was considered to be dehumanizing conditions and the denial of basic constitutional liberties to their inmates. Even severely disabled people were deemed to have the same basic rights as others.

The 1970s saw a resurgence in arguments for withholding treatment for patients with spina bifida, but researchers such as Dr. David Shurtleff provided a voice of reason in these confusing times. In 1977, disabled people staged the first public protest, a sit-in at the Old Federal Building in San Francisco. For 25 days, they occupied the building and ignited other protests across the country, which ended after Joseph Califano, then Secretary of Health, Education, and Welfare, signed regulations to begin enforcing Section 504 of the Rehabilitation Act. It was only after these protests, which were relatively mild by civil rights protest standards, that actual changes began to take place in the United States [10, p. 19].

Two universities had already taken steps to help disabled students on campus. The University of Illinois at Champaign-Urbana in 1950 and the University of California, Berkeley, in 1964 were the first to establish programs that facilitated campus life for disabled students. Following the University of California model, The Center for Independent Living was established in Berkeley, California, in 1972. The Center provided a wide range of practical services to encourage independent living for people with physical disabilities, and served as a stimulus for disabled people in other cities to establish their own programs for independent living [6, 7, 29]. The independent living movement marked the beginning of a more aggressive approach to life on the part of disabled people. They refused to accept the tradition of exclusion and dependency. They formed organizations made up of people with different medically based disabilities, and together they worked out solutions to the common environmental and social problems they faced when moving out into the community.

The 1980s: The Minority Model

By the beginning of the 1980s, the social position of physically disabled people had a great deal in common with other categories of socially devalued people [26]. They continued to be the recipients of unwanted and unfavorable identities and the objects of prejudice. However, the consciousness that grew out of the 1960s and the independent-living movement of the 1970s had changed the way disabled people viewed themselves. No longer were they prepared to accept the medical model which held that the pathology was localized in the individual, and the professional role consisted of making all the decisions and then informing the patients, who were expected to be passive recipients of treatments. According to the new view, the pathology was not in the person with the disability, but was in the political and economic environment that severely limited the options of people with disabilities. The thought was that if the environment could be changed, the disability would disappear, or at least be greatly diminished in its impact.

Disabled people came to think of themselves as a minority group that had been denied their civil liberties, and not as victims in need of benevolent oversight. They no longer tolerated the dependency and active exclusion that had denied them the opportunity to participate equally in society. From these ideas emerged a new way of thinking about disability that has become known as the minority model. This model defines the disability experience as a socially constructed identity, determined by stigmatized physical traits, and not an inevitable condition [20]. According to the minority group model, people with disabilities should not accept a stigmatized social identity. They should assert pride in themselves as humans; they should break out of limiting and subordinate roles, and they should actively pursue the elimination of artificial barriers to the full extent of the law. The model held that the goals for disabled persons should be the freedom to choose, to belong, to participate, to have dignity, and to have the opportunity to achieve [10, p. 33].

Perhaps the most difficult barrier faced by disabled people is the emotional barrier of able-bodied people who continue unconsciously to stigmatize and devalue disabled persons [21]. As a society, we continue to characterize people by their most obvious trait—skin color, malformed arm, limp. Today, overt rejection is socially unacceptable, so people tend to be more subtle. They hide their fear and anxiety by politely smiling, and then they go out of their way to avoid the disabled person.

The 1990s: The Disability Rights Movement

In the USA, the decade of the 1990s started out well for disabled people with the passage of The Americans with Disabilities Act of 1990 (Public Law 101-336), which expanded civil rights protection to include employment and complete access to all public accommodations and transportation. The spirit of the law was to bring all persons with disabilities into the "mainstream of American life" by the guarantee of equal treatment in all the routine events of life [27, p. 1].

The new laws against discrimination, plus the technological advances that improved mobility for the disabled, coupled with a critical mass of better-educated disabled students have greatly increased the participation of disabled people in American life. Advancing the cause of the disabled has reshaped the way people with disabilities view their world. The activists hold that a disability, of itself, is not tragic or pitiable, and they resent suggestions that they are sick, pitiful, dependent, or objects of admiration for dealing with their physical problems. People with disabilities do not want charity and pity. They want equal opportunity, free choice, and the chance to control their own lives [33, p. 14].

An Uncertain Future: Managed Care and the New Genetics

Currently, there are signs of a public backlash to the social gains that disabled people have achieved, particularly as regards the cost of making the environment more accessible, and the cost of medical care for people with disabilities. Some firms resent the financial burden of altering the office environment so that one disabled worker in an office of 25 people can work at a desk in a wheelchair. These financial considerations, plus a change in the health care economy, threaten to bring an attenuation of some of the hard-earned social gains.

Managed Care

Great changes are taking place within the American health system, and these changes have implications for disabled people. The health care marketplace is moving away from the traditional indemnity, fee-for-service payment system and embracing managed care as a way to control health care costs [9, 24]. The keystone of managed care economics is capitation as opposed to fee-for-service.

Capitation financing has some potentially troubling consequences for the health care of disabled people, because physicians' incomes are directly related to their success at minimizing hospitalizations, minimizing referrals, and decreasing the use of diagnostic tests. The problem is that disabled people require more health care services than the average person, making them known financial risks for any health maintenance organization (HMO). Both government and private HMOs are aware of the high medical costs of disabled people with chronic conditions and the disproportionate use of medical resources by this group [17]. Unfortunately, since disabled people are a minority, most members of any capitation plan probably would not object if the plan excluded seldom-used and expensive drugs, braces, prosthetics, and wheelchairs as a way to keep premiums lower.

In this fearsomely competitive, market-oriented health care system, parents of children with spina bifida may find it more difficult to obtain referrals to a specialist for extensive, and often expensive, surgery. The financial risk has shifted from the insurers to the physicians, and the payment system rewards the provision of less care, a situation which will put a disproportionate burden on those requiring more care, as children with spina bifida do. No matter how ethical the physician may be, it will be difficult to divorce medical decisions from the financial realities that penalize the physician for providing care.

Medical ethics dictates that all doctors act exclusively in the best interests of their patients [5], but many decisions being made today are no longer up to physicians, so the tenets of medical ethics are short-circuited. Commonly, decisions about referrals or diagnostic services are being made by corporate-employed nurses or businees people in the HMO headquarters, who follow the fine print of the HMO contracts. Public concern over the apparent denial of care to some HMO patients has led to the introduction of many bills in state legislatures and Congress to regulate HMO practices, but so far the legislative impact has been negligible [15].

The Human Genome Project

The goal of the Human Genome Project is to decipher the human genetic blueprint, which is the sequence of nucleotides in DNA that codes for the 100000 genes for the proteins and enzymes that are responsible for the development and maintenance of a human being. Using the powerful methods of biochemistry and molecular genetics, scientists have determined the exact chromosomal locus and the molecular defect causing a number of human diseases and deformities. Many human genes can now be manipulated in the laboratory and inserted into microorganisms or other eukaryocytic cells.

The project has spawned new findings and technologies that are challenging our capacity to deal with them. Genetic tests for diseases such as cystic fibrosis, breast cancer, colon cancer, and sickle cell anemia are already in use, and the Human Genome Project promises the delivery of tests for the identification of all inherited genetic diseases and deformities prior to birth. These tests can tell not only if an infant will have a certain condition at birth, but whether that infant will come down with the condition in the future, or whether that infant's children, or potential children, will come down with the condition: a medical crystal ball of sorts. This means that the risk of future disease, disability, and early death can be calculated from a buccal smear or a blood test.

The potential benefits from this technology are great, but the risks of abuse are also great, particularly for disabled people or for those at risk of becoming disabled. The prospect of reducing the frequency of congenital malformations seems to be in keeping with the promotion of health and well being. However, genetic tests could acquire the characteristic of "quality control" in the demand for perfect offspring [16].

The Need for Vigilance

Social acceptance has been elusive for people with disabilities. The divorce rate among couples with a disabled child is very high, due no doubt to familial and social pressures. Many disabled children grow up in single-parent homes, and these families often rely on welfare and MediCaid programs which are at risk from budgetary cutbacks. We live in a world of finite resources, but almost infinite demands. In our market economy, each dollar could be prudently spent for education, for defense, for health care, or for one of many other good causes. Within the field of health care, money could be spent for research and development, for preventive care, for hospital services, for physician services, for rehabilitation services, or in many other ways. Financial support for disability services, which are important for so many families, will have to compete with other areas of medical care, and the level of funding will depend on the strength of our social commitment to people with disabilities. Given the emotional currents and the long social history of prejudice against people with disabilities, our current commitment cannot be taken for granted. People with disabilities must be organized; they must remain visible, and they must be vigilant. A strong public presence must continue to fight against the pejorative myths and emotions that have historically surrounded people with disabilities.

References

1. Anderson T (1994) Evidence of birth deformities in 16th century Kent. Br Med J 309:1748
2. Bogdan R (1988) Freak show. Presenting human oddities for amusement and profit. University of Chicago Press, Chicago
3. Bowe FG (1978) Handicapping America. Barriers to disabled people. Harper and Row, New York
4. Burgdorf MP, Burgdorf R (1975) A history of unequal treatment. The qualifications of handicapped persons as a "suspect class" under the equal protection clause. Santa Clara Law Review 15:863–864
5. Council on Ethical and Judicial Affairs, American Medical Association. Ethical Issues in Managed Care (1995) J Am Med Assoc 273:330–335
6. Crewe NM, Zola IK (1983) Independent living for physically disabled people. Addison-Wesley, San Francisco
7. DeJong G, Lifchez R (1983) Physical disability and public policy. Sci Am 248:40–49
8. Finkelstein V (1980) Attitudes and disabled people: issues for discussion. World Rehabilitation Fund, New York
9. Fuchs VR (1993) No pain, no gain: perspectives on cost containment. J Am Med Assoc 269:631–633
10. Funk R (1987) Disability rights: from caste to class in the context of civil rights. In: Gartner A, Joe T (eds) Images of the disabled, disabling images. Praeger, New York, pp 7–30
11. Gallagher HG (1985) FDR's splendid deception. Dodd, Mead, New York
12. Garland R (1995) The eye of the beholder. Deformity and disability in the Graeco-Roman world. Cornell University Press, Ithaca
13. Goddard J, Savitz H (1918) Education of the mentally deficient. Department of Public Instruction, Trenton
14. Haffter C (1968) The changeling: history and psychodynamics of attitudes to handicapped children in European folklore. J Hist Behav Sci 4:55–61
15. Hellinger FJ (1996) The expanding scope of state legislation. J Am Med Assoc 276:1065–1069
16. Hepburn ER (1996) Genetic testing and early diagnosis and intervention: boon or burden? J Med Ethics 22:105–110
17. Hoffman C, Rice D, Sung H-Y (1996) Persons with chronic conditions. Their prevalence and costs. J Am Med Assoc 276:1473–1479
18. Kevles DJ (1995) In the name of eugenics. Genetics and the uses of human heredity. Harvard University Press, Cambridge
19. Livneh H (1980) Disability and monstrosity: further comments. Rehabil Lit 41:280–283
20. Longmore PK (1985) A note on language and the social identity of disabled people. Am Behav Sci 28:419–423
21. Longmore PK (1987) Elizabeth Bouvia, assisted suicide and social prejudice. Issues Law Med 3:141–168
22. Longmore PK (1987) Uncovering the hidden history of people with disabilities. Rev Am Hist 15:355–364

23. Longmore PK (1995) Medical decision making and people with disabilities. A clash of cultures. J Law Med Ethics 23:82–87
24. Lundberg GD (1994) United States health care system reform. An era of shared sacrifice and responsibility begins. J Am Med Assoc 271:1530–1533
25. Mackelprang RW, Salsgiver RO (1996) People with disabilities and social work: historical and contemporary issues. Soc Work 41:7–14
26. Murphy RF, Scheer J, Murphy Y, Mack R (1988) Physical disability and social liminality: a study of the rituals of adversity. Soc Sci Med 26:235–242
27. Americans with Disabilities Act of 1990 (Public Law 101-336), Legislative Summary Series, National Mental Health Association, Alexandria
28. Reed KL (1992) History of federal legislation for persons with disabilities. Am J Occup Ther 46:397–408
29. Rogers JC (1982) The spirit of independence: the evolution of a philosophy. Am J Occup Ther 36:709–715
30. Roth W (1983) Handicap as a social constraint. Society 20:56–61
31. Safilios-Rothschild C (1970) The sociology and social psychology of disability and rehabilitation. Random House, New York
32. Scotch R (1985) From goodwill to civil rights. Transforming federal disability policy. Temple University Press, Philadelphia
33. Shapiro JP (1993) No pity. People with disabilities forging a new civil rights movement. Time Books, Random House, New York
34. Stone D (1984) The disabled state. Temple University Press, Philadelphia
35. Wolfensberger W (1981) The extermination of handicapped people in World War II Germany. Ment Retard 19:1–7
36. Wolfensberger W (1995) The origin and nature of our institutional models. Human Policy Press, Syracuse

Moderator's Comments on Session—Gait Disturbance by J.G. Gamble

Malcom B. Menelaus

Thank you, Dr. Gamble, for the interesting and thought provoking address. It is clear that you have given a lot of thought to the problems of disability.

In answer to questions, Dr. Gamble indicated that all children in the United States now have to attend regular schools, and that special schools for those with a disability are no longer available and are regarded as less than ideal. There is commonly an aide to help a disabled child. It is illegal in the United States to prevent a child in a wheelchair from attending a normal school.

In answer to a question as to what might be done to improve the image of disability, Dr. Gamble suggested that we should be advocates for our patients.

In answer to a question about what is happening in Third World countries, Dr. Gamble said that we just have to turn back the clock when we look at Third World countries. Clearly management differs in different Third World countries, but in general they correspond to attitudes which were held elsewhere in the past.

Spina Bifida Clinic, Royal Children's Hospital, 25 Victoria Parade Collingwood, Victoria 3066, Melbourne, Australia

Deformity and Gait

Malcolm B. Menelaus

The Need to Keep Accurate Records

Unless we have accurate records, we cannot know whether our patients are getting better or worse, we cannot detect neurological deterioration, and we cannot assess the results of our procedures or carry out any basic research in this area.

The Patient Data Management System (PDMS) has been of tremendous value to us. This was developed by Dr. David Shurtleff and involves a computerized system whereby many hundreds of observable facts (in my case facts relating to gait and limb deformity) are recorded at 6-monthly intervals for the first 2 years of life and then annually indefinitely. The printout, on each occasion, includes all the previous readings. Changes in muscle power can be seen at a glance.

The use of these data has enabled us to carry out many studies, some in cooperation with Seattle and elsewhere. The same system of data collection is now used at many centers including the Children's Memorial Hospital, Chicago, and I can highly recommend it.

Using these data we studied 1061 children with myelomeningocele, and reviewed 3184 pelvic radiographs from 802 patients. Hip dislocation had occurred by the age of 11 years in 28% of children with a thoracic neurosegmental level, in 30% of those with an L1/2, in 36% of L3, in 22% of L4, in 7% of L5, and in only 1% of those with sacral levels. Our findings indicate that muscle imbalance is not a significant factor in the production of flexion deformity or dislocation of the hip; both are commonly seen in the absence of imbalance. We can only hypothesise that completely paralysed hips dislocate simply because they are not kept in place by normal muscle tone. In addition, both prolonged sitting and spinal deformity may encourage the development of flexion contracture and dislocation. Hip deformity cannot be predicted from a muscle imbalance about the hip.

General Principles

The principle that I would stress is the need to perform surgery that will meet the future demands of the child. The main goal of orthopaedic management is to allow the child to be mobile in the community. This does not necessarily imply walking, as many are more mobile

Spina Bifida Clinic, Royal Children's Hospital, 25 Victoria Parade Collingwood, Victoria 3066, Melbourne, Australia

in a wheelchair. However, we have shown that children who have walked for a period in childhood, even if they later cease walking, are better at many functions of daily living than those who have never walked.

Children should be given the best chance of walking by establishing stable posture. This means that they must have their centre of gravity directly over their feet, with minimal flexion deformity at hips and knees. Approximately 60% of spina bifida children have neurological deficiencies in their upper limbs, and often need the use of both hands for activities that can normally be carried out single-handed. For this reason also, we aim, whenever possible, to enable them to stand for long periods without using their hands for support.

Orthopedic surgery has different goals according to the level of the neurosegmental lesion. Most children with thoracic lesions will not continue useful walking into adult life. Children with lumbar lesions may continue useful walking in adult life if they have strong quadriceps muscles and do not develop significant flexion deformity at the hip.

Children who will not continue walking into adult life require simple surgery to provide a stable posture in childhood. Those who will continue walking require more sophisticated surgery to meet the demands of their way of life. Because the surgery necessary in children with high lesions is relatively minor, it can and should be performed at several levels and in both limbs under one anaesthetic. Although muscle imbalance is not the prime cause of deformity, it should be corrected when present, and this can be done by relatively simple surgery. Radical surgery is necessary to correct rigid, arthrogrypotic-type deformities, and care must be taken to avoid pressure on anaesthetic skin. There are other principles to be considered also, such as the need for a multiple disciplinary clinic including a coordinator, a neurosurgeon, an orthopaedic surgeon, a urologist, a paediatric surgeon, a psychiatrist and psychologist, a medical social worker, a physiotherapist and occupational therapist, an appliance specialist, and an orthotist.

If spasticity appears, it requires investigation. Those with spasticity walk less well than those without spasticity, but with the same level of lesion.

Local Principles

In the preceding section I referred briefly to extension posture—that is the need for the child's centre of gravity to lie directly over their feet with minimal flexion deformity. To achieve this posture requires surgery for flexion deformity at hip and knee, and for various deformities at the foot (although it is calcaneous deformity which mostly imposes a flexion posture).

The management of flexion posture at the hip [1] has been considered in great detail by hip specialists, and I will not expand on it further here.

Flexion deformity of the knee is well treated by soft tissue release. We recently published a prospective study of the surgical release of 45 knee flexion contractures in 28 patients [2]. The mean age of surgery was 6.4 years, and the mean period of follow-up was 13 years. The mean knee flexion contracture before surgery was 39°, which improved to 5° at maximum correction and to 13° at the latest follow-up. Recurrence of knee flexion contracture after surgical release is most common in those with thoracic lesions who do not achieve independent walking. It would, like the hip situation, seem to be that sitting is bad news for the knee.

One problem at the knee which demands attention, and I know that Dr. Dias is giving it detailed attention in his Gait Laboratory, relates to knee pain in adults. Of 72 community ambulators in adulthood, 24% had significant knee symptoms [3]. We identified a specific gait pattern in symptomatic patients with low lumbar lesions which may be explained on the basis of hip and abductor and calf weakness. These patients have a characteristic gait which places abnormal stresses on the knee, leading to medial and anteromedial rotary instability and eventually degenerative change. It seems likely that disability resulting from knee symptoms will be the factor precluding independent ambulation in these patients. They walk with their hip internally rotated and with the tibia in external rotation. Gross degenerative changes are seen radiologically as early as 25 years of age.

Use of Circular Frames

Professor Kerr Graham, who came to our department from Belfast about 4 years ago, has had considerable experience in the use of circular frames for spina bifida patients. He has used them in the management of difficult foot deformities, for angular and rotary deformities in the tibia, and in the management of gross limb length inequality.

Absence of sensation in the limb, which is a disadvantage in most circumstances to those patients who have spina bifida, becomes an advantage when this method of management is employed.

Very gross foot deformities presenting in the latter part of the first decade and through to maturity have been treated by this means with excellent results. The foot is exposed throughout treatment so there are no problems with pressure sores. Twelve feet have been treated in this way.

Frames have been used in the management of six rotary deformities in the tibia. The frame is also of value in the management of delayed union and nonunion of supramalleolar osteotomy. The small fragment of lower tibia can readily be controlled with wires and compression.

Limb-length inequality in patients with spina bifida is generally mild and may not require treatment, although a few patients require a raise. Growth plate arrest is rarely necessary.

Recently, more patients with hemimyelomeningocele have survived. The limb length inequality has been gross, and has been corrected by the use of circular frames.

Gait Analysis

Kerr Graham has provided very useful information on spina bifida patients in our Gait Laboratory. He has shown that pelvic rotation is associated with high oxygen cost. Patients who had ileopsoas transfer have very gross pelvic rotation and very high oxygen cost, and there are good reasons why this procedure should not continue to be performed. The determination of oxygen cost in the Gait Laboratory offers the possibility of determining whether a child will continue walking into adulthood, so that we can give realistic aims to parents and realistic management to such children.

References

1. Broughton NS, Menelaus MB, Cole WG, Shurtleff DB (1993) The natural history of hip deformity in myelomeningocele. J Bone Joint Surg 75-B:760–763
2. Marshall PD, Broughton NS, Menelaus MB, Graham HK (1996) Surgical release of knee flexion contractures in myelomeningocele. J Bone Joint Surg 78-B:912–916
3. Williams JJ, Graham GP, Dunne KB, Menelaus MB (1993) Late knee problems in myelomeningocele. J Pediatr Orthop 13:701–703

Moderator's Comments on Session—Gait Disturbance by M.B. Menelaus

Nobuhiko Haga

Dr. Menelaus, a famous and experienced orthopedic surgeon, gave us an impressive lecture about the orthopedic management of patients with spina bifida. "Less surgery" and "condensed surgery" were the keywords. His principles were to select surgery appropriate to later walking ability to avoid the repetition of complicated procedures, and to condense surgery by correcting deformities of the hips, knees, and feet at the same time, if necessary. For hip dislocations, especially if both hips are involved, he said that correction of deformities is more important than reducing dislocations, and reduction is incidental. He also showed us the usefulness of gait analysis in assessing the preoperative and postoperative gait patterns of patients. To perform less surgery and condensed surgery is not easy. We must have the ability to assess the present and future status of each patient, and understand what changes will occur after surgery.

The Application of Gait Analysis to the Treatment of Children with Spina Bifida: A Look Back and as We Move Forward

Luciano Dias and Stephen J. Vankoski

Children with spina bifida present the orthopedic surgeon, therapist, orthotist, and bioengineer with a wide array of challenges. Some of the orthopedic problems, such as clubfoot and hip dislocation, are present at birth, but many develop with growth during childhood because of unbalanced muscle groups and each child's unique gait pattern. The muscle imbalance is most evident around the hip, as the gluteus maximus and gluteus medius are weak relative to the antagonist flexor and adductor muscle groups. Neural innervation of the ankle dorsiflexors and plantar flexors also originates from the sacral level of the spinal cord, and therefore these muscle groups are typically weak or absent. The muscle weakness induces certain compensatory movements at the pelvis and hip to facilitate forward progression and maintain independent ambulation. This unique gait pattern is characterized by an exaggerated dynamic range of pelvic rotation and pelvic obliquity, increased stance-phase hip abduction, increased stance-phase knee flexion, and increased ankle dorsiflexion [1–3]. Park et al. [4] recently examined the electromyographic activity of muscle groups around the hip, knee, and ankle of patients who walked with and without solid ankle, foot orthosis (AFO). As the AFO substituted for plantar flexor weakness and restrained tibial advancement, the prolonged quadriceps activity ceased earlier during stance due to decreased knee flexion amd decreased internal knee extension moment. Hullin et al. [5] similary showed improved ankle and knee kinematics and kinetics. They also demonstrated how gait analysis can be used to document the profound effect that orthotic design can impose on the gait of patients with myelomeningocele, which is particularly noteworthy since a number of orthotic options are available, including knee, ankle, foot orthosis (KAFO), various crouch control AFO designs, and the classic solid AFO. Many high-sacral and low-lumbar patients use crutches for some or all of their walking. Crutch use is often an issue, particularly with adolescent patients concerned with the stigma which crutches carry. Vankoski et al. [6] documented the benefits of crutch use, since the kinematics improved with crutch use for many patients with high-sacral-level lesions. Patients with thoracic-level lesions use reciprocating gait orthosis (RGO), hip guidance orthosis or hip, knee, ankle, foot orthosis (HKAFO). Mazur et al. [7] documented the differences in temporal parameters between the RGO and the HKAFO. Most of the higher braces permit only flexion and extension of the hip and limit pelvic movement, but these patients adopt exaggerated coronal and transverse plane motions to compensate for muscle weakness. Armed with knowledge of the magnitude of compensatory motions, perhaps

Department of Orthopaedic Surgery, Northwestern University, 680 N. Lakeshorf Dr. Suite, and Gait Analysis Laboratory, Children's Memorial Hospital, Chicago, IL, USA

orthotic design modifications to accommodate the compensatory motion, or actively assist the motion, may improve walking for these patients. With improving technology, gait analysis will play a vital role in potential advances in orthotic and assistive device design, such as externally powered AFOs, electronically controlled tree knee joint KAFOs, and ultimately CAD–CAM fabrication to benefit these patients.

Williams et al. [8] reported a 24% incidence of late knee pain in patients with lumbosacral level lesions, and described a knee valgus and flexion deformity. Most often, this appearance of knee valgus is in fact "apparent" knee valgus which results from a combination of internal pelvic and hip rotation, external tibial rotation, and stance-phase knee flexion. Over time, the constant proximal swivel movement of the pelvis and hip over the planted stance foot often induces rotational deformity. Lim et al. [9] documented the possible source of this high incidence of knee pain by showing an excessively high internal knee varus moment related to the magnitude of external tibial torsion in association with increased pelvic rotation and lateral trunk sway. Early attention to these patients is usually directed to the hips and feet, but knee problems may preclude long-term ambulatory status. The use of gait analysis for early detection of abnormal knee moments, followed by treatment with tibial derotational osteotomy or KAFO to avoid later knee pain holds promise.

Patients with sacral- and lumbar-level lesions tend to be quite active individuals despite the greater energy demands placed upon them. The functioning muscle mass in children with myelomeningocele is reduced, and hence they have a lower aerobic capacity. When this physiological change is compounded with excessive pelvic movements, oxygen cost during walking is elevated [10, 11]. As energy consumption analysis becomes a staple procedure in clinical gait laboratories, more research will be performed on these patients to help direct physical therapy and structured exercise programs to improve their long-term walking potential. The introduction of elegant musculoskeletal modelling techniques and the use of artificial intelligence technology promises to further enhance our understanding of orthopedic deformity. The beneficiaries will be the children who receive improved intervention to prevent and treat musculoskeletal deformity.

Gait analysis has played a prominent role in the evolution of treatment for patients with cerebral palsy. This has led to selective intramuscular tenotomies to preserve muscle function, classification of spastic gait patterns to focus treatment plans, and improved surgical planning, particularly when multilevel simultaneous surgery is considered. The use of gait analysis in the treatment of children with myelomeningocele has certainly progressed more slowly. Nonetheless, its significant influence in cerebral palsy treatment offers much hope for clinicians who treat ambulatory children with spina bifida to address issues such as relocation of subluxed or dislocated hips, rotational abnormalities, and efficacy of therapeutic electrical stimulation. This hope will become reality only through well-designed, multidisciplinary studies, diligent requests for pre- and posttreatment evaluations, multicenter collaborations, now made easier with the information superhighway, and as much hard work and motivation as the children demonstrate.

References

1. Selber P, Pauleto AC, Dias L (1997) The sacral and low lumbar level adult myelomeningocele patient. American Academy of Orthopaedic Surgeons 1997 Annual Meeting
2. Vankoski SJ, Sawark JF, Moore C, Dias L (1995) Characteristic pelvic, hip and knee patterns in children with lumbosacral myelomeningocele. Gait Posture 3:51–57
3. Duffy CM, Hill AE, Cosgrove AP, Corry IS, Mollan RAB, Graham HK (1996) Three-dimensional gait analysis in spina bifida. J Pediatr Orthop 16:786–791

4. Park BK, Song HR, Vankoski SJ, Moore CA, Dias L (1997) Gait electromyography in children with myelomeningocele at the sacral level. Arch Phys Med Rehabil in press
5. Hullin MG, Robb JE, Loudon IR (1992) Ankle-foot orthosis function in low-level myelomeningocele. J Pediatr Orthop 12:518–521
6. Vankoski S, Moore C, Statler K, Sarwark JF, Dias L (1995) The influence of forearm crutches on pelvic and hip kinematic parameters in childhood community ambulators with low-level myelomeningocele–Don't throw away the crutches. Dev Med Child Neurol 37(Suppl 75):5–6
7. Mazur JM, Sienko-Thomas S, Wright N, Cummings RJ (1990) Swing-through vs. reciprocating gait patterns in patients with thoracic level spina bifida. Z Kinderchir 45(Suppl 1):23–25
8. Williams JJ, Graham GP, Dunne KB, Menelaus MB (1993) Late knee problems in myelomeningocele. J Pediatr Orthop 13:701–703
9. Lim R, Moore CA, Dias LS, Vankoski SJ, Sarwark JF (1996) Valgus stress at the knee in lumbosacral myelomeningocele: a gait analysis evaluation. POSNA 1996 Annual Meeting
10. Duffy CM, Hill AE, Cosgrove AP, Corry IS, Graham HK (1996) The influence of hip abductor weakness on gait in spina bifida. Gait Posture 4:34–38
11. Vankoski S, Bare A, Dias L, Danduran M, Boas S (1997) Energy expenditure in children with myelomeningocele. What's the cost of walking? NASGCMA 1997 Annual Meeting

Moderator's Comments on Session—Gait Disturbance by L. Dias and S.J. Vankoski

James G. Gamble

Drs. Dias, Sarwark, and Vankoski, and members of the Chicago group are pioneers in the application of quantitative methods of motion analysis to the decision-making process for patients with spina bifida. They have shown the importance of considering three dimensions when evaluating gait problems in these patients. The goals in studying patients with spina bifida in the laboratory are to determine pelvic, hip, knee, and ankle kinematics in order to devise treatments that reduce the energy expenditure of walking, increase indurance, and improve the cosmetics of gait, which is the aspect that often concerns parents and patients the most.

Recently, Dr. Dias and co-workers demonstrated the value of gait analysis in the evaluation and treatment of valgus knee stress in patients with spina bifida. They also showed that the use of forearm crutches by some patients greatly improves pelvic and hip kinematics. The data from the Chicago group indicate that even in the high-tech world of the 1990s, Dr. Walter Blount's admonition, "Don't throw away the cane," is still valuable advice.

Ability in Walking is a Predictor of Bone Mineral Density and Body Composition in Prepubertal Children with Myelomeningocele

E. Salvaggio[1], G. Mauti[2], P. Ranieri[2], L. Venuti[1], S. Pulitanò[1], P. Ferrara[1], and P. Caradonna[2]

Summary. This study investigates the relationship in myelomeningocele patients between body composition and bone mineral density in 18 nonambulatory and 23 ambulatory prepubertal children. Fat mass (FM) and fat-free-mass (FFM) were calculated by anthropometry. The bone mineral content (BMC) and density (BMD) were evaluated by dual-energy X-ray absorptiometry. A scattergram of weight and height for age in females and males showed a significant reduction, which was more evident in the nonambulatory group. Percentage body fat was greater than expected, without a difference between groups. The BMD (as the *Z*-score) was low, but was lower in nonwalking patients. Multivariate analysis indicated that the best predictor for BMD in the nonwalking group was height and forearm circumference. In the walking children, only mid-thigh circumference and weight explained the BMD variation. In conclusion, the ability to walk was a highly significant determinant of bone density, and the development of muscle mass was important in promoting bone and body growth.

Key words. Myelomeningocele, Body composition, Bone mineral density

Introduction

Myelomeningocele (MMC), or spina bifida, is an important congenital physically disabling disease of childhood. It is a cause of serious locomotor disability. Moreover, spinal deformities are present, i.e. abnormalities of the vertebra and smaller lower extremities. Weight and stature can also be lower than expected for age and sex.

Particular attention must be given to the problems of growth in children with MMC. Thus body composition, which is an increasingly important measurement in paediatric clinical practice, can be assessed to evaluate changes in fat mass (FM), fat-free mass (FFM), and bone mineral density (BMD).

Previous studies of children from different ethnic groups have not shown male/female differences in whole body bone mass and bone density before puberty [2, 4]. Body weight and pubertal status account for changes in BMD. In recent years, it has been possible to measure BMD quantitatively by dual-energy X-ray absorptiometry (DEXA), which, due to its short

[1] Paediatric Department, Centro Spina Bifida, [2] Department of Internal and Geriatric Medicine, Centro per l'Osteoporosi, Università Cattolica del Sacro Cuore, Policlinico "A. Gemelli," Rome, Italy

time and low dose radiation, is suitable for use in children [3]. The assessment of body composition by anthropometry is reputed to be the primary measurement method in infancy and childhood.

In the present study, we used cross-sectional data to investigate the prevalence of a low BMD and changes in FM and FFM in prepubertal children with MMC. The relationship between body composition and BMD was assessed.

Materials and Methods

Forty-eight children with MMC (21 females and 27 males, aged 2–10 years) were studied. The patients were under regular care in our spinal disabilities clinic. Ventriculo-peritoneal shunt implantation was performed on all children. The patients were classified in two groups: nonambulatory (5 female and 9 male wheelchair users) and ambulatory (16 females and 18 males walking with aid or unaided). The children with precocious or early puberty were recorded. The diagnosis was based on the appearance of secondary sex characteristics in girls before the age of 8 years (Tanner B_2) and in boys before the age of 9 years (testicular volume ≥4 ml). All our children had normal basal levels of testosterone, 17-β-estradiol, and deidroepiandrosterone measured by routine RIA methods, and there were no signs of puberty.

Anthropometry was performed using standard techniques (measurement of skinfolds by a calliper, and of waist, hip, upper and middle thigh, and calf circumferences with a tape), and thrice-repeated measurements were averaged. Body fat as a percentage of body weight was calculated from a 4-skinfold thickness using Brook's method [1].

The bone mineral content (BMC) and BMD were evaluated by DEXA Hologic QDR 1000. The BMD was expressed as a *Z* score in order to correct values for age and sex. The *Z*-score is (OV − EV)/SD (OV = observed value, EV = expected value, SD = standard deviation for expected value). For reference values of BMD we used data from Zanchetta et al. [5].

For the statistical analysis was used the software STATISTICA for Windows. A detailed descriptive analysis was first performed to obtain information about the distribution of the variables, then an ANOVA test was performed in order to evaluate the variability in the different groups (sex and ability in walking), and some variables were analysed by the Kolmogorov–Smirnov test since there was no normal distribution for them. A Spearmann correlation test showed the influence of measured variables and walking ability on BMD. A multiple regression forward stepwise analysis was performed in order to evaluate which was the best predictor of bone density among the variables that showed significant correlation with BMD in the Spearmann analysis.

Observations and Results

A scattergram of weight for age in females (36th percentile) and males (48th percentile) showed that these subjects were underweight compared with reference data. Similarly, height for age was reduced compared with reference values (males 19th percentile, females 15th percentile). The reduction of weight and height was significantly ($P = 0.01$) more evident in the nonambulatory group (33th and 9th percentile, respectively). There were no differences in age among groups (Table 1).

Body fat as a percentage of body weight (%BF) was greater than expected, ranging from 10.6 to 40.2%, without any difference between the ambulatory group (24.9%) and the wheelchair users (23.4%). The mean *Z*-score at the lumbar (−0.55 ± 0.90) and femoral (−1.04 ± 0.91)

TABLE 1. Descriptive statistics and significant differences between means

	Weight percentile[a]	Height percentile[a]	%BF	Lumbar *Z*-score*	Neck *Z*-score**	Thigh circumference	Hip circumference
Walking	53th	26th	24.9	−0.32 ± 0.78	−0.66 ± 0.79	35.1 ± 6.4	66.1 ± 10.3
Nonwalking	33th	9th	23.4	−1.02 ± 0.99	−1.69 ± 0.73	30.2 ± 3.1	63.4 ± 7.9

[a] P = 0.01.
* P < 0.01; ** P < 0.001.
%BF, body fat as a percentage of body weight.

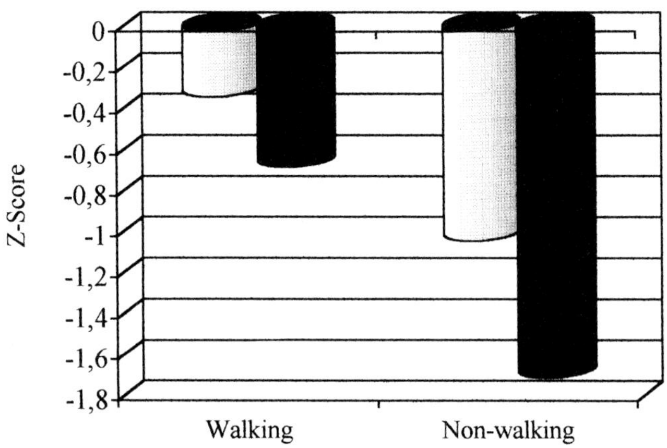

FIG. 1. Difference in *Z*-score at lumbar and femoral sites between walking and non-walking children. *Open bar*, lumbar; *solid bar*, neck

sites was low, and was lower in the nonwalking than in the walking group both at the lumbar ($P < 0.01$) and femoral ($P < 0.001$) sites (Fig. 1).

No significant difference was observed between males and females. In the nonwalking group, a simple regression was unable to show any correlation between lumbar BMD and anthropometry, although femoral BMD was correlated with age, weight, height, FFM, waist, and upper and middle thigh circumferences. Multivariate analysis indicated that the best predictor of femoral BMD in this group was height, forearm circumference (positive), and hip circumference (negative).

In the walking group, simple regression showed that lumbar and femoral BMD was highly correlated with age, waist, height, FFM, FM, upper and middle thigh circumferences, hip circumference, and subscapular skinfold. When a multivariate analysis was performed with these variables, only middle thigh circumference and weight significantly explained the BMD variation at the lumbar site. Bone density at the femoral neck site showed a high correlation with weight, age, and upper and middle thigh circumferences (Fig. 2).

Discussion and Conclusion

We conclude that prepubertal children with spina bifida are shorter than normal children. The nonwalking group was underweight compared with reference values. All subjects showed an excess of fat as percentage of body weight. They also showed a low BMD, with no difference between males and females. The effect of age on BMD was significant at two sites. After controlling for this, the neurological level (walking/nonwalking) was a highly significant

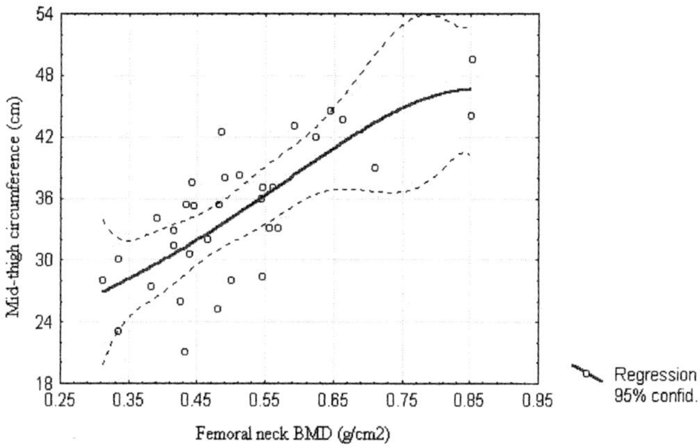

FIG. 2. Femoral neck BMD vs. middle thigh circumference in walking subjects. Middle thigh = 14.558 + 39.116, $P < 0.01$; neck BMD, Pearson's correlation: $r = 0.746$, $P < 0.001$

determinant of bone density. The ability to walk, along with the development of muscle mass (expressed by hip and thigh circumferences), is important in promoting bone and body growth.

References

1. Brook CGD (1971) Determination of body composition of children from skinfold measurement. Arch Dis Child 46:182–184
2. Glastre C, Braillon P, David L, Cochat P, Meunier PJ, Delmas PD (1995) Measurement of bone mineral content of the lumbar spine by dual energy X-ray absorptiometry in normal children: correlation with growth parameters. J Clin Endocrinol Metab 79:775–779
3. Lapillonne A, Braillon PM, Delmas PD, Salle BL (1997) Dual-energy X-ray absorptiometry in early life. Horm Res 48(suppl):43–49
4. Nelson DA, Simpson PM, Johnson CC, Barondess DA, Kleerekoper M (1997) The accumulation of whole body skeletal mass in third- and fourth-grade children: effects of age, gender, ethnicity, and body composition. Bone 20:73–78
5. Zanchetta JR, Plotkin H, Alvarez FML (1995) Bone mass in children: normative values for the 2–20-year-old population. Bone 16(Suppl.):393S–399S

Magnetic Resonance Imaging of Hip Extensor and Knee Flexor Muscles in Patients with Spina Bifida

N. Haga[1], S. Nakamura[1], K. Taniguchi[1], T. Akune[1], K. Yoshida[2], and T. Iwaya[2]

Summary. In patients with spina bifida, ambulatory status has been reported to be related to the power of the knee extensor, knee flexor, and hip extensor muscles. We performed a magnetic resonance imaging (MRI) study of the thigh muscles of 16 spina bifida children aged 5 to 16 years. We wanted to know if the MRI findings were related to the manual muscle testing (MMT) score and the ambulatory status. The results showed that the signal density of the semimembranous (SM) muscle in MRI was related to the MMT scores of knee flexion and hip extension. The signal density of the biceps femoris and glutus maximus muscles showed a weaker relationship with these MMT scores. The signal density of the SM muscle was also related to ambulatory status. We concluded that the status of the SM muscle is important for the function of hip extension and knee flexion, and therefore influences the ambulatory status in patients with spina bifida.

Key words. Spina bifida, Magnetic resonance imaging, Thigh muscle, Ambulatory status

Introduction

In patients with spina bifida, ambulatory status has been reported to correlate with neurosegmental level. The neurosegmental level of a specific patient is usually determined by comparing the observed amd measured leg motion with the chart of segmental innervation of lower-limb muscles described by Sharrard in 1964 [6]. In our study, the strength of the knee flexor and hip extensor muscles measured by manual muscle testing (MMT) was correlated with the patient's ambulation status. However, MMT needs the patient's cooperation, and is not suitable for infants, measures only one group of muscles, and is not quantitative. Conversely, magnetic resonance imaging (MRI) does not need the patient's cooperation and can differentiate each muscle. Whether MRI can provide quantitative information is not clear. The objective of this study was to know if the MRI of hip extensor and knee flexor muscles correlate with corresponding MMT scores and the patient's ambulation status, and to clarify whether MRI can provide information additional to MMT scores.

[1] Department of Pediatric Orthopedics, Shizuoka Children's Hospital, 860 Urushiyama, Shizuoka 420, Japan

[2] Section of Rehabilitation Medicine for the Physically Disabled, Tohoku University Graduate School of Medicine, 2-1 Seiryo-cho, Aoba-ku, Sendai 980-77, Japan

Materials and Methods

The study was carried out on 16 patients with spina bifida. Thirteen patients had myelomeningocele and three had spinal lipoma. Six males and 10 females were included, and their age range was from 5 to 16 years, with a mean of 10 years. Using the spin echo method, T1 weighted axial images were obtained between the iliac crest and the knee joint. The signal intensities of semimembranous (SM) muscle, biceps femoris (BF), and gluteus maximus (GM) were estimated.

We expressed the signal intensity of each muscle as normal (n) or diminished (d). Figure 1 shows the axial image at the junction of the middle and distal one-third of the femur, and Fig. 2 shows the axial image at the level of the hip joint.

We first studied the relationship between the MRI findings and the MMT score. MRI findings of SM and BF were compared with the MMT scores of knee flexion and hip extension, and those of GM were compared with MMT scores of hip extension. We then studied the relationship between the MRI findings and ambulation. We classified ambulation status into two groups according to the ability to walk without crutches.

a 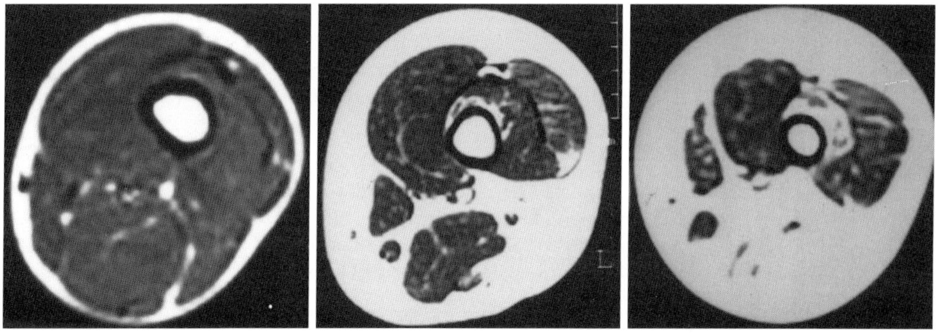 b,c

FIG. 1a–c. Axial images at the junction of middle and distal one-third of the femur. **a** The intensity of semimembranous (SM) muscle and biceps femoris (BF) seems normal. **b** SM muscle is normal, but BF is diminished and replaced by the density of fat. **c** Both SM muscle and BF are diminished

a 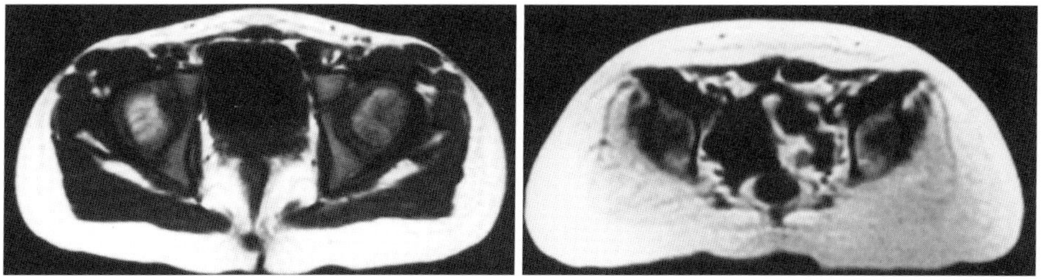 b

FIG. 2a,b. Axial imagea at the level of the hip joint. **a** The intensity of gluteus maximus (GM) seems normal. **b** GM is diminished

Observations and Results

MRI findings of SM muscle and BF were classified into three groups, one with normal SM muscle and BF, one with normal SM muscle and diminished BF, and one with diminished SM muscle and BF. There was no MR image with diminished SM muscle and normal BF.

The results of the relationship between MRI findings and MMT score were as follows. If SM muscle was normal in MRI, MMT scores of knee flexion were 5–4 in most cases, in spite of the MRI finding of BF. If SM muscle was diminished, MMT scores were distributed from 4 to zero. The relationship between the MRI of SM muscle, normal or diminished, and the knee flexion MMT, 5–4 or 3–0, showed significant independence by Fisher's exact probability test (Table 1). If SM muscle was normal in MRI, MMT scores of hip extension were 5–3 in most cases, in spite of the MRI finding of BF. If SM muscle was diminished, MMT scores were 1–0 in five cases out of seven. The relationship between the MRI of SM muscle, normal or diminished, and the hip extension MMT, 5–2 or 1–0, also showed significant independence (Table 2). The distribution of MMT scores of hip extension and MRI findings of GM showed no significant independence (Table 3).

The results of the relationship between the MRI findings and ambulation were as follows. If SM muscle was normal in MRI, all patients walked without crutches. If SM muscle was diminished, one patient out of three walked without crutches. There was significant independence between the normal and diminished SM muscle groups as to ambulation status (Table 4). If GM was normal in MRI, all patients walked without crutches. If GM was diminished, 10 out of 12 patients walked without crutches. There was no significant independence (Table 5).

Table 1. The relationship between magnetic resonance imaging (MRI) findings of SM muscle and manual muscle testing (MMT) scores of knee flexion[a]

	MMT	
SM	5–4	3–0
Normal	23	2
Diminished	3	4

[a] $P < 0.05$.

Table 2. The relationship between MRI findings of SM muscle and MMT scores of hip extension[a]

	MMT	
SM	5–2	1–0
Normal	23	2
Diminished	2	5

[a] $P < 0.05$.

Table 3. The relationship between MRI findings of GM and MMT scores of hip extension[a]

GM	MMT 5–2	MMT 1–0
Normal	7	2
Diminished	18	5

[a] n.s.

Table 4. The relationship between MRI findings of SM muscle and ambulation status[a]

SM	Walk without crutches	Others
Normal	13	0
Diminished	1	2

[a] $P < 0.05$.

Table 5. The relationship between MRI findings of GM and ambulation status[a]

GM	Walk without crutches	Others
Normal	4	0
Diminished	10	2

[a] n.s.

Discussion and Conclusions

In 1983 [2], Asher reported that among the 16 different factors, the most significant single factor affecting walking ability was the level of neural involvement. He also found that 4th lumbar paraplegics, with grade-3 knee flexion strength, were usually functional ambulators. In 1991 [4], McDonald et al. modified Sharrard's description of neurosegmental innervation, and reported that medial hamstring strength more frequently correlated with iliopsoas and quadriceps, and glutei with anterior tibialis. As for the correlation with ambulation status, he found that iliopsoas strength was the best predictor of ambulation, with the quadriceps, anterior tibialis, and glutei also contributing significantly, and that grade 4–5 gluteal and anterior tibialis function was associated with community ambulation, without aids or braces [4].

Our previous studies [1, 5] showed that 4 or more knee flexion strength and 2 or more hip extension strength were related to the patient's ability to walk without crutches, but each joint motion is performed by a group of muscles. For flexion of the knee, SM muscle, BF, and semitendinous muscles do most of the work, and some other muscles assist. For extension of the hip, GM, SM muscle, BF, and semitendinous muscles work together.

The present study showed that MRI findings of SM muscle were related to the MMT scores of knee flexion and hip extension, but MRI findings of BF and GM were not related to the corresponding MMT scores. This study also showed that MRI findings of SM muscle were related to the patient's ambulation status. The only patient who could walk without crutches, even though her SM muscle is diminished in MRI, walks with a pair of AFO, swaying her body markedly.

From the results of this study, we consider that MRI is useful in assessing patients with spina bifida for the following reasons.

1. As MRI can estimate the status of muscles without the patient's cooperation, it can be used to predict future ambulation status in the infantile period.
2. As MRI can differentiate each muscle, it can inform us of changes in the neurological status of a patient.

Whether MRI can provide quantative information about muscles is not clear from this study.

In conclusion, the signal density of SM muscle in MRI is related to the MMT scores of knee flexion and hip extension. The signal density of SM muscle is related to ambulation status. MRI can provide information additional to MMT because the patient's cooperation is unnecessary, and it can assess each muscle group.

References

1. Akune T, Haga N, Iwaya T, Yoshida K, Nakamura S (1996) Ambulatory status of children with spina bifida and findings by magnetic resonance imaging of the hip extensor muscles (in Japanese). J Jpn Paediatr Orthop Assoc 6:100–103
2. Asher M, Olson J (1983) Factors affecting the ambulatory status of patients with spina bifida cystica. J Bone Joint Surg 65-A:350–356
3. McDonald CM, Jaffe KM, Mosca VS, Shurtleff DB (1991) Ambulatory outcome of children with myelomeningocele. Effect of lower-extremity muscle strength. Dev Med Child Neurol 33: 482–490
4. McDonald CM, Jaffe KM, Shurtleff DB, Menelaus MB (1991) Modifications to the traditional description of neurosegmental innervation in myelomeningocele. Dev Med Child Neurol 33: 473–481
5. Nakamura S, Haga N, Nakajima K, Iwaya T, Yoshida K, Taniguchi K (1995) Magnetic resonance imaging of thigh muscles of patients with spina bifida (in Japanese). J Jpn Paediatr Orthop Assoc 5:1–4
6. Sharrard WJW (1964) Posterior iliopsoas transplantation in the treatment of paralytic dislocation of the hip. J Bone Joint Surg 46-B:426–444

Bracing for Ambulation: Basic Principles, Brace Alternatives by Motor Level and Predictive Long-Term Goals

John V. Banta

The first basic principle of bracing a child with paralytic residuals of myelomeningocle is to conduct a thorough clinical examination to determine their functional motor level. This is defined as the lowest motor level showing grade three (i.e., antigravity strength through a full range of motion). Failure to do so will ultimately result in either overbracing, providing the child with more cumbersome, heavy, and nonfunctional apparatus which will encumber mobility, or underbracing, which will inhibit function and lead to further orthopedic deformity. It is essential to differentiate spastic versus flaccid paralysis. Fully one-third of affected children will present with an upper motor neuron component to their neurologic pattern, and the spastic component may be reflected in overt spasticity, subtle alteration in the tone of the muscle, or purely reflexive motor activity or synergistic motor activity in which the child can only move a limb through synergistic patterned movements. Additionally, the examiner must note the presence or, more importantly, the absence of protective sensation and equilibrium reactions which greatly influence the child's ability to react to position in space and the effects of gravity.

Using the above definition, the functional level of the child can best be determined by referring to the functional classification popularized by Lindseth [10] (Table 1). Walking or ambulatory function was best defined by Hoffer et al. [6] at Rancho los Amigos Hospital in 1982, with strict definitions which for the first time allowed clinicians to relate the walking abilities of patients to the treatment objectives, and form a definition for outcome analysis of therapeutic treatments. A child who is a community ambulator may or may not use crutches and orthoses to walk outdoors, but may use a wheelchair for long distances. A household ambulator, by definition, walks within the home or school with orthoses, can self-transfer, and uses a wheelchair part time in the home and for all outdoor activities. A nonfunctional walker uses walking purely for a therapeutic exercise in the home only, and a nonambulator is wheelchair-bound.

The goals of orthoses are clear and concise. To provide an upright position with mobility through space leading to independence in activities of daily living, access to the community, school achievement, and the enhance self-image [18]. In the past, the orthopedic community mistakenly assumed that the surgical interventions devised to assist children afflicted with poliomyelitis would be of equal benefit for the child with spina bifida, failing to realize that the sensory and proprioceptive loss in myelomeningocele would result in a significantly lower

---

Newington Department of Orthopaedic Surgery, Connecticut Children's Medical Center, 282 Washington Street, Hartford, CT 06106, USA

TABLE 1. Functional motor level

Level	Muscles	Function
Thoracic	Flail	Static contractures
L-1	Iliopsoas	Weak hip flexion
L-2	Psoas + sartorius	Strong hip flexion
L-3	Quadriceps	Knee extension
L-4	Medial hamstrings	Knee flexion
L-5	Anterior tibialis	Foot dorsiflexion
	Peroneals	Strong knee flexion
	Lateral hamstrings	
Sacral	Gastrocnemius + posterior tibialis	Plantar flexion

level of ambulatory skill [21]. Recent long-term studies by Brinker et al. [4] and Lias et al. [8] have confirmed the clinical impression that slow deterioration in not uncommon in these children.

Since the child with spina bifida has sensory and proprioceptive loss in addition to motor weakness, long-term walking ability is directly related to the strength of the remaining active muscles, which are under voluntary control of the motor cortex (i.e., not reflexive or synergistic), and this directly relates in the long term to what may best be termed "the law of mass". The weight of the body is measured by the cube and increases proportionally to the volume that it occupies, whereas the strength of the muscle units within the body are directly related to the cross-sectional diameter of the muscle. It follows that with increasing age, the child's mass increases by the cube whereas its strength increases only by the square, with the inevitable result that by the second decade of life, as the child enters the adolescent growth spurt, walking efficiency drops off as the energy demands become greater, so that the child often self-selects the most energy-efficient means of mobility, i.e., the wheelchair, particularly as the demands of school and social obligations demand more mobility within increasing time constraints [2].

The choice of orthotic prescription is influenced by two conflicting philosophical options; namely, either to brace the child initially to a high level and let the child demonstrate that there is sufficient motor control to progressively lower the level of bracing, or only to provide a minimal support and progressively increase the level of orthotic control as the child demonstrates an inability to control the body in space. I have personally developed the former approach as being more effective, since the child is immediately upright at the appropriate developmental age without unnecessary energy expenditure, as well as preventing early joint contractures. As the child develops, one can then more accurately assess the true neurologic level and rapidly lower the level of bracing as the child demonstrates functional control of the spine, pelvis, and lower extremities. It is also important to realize that the orthopedist is faced with a dilemma in prescribing braces: there is an invariable trade-off between mobility and stability. For example, adding a pelvic band to a knee–ankle orthosis will promote greater stability at the pelvis, but will also interfere with rotation of the lower extremities.

Brace alternatives are best considered by motor level, and the following generic orthotic devices should be considered within the context of not only the child's motor loss, but also the functional expectations. The best initial treatment is obtained when the physician, orthotist, *and the child's family* all participate in the decision. At the thoracic level with flail lower extremities, the goal is to maintain a straight spine, level pelvis, and symmetric lower limbs. This is also the level at which the risk of spinal deformity is greatest! A parapodium is an excellent first standing device but it lacks mobility, and children who have the developmental motor skills are best advanced to a swivel walker, conventional HKAFO (hip, knee, ankle, foot orthosis) or reciprocating orthoses. The swivel walker lacks mobility and requires donning and doffing by another person. HKAFOs are traditional, but are inefficient and require frequent modifications to maintain proper alignment.

Reciprocating orthoses have gained a great deal of popularity in the past decade, and can be referred to as hip guidance orthoses (Parawalker), reciprocating gait orthoses (RGO), isocentric reciprocating orthoses, and RGOs accompanied by the application of surface electrical stimulation [17, 22]. The problems inherent in *all* these orthotic devices include expense, donning and doffing, (toileting), energy cost, and limited long-term clinical use (i.e., there are no long-term clinical studies to confirm their use into the second decade) [19, 20].

At the Lumbar 2 level, the child has weak hip flexion which can initiate hip flexion, making all RGOs more functional as the energy demands begin to decline. Hip rotational control is still necessary, and a pelvic band is necessary. At the Lumbar 3 level, knee extension is present, albeit weak compared with the Lumbar 4 level, but the child exhibits hip adduction. However, there is no knee extension, resulting in absent knee flexion, weak to absent hip extension, and heavy reliance upon the upper extremities with crutches, with the resultant increased lumbar lordosis with the trunk tilted forward to the ground reaction force, often accompanied by hip instability [9, 21]. At the Lumbar 4 level, knee flexion is present and the medial hamstrings provide weak hip extension, but no biceps femoris is active and knee instability can result from inadequate support. For this reason, the use of a KAFO is recommended until the motor control about the knee includes not only the quadriceps, but also both medial and lateral hamstring function.

At the mid-lumbar level, the child is subject to the "physiological curse of the crouch gait". Perry et al. [15], in experiments on cadaver specimens, showed that there is a rapid rise from 22% to 51% of the maximum quadriceps force across the knee joint with an increase of between 15 and 30 degrees of knee flexion. The mechanical work increases progressively with increased knee flexion. Ounpuu et al. [14] analyzed the joint kinetic, demonstrating that the hip provides 54% of the mechanical work in normal gait, whereas the ankle provides only 30%. Therefore control of the ankle is essential to the proper alignment of the body to the ground reaction force.

The orthotic choices for control of the foot and ankle include floor reaction orthoses to prevent cancaneal crouch gait. They reduce the external knee moment by aligning the knee with the ground reaction force [11]. In clinical use, however, these orthoses, which require an intimate fit in the malleolar and tibial areas, are inclined to cause pressure on the insensate soft tissues and must be fitted expertly, and the child's foot and ankle must be checked carefully for skin irritation. The conventional AFO (ankle, foot orthosis) is widely used, but is subject to deformation of the plastic and may result in an external foot progression angle if no third rocker is provided for the end of the stance phase of gait [7]. Therefore, the use of a rocker bottom sole to the shoe is often advisable.

The choice between an AFO and a KAFO is best answered by assessing the following factors. Does isolated medial hamstring function adequately control the knee? Is the patient skeletally mature, with strong collateral ligaments and no deformation of the femoral condyles or the tibial plateaus? A major unresolved question has been whether the KAFO improves the saggital alignment of the knee and prevent valgus thrust? Recent studies of gait in these patients suggest that the apparent knee valgus thrust may result from a combination of (1) excessive and prolonged internal pelvic rotation in the transverse plane, (2) excessive and persistent knee flexion, and (3) external foot rotation during the loading phase of gait [14].

The Lumbar 5 level is the best candidate for community ambulation as a child *and as an adolescent*! Therefore, a KAFO prescribed early is appropriate to promote proper alignment and then reduce bracing as the child matures. An AFO in late childhood is adequate once the child demonstrates hip stability and adequate knee stability. At the sacral level, all patients should have unrestricted community ambulatory skills *but their feet are insensate*! This group of patients must be monitored closely for neurological loss, as was described in the report by Brinker et al. [4]. An AFO, with its solid ankle support, is the best first choice, and this can then be ground away at the ankle angle to convert it to a posterior leaf spring (PLS) for those few patients who only require a modest dorsiflexion assistance to clear their foot in the swing phase of gait. Articulated AFOs provide more mobility at the ankle joint but are more subject to wear and breakdown. I do not believe that the supramalleolar orthosis (SMO) is ever indicated for treatment of patients with insensate skin. This orthosis fails to provide any control of the tibia over the ankle, and in reality only functions as a control of the hindfoot, much as the UCBL (University of California Berkeley Laboratories) heel cup. For the rare child with excellent motor control through the sacral level but with a hind foot valgus, the UCBL is an excellent device.

As indicated earlier, any child can be fitted with an orthosis, but the critical issues are the long-term goals and objectives of orthotic management during growth. Predictive indications for continued ambulation include the following factors which all *adversely* affect walking ability: motor level, obesity, scoliosis, lower extremity deformity, motivation, and perhaps intelligence as it relates to the degree of hydrocephalus [1, 20]. Of these factors, most clinicians agree that the *functional motor level* is the most critical. The second is age. By the second decade of life, most children who are not competitive walkers will self-select a wheelchair for one major reason: *energy cost* [1]!

As indicated earlier, the neurological level is not always static. Younger children with synergistic or reflexive motor function can often utilize braces, but they may loose function with growth. With the advent of MRI, it is now recognized that most, if not all, repairs of the myelomeningocele lesions will result in radiological evidence of adherence of the underlying nerve elements to the site of the repair. This so called "tether"may result in a slow, insidious deterioration of function, but conversely there are no long-term analyses of detethering and the operation is not without the risk of causing neurological loss. Finally, overuse of insensate joints without adequate support can result in Charcot arthropathy involving not only the foot and ankle, but also the knee and hip [12]. Finally, data confirm that the last intact laminar arch is a valuable predictive indicator of scoliosis [16]. Spinal orthoses are a valuable adjunct in providing stability of the spine for the child with a high-level paralysis with collapsing or functional scoliosis, but they serve no purpose in congenital spinal deformity. However, once the coronal deformity reaches 45–50 degrees, most authors recommend surgical stabilization of the spine. This is a complete topic in itself and is beyond the scope of this presentation.

In summary, by performing a through physical examination of the child and applying the basic principles outlined above, the clinician can provide the optimum functional support for the child with myelomeningocele, thereby allowing the child optimum growth and the potential for attaining realistic mobility goals consistent with their neurologic lesion and age.

References

1. Asher M, Olson J (1983) Factors affecting the ambulatory status of patients with spina bifida cystica. J Bone Joint Surg 65A:350–358
2. Banta JV (1996) The orthopaedic history of spinal dysraphis. Review article II. The modern surgical treatment. J Dev Med Child Neurol 38:954–960

3. Beaty JH, Canale ST (1990) Current concepts review: orthopaedic aspects of myelomeningocele. J Bone Joint Surg 72A:626–630
4. Brinker MR, Rosenthal SR, Feiwell E, Granger SP, Mitchell DC, Rice JC (1994) Myelomeingocele at the sacral level: long-term outcomes in adults. J Bone Joint Surg 76A:1293–1300
5. Feiwell E, Sakar D, Blatt T (1978) The effects of hip reduction on function in patients with myelomeningocele: potential gains and hazards of surgical care. J Bone Joint Surg 60A:169
6. Hoffer MM, Feiwell D, Perry R, Perry J, Bonnet C (1982) Functional ambulation in patients with myelomeningocele. J Bone Joint Surg 64A:841–850
7. Hullin MG, Robb JE, Loudion IR (1992) Ankle foot orthosis function in low-level myelomeningocele. J Pediatr Orthop 12:518–521
8. Lais A, Kasabian NG, Dryo FM, Scott RM, Kelly MD, Bauer SB (1993) The neurosurgical implications of continuous neurological surveillance of children with myelodysplasia. J Urol 150:1897–1883
9. Lee EH, Arroll NC (1985) Hip stability and ambulatory status in myelomeningocele. J Pediatr Orthop 5:522–525
10. Lindseth RE (1976) Treatment of the lower extremities in children paralyzed by myelomeningocele (birth to 18 months). Instruction Course Lecture AAOS XXV, pp 76–82
11. Lindseth RE, Clance J (1979) Polypropylene lower extremity braces for paraplegia due to myelomeningocele. J Bone and Joint Surg 56A:566–570
12. Nagrakatti D, Banta JV, Thomson J Neuropathic joints in myelomeningocele. (In press)
13. Ounpuu S, Gange JR, Dabis RB (1991) Three-dimensional lower extremity joint kinetics in normal pediatric gait. J Pediatr Orthop 11:341–349
14. Ounpuu S, Davis RB, Banta JV, DeLuce PA (1992) The effects of orthotics on gait in children with low-level myelomeningocele. Proceedings of the North American Congress on Biomechanics, Chicago, IL, pp 323–324
15. Perry J, Antonelli D, Ford W (1975) Analysis of knee joint forces during flexed knee stance. J Bone Joint Surg 57A:961–976
16. Piggott H (1980) The natural history of scoliosis in myelomeningocele. J Bone Joint Surg 62B:54–59
17. Rose GK, Stallard J, Sankarankutty M (1981) Clinical evaluation of spina bifida patients using hip guidance orthosis. Dev Med Child Neurol 23:30–40
18. Rose GK, Sankarankutty M, Stallard J (1983) A clinical review of the orthotic treatment of myelomeningocele patients. J Bone Joint Surg 65B:242–248
19. Samuelson C, Skog M (1988) Ambulation in patients with myelomeningocele. A multivariate statistical analysis. J Pediatr Orthop 8:569–575
20. Stillwell A, Menelaus MB (1983) Walking ability in mature patients with spina bifida. J Pediatr Orthop 3:184–190
21. Stillwell A, Menelaus MB (1984) Walking ability after transplantation of the iliopsoas—a long-term follow-up. J Bone Joint Surg 66B:656–659
22. Yngve D, Douglas R, Roberts J (1984) The reciprocating gait orthosis in myelomeningocele. J Pediatr Orthop 4:304–310

Comprehensive Rehabilitation of Adults with Spina Bifida

TETSUO SUYAMA[1], RYUICHI NIHEI[2], TETSUHIKO KIMURA[3], and YASUHIRO HATSUYAMA[3]

Summary. Spina bifida is often complicated by physical and mental disabilities of various forms. Long-term rehabilitation is necessary not only to inhibit the occurrence of the disabilities, but also to develop the faculty of ambulation, to establish independence in the activities of daily life (ADL), to train patients efficiently and systematically, to encourage them to acquire the knowledge and techniques required in social life, and to promote their social independence. Many studies of infants have been reported in the literature, but unfortunately we have never found one on the rehabilitation of adults with spina bifida.

Between 1981 and 1997 we studied 50 patients. Their ages varied from 18 to 47 years, with a mean age of 20.3 years, and there were 18 men and 32 women. Their spinal cord lesion ranged from T5 to S2. Patients with spinal cord lesion L3 were the largest group, and most patients (80.5%) ranged from L2 to S1. There were 13 cases of community ambulators with spinal cord lesion L4 to S2; there were 20 household ambulators using crutches or apparatus, and 17 nonambulators in wheelchairs. The spinal cord lesion of most of them ranged from T5 to L2. More than half the patients (53%) urinated by self-catheterization, and the others urinated naturally with urine bags or tapping. According to intravenous pyelography (IVP) findings on admission, hydronephrose or renal atrophy was found in 48% of patients. As a result of intelligence tests measured by WAIS-R, it was found that patients' IQ ranged from 61 to 124, and the mean was 88.6. After the rehabilitative training, 37 patients (74%) were employed in ordinary paid jobs, nine (18%) were in sheltered workshops or welfare factories, and two did business on their own. The others did not find jobs. The IQs of those employed in paid jobs and those employed in sheltered workshops were 92 and 87, respectively. Compared with the general employment rate of patients with thoracic or lumbar injury, which is 80% or more, the employment rate of those with spina bifida was low.

From these findings, we believe that the following steps are necessary for the promotion of rehabilitation of patients with spina bifida: the prevention of a decline of IQ and the progress of hydrocephalus; the control of urination; the prevention of the occurrence of decubitus; retraining and the establishment of ADL, which declines with aging; the provision of a general education, and training for employment for re-entry into society.

[1] Department of Rehabilitation, Saitama Medical Center and Medical School, Iruma, Saitama 350-0495, Japan
[2] Nihon Rehabilitation College
[3] National Rehabilitation Center for the Disabled

Introduction

Spina bifida is often complicated by physical and mental disabilities of various forms. Long-term rehabilitation [1] is necessary not only to keep the occurrence of the disabilities to a minimum, but also to develop the faculty of ambulation, to establish independence in the activities of daily life (ADL), to train patients efficiently and systematically [3], to encourage them to acquire the knowledge and techniques required in social life, and to promote their social independence [2, 11].

We now report on a study of the physical condition of adults with spina bifida, their ambulation and apparatus, and other important factors necessary for their rehabilitation.

Subjects

The subjects were 50 patients who had been treated and trained in the hospitl and in the rehabilitative training center of the National Rehabilitation Center for the Disabled between 1981 and 1997.

Their ages varied from 18 to 47 years, with a mean age of 20.3 years, and there were 18 men and 32 women.

Their educational background before their admission to the center was that 45 (90%) had graduated from ordinary high schools, and the other two (4%) were from special schools for the handicapped and both undertook self-education.

Their spinal cord lesion ranged from T5 to S2; patients with spinal cord lesion L3 were the largest group, and most patients (80.5%) ranged from L2 to S1.

Forty cases (80%) with spinal bifida had neurosurgical operations between birth and 4 years of age. Five patients had operations for hydrocephalus before 1969, while 21 patients (66%) had that operation after 1970. Many patients had other operations after 1970.

Thirteen patients had severe scoliosis, and one of them had spinal surgery with the use of a Harrington rod. After the operation, paralysis with the spinal cord lesion below T5 occurred.

Assessment Areas

Lower Limb Deformity

In ankle joint deformities, there were 22 cases of varus deformity, which was the largest group, and other cases of equinus, flaccid paralysis, or talipes cavus. In knee deformities, there were two cases of contracture in flexion, while in hip joint deformities, there were congenital dislocation of the hip (CDH) and contracture in flexion.

Operations for tendon lengthening and transfer were performed for varus deformity, and RAO was performed for congenital dislocation of the hip (Table 1).

TABLE 1. Foot operations

Deformity	Patients	Operations
Varus	22	11
Equinus	4	2
Excavatus	2	
Paralytic foot	4	

Upper Limb Deformity

There were three cases of upper limb deformity, such as Chiari II type and syringomyelia.

Ambulation

There were 13 cases of community ambulators with the spinal cord lesion L4–S2; there were 20 household ambulators using crutches or apparatus, which was the largest group. There were 17 nonambulators in wheelchairs, and the spinal cord lesion of most of them ranged from T5 to L2. Their ambulation is up to their spinal cord lesion; those with the lesion level T to L2 used a wheelchair, those with the lesion L2 to 3, used crutches and a wheelchair, those with the lesion L4 walked using apparatus, and those with the lesion L5–S2 walked without apparatus (Tables 2 and 3).

Decubitus

The most patients had a history of decubitus. There were 15 nonambulators, 15 household ambulators, and 2 community ambulators on admission, and decubitus was found in many wheelchair users. The prevention of the occurrence of decubitus is an urgent necessity.

Urination

More than half the patients (53%) urinated by self-catheterization, and the others urinated naturally with urine bags or with tapping. Cystectasia or ileal catheterization was used on 11 patients (22%). Of the female patients, 86% needed diapers.

TABLE 2. Ambulation ability

1. Community ambulator	
(a) Without support	3 patients
(b) With cane	10 patients
2. Household ambulator (with crutches and wheelchair)	20 patients
3. Nonfunctional ambulator	10 patients
4. Nonambulator	7 patients

TABLE 3. Correlation between paralysis level and orthosis

1. Group T_{12}	Nonambulator	Wheel chair
2. Group L_2	Nonfunctional ambulator	LLB + two crutches (exercise) Wheelchair
3. Group L_4	Household ambulator	LLB or SLB + two crutches Wheelchair
4. Group L_5	Community ambulator	SLB + Lofstrand crutch
5. Group S2	Community ambulator	SLB, shoes (with or without)

Passage

Twenty-eight cases evacuated by abdominal pressure, while 13 cases did so naturally. Although there were some cases of incontinence, most patients controlled their passage fairly well.

Uropathy

According to intravenous pyelography (IVP) findings on admission (Table 4), hydronephrose or renal atrophy was found in 48% of patients, and the degree in five of these cases was serious. One of these five patients was given renal dialysis at age 20.

Men's Sexual Function

While erection was found in 10 (71.4%) of 14 cases, ejaculation was found in five cases (35.7%).

Intelligence Quotient (IQ)

As a result of intelligence tests measured by WAIS-R, it was found that patients' IQ ranged from 61 to 124, and the mean was 88.6. The IQs of patients with spina bifida were higher than those of patients with cerebral palsy who were disabled since birth and who also required special training and care, and were lower than those of patients with osteogenesis imperfecta (Table 5).

Employment

After the rehabilitative training, 37 patients (74%) were employed in ordinary paid jobs, nine (18%) were in sheltered workshops or welfare factories, and two did business on their own. The others did not find jobs. Compared with the general employment rate of patients with thoracic or lumbar injury, which is 80% or more, the employment rate of those with spina bifida was low (Table 6). The IQs of those employed in paid jobs and those employed in sheltered workshops were 92 and 87, respectively. Driving was possible for two-thirds of the total number of spina bifida patients.

TABLE 4. Intravenous pyelography findings

	Severe	Moderate	Slight	Nothing	Rate of changes
Kidney	5	2	6	14	48.1%
Ureter	1	1	1	24	11.1%
Bladder	6	2	6	13	51.9%

TABLE 5. TIQ measured by WAIS-R

Spina bifida (n = 41)	61–124 (mean = 88.6)
Cerebral palsy (n = 69)	55–110 (mean = 79.3)
Osteogenesis imperfecta (n = 21)	62–130 (mean = 100.7)

TABLE 6. Places of employment

General work	30 patients	(60%)
Work center	9 patients	(8%)
Independent enterprise	2 patients	(4%)
House support	1 patient	(2%)
None (training center)	8 patients	(16%)
		(n = 50)

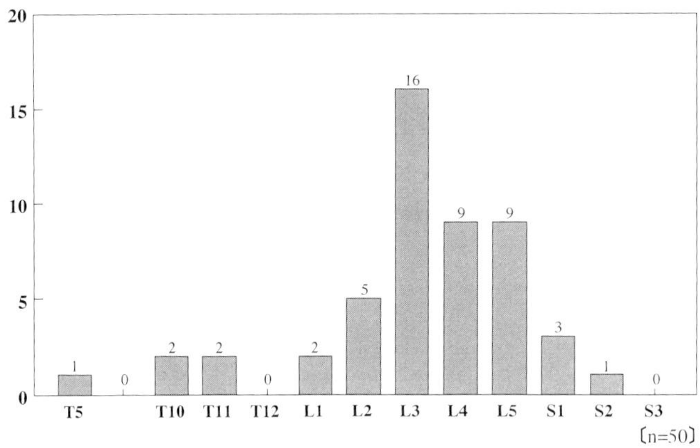

FIG. 1. Level of paralysis

Findings

One of the physical characteristics of spina bifida is paralysis in the lower limbs. If the spinal cord itself and the nerve root are injured, spastic paralysis and flaccid paralysis, respectively, occur. For the evaluation of ambulation, the classifications of Sharrard [9] and Hoffer et al. [5] are available. These classifications are according to the spinal cord lesion.

Crutches, sticks, and other apparatus for long or short lower limbs are used for paralyzed limbs, and an operation is sometimes performed to correct a deformity [7, 8]. However, the ambulation of patients often declines with aging or for many other reasons [10]. To prevent this decline, the prevention of obesity [4] and training of the musculi quadriceps femoris are important (Fig. 1).

Conclusions

From these findings, it can be seen that for the promotion of rehabilitation of patients with spina bifida, the following steps are necessary: the prevention of a decline in IQ [6] and the progress of hydrocephalus; the control of urination; the prevention of the occurrence of decubitus; retraining and the establishment of ADL, which declines with aging; the provision of a general education, and training for employment for re-entry into society.

References

1. Barden GA, Meyer LC, Stelling FH (1975) Myelodysplastics—fate of those followed for twenty years or more. J Bone Joint Surg 57-A:643–647
2. Bunch WH (1972) Modern management of myelomeningocele. Warren H. Green, St. Louis

3. Curtis BH (1970) The team approach. Symposium on myelomeningocele (A.A.O.S.). Mosby, St. Louis, pp 301–305
4. Hayes-Allen MC (1972) Obesity and short stature in children with myelomeningocele. Dev Med Child Neurol 14 (Suppl 27):59–64
5. Hoffer MM, Feiwell E, Perry R, Perry J, Bonnet C (1973) Functional ambulation in patients with myelomeningocele. J Bone Joint Surg 55-A:137–148
6. Hunt GM, Holmes AE (1975) Some factors relating to intelligence in treated children with spina bifida. Dev Med Child Neurol 17 (Suppl 35):65–70
7. Kopits SE (1974) Orthopedic aspects of meningomyelocele. In: Freeman JM (ed) Practical management of myelomeningocele. University Park Press, Baltimore, pp 106–165
8. Rose GK, Sankarankutty M, Stallard J (1983) A clinical review of the orthotic treatment of myelomeningocele patients. J Bone Joint Surg 65-B:242–246
9. Sharrard WJW (1964) Posterior iliopsoas transplantation in the treatment of paralytic dislocation of the hip. J Bone Joint Surg 46-B:426–444
10. Stauffer ES, Hoffer M, Nickel VL (1972) Ambulation in thoracic paraplegia. J Bone Joint Surg 54-A:1336–1337
11. Zachary RB (1968) Ethical and social aspects of treatment of spina bifida. Lancet ii:274–276

Abstract

The Energy Cost of Walking in Children with Spina Bifida

Kazunari Yoshida[1], Kuniko Shirane[1], Keigo Kumamoto[1], Tsutomu Iwaya[1], Shigeru Nakamura[2], and Nobuhiko Haga[3]

We carried out a longitudinal study of 16 children with spina bifida, 11 girls and 5 boys, aged 7–17 years. Seven of them had L3- or L4-level lesions (group 1) and nine had L5-level or below S1-level lesions (group 2). All the children could walk independently, with or without walking-aids or braces, in the community. Oxygen uptake, heart rate, and walking speed were measured during walking at their self-selected speed in consecutive walkways on a flat floor using K2 system equipment. The oxygen uptakes were normalized by dividing by the patient's body weight, and were expressed two ways: oxygen cost (ml/kg/m) and oxygen consumption (ml/kg/min). We also calculated the physiological cost index (PCI) based on the method described by McGregor (1979). PCI = $HR_w - HR_r$/average walking speed (bts/m), where HR_r is heart rate during rest and HR_w is heart rate during walking. Each child was retested after a period of 1 or 2 years. The values of the initial examinations were compared with those of the second examinations. Statistical analyses were performed using Student's *t*-test, and a *P* value of less than 0.05 was considered to be statistically significant.

No significant change in walking speed, heart rate, and PCI with age was seen. Oxygen consumption and oxygen cost measured at the second examinations were significantly higher than those at the first examinations. In the group 1 patients, both oxygen consumption and PCI increased with age, whereas the oxygen cost increased with age, but not significantly. In the group 2 patients, oxygen consumption and oxygen cost increased with age, but there was no difference in PCI.

These results suggest that the older the spina bifida children, the more oxygen is needed during walking, and the deterioration in energy cost may influence locomotor performance.

[1] Section of Rehabilitation Medicine for the Physically Disabled, Tohoku University Graduate School of Medicine, Sendai, Japan

[2] Department of Orthopedic Surgery, Teikyo University School of Medicine, Tokyo, Japan

[3] Department of Orthopedics, Shizuoka Children's Hospital, Shizuoka, Japan

Moderator's Comments on Sessions—Gait Disturbance

John V. Banta

Elio Salvaggio presented anthropomorphic measurements taken with e-ray scintigraphy of a group of nonambulatory children who were using wheelchairs for their mobility. All were short, with excessive weight and reduced bone mineral density. No correlations were made as to how much weight-bearing activity these children would require to alter the adverse findings.

Nobuhiko Haga presented interesting data on the MRI signal from three select muscles, the semimembranosis, the biceps femoris, and the gluteus maximus, and related the findings to the patients' ambulatory function. The semimembranosis had the most significant correlation with ambulatory function in children whose average age was 10 years. Of great interest was the fact that the MRI correlation was valid at a young age when the manual muscle test is notoriously difficult to elicit. Walkers were divided into those who did or did not require crutches. Of note is that the correlation with the gluteus maximus was not of value compared with that of the cross-sectional area of the semimembranosis. The cost of the test was a factor which would limit its use in routine examination, but it may be of value in the young child to project potential ambulatory function.

Banta presented the key concepts necessary prior to prescribing braces, which included meticulous physical examination to define the functional motor level, establish realistic goals, recognize mobility as being more valuable than walking per se, and called attention to the law of mass in which the body increases in weight by volume, or by the power of three, whereas muscle strength increased as the cross-sectional diameter of the muscle mass or by the power of two, which inevitably leads to diminished function in patients with paraparesis with increasing age.

Virginia Bins highlighted the results of compliance with orthoses in a population of 111 patients and their families. Major problems centered around the patients' response to heat, discomfort, and the esthetics of the brace. Families were concerned with the maintenance or repair factors, ease of measurement and delivery, cost, and the universal problem of obtaining properly fitting shoes. Lastly, the issue of the child's inevitable dilemma of being braced for mobility yet being hindered in their ability to play with their peers, which often required frequent changes of position from upright to sitting or crawling activity.

Kazumari Yoshida reviewed a group of 16 children of 12 years of age who were the subjects of a study of the energy cost of ambulation. This was assessed using the physiological cost index (PCI) and expired oxygen, and their relation to walking speed. All children

The Newington Department of Orthopaedic Surgery, Connecticut Children's Hospital, Hartford, CT, USA

self-selected their most efficient speed of walking, but all demonstrated increased oxygen consumption in tests 1 year later in a second assessment session. There was no good explanation for the less efficient ambulation except that deconditioning with age may have been a factor.

Tetsua Suyama related detailed findings about 50 adults with spina bifida evaluated in a rehabilitation center. The goal was to provide maximum re-entry to society for all persons. The study covered the years 1981 to 1997, and the mean age of the subjects was 20 years. Ninety-five percent had graduated from high school. The major goals were to prevent further neurological deterioration, prevent pressure ulcerations, control urinary continence, and establish realistic goals for the activities of daily living. Unfortunately, in the authors experience, only 60% of the subjects were able to achieve re-entry into society. Many of the cultural and socioeconomic factors faced by these patients were also common in the countries of many of the conference attendees from around the world.

Banta related the problem of scoliosis in myelomeningocele, and stressed that the child must be watched until the end of growth, which was approximately 15 years of age in his series, and emphasized that bracing beyond the age of 10 years did not prevent further curve progression. Predictive factors for scoliosis included the last intact laminar arch of the spine, the functional motor level, mobility, and the presence of motor asymmetry.

The Management of Hip Pathology in Spina Bifida

Luciano Dias

Neary one-third to one-half of children with spina bifida will present at some time during their growth with either a hip dislocation or subluxation. Hip contractures, such as abduction, adduction, external rotation, and flexion, can be more of a problem, interfering with bracing and ambulation. Treatment of these deformities should have the objective of improving function and mobility.

It is well known that the motor level is the main factor in the walking ability of a spina bifida child. Our experience has shown that only 4% of high-level children with no quadriceps retain a community ambulation level in adult life. In these children, it is well accepted that a hip subluxation or dislocation will not interfere with function.

The approach to hip problems in myelomeningocele has evolved in the last 20 years, and more recently, with the advent of gait analysis, more effective determinations regarding surgical intervention can be made. Surgical correction of orthopedic deformities, including hip contractures and dislocation, should be performed during the second year of life or after.

Indications for treatment of hip dislocation related to motor level are as follows: high level (never need reduction, but treat contractures); low lumbar level (selection, using gait analysis); sacral level (always treat). The use of the gait analysis tool in the decision-making process will be touched on in this session, and covered more fully in other sessions devoted specifically to its use. Surgical options for the management of hip subluxation / dislocation, contractures, etc., will also be discussed.

References

1. Canal ST, Beaty JH (editors) (1995) Operative pediatric orthopaedics, 2nd edn. Myelomeningocele. Mosby, St. Louis, p 739
2. Caroll NC (1978) Hip instability in children with myelomeningocele. Orthop Clin N Am 9:403
3. Drummond DS, Moreau M, Cruess RL (1980) The results and complications for surgery for the paralytic hip and spine in myelomeningocele. J Bone Joint Surg 62:49
4. Feiwell E (1980) Surgery of the hip in myelomeningocele as related to adult goals. Clin Orthop 148:87

Department of Orthopaedic Surgery, Northwestern University, 680N. Lakeshorf Dr. Suite Chicago, IL 60611, USA

5. Lee EH, Caroll NC (1985) Hip stability and ambulatory status in myelomeningocele. J Pediatr Orthop 5:522
6. Schafer MF, Dias LS (1983) Myelomeningocele: orthopaedic treatment. Williams & Wilkins, Baltimore

Paralytic Dislocation and Subluxation of the Hip in Myelomeningocele—Comparison of Surgical and Nonsurgical Groups

M. Kamegaya[1], Y. Shinohara[1], K. Yoh[1], H. Moriya[1], K. Yoshinaga[2], T. Yamane[3], and T. Yamashita[4]

Summary. We reviewed 28 patients (44 hips) who suffered from spina bifida cystica, with the following three conditions: the ages were 6 years or more at follow-up, the hips were dislocated or subluxated, and the motor function levels were L3 or lower. A comparison of an operative group (12 patients, 17 hips) with a nonoperative group (16 patients, 27 hips) was performed in relation to the following four points: transfer ability (Hoffer's criteria), range of hip motion, sitting balance, and hip pain. The operative group was studied separately in relation to recurrence rate of dislocation or subluxation after surgery, in terms of preoperative conditions and surgical procedures.

We could not find any difference in any of the four points between the two groups. Surgical results were well observed in subluxated hips before surgery, rather than in dislocated hips. The postoperative recurrence of dislocations or subluxations was much lower in patients who had preoperative subluxated hips and underwent combined surgery with derotation varus osteotomy (DVO) of the femur as compared to patients who had preoperative dislocated hips and underwent surgery without DVO.

We concluded that hip dislocation and subluxation in myelomeningocele patients does not seriously affect their activities in daily life. Regarding operative indication, a progressive subluxation would be a reliable indication to expect a successful result with minimum surgical intervention.

Key words. Operative treatment, Activities of daily life, Paralytic dislocation and subluxation of the hip

Introduction

There is some controversy about surgical indications or procedures for paralytic hip dislocation or subluxation in spina bifida patients [2, 5, 8]. Many papers have been published about problems in the orthopedic field [1–3, 5, 8]. The purpose of this paper is to clarify whether

[1] Division of Orthopedic Surgery, Chiba Childrens' Hospital, 579-1 Heta-chou, Midori-ku, Chiba 266-0007, Japan
[2] Department of Orthopedic Surgery, School of Medicine, Chiba University, 1-8-1 Inohana, Chuou-ku, Chiba 260-0856, Japan
[3] Department of Orthopedic Surgery, School of Medicine, Teikyo University, 2-11-1 Kaga, Itabashi-ku, Tokyo 173-0003, Japan
[4] Department of Orthopedic Surgery, Chiba Municipal Hospital, 827 Yahagi-chou, Chuou-ku, Chiba 260-0851, Japan

or not surgical effects are observed in spina bifida patients, in terms of four points related to their activities in daily life.

Materials and Methods

We reviewed 28 patients (44 hips) who suffered from spina bifida cystica, with the following three conditions: the ages were 6 years or more at follow-up, the hips were dislocated or subluxated, and the motor function levels were L3 or lower. We divided them into two groups, a surgical group (12 patients, 17 hips) and a nonsurgical group (16 patients, 27 hips). In the surgical group, the average age at surgery was 6 years (ranging from 1.3 to 12.3 years). The average age of follow-up was 13 years (from 8.2 to 21.6 years). Preoperative conditions were 12 dislocated hips and 5 subluxated hips, and motor function level was L3 in 8 patients, L4 in 2, and L5 in 2. In the nonsurgical group, the average age at follow-up was 12.4 years (from 6.0 to 21.3 years). Their follow-up conditions were 10 dislocated hips and 17 subluxated hips, and motor function level was L3 in 9 patients, L4 in 6, and L5 in 1.

The surgical procedures were Salter innominate osteotomy + derotation varus osteotomy (DVO) in 9 hips, Sharrard's method in 5 hips, DVO in 2 hips, and adductor tenotomy in 1 hip.

We compared these two groups on the following four points: ability of transfer by Hoffer's criteria, range of hip motion, sitting balance measured by a foot plate, and hip pain at rest or in motion. If the surgical group patients suffered from redislocation or subluxation after surgery, we utilized the data which had been evaluated before those events occurred.

Results

Ability of Transfer

There were 6 community ambulators, 1 household ambulator, and 5 nonambulators (including nonfunctional) in the operative group, compared with 7, 2, and 7, respectively, in the nonoperative group. Both groups had almost the same distribution in the classifications (Fig. 1).

Range of Hip Motion

The range of hip motion was almost the same in both groups in each direction of motion. In the patients who underwent DVO, the range of abduction was somewhat limited (Fig. 2).

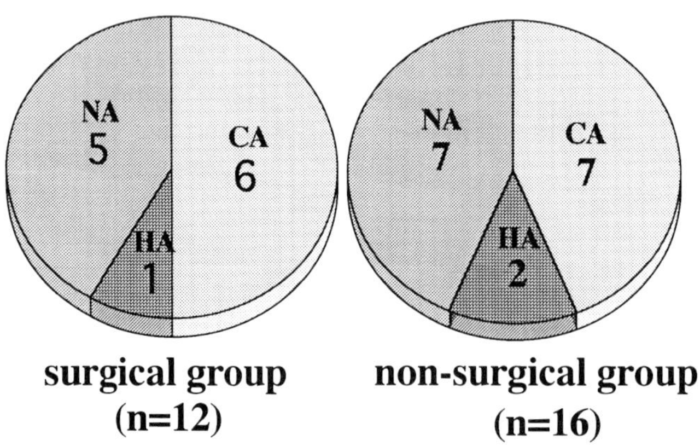

FIG. 1. Ability of transfer (Hoffer's criteria). *CA*, community ambulator; *HA*, household ambulator; *NA*, nonambulator

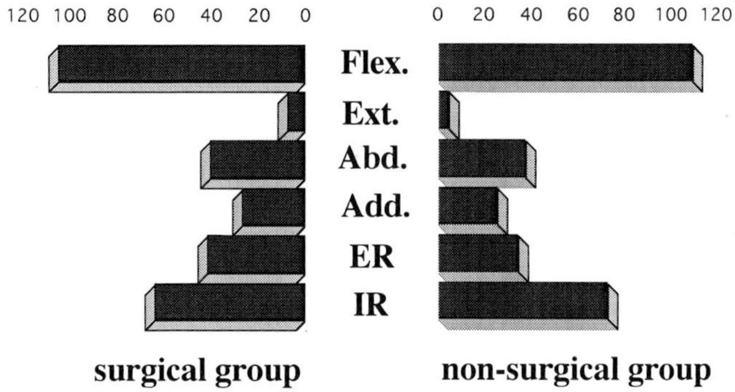

FIG. 2. Range of hip motion

TABLE 1. Sitting balance

	Pelvic obliquity	Asymmetry of sciatic pressure
Surgical group ($n = 12$)	2	2
Nonsurgical group ($n = 16$)	1	2

Sitting Balance

We evaluated the pelvic obliquity on a plain radiograph taken in the sitting position, and asymmetry of sciatic pressure using a foot plate. In the surgical group, 2 patients had positive signs of pelvic obliquity, and 2 patients had positive signs of asymmetry of sciatic pressure. In the nonsurgical group, one patient had positive signs of pelvic obliquity and 2 patients of asymmetry of sciatic pressure. There was no difference in sitting balance between the groups (Table 1).

Hip Pain

All patients in both groups had no hip pain at rest or in motion.

In the surgical group, 6 of 12 dislocated hips before surgery had redislocations after surgery. On the other hand, 1 of 5 subluxated hips before surgery had a resubluxation after surgery (Table 2). Surgery combined with DVO had 2/11 recurrences, which was much less than 5/6 without DVO (Table 3).

Discussion

Paralytic hip dislocation or subluxation is caused by a muscle imbalance around the hip joint. Some surgical procedures have been reported to correct the mechanical disorder, and Sharrard's iliopsoas tendon transfer is well known [6, 7]. However, several authors reported follow-up studies of this surgery and concluded that the transferred tendon did not functionally work as an abductor and extensor muscle, in spite of the theory [2, 7, 8]. Bunch and Hakala [2] reported weakness of hip flexion as one of the disadvantages of the surgery, due to transferring the iliopsoas tendon which did the work of a hip flexor muscle. On the other hand, Feiwell et al. [3] reported that hip dislocation in spina bifida patients did not affect

Table 2. Surgical results 1

Preoperative condition	Recurrence rate
Dislocation	6/12 (50%)
Subluxation	1/5 (20%)

Table 3. Surgical results 2

Surgical procedure	Recurrence rate
+DVO	2/11 (18%)
−DVO	5/6 (83%)

DVO, derotation varus osteotomy.

their transfer and movement ability. According to our results, surgical benefits were also unlikely to be expected in daily life. However, some questions still remain. Do we overlook the progressive subluxation which could lead to dislocation? It is very difficult to answer that at the moment. It might be said that a few, but not all, patients would need some surgery to obtain some extra benefit which cannot yet be guaranteed. In this situation, we would recommend DVO alone, or with other surgery, for preoperative subluxated hips.

Conclusions

We concluded that hip dislocation and subluxation in myelomeningocele patients do not significantly affect their activities in daily life. Regarding operative indications, a progressive subluxation would be a reliable indication to expect a successful result with minimum surgical intervention.

References

1. Barden GA, Meyer LC, Stelling III FH (1975) Myelodysplastic: fate of those followed for twenty years or more. J Bone Joint Surg 57-A:643–647
2. Bunch WH, Hakala MW (1984) Iliopsoas transfer in children with myelomeningocele. J Bone Joint Surg 66-A:224–227
3. Feiwell E, Sakai D, Blatt T (1978) The effect of hip reduction on function in patients with myelomeningocele. J Bone Joint Surg 60-A:169–173
4. Hoffer MM, Feiwell E, Perry R, Perry J, Bonnett C (1973) Functional ambulation in patients with myelomeningocele. J Bone Joint Surg 55-A:137–148
5. Rueda J, Carroll NC (1972) Hip instability in patients with myelomeningocele. J Bone Joint Surg 54-B:422–431
6. Sharrard WJW (1959) Congenital paralytic dislocation of the hip in children with myelomeningocele. J Bone Joint Surg 41-B:622
7. Sharrard WJW (1964) Posterior iliopsoas transplantation in the treatment of paralytic dislocation of the hip. J Bone Joint Surg 46-B:426–444
8. Weisl H, Fairclough JA, Jones DG (1988) Stabilization of the hip in myelomeningocele: comparison of posterior iliopsoas transfer and varus-rotation osteotomy. J Bone Joint Surg 70-B:29–33

Radical Hip Release in Spina Bifida Patients—an Aid to Improving Mobility

Richard D. Beauchamp[1], Bonita J. Sawatzky[1], Carol E. King[2], and Beverly Irwin[3]

Summary. The Spina Bifida Clinic at British Columbia's Children's Hospital has supported the theory that mobility for children with spina bifida is our primary goal in orthopaedic treatment. We have reviewed both the radiographic appearance of hips and the functional use of orthotics in children with spina bifida with thoracolumbar-level lesions, and determined that hip and other joint mobility are the primary factors that determine the daily motor functional level of these children. We have found this to be effectively achieved by performing, when indicated, radical hip release to maintain hip joint mobility. This may at times include a radical hip capsulectomy, and even the production of an iatrogenic hip dislocation. This ensures maintenance of the patients' hip mobility and, in spite of 40% of the patients showing worsening of their hips on X-ray, 75% of the patients actually improved their functional use of orthotics following radical hip release.

Key words. Spina bifida, Surgery, Hip, Orthotics, Function

In order that patients with meningomyelocoele can assume an upright posture and be mobile, they must be relatively free of contractures of their hips, knees, and ankles. Those children with a high level of involvement (L1 and above) may at times require extensive bracing or orthotic support to supplement their absent voluntary antigravity muscles. Orthotists are able to fabricate custom standing devices and mobility aids to within a certain level of tolerance for contractures. With thoracolumbar levels of involvement, excessive pressure on insensitive skin due to unacceptable joint contractures can lead to tissue necrosis and the development of decubitus ulcers. These pressure sores can typically be seen on the lateral borders of the foot and ankle with children in an equinovarus foot position.

With excessive knee flexion contractures, the proximal tibia may be forced to absorb the majority of the body weight. Unless a hip flexion contracture is less than 15°, patients in upright devices will develop compensatory knee flexion contractures and increased lumbar lordosis from standing. Children will not be effective users of reciprocating gait orthoses (RGO) unless their hip flexion contracture is minimal (ideally 0, but at least less than 15°). In order to assess our results of maintaining "ambulation" in our spina bifida population with high neurological levels, we have retrospectively analyzed those patients who required surgical correction of their hip flexion contractures, assessing inital preoperative hip flexion con-

[1] Department of Orthopaedics, [2] Physiotherapy Department, [3] Department of Nursing, British Columbia's Children's Hospital, 4480 Oak Street Vancouver, British Columbia V6H3V4, Canada

tractures, operative technique, postoperative contractures, and change in orthotic usage. Radiographic analysis was also undertaken.

The orthopaedic literature contains numerous articles about maintaining hips in their reduced position through various operative techniques [5, 8, 10, 12, 13]. However, clinical reviews are now contradicting what was proposed several years ago about the importance of maintaining hips in their joints [4]. Lee and Carroll [7] stated that "children with myelodysplasia who have strong quadriceps and stable neurological status can therefore have surgical stabilization of their hips with good results." On discussing iliopsoas transfers in children with myelomeningocoele, Bunch and Hakala [5] "concluded that the procedure has value, but it does not produce a normal hip." It has long been recognized that the level of neural deficit was the most important factor in determining ambulatory function [1–3, 6, 9–11]. Samuelsson and Skoog [9] reviewed factors determining ambulation in 163 patients with myelomeningocoele by a multivariate statistical method. They concluded that "severe scoliosis was closely, age moderately, and hip flexion contracture slightly related to the inability of the other non-ambulators to walk, while pelvic obliquity, hip dislocation, or knee flexion contracture was not." It has therefore become quite apparent to us that maintaining hip stability was NOT a goal in our treatment of these patients, and would not be a factor influencing the patients ultimate function. Therefore, we have taken the opposite path, and suggest that releasing hip contractures in order to allow these children to be placed in their standing and mobility devices might also include actually releasing enough of their hip capsule to allow the hip to subluxate or even, frankly, to dislocate. This might then lead to a much more effective and permanent hip release into adolescence, as reflected in maintenance of their particular orthotic usage.

Patients and Methods

Clinical and radiographic analysis of all those patients who underwent radical hip releases at BCCH were reviewed. There were 16 patients available for review (17 hips): 10 males and 6 females. The mean age at the time of surgery was 5 years 7 months, ranging from 1 year 5 months to 9 years 10 months. The mean follow up was 39 months (range 4–84 months).

Hip Flexion Contracture. This was measured using the standard Thomas test and recorded in degrees. The maximum amount of hip flexion was also recorded.

Neurological Level. This was determined by describing the last functioning motor unit, and generally ascribing active hip flexion as L1, active knee flexion as L3, and absent hip flexion as thoracolumbar level.

Orthotic Use. This included standing frames, parapodia, reciprocating gait orthoses (RGO), and knee ankle foot orthoses (KAFO). The use of orthotic devices was graded as follows:

0. no orthotics/no standing;
1. standing frame;
2. reciprocating gait orthosis (RGO);
3. knee-ankle-foot orthotic (KAFO);
4. ankle-foot orthotic/walker.

Radiographic Analysis. All available pelvic radiographs, both preoperative and postoperative, were reviewed. For our purposes, the CE angle of Wiseberg was chosen to measure hip joint coverage, but for ease of analysis the CE angles were grouped as follows:

0. hip dislocated (CE –20 or lower);
1. hip subluxated (CE –20 to +20);
2. hip located (CE +20 or higher).

Surgical Procedure

The patients all underwent radical hip releases under general anaesthesia. They were positioned with the operative hip elevated 45°. The leg was free-draped. The incision was a standard "bikini" incision 1 cm below the iliac crest and parallel to it. The incision extended from the mid-axillary line to the mid-point of the inguinal ligament. The interval between the tensor and the sartorius was identified. The sartorius was completely divided from its origin at the ASIS and the fascia lata was divided transversely. The heads of the rectus femoris were identified over the hip capsule and divided completely. The precapsular fat was dissected off the hip capsule. The abductors were palpated at their insertion in the greater trochanter and divided. The iliopsoas tendon was palpated at its insertion in the lesser trochanter by externally rotating and flexing/extending the hip. A retractor was placed around the tendon and it was divided in its entirety. The capsule of the hip was now visualized and a complete transverse incision made from the inferior acetabular ligament to as far posteriorly as one could palpate. The hip would then often anteriorly subluxate or dislocate when the hip was placed in full extension. Closure was then done to the subcutaneous tissue and the skin. The patients were then placed either in extension skin traction on both legs or in a bilateral hip spica cast.

Postoperatively. The patients were maintained in their cast for approximately 3 weeks and then begun on passive stretching exercises, often utilizing a resting night splint to hold the pelvis/hips in full extension for 3 months. Traction was maintained in hospital for 3–4 days and then at home for 3 weeks, with active stretching exercises daily. A resting extension orthosis was used following discontinuation of the traction for 3 months. Approximately 3 weeks following surgery, the patients were fitted for their new standing devices and standing therapy commenced.

Results

Hip Flexion Contractures

The patients meningomyeocoele clinic notes were reviewed retrospectively, and the hip flexion contracture was recorded preoperatively and postoperatively. Preoperatively the hips had an average flexion contracture of 42.5° (range 30–70°). The postoperative measurement was 13.8° (range 0–45°) The patient (TC) who had the 45° flexion contracture postoperatively at follow-up after 7.3 years had previously had several unsuccessful attempts at surgical correction of his contracture. His preoperative contracture had been 60°, so there was still an improvement of 15° following his most recent radical hip release some 7 years earlier. Eliminating this patient's figures would have given us an average FD at follow-up of only 10.3°.

Radiographic Analysis

There was very little change in the average postoperative CE angle at follow-up 39 months later when compared with the CE angle of the same hip preoperatively (6.9° pre-op and 7.2° post-op). If individual hips are analyzed according to the numerical score, 4 hips fell a grade following surgery (i.e., went from subluxated to dislocated or from normal to subluxated) and 10 hips remained the same. One hip actually improved in radiographic grade from subluxated to concentrically reduced (TC).

Orthotic Usage (Functional Change)

In accordance with the grading format for orthotic usage pre- and postoperatively, we see that 2 patients lost a level of orthotic usage following surgery. One patient (TC) had a residual hip FD of 45° and could not be maintained in his standing frame, and at follow-up 7 years later was not standing at all. This could also be related to other factors than his residual hip flexion contracture (older age, increased weight, other contractures). The other patient who was no longer standing at follow-up has also had a long follow-up period (7 years) but has not shown any recurrence of her hip contracture. Five patients have shown no change in their orthotic use postoperatively, but 3 of the 5 have shown improved ease of applying their orthotics and are probably utilizing the orthotics on a more regular, consistent basis. One patient (JM) progressed from a standing frame before his hip release to using AFOs and a walker at follow-up. He has no flexion contracture 3 years after surgery. One patient (DG) had a preoperative hip FD of 40°, and following his radical hip release (which in this situation included proximal femoral resection) became able to ambulate using AFO and a walker.

The majority of patients (10), however, showed a significant improvement in their orthotic usage. The average improvement was +2 functional points. This ranged from a patient who had utilized only a standing frame and who became a very successful "ambulator" with a pair of AFOs and a walker (grade 1 to grade 4), to another patient (DG) who went from being a nonambulator and nonbracer grade 0 to being a functional ambulator grade 4 after a proximal femoral resection.

Combined Variables

The indications for proceeding with radical hip releases include the prospect of improved standing ability and hence improved overall function, both physically and psychologically. Of the four children who demonstrated deterioration in their radiographic parameters (i.e., dropped at least one grade in the scoring), three showed improved function and required less orthotic support in order to mobilize. (Hence, hips located in joint do not equal improved function.) The only two patients who showed decreased orthotic use at follow-up and hence poorer functional gains (one had a lower X-ray grade and the other had an improved X-ray grade) were assessed on the basis of a 7-year follow-up when both of the children were well into their adolescent years. As has been shown, adolescents with high level spina bifida lesions are not functional ambulators in any event.

Discussion

The Spina Bifida Clinic at British Columbia's Children's Hospital in Vancouver, Canada, is very PRO-active in promoting the maintenance of being upright and mobile for those children with high-level spina bifida lesions who wish to do so and who are motivated with supportive therapists and family. We believe the beneficial effects of standing and "walking" are enormous, and lead to an improved quality of life. However, in order to be placed in some of these mobility and ambulatory devices, the patient should have an adequate range of movement of their joints, with minimal hip contractures. In reviewing our treatment of hip flexion contracture releases at BCCH, we have found that by including a radical hip capsulectomy in the surgical technique, we have prevented recurrence of the contracture. At times, some of the patients' hips have been surgically dislocated during surgery and also at follow-up X-ray. We have also had occasion to include a proximal femoral resection as our extreme form of radical hip release. There have been no deleterious effects with the production of a dislocated hip, and in fact there has been sustained maintenance of the releases following surgery with only minimal evidence of recurrence.

Conclusion

In spite of 40% of patients showing worsening of their hip parameters on radiographic analysis, 75% of them have improved their functional use of orthotics following radical hip releases. This procedure was once associated with a high recurrence rate in spina bifida patients. We feel that if a hip flexion contracture release is done, then it should be accompanied by a radical anterior hip capsulectomy—even to the extent of producing an anterior dislocation of the hip joint with hip extension. This will ensure maintenance of the hip release and, as seen in our series, improves mobility and leads to a functional maintenance of hip mobility.

In order to keep children as functionally ambulatory as possible in spite of a high-level neurological lesion, radical release of their hip flexion contractures can be done. This further supports the theory that hip stability is *not* associated with improved ambulatory function, and, conversely in the case of a dislocated hip in these high neurological level patients, their function is better with the hip out of joint (dislocated) than with it in joint (located).

The primary long-term goal in managing children with spina bifida should be to maintain and maximize overall mobility regardless of joint stability.

References

1. Alumna BA, Bandar M, Write JG (1996) Function of dislocated hips in children with lower level spina bifida. J Bone Joint Surg (Br) 78:294–298
2. Bazih J, Gross RH (1981) Hip surgery in the lumbar level myelomeningocele patient. J Pediatr Orthop 1:405–411
3. Birkebak RC, Winter RB (1989) The role of hip dislocation in the functional status of the myelodysplastic patient. A review of 100 patients. Orthopedics 12:675–684
4. Broughton NS, Menelaus MB, Cole WG, Shurtleff DB (1993) The natural history of hip deformity in myelomeningocoele. J Bone Joint Surg (Br) 75:760–763
5. Bunch WH, Hakala MW (1984) Iliopsoas transfers in children with myelomeningocele. J Bone Joint Surg (Am) 66:224–227
6. Fraser RK, Bourke HM, Broughton NS, Menelaus MB (1995) Unilateral dislocation of the hip in spina bifida. A long-term follow-up. J Bone Joint Surg (Br) 77:615–619
7. Lee EH, Carroll NC (1985) Hip stability and ambulatory status in myelomeningocele. J Pediatr Orthop 5:522–527
8. Menelaus MB (1980) Progress in the management of the paralytic hip in myelomeningocele. Orthop Clin N Am 11:17–30
9. Samuelsson L, Skoog M (1988) Ambulation in patients with myelomeningocele: a multivariate statistical analysis. J Pediatr Orthop 8:569–575
10. Sherk HH, Melchjionne J, Smith R (1987) The natural history of hip dislocations in ambulatory myelomeningocoeles. Z Kinderchirurgie. 42, Suppl 1:48–49
11. Sherk HH, Uppal GS, Lane G, Melchionni J (1991) Treatment versus non-treatment of hip dislocations in ambulatory patients with myelomeningocoele. Dev Med Child Neurol 33:491–494
12. Tachdjian MO (1972) Pediatric orthopedics, vol 2. Saunders, Toronto
13. Tosi LL, Buck BD, Nason SS, McKay DW (1996) Dislocaiton of the hip in myelomeningocoele. The McKay hip stabilization. J Bone Joint Surg (Am) 78:664–673

Surgical Correction of Myelomeningocele Hip

Toshio Fujii, Haruhisa Yanagida, Akihiko Takashima, and Kazuyuki Takamura

Summary. We reviewed 35 hips in 24 children with myelomeningocele who had undergone surgery to stabilize a hip between 1980 and 1995. The age at surgery ranged from 2 years 11 months to 13 years 5 months, and age at follow-up ranged from 9 years 2 months to 22 years 5 months. The surgical procedures we used changed over time. Six hips underwent the hip release procedure alone for flexion contracture, and seven hips underwent Sharrard's iliopsoas transfer (ST) alone for subluxation or dislocation. Seven hips underwent ST and Pemberton's osteotomy (PO) simultaneously, and 3 hips had ST combined with PO and detorsion-varus osteotomy (DVO). Three hips had ST, shelf procedure, and DVO. The original ST procedure was used in the first eight cases, and the modified procedure in which only the psoas muscle was transfered was used in the later 12 cases. From 1994, three hips underwent external oblique muscle transfer (EOT) and PO. Six hips had EOT, PO, and DVO simultaneously. Most of the children had capsulorrhaphy, and some of them had open reduction at the same time. The patients who underwent ST alone showed both good and bad results, but the major factor influencing the results was unclear. The patients who underwent the combined procedure with muscle transfer and osteotomy showed better results. The patients who underwent EOT and osteotomy maintained concentric reduction after surgery better than those who had the other two procedures. The patients who underwent ST alone improved in walking after surgery for a period of time, but in half of the patients this improvement was not maintained at the time of follow-up, and the acetabular dysplasia remained. The patients who underwent muscle transfer and osteotomy were encouraged to walk from infancy using HKFO or reciprocating gait orthosis, and most of them maintained the improved ambulatory status after surgery. Hip abduction muscle force was more powerful in the patients who underwent EOT than in those who had ST. There was no significant correlation between ambulatory status and the concentricity of the hip. Mental retardation, obesity, and hip and knee contracture caused deterioration in walking ability after surgery.

Key words. Myelomeningocele, Hip, Dislocation, Surgery

Department of Orthopedic Surgery, Fukuoka Children's Hospital, 2-5-1 Tojin-Machi, Chuo-Ku, Fukuoka 810-0063, Japan

Introduction

The dislocation of the hip in myelomeningocele may lead to a poor sitting balance and poor gait due to a leg length discrepancy and pelvic obliquity. We reviewed the clinical and radiographic results of our surgical corrections of myelomeningocele hips over a period of 15 years.

Materials and Methods

We reviewed 35 hips in 24 children with myelomeningocele who underwent surgery at Fukuoka Children's Hospital between 1979 and 1994. The age at surgery ranged from 2 years 11 months to 13 years 5 months (mean, 6 years 11 months) and age at follow-up ranged from 9 years 2 months to 22 years 5 months (mean, 14 years 2 months). The neurosegmental level of the patients ranged from the lower thoracic region to the lower lumbar region. L3 and L4 were most frequent (Fig. 1).

Surgical procedures have changed over time and they also differed depending on the patient's age and hip condition. If the patient had severe coxa valga and was over 6 years of age, we performed femoral detorsion varus osteotomy (DVO). Six hips underwent a hip release procedure alone, which was mainly for flexion contracture, and seven hips underwent Sharrard's iliopsoas transfer alone for subluxation or dislocation. The original Sharrard's iliopsoas transfer was used in the first eight cases. A modified Sharrard's procedure in which only the psoas muscle was transfered was used in the later 12 cases. Seven hips underwent Sharrard's transfer and Pemberton's osteotomy simultaneously, and three hips had Sharrard's transfer combined with Pemberton's osteotomy and DVO. Three hips had Sharrard's transfer, shelf procedure, and DVO.

From 1994, three hips underwent external oblique muscle transfer and Pemberton's osteotomy. Six hips had external oblique muscle transfer, Pemberton's osteotomy, and DVO simultaneously. External oblique muscle transfer was an easier technique to perform than Sharrard's transfer. Most of the children had capsulorrhaphy, and some of them had open reduction at the same time.

Results

Radiographic Status of the Hips after Surgery

The patients who underwent Sharrard's transfer alone showed both good and bad results. The patients who underwent the combined procedure with muscle transfer and osteotomy showed better results than the patients with Sharrard's transfer alone. The patients who

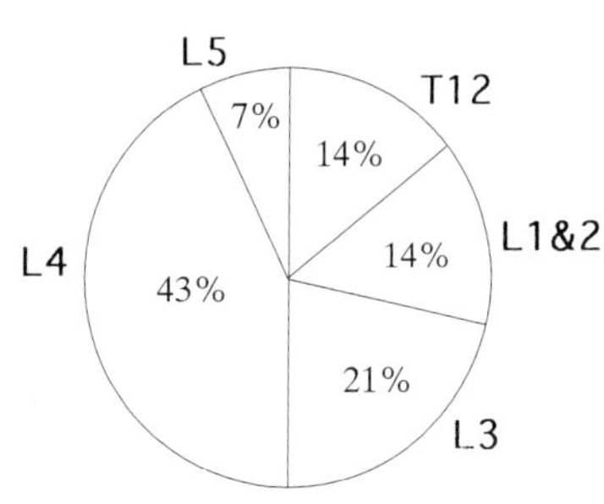

FIG. 1. Neurolosegmental level

underwent external oblique muscle transfer and osteotomy maintained concentric reduction after surgery better than those who underwent the other two procedures (Fig. 2).

There was a significant difference in the Sharp angle between the patients who underwent Sharrard's muscle transfer alone and those who underwent muscle transfer and osteotomy. The acetabular dysplasia of the myelomeningocele hip did not improve much after the Sharrard's muscle transfer alone, and that is one of the main reasons why we subsequently did not expect good results in every patient undergoing Sharrard's transfer alone (Fig. 3).

Among the patients who underwent Sharrard's transfer alone, some hips maintained the increased CE angle after surgery, but others did not. Conversely, most of the patients who underwent the combined procedure with muscle transfer and osteotomy maintained the improved CE angle after surgery. However, in the older children with highly dysplastic hips, the CE angle decreased again after surgery (Fig. 4).

An investigation of acetabular head index (AHI) after surgery showed the same results as for CE angle. AHI decreased again in most of the patients who underwent Sharrard's muscle transfer alone, but was maintained in the patients who underwent the combined procedure with muscle transfer and osteotomy (Fig. 5).

The patients who underwent external oblique muscle transfer and osteotomy showed better radiographic results than the patients who underwent Sharrard's transfer and osteotomy (Table 1).

Ambulatory Status

The patients who underwent Sharrard's transfer alone could hardly walk before surgery. Their walking improved after surgery for a period of time, but in half of the cases this improve-

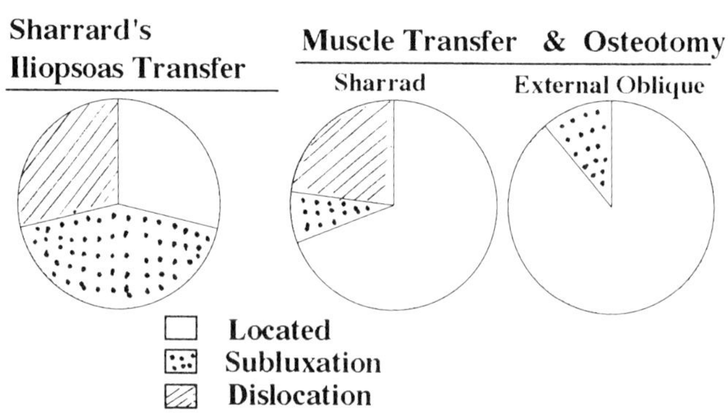

FIG. 2. Radiographic status of the hip after surgery

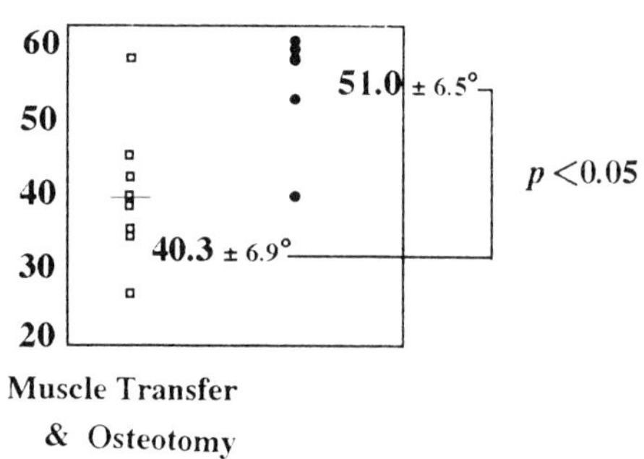

FIG. 3. Sharp angle

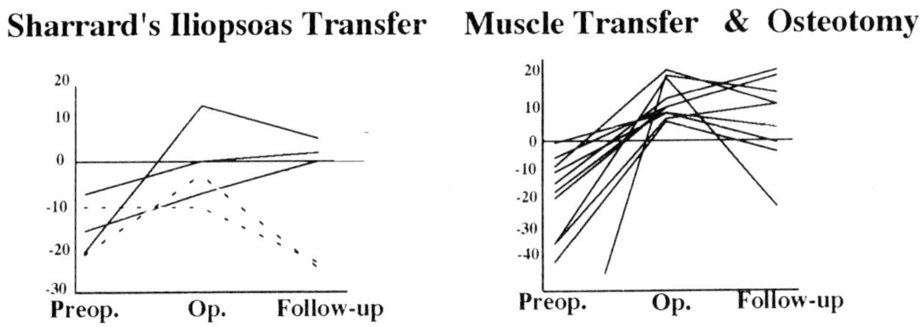

FIG. 4. CE angle

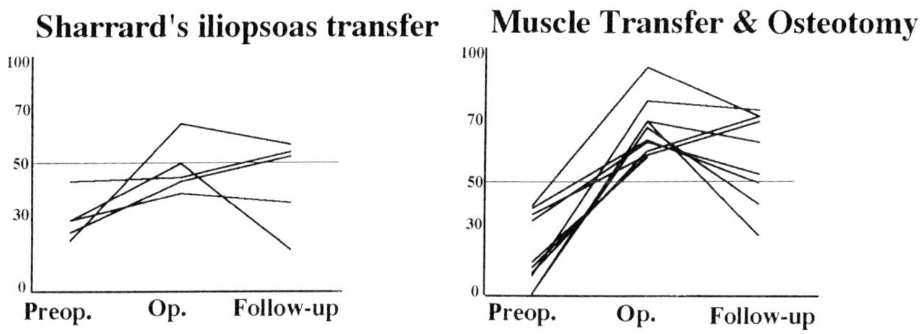

FIG. 5. Acetabular-head index (AHI)

TABLE 1. X-ray results

Procedure	Hips	CE	AHI	Sharp	Procedure	Hips	CE	AHI	Sharp
S + P	7	8	78	40	E + P	2	18	70	40
S + P + F	6	7	61	39	E + F	1	20	81	35
					E + P + F	6	27	92	41

S, Sharrard's transfer; P, Pemberton's osteotomy; F, detorsion-varus osteotomy; E, external oblique muscle transfer; P, Pemberton's osteotomy; F, detorsion-varus osteotomy.

ment was not maintained at the time of follow-up. The patients who underwent muscle transfer and osteotomy were encouraged to walk from infancy using HKFO or reciprocating gait orthosis, and most of them maintained the improved ambulatory status after surgery. Hip abduction muscle force was more powerful in patients who underwent the external oblique muscle transfer rather than the Sharrard's iliopsoas muscle transfer (Fig. 6). There was no significant correlation between ambulatory status and the concentricity of the hip.

We investigated the factors related to ambulatory status after surgery. In the patients of the nonfunctional ambulator and nonambulator groups, we found a high incidence of obesity, mental retardation, flexion contracture of the hip and knee, and pelvic obliquity. These factors caused significant deterioration in walking ability after surgery (Fig. 7).

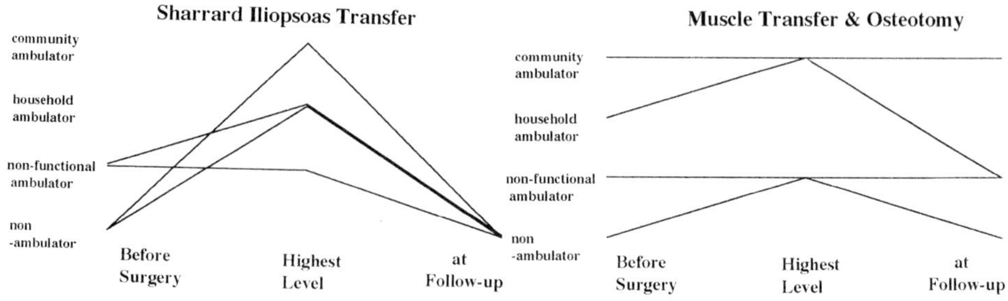

FIG. 6. Ambulation

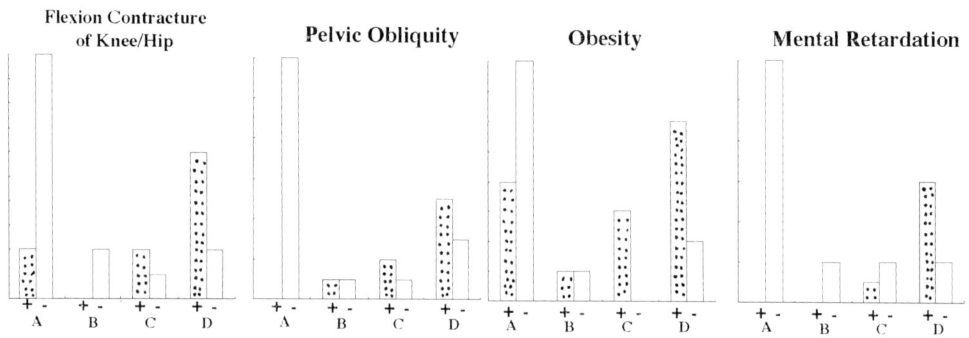

FIG. 7. Factors related to ambulatory status. *A*, community ambulator; *B*, household ambulator; *C*, non-functional ambulator; *D*, nonambulator

Discussion

The muscle imbalance of the hip of myelomeningocele patients can result in hip instability, an awkward gait, impaired ambulation, and hip dislocation [1–4]. A variety of procedures has been used to stabilize the hip, such as muscle transfers and osteotomies.

We used the original Sharrard's iliopsoas transfer in the first eight cases, but we found iliacus muscles atrophied at the time of surgery in most cases, so we modified the procedure to transfer the psoas muscle alone in the later 12 cases. However, we found only a few patients with good hip abduction muscle power after Sharrard's transfer, in addition to the inevitable loss of hip flexor power.

As a result of this, we adopted McKay's external oblique muscle transfer procedure, which resulted in better muscle balance around the hip than in our iliopsoas-transfer patients.

With regard to the concentricity of the hip, Sharrard's iliopsoas transfer alone improved the concentricity of the hip for a period of time after surgery, and acetabular dysplasia remained in half of the patients, which caused a recurrence of subluxation of the hip after surgery. We therefore began to combine the muscle transfer with Pemberton's osteotomy, with or without detorsion-varus osteotomy, and this combined procedure resulted in the unstable hips being maintained in good concentricity after surgery.

Many factors influence the ambulatory potential of myelomeningocele patients. Neurological level is the most important factor in the ability to walk [2]. In addition, mental retardation, obesity, and hip and knee contracture cause deterioration in walking ability after surgery. An improvement in walking ability occured over the first 1–2 years after surgery, but gradually decreased after the patients entered junior high schools. This was due to obesity and the need to move faster and more frequently at school, which often results in the overuse of wheelchairs, which in turn creates a vicious circle.

The ability to walk independently without the assistance of crutches and AFOs with attached leather shoes is extremely important for Japanese patients owing to their lifestyle. In Japanese homes, shoes must be removed before entering. This means that crutches are not usually used indoors, and the AFOs with attached shoes must also be removed before entering a house and replaced upon leaving the house. This all creates a great deal of inconvenience for the patient. The same can also be said for the use of wheelchairs in Japanese houses.

Conclusions

1. Sharrard's iliopsoas transfer alone improved the concentricity of the hip for a period of time, but acetabular dysplasia remained in half of the patients.
2. Muscle transfer combined with Pemberton's osteotomy, with or without detorsion-varus osteotomy, maintained unstable hips in good concentricity.
3. Mental retardation, obesity, and hip and knee contracture caused deterioration in walking ability after surgery.

References

1. Broughton NS, Menelaus MB, Cole WG, Shurtleff DB (1993) The natural history of hip deformity in myelomeningocele. J Bone Joint Surg (Br) 75:760–763
2. Lee EH, Carroll NC (1985) Hip stability and ambulatory status in myelomeningocele. J Pediatr Orthop 5:522–527
3. Samuelsson L, Eklof O (1990) Hip stability in myelomeningocele. Acta Orthop Scand 61:3–6
4. Shurtleff DB, Menelaus MB, Staheli LT et al. (1986) Natural history of flexion deformity of the hip in myelomeningocele. J Pediatr Orthop 6:666–673

The Hip—Current Treatment

Malcolm B. Menelaus

For each child who has a hip abnormality, we should think very hard about whether treatment for the hip condition is necessary or not [1, 3]. There is the potential to do a lot of harm by unnecessary surgery on the hip. Dislocation of a hip, which was always treated in the past, seldom needs reduction. On the other hand, fixed flexion deformity at the hip does cause a lot of harm and does require treatment. Seldom should a decision be made before the age of 3–3.5 years, as until that age the degree of flexion deformity is commonly altering quite rapidly.

For each child we should consider whether there is a deformity, whether there is dislocation, and whether there is a muscle imbalance that requires treatment. We should consider this for each hip, so there are six questions to ask ourselves. In addition, we have to take into account the general condition of the child, and there are many variable factors which could affect our decision-making process—i.e., many factors affecting the general health of the child which are quite independent of the hip condition. Thus what follows represents general guidelines only.

Hip Deformity [2]

The major common and troublesome hip deformity is hip flexion contracture. Hip flexion contracture is commonly seen in normal neonates and in spina bifida neonates with all neurosegmental levels. The deformity decreases during the first years of life, but improves least in thoracic neurosegmental levels and, in these patients, has a strong tendency to increase again with advancing years.

Where hip flexion deformity is interfering with a child's ability to walk—generally this occurs when the deformity is more than 20°—a soft tissue release should be performed. The procedure is best performed through the incision described by Salter [4] for innominate osteotomy. Sweep the muscles off both inner and outer surfaces of the ilium, divide the psoas tendon (for those with high-level lesions), release the sartorius and rectus femoris, and, if necessary, divide the anterior capsule of the hip joint transversely. For those with low lumbar lesions, the psoas is lengthened in the pelvis. At the conclusion of the operation, the anterior superior iliac spine and adjacent portions of the iliac crest will protrude forward and should

Department of Orthopaedics, Royal Children's Hospital, 25 Victoria Parade Collingwood, Victoria 3066, Melbourne, Australia

be removed. Drape the patient so that Thomas' test can be performed throughout the procedure. Our results after long-term follow-up are satisfactory. If the hip is also dislocated, consideration may be given to reducing the hip along the lines described in the next section, but it is seldom that the decision will be made to reduce the hip.

Postoperatively, the child is nursed on a Bradford frame for 6 weeks, lying alternately prone and supine with the hips extended.

Hip Dislocation

The presence of hip dislocation is not an indication to attempt reduction. Reduction should be attempted only where the child will derive considerable benefit from the procedure. Attempts at operative reduction are not always successful, may result in stiff painful hips, and are sometimes associated with heterotopic calcification, and these complications generally reduce the child's ability to walk. An untreated dislocated hip is rarely painful, but if it is unilateral it may give rise to limb-length inequality.

Children with hip dislocation who would benefit from surgery to reduce the hip are those with lesions at L3 and below, who therefore have strong quadriceps muscles and do not require bracing above the knee, and will probably be good walkers. In this group, unilateral hip dislocation should generally be reduced. In general, bilateral hip dislocations in this group do not benefit from attempts at reduction. Reduction is occasionally performed if surgery is necessary for the management of flexion contracture. In children with high lesions (thoracic L1 and L2) and therefore without quadriceps, we seldom reduce either bilateral or unilateral dislocations.

If hip dislocation is present at birth and is irreducible, attempts at reduction should not be made. If a hip is unstable but can easily be reduced by Ortolani's test, and if the lesion is low, it is worthwhile using an abduction brace to encourage acetabular development. However, this should not interfere with closure of the spinal defect and its postoperative management, and if there are any problems resulting from the use of a brace, then the management should be abandoned until the child gets to about the age of 3 years. Then a decision will be made as to whether operative treatment for dislocation is necessary. This decision is based on the principles outlined in the preceding paragraphs. Operative reduction should aim for correction with the minimum of postoperative immobilization. The principles of the operation are to achieve a concentric reduction of the femoral heads with capsulorrhaphy and surgery to intraarticular structures, correction of muscle imbalance by flexor and adductor releases, and improvement in the acetabular coverage, generally by a Pemberton osteotomy. Plaster immobilization is necessary for only 6 weeks postoperatively.

Provision of Abductor and Extensor Power at the Hip

Muscle transfers about the hip were popular for spina bifida when it was thought that muscle imbalance caused hip dislocation and contractures. Because we now know that the relationship between muscle imbalance and hip deformity is less clear, and because we know that dislocation occurs in the absence of muscle imbalance, we believe there is no place for the use of prophylactic muscle transfers.

Some believe that there is a place for muscle transfers in selected circumstances, but most now agree that there is no place for posterior ileo psoas transfer as described by Sharrard [5]. Gait analysis has established that the energy cost following this procedure is unacceptably high. We had abandoned this procedure before we had this knowledge, because we had observed on clinical grounds that children who had undergone the procedure walked with gross pelvic rotation, and that the procedure had carried no advantage. Triple transfer, described by Yngve and Lindseth [6], or external oblique transfer alone might be of value for a specific patient with a low lumbar lesion.

Conclusion

Hip flexion contracture and hip dislocation have previously been thought to be due entirely to muscle imbalance across the hip. We have shown that the hip flexion contracture is most common and most severe in children with thoracic neurosegmental levels. Dislocation of a hip is also common in thoracic neurosegmental levels, whereas in children with innervation to L4, who presumably have maximum muscle imbalance, only a third develop hip dislocation or require hip surgery. Muscle imbalance is therefore one of a number of factors implicated in the development of hip flexion contracture and hip dislocation, and the management described above takes these important developments into account.

References

1. Fraser RK, Bourke HM, Broughton NS, Menelaus MB (1995) Unilateral dislocation of the hip in spina bifida—a long-term follow-up. J Bone Joint Surg 77-B:615–619
2. Frawley PA, Broughton NS, Menelaus MB (1996) Anterior release for fixed flexion deformity of the hip in spina bifida. J Bone Joint Surg 78-B:299–302
3. Heeg M, Broughton NS, Menelaus MB (1998) Bilateral dislocation of the hip in spina bifida. A long-term follow-up study. J Paediatr Orthop 18:434–436
4. Salter RB (1961) Innominate osteotomy in the treatment of congenital dislocation and subluxation of the hip. J Bone Joint Surg 43-B:518–539
5. Sharrard WJW (1964) Posterior iliopsoas transfer in the treatment of paralytic dislocation of the hip. J Bone Joint Surg 46-B:426–444
6. Yngve DA, Lindseth RE (1982) Effectiveness of muscle transfers in myelomeningocele hips measured by radiographic indices. J Paediatr Orthop 2(2):121–125

Abstract

External Oblique Abdominal Muscle Transfer

Junichi Monji

Hip dislocation and subluxation in spina bifida children were treated with external oblique abdominal muscle transfer, adductor release or transfer, or detorsion-varus femoral osteotomy. From May 1990 to April 1997, 16 cases (27 hips) were operated on with this method. The indication for this surgery was that a spina bifida child with hip dislocation or subluxation has the ability to stand and/or the possibility of walking. These children have more than fair knee extensor power.

Fifteen hips were good in reduction, 3 were subluxated, and 2 are now redislocated. In this series, no acetabular plasty was performed which might lead to redislocation. Three subluxated hips resulted from improper surgical methods (2 hips) and spastic paresis (1 hip).

This method is easier than Sharrard's iliopsoas transfer, and the postsurgical physiotherapy is easy to motivate. There is no loss of hip flexor power, but the influence on spinal deformity should be carefully observed.

Department of Orthopaedic Surgery, Clark Hospital, Sapporo, Japan

Moderator's Comments on Sessions—Hip Pathology

Malcolm B. Menelaus

A consensus was reached that fixed flexion deformity is bad news and generally should be corrected.

There was general agreement that hip dislocation is unimportant in children who do not have acting quadriceps muscles and are unlikely to remain walkers into adult life. Those children with high-level lesions should not have treatment for dislocation of the hip, and it would be exceptional to find an indication for operative treatment for dislocation in this group. It was generally agreed that there is usually little advantage in reducing hip dislocation in children with bilateral dislocation in low-level lesions. However, it was felt that unilateral dislocation in low-level lesions should be treated.

It was generally felt, particularly among those who have the advantage of a gait laboratory, that ileo psoas transfer leads to high energy expenditure and there is little advantage to be gained from this procedure.

In answer to questions, Dr. Dias pointed out that some recurrence of fixed flexion deformity of the hip was common following surgery, as was confirmed by a review of mature patients.

In answer to a question about the best way to retain correction of fixed flexion deformity, Dr. Menelaus felt that all one could do was to encourage standing and walking. Dr. Dias agreed with this.

In answer to a question about whether any action can be taken when a young child is seen to have subluxation of the hip, Dr. Menelaus felt that it was best to watch and wait. He pointed out that many children with spina bifida have lax capsules and floppy hips, and it is hard to be sure whether subluxation is present or not. Serial X-rays would disclose whether the hips dislocated, and if they did then they required management along the lines that Dr. Menelaus has discussed in his paper.

Department of Orthopaedics, Royal Children's Hospital, 25 Victoria Parade Collingwood, Victoria 3066, Melbourne, Australia

Moderator's Comments on Sessions—Hip Pathology

Toshio Fujii

Hip dislocation or subluxation in myelomeningocele has been a very fascinating problem for orthopedic surgeons for a long time. We had believed that muscle imbalance around the hip was the main cause of hip dislocation and should be corrected by surgical procedures. Thus, we expected Sharrard's iliopsoas transfer to restore the muscle imbalance and to improve hip stability. However, the results of Sharrard's procedure alone were not as good as expected in all cases, as Fujii (Fukuoka, Japan) and Kamegaya (Chiba, Japan) reported in this session. Fujii said that Sharrard's procedure alone improved the concentricity of the hip for a period of time, but acetabular dysplasia remained in half of the patients which resulted in a recurrence of hip subluxation. Both of the authors also reported combined procedures, such as Sharrard's iliopsoas transfer and Pemberton's osteotomy or Salter's osteotomy, with or without detorsion varus osteotomy, which maintained unstable hips in good concentricity. Monji (Sapporo, Japan) reported the good results obtained by detorsion varus osteotomy with external oblique muscle transfer. These Japanese authors presented the long-term results of their surgical experiences.

Dias (Chicago, USA) reported his recent approach to hip problems in myelomeningocele through his gait analysis results. He stated that hip contractures can be more of a problem, by interfering with bracing and ambulation, and should be treated to improve function and mobility. Indications for treatment of hip dislocation in lower lumbar level patients were set using his gait analysis.

Menelaus (Melbourne, Australia) talked on the current treatment of the hip. He reviewed a number of Patients Data Management System (PDMS) statistical studies done by Menelaus and Dias and their groups. Hip dislocation and deformities in myelomeningocele patients were prevalent even in the absence of demonstrable muscle imbalance. The muscle imbalance itself was not the cause of hip dislocation, and therefore there was no need to treat it. This was a drastically different finding from the studies of Sharrard's age. Menelaus now generally reduces unilateral dislocation, and occasionally bilateral dislocation, in patients who have a strong quadriceps muscle. He performs open reduction combined with anterior hip release, lengthening of the psoas muscle, and a Pemberton osteotomy, with or without a femoral detorsion varus osteotomy. Beauchamp (Vancouver, Canada) stated that their radical hip release improved ambulation, mobility, and independence. Fujii and Beauchamp men-

Department of Orthopaedic Surgery, Fukuoka Children's Hospital, 2-5-1 Tojin-Machi, Chuo-Ku, Fukuoka 810-0063, Japan

tioned that mental retardation, obesity, and hip and knee contracture caused deterioration in walking ability, and that there was no significant correlation between ambulatory status and the concentricity of the hip.

The discussion of this session clearly showed some current solutions to the long and difficult problem of hip pathology in myelomeningocele. The approach to hip problems, especially dislocations or subluxations, has recently changed. Unilateral hip dislocations in lower lumbar level patients show pelvic obliquity which decreases walking ability, and thus they should always be reduced. However, bilateral dislocations do not interfere with walking except when they are accompanied by severe contractures. Therefore, it is not always necessary to reduce bilateral dislocations.

We should now use the fruitful results of this session to minimize excessive hip surgery in myelomeningocele children.

The Natural History of Scoliosis in Myelomeningocele

John V. Banta, Joseph Slakey, and Jefrey Thomson

The incidence of myelomeningocele in North America is estimated at approximately 0.5–1% live births annually. The prevalence of scoliosis is variably estimated at from 62% to 90% in current literature. An early study at our institution in 1972 by Raycroft and Curtis distinguished between congenital and paralytic spinal deformities, but did not separate coronal from saggital plane deformities. They concluded that 50% of patients developed deformity, and all but two did so by 10 years of age.

The definition of scoliosis is variable in the literature, varying from 10° to 20°, and few authors distinguish between curves of congenital or developmental origin. Few reports evaluate an index population beyond the first decade of life. The details and end results of brace management are poorly defined. The present report consists of a review of 209 patients, of whom 141 met the criteria of:

Diagnosis of myelomeningocele;
Age 10 years or over at the time of evaluation;
Documented serial manual motor testing;
Noncongenital coronal plane deformity;
Adequate radiographs throughout growth.

The definition of scoliosis is a curve of at least 20°, as many smaller curves were positional and variable without progression until they reached at least 20°, when they became fixed and curve progression was usually observed.

Population age of 141 patients was 19 years, with a range of 10–40 years.
Incidence of developmental scoliosis was 52% (74 patients).

Curve patterns were:		
	lumbar	38
	double major	18
	thoracolumbar	14
	thoracic	4

Clinical motor level was based upon the functional motor level of the lowest nerve root showing antigravity grade 3 or more which was under voluntary control. Patients with synergistic motor activity (i.e., recruiting movement through movement of the opposite limb)

The Newington Department of Orthopaedic Surgery, Connecticut Children's Hospital, Hartford, CT, USA

or showing obvious alteration of tone were considered to have spastic or reflexive activity. Motor asymmetry was defined as at least a two motor-level difference between the right and left sides of the body.

Periodic manual muscle testing was mandatory in order to properly assess the neurological status of the patient. Since many patients were over 10 years of age at examination, they had not, in their first decade, had access to magnetic resonance imaging technology, and hence information concerning a possible tethered cord was not available for the older patients.

Motor level distribution and the development of scoliosis

Motor level	No. of patients	% with scoliosis
Thoracic	41	93
L1–2	8	75
L3–4	29	59
L5	21	43
Sacral	42	10

The importance of the last intact laminar arch, first reported by Piggot, was confirmed in this study, which emphasizes the fact that, irrespective of the apparent motor function observed in the lower extremities in the neonate, if the dysraphic vertebral arch is at the thoracolumbar junction or higher, the risk of developing scoliosis is significant. In other words, cord pathology is frequent at and below the level of the bony dysraphism!

Last intact laminar arch distribution vs. scoliosis

LILA	No. of patients	% scoliosis
Thoracic	42	86
L1–2	26	58
L3–4	47	26
L5	12	8
Sacral	2	0

Of 74 patients with developmental scoliosis, 43 developed curves before the age of 9, and 31 developed scoliosis after 9 years of age. The functional level had a positive predictive value of 85%, with a specificity of 85%. With regard to spasticity, the positive predictive value was 83%, with a specificity of 94%. Hip instability had a positive predictive value of 79%, with a specificity of 90%.

The use of bracing to restrict the progression of neuromuscular spinal deformity has been controversial, especially once the curve develops structural changes. In this population the use of a total contact orthosis delayed the age of fusion by 2 years compared with those children not continued in an orthosis for further spinal growth. Comparing the 11 braced patients with 13 unbraced patients, the rate of curve progression was identical for each group at 8° of progression per year, yet the average curve at the time of fusion was 90° in the prolonged brace group versus an average cure of 62° in those not braced.

We concluded from this analysis that curves over 20° become true structural curves. Scoliosis continues to progress in children up to the age of 15 years. The predictive factors be fore the development of scoliosis are, in decreasing order of importance, functional motor level, the last intact laminar arc of the spine, the child's functional mobility, and lastly the presence of motor asymmetry.

Bibliography

1. Banta JV (1986) Natural history of scoliosis in myelomeningocele. Orthop Trans 10:18
2. Barden GA, Mayer LC, Stelling FH (1975) Myelodysplastics: fate of those followed for 20 years or more. J Bone Joint Surg 57A:643
3. Drummond DS, Moreau M, Cruess RL (1980) The results and complications of surgery for the paralytic hip and spine in myelomeningocele. J Bone Joint Surg 62B:49
4. Esyel P, Hopf C, Schwartz M, Voth (1993) Development of scoliosis in myelomeningocele. Differences in the history caused by the idiopathic pattern. Neurosurg Rev 16:301
5. Hoffer M, Feiwell E, Perry R, Perry J, Bonnet C (1973) Functional ambulation in patients with myelomeningocele. J Bone Joint Surg 55A:137
6. Keggi JM, Banta JV, Walton C (1992) The myelodysplastic hip and scoliosis. Dev Med Child Neurol 34:240
7. Knox EG (1967) Spina bifida in Birmingham. Dev Med Child Neurol Suppl 13:14
8. Lindseth RE (1994) Myelomeningocele spine. In: The pediatric spine: principles and practice. Raven, New York
9. McLaughlin TP, Banta JV, Gahm NH, Raycroft JF (1986) Intraspinal rhizotomy and distal cordectomy in patients with myelomeningocele. J Bone Joint Surg 68A:88
10. Muller EB, Nordwall A (1992) Prevalence of scoliosis in children with myelomeningocele in Western Sweden. Spine 19:1097
11. Muller EB, Nordwall A (1994) Brace treatment of scoliosis in children with myelomeningocele. Spine 19:151
12. Osebold WR, Mayfield JK, Wintger RB, Moe JH (1982) Surgical treatment of the paralytic scoliosis associated with myelomeningocele. J Bone Joint Surg 64A:841
13. Piggot H (1982) The natural history of scoliosis in myelodysplasia. J Bone Joint Surg 62B:54
14. Raycroft JF, Curtis BH (1972) Spinal curvature in myelomeningocele: natural history and etiology. In: The American Academy of Orthopaedic Surgeons Symposium on Myelomeningocele. Mosby, St. Louis
15. Siram K, Bobetchko WT, Hall JE (1972) Surgical management of spinal deformities in spina bifida. J Bone Joint Surg 54B:666

Scoliosis Associated with Syringomyelia

Toshinobu Onomura and Kohji Iwai

This chapter describes our experience of cases with syringomyelia, with special reference to the features of their spinal deformities. Because of the advancement of image diagnosis and peoples' concern about posture, which has been increasing since the school screening program for scoliosis started in Japan, the figures show that orthopedic surgeons meet syringomyelia in the clinic more frequently than before.

Thirty-one cases of syringomyelia were hospitalized in the Department of Orthopedic Surgery of Osaka Medical College in the last 15 years. Genders and age distributions are as shown in Table 1, and 20 patients were under 20 years of age.

The pathologies combined with syringomyelia were Arnold–Chiari malformation (ACM) in 19 cases, spinal cord tumor in five cases, and spinal injury, archnoiditis, and spina bifida in two cases each. The clinical pictures of the syringomyelia patients varied according to the case. Because they were different from classical symptoms of syringomyelia, the most frequent main symptom of the patients in our orthopedic clinic was scoliosis (15 cases), followed by paraplegia, tetraplegia, sensory disturbance, and foot deformity (Table 2). In our series, spinal deformity was found only in ACM cases.

Regarding the location of the syrinx in ACM cases, the cervical spinal cord was always involved, and the extent of the syrinx was from only one spinal segment to almost the entire spinal cord. The size of the syrinx also varied. Neurological impairment was not necessarily affected by the size or extent of the syrinx. A 12-year-old girl (Fig. 1), whose scoliosis was first noticed at the age of 4 years, had a syrinx extending from C-1 to L-1. The cavity was huge and she had paraparesis, but the effect on her daily activity was rather mild and she could still walk and trot.

Out of 19 ACM cases, scoliotic curve was found in 16 (9 males and 7 females), and the curve measured from 18° to 102° (average 64°). Regarding the pattern of spinal curvature, 9 cases had curves similar to the idiopathic scoliosis pattern, i.e., young female, right thoracic curve, etc. In the remaining 7 cases, however, the clinical picture differed from that of idiopathic scoliosis, e.g., young male patient, left thoracic curve, etc. Because spinal deformity is often the initial abnormality noticed by patients or their family without any neurological deficit being recognized, it is thought that this fact is very important in a general orthopedic clinic in order not to miss syringomyelia in the early stage of the disease. We are afraid that a considerable number of syringomyelia cases are still classified as idiopathic scoliosis. The value

Department of Orthopedic Surgery, Osaka Medical College, 14-26 Kitashowa, Nishinomiya, Hyogo 662, Japan

TABLE 1. Cases with syringomyelia hospitalized in the department of orthopedic surgery, osaka medical college, since 1980

Sex	Male	21
	Female	10
Age (years)	Under 10	10
	11–20	10
	21–30	2
	31–40	1
	41–50	4
	51–60	4
Total		31

TABLE 2. Principal symptom

Scoliosis	15
Paraplegia	7
Tetraplegia	4
Sensory disturbance	3
Foot deformity	2
Total	31

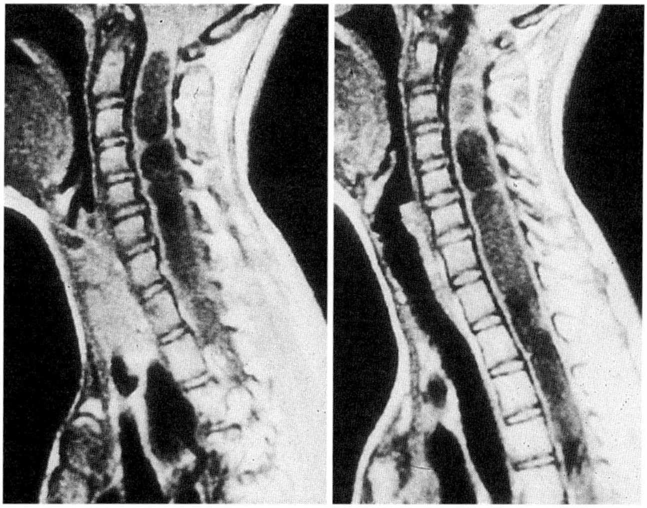

FIG. 1. A girl aged 12 years 7 months with Arnold–Chiari malformation. TR/TE = 600/200

of school screening programs for scoliosis is controversial, because it not only consumes a lot of time and money, but it also picks up many false-positive and false-negative cases. In addition, after the introduction of school screening programs, the number of patients with anxieties about postural problems has increased. When taking a spinal X-ray of these patients at the first consultation, the inclusion of the cervical spine in the lateral view can also contribute to a check for the presence of a wide cervical canal, which is an important sign in the differential diagnosis of syringomyelia. We have picked up several patients with syringomyelia from school screening in this way.

Sensory disturbance was not the chief complaint of ACM cases except for 3 patients, but on physical examination, sensory disturbance was detected in 18 patients out of 19. The pattern of sensory deficit was the unilateral type in 13 cases, the dissociated type in 14 cases, and the facial type in 3 cases. It was interesting and noticable that the convexity of the scoliotic curve was toward the dominant side of the sensory disturbance in 15 out of 17 cases in our ACM series. This fact suggests that sensory disturbance is related to, or may play an important role in, the initiation or progression of lateral curvature of the spine.

Selecting the treatment for scoliosis associated with syringomyelia caused by ACM is not simple, because even now predicting the natural course of both syrinx and scoliosis is a difficult problem. In cases where the neurological deficit is evident or deteriorating, surgery for ACM and/or syrinx is preferantially performed. An operation for scoliosis is performed in cases where the spinal curvature is more than moderate or is progressive (Tables 3 and 4). In cases where the scoliosis needs surgical correction and both the syrinx and the neurological deficit are minimum, scoliosis surgery is performed first.

The treatments for syrinx used in our 19 ACM are listed in Table 3. Suboccipital decompression was performed in 7 cases; this was combined with S–P shunt in 3 cases, with S–S shunt in 2 cases, and with S–P shunt and terminal ventriculostomy in 1 case. Terminal ventriculostomy alone was performed in 1 case. Eleven cases were treated conservatively.

A 12-year-old girl (Fig. 1) had paraparesis and spinal deformity, and received suboccipital decompression and a syringoperitoneal shunt operation. After the operation the syrinx decreased considerably in size, the tonsils were elevated, and her neurological symptoms improved. Eight months after the operation, shunt tube trouble occurred and the syrinx began to increase in size. However, 2 years after the operation her neurological status remained at the improved level (Fig. 2).

The clinical results for 6 patients who received suboccipital decompression and a shunt operation are satisfactory (Table 5). Tonsillar herniation had improved in 4 cases, and both

TABLE 3. Treatment for syringomyelia associated with ACM

Suboccipital decompression	1
Suboccipital decompression + S–P shunt	3
Suboccipital decompression + S–S shunt	2
Suboccipital decompression + S–P shunt + terminal ventriculostomy	1
Terminal ventriculostomy	1
No operation	11
Total	19

TABLE 4. Treatment for scoliosis associated with syringomyelia

Instrumental correction and fusion	7
With syrinx operation	3
Without syrinx operation	4
Conservative treatment	9
Total	16

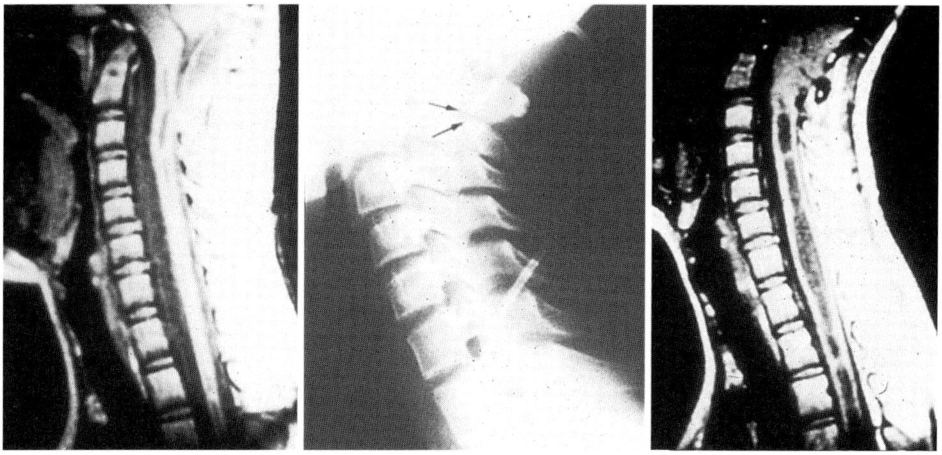

a,b c

FIG. 2. A 12-year-old girl who was treated by suboccipital decompression + S–P shunt. **a** One month after the operation. **b** Eight months after the operation shunt tube trouble occurred. **c** Two years after the operation

TABLE 5. Results of surgery for ACM (suboccipital decompression + shunt operation)

	Improved	No change
Tonsillar herniation	4	2
Size of syrinx	6	0
Neurological symptoms	6	0

the size of the syrinx and the neurological impairment had improved in all cases. However, terminal ventriculostomy did not bring any significant improvement.

Of the 16 cases with scoliosis, surgical correction and spinal fusion were performed in 7 cases. In 3 of these cases a syrinx operation was also performed, while in 4 cases it was not (Table 4). In the remaining 9 cases the spinal deformity was mild and did not show any progression during the period of observation, and conservative treatment was indicated. The results of these correction and fusion operations for scoliosis were satisfactory and did not cause any neurological worsening.

Summary

1. Spinal deformity was the initial complaint of young patients with syringomyelia in the majority of cases.
2. In many patients, the scoliosis pattern was different from that of an idiopathic curve.
3. The convexity of the scoliosis was towards the dominant side of the sensory disturbance in most cases.
4. Surgical treatment was carried out for 47% of cases with a syrinx with ACM, and for 44% of scoliosis cases.

Experience with Decancellation Kyphectomy for the Correction of Kyphosis in Children with Myelomeningocele

JOHN F. SARWARK, TODD SIMMONS, JEFFERY VANFLANDERN, and JOHN GRAYHACK

Summary. We reviewed the early results of the operative treatment of kyphosis (flexible, nonangular) in juvenile myelomeningocele patients. We utilized the decancellation kyphectomy procedure recently described by Lindseth with two fixation methods: tension bend wiring and a pedicle screw, hook, and rod construct. The decancellation methods combined with stable instrumentation in the sagittal neutral plane as a way to control these difficult curves, at least for a period of time sufficient to allow adequate spinal growth prior to definitive treatment, appears effective.

Key words. Myelomeningocele, Spine, Kyphosis

Introduction

Kyphosis spine deformity is associated with significant disability [1, 10, 14, 15]. Surgical correction and lasting stability of the corrected spine is the goal in each child [3–5, 8, 12]. Further improvements in surgical techniques have allowed surgery to come closer to these goals. A procedure is described here for spinal reconstruction which is associated with lower morbidity and improved results.

Materials and Methods

Nine patients with a flexible C-shaped kyphosis were treated with the decancellation procedure over the 2-year study period. Four patients had tension banding and five patients had a pedicle-screw/rod construct. Indications for surgery were persistent skin breakdown in two patients, and progressive, uncontrollable kyphosis in seven. The average age at surgery was 6 years. The mean follow-up was 22 months (range 12–31 months).

Observations and Results

Overall, the preoperative kyphosis measured 91° (range 75°–125°). The curves overall were corrected to an average of 29° at surgery. At final follow-up, the kyphosis measured 65° (range 22°–120°). All were managed postoperatively with TLSO or TLSO–thigh extension for at least 1 year.

Northwestern University Medical School and Children's Memorial Hospital, Division of Orthopaedic Surgery, No. 69, 2300 Children's Plaza, Chicago, IL 60614, USA

We noted a significant difference between results when we compared the fixation methods. All four patients in the tension-banded group had a significant loss of correction that measured 55°. At final follow-up, the kyphosis measured 91°, which was similar to the preoperative average of 101° in spite of an average correction to 36°. Two patients had radiographic evidence of fixation failure.

The five patients in the pedicle fixation group performed much better. The average kyphosis at final follow-up measured 44°, compared with 83° preoperatively, and represented only a 20° average loss of correction. No fixation failures were evident in radiographs.

At this very early follow-up, there has been no evidence of premature disc space closure or anterior spinal growth arrest. Biological restoration of lordosis due to growth has not been seen in either group.

Discussion and Conclusions

On the basis of these results, we feel that tension-band wiring does not sufficiently stabilize the kyphosis deformity after decancellation for long-term stability in spite of good posture and kyphosis correction initially. We have abandoned this wiring technique while retaining the decancellation concept. Instrumentation is required in the complete sagittal contour [2, 6, 7, 9, 11, 13, 16–18].

References

1. Banta JW, Hamada JS (1976) Natural history of the kyphotic deformity in myelomeningocele. J Bone Joint Surg 58A:279
2. Christofersen MR, Brooks AL (1985) Excision and wire fixation of rigid myelomeningocele kyphosis. J Pediatr Orthop 5:691–696
3. Duncan JW, Lovell WW, Bailey SC, Ranson D (1976) Surgical treatment of kyphosis in myelomeningocele. J Bone Joint Surg (Am) 58:155
4. Eckstein HB, Vora RM (1972) Spinal osteotomy for severe kyphosis in children with myelomeningocele. J Bone Joint Surg (Br) 54:328–333
5. Hall JE, Poitras B (1977) The management of kyphosis in patients with myelomeningocele. Clin Orthop 128:33–40
6. Heydemann JS, Gillespie MD (1987) The management of myelomeningocele kyphosis in the older child by kyphectomy and segmental spinal instrumentation. Spine 12:37–41
7. Hoppenfeld S (1967) Congenital kyphosis in myelomeningocele. J Bone Joint Surg 49B:276–280
8. Hull WJ, Moe JH, Winter RB (1974) Spine deformity in myelomeningocele: natural history, evaluation, and treatment. J Bone Joint Surg 56A:1767
9. Leatherman KD, Dickson RA (1978) Congenital kyphosis in myelomeningocele: vertebral body resection and posterior spine fusion. Spine 3:222–226
10. Lindseth RE (1991) Spine deformity in myelomeningocele. Instrum Course Lect 40:273–279
11. Lindseth RE, Steltzer L (1979) Vertebral excision for kyphosis in myelomeningocele. J Bone Joint Surg 61A:699–704
12. Lowe GP, Menelaus MBL (1978) The surgical management of kyphosis in older children with myelomeningocele. J Bone Joint Surg (Br) 60:40–45
13. McCarthy RE, Dunn F, McCullough FL (1989) Luque fixation to the sacral ala using the Dunn–McCarthy modification. Spine 14:281–283
14. Mintz LJ, Dias LS, Sarwark JF, Schafer MF (1990) A challenging problem in myelodysplasia: the child with severe kyphosis. Problems, prognosis and outcome. Orthop Trans 14:590
15. Mintz LJ, Sarwark JF, Dias LS, Schafer MF (1991) The natural history of congenital kyphosis in myelomeningocele: a review of 51 children. Spine (Suppl) 16(8):348–350

16. Sharrard WJW (1968) Spinal osteotomy for severe kyphosis in children with myelomeningocele. J Bone Joint Surg 50B:466–471
17. Sharrard WJW, Drennan JC (1972) Osteotomy-excision of the spine for lumbar kyphosis in older children with myelomeningocele. J Bone Joint Surg 54B:50–60
18. Walker GA, Cheong-Leen P Spinal excision osteotomy in myelomeningocele with special reference to internal fixation. Postgrad Med J 50:145–149

Abstract

The Surgical Correction of Myelomeningocele Kyphosis

Nobuaki Tsunoda[1], Toshio Fujii[2], Akihiko Takashima[2], Kazuyuki Takamura[2], Haruhisa Yanagida[2], and Yutaka Oketani[2]

Myelomeningocele kyphosis is a very rigid deformity, and progresses rapidly during infancy. The surgical correction of kyphosis is extremely difficult, and the stabilization techniques for preventing recurrence are controversial. From 1987, 5 patients with this deformity were treated using resection of the lordotic segments, cephalad and apical vertebrae, and fixation of proximal and distal vertebrae employing several fixation instruments. The first 3 patients, whose ages were 2.3, 3.5, and 1.2 years, were treated using the Lindseth technique with stainless steel wire for fixation. Loss of correction occurred in 2 patients soon after surgery; one due to a fracture of the upper fixed level, and the other by infection. The Lindseth technique (fixation with wire) did not maintain the correction curve during surgery in the 4th and 5th patients, a 6-year-old girl and a 3.6-year-old boy, respectively. Owing to the loss of correction in previous patients and the difficulty of correction in these 2 patients, we performed bilateral long plate vertebral fixation on the 4th and 5th patients, which subsequently resulted in satisfactory curve maintenance.

[1] Tsunoda Orthopaedic Clinic, Fukuoka, Japan
[2] Department of Orthopaedic Surgery, Fukuoka Children's Hospital and Medical Center, Fukuoka, Japan

Moderators' Comments on Sessions—Spine Pathology

John F. Sarwark

Dr. Banta describes the natural history of scoliosis in myelomeningocele and its association with neurosegmental level. Neurosegmental motor level is most closely approximated by the last intact laminar arch (LILA). Progressive severe curves require surgical stabilization, while moderate curves do not generally benefit from bracing.

Prof. Onomura considered scoliosis associated with syringomyelia, and gave a detailed summation of his surgical experience. Spinal deformity is often the initial presentation of syringomyelia and not the neurological findings. Inclusion of the cervical spine in a lateral radiograph of the spine is recommended to increase the number of positive results. A complaint of headache may also be significant in diagnosing syringomyelia. The clinical significance of the lesion will determine the need for surgical intervention

Prof. Tsunoda described surgical correction of myelomeningocele kyphosis by vertebral resection. Postoperative immobilization in a cast (4 weeks) and brace (6 months) is then necessary. Techniques of internal fixation are discussed. The long-term follow-up of cases illustrates the effectiveness of these techniques.

Prof. Sarwark reported his experience with decancellation kyphectomy for the correction of kyphosis in children with myelomeningocele. Decancellation kyphectomy is a surgical technique for the reconstruction of pediatric myelomeningocele deformity that allows lower morbidity and improved correction. Instrumentation of the entire sagittal plane deformity is required for both short- and long-term stabilization.

Northwestern University Medical School and Children's Memorial Hospital, Division of Orthopaedic Surgery, No. 69, 2300 Children's Plaza, Chicago, IL 60614, USA

The Incidence of Foot Deformity in Japanese School-Age Patients with Spina Bifida

HARUHISA YANAGIDA, TOSHIO FUJII, AKIHIKO TAKASHIMA, and KAZUYUKI TAKAMURA

Introduction

Deformities of the foot are common in spina bifida. We studied the incidence of foot deformities in Japanese school-age patients with spina bifida.

We studied 103 spina bifida patients who had been treated at Fukuoka Children's Hospital. Both spina bifida occulta and spina bifida cystica cases were included. There were 48 males and 55 females, and the average age at examination was 9.4 years.

Regarding the neurosegmental level of the lesion, there were three patients with lesions above level T12, 18 between L1 and L3, 32 at L4, 22 at L5, and 28 at the sacral level.

Results

Foot deformities were recognized in 84% of the patients, and 16% had no foot deformity. Of the patients who had foot deformities, 48.8% were pes varus or equinovarus, 17.4% were pes calcaneovalgus, 10.5% were pes cavus, 9.3% were pes calcaneus, 5.8% were pes calcaneovarus, 4.7% were pes valgus or equinovalgus, and 3.5% were equinus.

We also studied foot deformities according to lesion level. There were only three patients with lesions above T12, of which two had pes equinus and one had equinovarus deformities. Of the patients whose lesions were between L1 and L3, 88.9% had pes varus or equinovarus, and 11.1% had calcaneovalgus deformities. Of the patients with level L4 lesions, 50% had pes varus or equinovarus, 21.9% had calcaneovalgus, 12.5% had calcaneus, 6.3% had calcaneovarus, and 9.4% had no deformity. Of the patients with level L5 lesions, 36.4% had pes varus or equinovarus deformities, 18.2% had calcaneus deformities, and calcaneovalgus, valgus or equinovalgus, calcaneovarus, cavus, and no deformity cases each accounted for 9.1% of the total. Of the deformities of patients with sacral level lesions, 25% were pes cavus, 14.3% were calcaneovalgus, 7.1% were varus or equinovarus and valgus or equinovalgus, 3.6% were calcaneovarus, and 42.9% had no deformity.

Sharrard and Grosfield, in a study of 296 feet, found that 81.4% had foot deformities. Shafer and Dias found 89.8%, Lindseth found 66.6%, and in our series, we found that 83.5% had foot deformities. These results indicate that foot deformities occur in approximately 80% of all

Department of Orthopaedic Surgery, Fukuoka Children's Hospital, 2-5-1 Tojin-machi, Chuo, Fukuoka 810, Japan cases of spina bifida. Sharrard and Grosfield observed no correlation between spontaneous motor activity and the type of deformity, but in our series, the foot deformities were well correlated with the neurosegmental level of the lesion.

In addition to muscle imbalance, spasticity, and teratologic factors which affect the severity of the deformity before and after birth, the foot deformities of school-age children are further influenced by an increase in body weight and tethered cord syndrome. For this reason, the foot deformities of school-age children should be observed with extreme care.

Conclusions

We found a high incidence (83.5%) of foot deformities in Japanese school-age patients with spina bifida. These deformities of the foot were also well correlated with the neurosegmental level of the lesion.

References

1. Sharrard WJW, Grosfield I (1968) The management of deformity and paralysis of the foot in myelomeningocele. J Bone Joint Surg 50-B:456
2. Shafer MF, Dias LS (1983) Myelomeningocele. Orthopaedic Treatment. Baltimore, Williams & Wilkins
3. Lindseth RE (1976) Treatment of the lower extremity in children paralyzed by myelomeningocele. A.A.O.S Instr Course Lect 25:76

Orthopedic Operative Management in Spina Bifida

Kokuji Yoh[1], Makoto Kamegaya[1], Yuhji Shinohara[1], Hideshige Moriya[2], Katsunori Yoshinaga[2], Tomojiro Yamane[3], and Takehiro Yamashita[4]

Summary. We reviewed orthopedic operative management in spina bifida patients. A group of 46 patients, with 78 feet undergoing surgery, were enrolled in the study. There were 30 cysticae and 16 occultae, 15 boys and 31 girls. A comparison between cystica and occulta showed a high percentage of L5 or lower motor lesion in occulta. More equinus and equinovarus deformities of the feet were found in cystica, while more varus and cavovarus were found in occulta. The most frequent surgery was tendon transfers to correct the muscle imbalance, which was performed on more than half the cases. Soft tissue release and bone surgery were the next most common. All of the equinovarus, varus, and valgus cases still needed orthoses after tendon transfers, but some of the calcaneus and cavovarus cases needed no orthotic treatment to attain stable walking.

Key words. Foot deformity, Occulta, Cystica, Orthopedic operative management

Introduction

Sharrard and Grosfield [5] reported that approximatedly 85% of spina bifida children develop paralytic malformation secondary to neuromuscular imbalance. A major problem in treatment is the provision of a plantigrade foot on which a brace can be fitted and a shoe worn. The purpose of this study was to evaluate the orthopedic operative management of foot deformities of spina bifida patients attending the Chiba Children's Hospital.

Materials and Methods

A group of 46 patients (78 feet) were enrolled in this study. Among them were 30 cysticae and 16 occultae, 15 boys and 31 girls. The average age at operation was 7 years and 8 months (ranging from 11 months to 20 years). The mean follow-up period was 6 years and 4 months. Patients were classified according to a modification of the functional categories proposed by

[1] Division of Orthopaedic Surgery, Chiba Children's Hospital, 579-1 Heta-cho, Midori-ku, Chiba 266, Japan
[2] Department of Orthopaedic Surgery, Chiba University School of Medicine, Chiba, Japan
[3] Department of Orthopaedic Surgery, Teikyo University School of Medicine, Tokyo, Japan
[4] Department of Orthopaedic Surgery, Chiba Municipal Hospital, Chiba, Japan

Hoffer et al. [3] as follows: IA, independent ambulator; CA, community ambulator; HA, household ambulator; NFA, nonfuntional ambulator; NA, nonambulator. The pattern of foot deformities was divided into equinus, equinovarus, varus, valgus, calcaneus, and cavovarus. Thirty-nine cases of tendon transfer, 29 cases of soft tissue release, and 15 cases of bone surgery were performed to correct the foot deformities caused by muscle imbalance.

Observations and Results

There were no surgical complications such as infection and skin sloughing, although repeat operations were necessary in 4/46 (9%) of the patients as compared with the 14% reported by Sharrard and Grosfield [5].

Regarding the relationship between motor level and ambulation (Table 1), all patients except one with a neurological level at L3 or lower belonged to either the IA or CA group. On the other hand, patients with a neurological level of L2 or higher were classified as NFA or NA.

Spina bifida children develop various paralytic foot deformities. In our study, equinus and equinovarus were mostly found at L3 or a higher level. Varus and valgus showed a broad distribution. Calcaneus and cavovarus appeared at a lower level (Table 2).

Patients were categorized into either cystica or occulta to assess their relationship with motor level and foot deformity. Regarding the distribution of motor level between these groups, only 12/53 cystica patients had L5 or lower residual motor level, while this was up to 17/25 in occulta patients. This meant that patients with cystica had much more neurological impairment (Table 3).

As expected, equinus, equinovarus, and calcaneus foot deformities were dominant in cystica patients. However, more varus, valgus, and cavovarus developed in occulta patients because of the high incidence of lower motor level paralysis in occulta itself (Fig. 1).

Table 1. Motor level and ambulation (Hoffer's criteria)

	L2≦	L3	L4	L5	S1≧
IA		1	15	8	17
CA		10	13	2	1
HA			1		
NFA	4				
NA	6				
Total	10	11	29	10	18

IA, independent ambulator; CA, community ambulator; HA, household ambulator; NFA, nonfunctional ambulator; NA, nonambulator.

Table 2. Motor level and foot deformity (total 78 feet)

	L2≦	L3	L4	L5	S1≧	Total
Equinus	6	2				8
Equinovarus	1	5	5	2		13
Varus	2	1	3	3	4	13
Valgus	1	2	8	1		12
Calcaneus			13	2	4	19
Cavovarus					9	9

TABLE 3. Motor level and types of spina bifida

	L2≦	L3	L4	L5	S1≧	Total
Cystica	9	9	23	8	4	53
				12/53		
Occulta	1	2	5	2	15	25
				17/25		

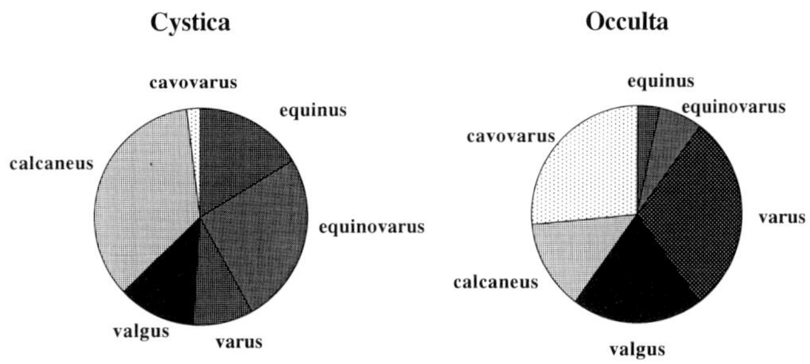

FIG. 1. Foot deformity

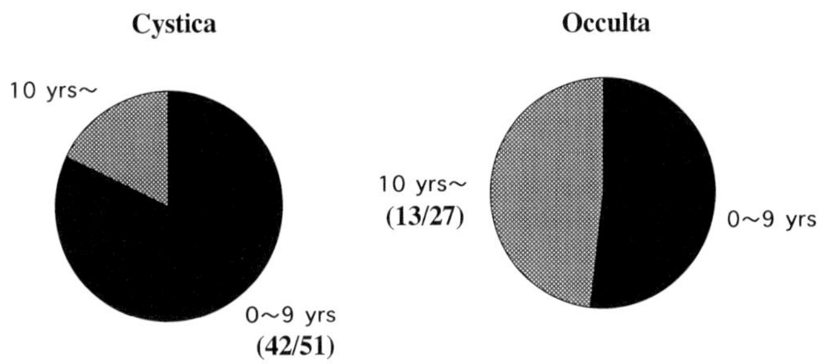

FIG. 2. Age at operation

Regarding the patient's age at operation, 42/51 of the foot surgery cases were indicated before the age of 9 years in cystica patients, but the timing of surgery tended to be delayed in occulta cases. There were 13/27 cases above the age of 10 years in the occulta group. This is because foot deformities develop in occulta patients as the children gradually begin to walk more and gain body weight (Fig. 2).

In our surgical management study there were 39 tendon transfers. We also prefer to do soft tissue release (29 cases) to the equinus, equinovarus, and varus cases. In the bone surgery patients, 4 cases of varus were treated with Evans procedure [1]. For valgus, we performed the Grice-Green procedure [2], but one case needed a further operation, i.e., triple arthrodesis, and for patients with cavovarus, we try to do 1st metatarsal osteotomy (Table 4).

Regarding orthotic requirements after surgery, all of the equinovarus, varus, and valgus cases still need orthoses (AFO), but 11/19 of the calcaneus cases and 6/9 of the cavovarus cases showed no orthotic requirements (Table 5).

TABLE 4. Operative method

	Soft tissue release	Tendon transfer	Bone surgery
Equinus	8		
Equinovarus	9	3	
Varus	4	10	4
Valgus		3	7 (1)[a]
Calcaneus		19	
Cavovarus	8	4	4[b]
Total	29	39	15

[a] Triple arthrodesis.
[b] Osteotomy.

TABLE 5. Orthoses

		AFO	With cane
Equinus	$n = 8$	2	2
Equinovarus	$n = 12$	12	3
Varus	$n = 13$	13	1
Valgus	$n = 10$	10	
Calcaneus	$n = 19$	8	
Cavovarus	$n = 9$	3	

Discussion and Conclusions

The goals of orthopedic operative management should be to upgrading function not to correct the deformity. The patients should be treated according to whether they are ambulatory or nonambulatory. Orthopedic surgery is probably most beneficial in the treatment of foot problems in spina bifida patients. The objectives of surgical treatment are to obtain an easier fitting of orthoses and a stable walking pattern with plantigrade feet and muscle balance. In patients of L2 or higher level, the indication for foot surgery was uncontrolled rigid equinovarus, where it is difficult to put the foot on the footplate of a wheelchair. The lower lumbar and sacral roots, which innervate the muscles of the foot and ankle, are the most common levels of paralysis. The muscle imbalance creates various foot deformities. We operate to correct deformities or muscle imbalance, to get a brace or shoe on a plantigrade foot, and to keep it comfortable and free from pressure sores, or eventually to get rid of the brace.

Menelaus recommended that surgery to correct muscle imbalance and limb deformity should be carried out around the age of two years, but said that surgery at a later age is frequently necessary either because new deformities have appeared or because previously treated deformities have recurred [4]. Our study showed the same result.

A comparison between cystica and occulta showed that the operation rate in L5 or lower lesions of cystica was 12/53, but it was up to 17/25 in occulta. More equinus and equinovarus deformities were found in cystica cases, but there was more cavovarus in occulta cases. Also, 42/51 of the foot surgery cases were indicated before the age of 9 years in cystica patients, but the timing of surgery tended to be delayed in occulta cases, and 13/27 of the cases were after the age of 10 years.

Tendon transfers to correct muscle imbalance were performed on 39 cases. All of the equinovarus, varus, and valgus patients still needed some orthoses after the operation, but some of the calcaneus and cavovarus patients had no orthotic requirements.

References

1. Evans D (1975) Calcaneo-valgus deformity. J Bone Joint Surg 57B:270–278
2. Grice DS (1952) An extra-articular arthrodesis of the subastragalar joint for correction of paralytic flat feet in children. J Bone Joint Surg 34A:927–940
3. Hoffer MM, Feiwell E, Perry R, Perry J, Bonnet C (1973) Functional ambulation in patients with myelomeningocele. J Bone Joint Surg 55A:137–148
4. Menelaus MB (1980) The orthopaedic management of spina bifida cystica. 2nd edn. Churchill Livingstone, New York
5. Sharrard WJW, Grosfield I (1968) The management of deformity and paralysis of the foot in myelomeningocele. J Bone Joint Surg 50B:456–465

Delayed Neurological Disorders of the Lower Extremities in Patients with Spina Bifida

HIRONORI ITO and TAKASHI OKI

Summary. In order to clarify the delayed onset of neurological disorders in patients with spina bifida, 70 patients who had been followed for at least 15 years from infancy were assessed retrospectively. There were 51 myelomeningoceles, 17 lipomeningoceles, and 2 meningoceles. Cavus deformity was seen in 26 patients (50 feet) (age range 2–17 years), spastic paralysis of a lower limb was found in 9 patients (age range 3–10 years), and an increase of flaccid paralysis was found in 4 patients (age range 6–14 years). Tethered cord syndrome was one of the major causes of delayed dysfunction in lower extremities. It was thought that the appearance or exacerbation of neurological disorders were seen in their growth period. In our study, 70% of the cavus deformities seen were in patients below 8 years old. In the spastic and flaccid paralysis group, dysfunction was seen between 5 years and 8 years of age in more than 50% of the patients.

Key words. Spina bifida, Delayed neurological disorder, Cavus deformity, Paralysis, Lower extremities

Introduction

Reports of deformity or paralysis of the lower extremities which occurs during or after childfood are rare. The purpose of this study was to clarify the relationship between patients' age and the manifestation of disorders.

Material and Methods

We retrospectively assessed 70 patients with spina bifida who had been followed for at least 15 years from infancy. There were 39 males and 31 females. The diagnoses of the patients were as follows: myelomeningocele, 51 (73%); lipomeningocele, 17 (17%); meningocele, 2 (3%). The level and number of the motor lesion were: thoracic, 4 legs; L1, 3; L2, 14; L3, 19; L4, 33; L5, 33; S1, 19; S2, 9; S3, 6.

Department of Orthopaedic Surgery, Central Hospital, Aichi Prefectural Colony, 713-8 Kagiya-cho, Kasugai, Aichi 480-0392, Japan

In this study, we evaluated neurological disorders of the lower extremities which were not observed at birth. These were pes cavus, talipes equinus, and spastic and flaccid paralysis of lower extremities.

Results

Cavus deformity was seen in 50 feet of 26 patients, 36% of total cases. There were 20 patients with myelomeningocele, 4 with lipomeningocele, and 2 with meningocele. They were all community ambulators except for one household ambulator. Their ages when the symptoms appeared ranged from 2 years to 17 years 7 months (mean 8 years 1 month; Table 1). The levels of motor lesion were L3 in 3 feet, L4 in 9, L5 in 16, S1 in 12, S2 in 6, and S3 in 4. The relationship between the motor lesion level and cavus deformity is shown in Fig. 1. This reveals that the incidence of cases with cavus are high in the group with lesion below L5. The deformities of talipes equinus associated with, or manifested after, cavus deformity were seen in 19 feet of 11 patients, i.e., 38% of cavus deformities. There were 7 patients with myelomeningocele, and 2 with lipomeningocele and meningocele. The ages when symptoms appeared ranged from 2 years 10 months to 15 years 2 months (mean 8 years 7 months; Table 1). The levels of motor lesion were L4 and L5 in 3 feet, S1 in 6, S2 in 4, and S3 in 3 (Fig. 1).

Spastic paralysis of a lower extremity was seen in 9 patients. There were 8 patients with myelomeningocele and 1 with meningocele. The ages when the symptoms appeared ranged from 3 years 4 months to 10 years 1 month (mean 6 years 9 months). We diagnosed spasticity mainly by the stretch reflex of the leg muscle and the tendon reflex. Evaluations of each patient are shown in Table 2. Spasticity of the hamstrings and adductor muscles was remarkable in cases with lumbar lesion. An increase in the patellar tendon reflex and the Achilles tendon reflex, and the appearance of ankle clonus, were remarkable in cases with sacral lesions. In this group, 7 of 9 patients had cavus deformity.

An increase in flaccid paralysis was seen in 4 patients; there were 2 with myelomeningocele and one with lipomeningocele. Their ages when the symptoms appeared ranged from 6 years 11 months to 14 years 4 months (mean 9 years 11 months). Their motor disturbance and symptoms are shown in Table 3. The cause of disorders in patients with a lesion of L1 was invasion of the lipoma and traction of the filum terminale. The cause of the disorder in

Table 1. Age of symptom appearance

Age (years)	Cavus deformity (No. of feet)	Equinus with cavus (No. of feet)
2	3	1
3	2	0
4	2	3
5	7	4
6	5	2
7	6	0
8	10	2
9	3	2
10	2	0
≧11	10	5

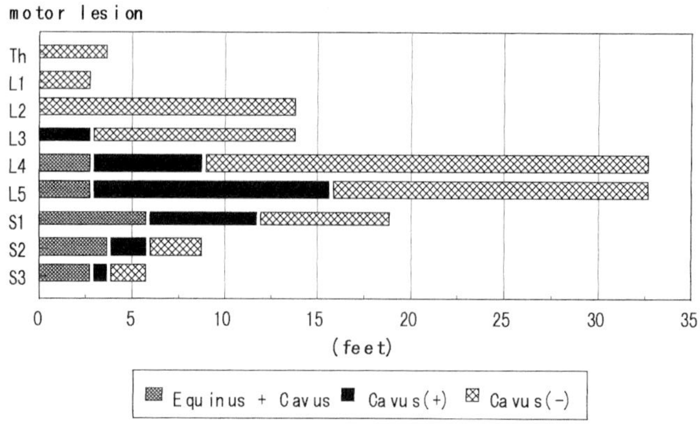

FIG. 1. Relationship of the motor lesion level and foot deformity

TABLE 2. Patients with spastic paralysis

Case level/sex	Age[a] (years/months)	Ham.[b] ↑	Add.[c] ↑	PTR[d] ↑	ART[e] ↑	Ankle clonus
L2 M	6/1	+				
L3 F	10/1	+	+			
L4 M	3/4	+	+	+		
L5 M	10/1	+		+		
L5 M	5/3	+	+			
S1 M	8/10			+		
S2 M	5/0			+	+	+
S2 M	6/7				+	+
S3 F	7/2			+		

[a] Age of symptom appearance.
[b] Stretch reflex of hamstrings.
[c] Stretch reflex of adductor muscles.
[d] Patellar tendon reflex.
[e] Achilles tendon reflex.

TABLE 3. Patients with flaccid paralysis

Case level/sex	Age of symptom appearance (years/months)	MMT hip	MMT knee
L1 M	7/4	Ext 3 → 0–2	Ext 4 → 2
L2 F	11/0	Ext/abd 2 → 0	Ext 3 → 2
L2 F	6/11		Ext/flex 4–3 → 2
L4 F	14/4		Ext 4 → 3

MMT, Manual muscle testing.

the patient with L4 lesion was traction of the filum terminale. In other patients, the causes of their symptoms were uncertain. In this group, no patient showed cavus deformity.

Discussion

The activity of patients with spina bifida often decreases during their growth period, and there is the possibility of the appearance of neurological disorders as they grow. The major neurological disorders seen during childhood or adolescence are deformity or paralysis of the lower extremities, pain in the lumbus or lower extremities, and dysfunction of the bladder and bowel. In our cases, however, there were few patients who complained of these problems. There are many pathogenetic causes affecting nerve function. Tethered cord syndrome is one of the major causes of decreased nerve function, especially in the lower extremities. Although all children with spina bifida have the possibility of the complication of a tethered cord, only a few actually have symptoms [3]. For these patients, surgical release of the tethered cord provides recovery of lost function. In our cases the existence of a tethered cord was uncertain, and therefore brace treatment and surgery for foot deformities were the main procedures. The second cause of decreasing nerve function is a developing lipoma. This may disturb the lumbosacral roots by direct pressure on, or invasion upon, the nerve elements. The third factor is syringomyelia. In our series, there was one patient with spastic paralysis caused by syringomyelia. Arnord-Chiari malformation and hydrocephalus may produce dysfunction not only in the lower extremities but also in the upper extremities.

The age of appearance or exacerbation of neurological disorders is generally thought to be in the growth period [4]. However, the ages reported in the past have varied. James [2] reported that it was between 2 years and 6 years, while Anderson [1] said it was between 1 year 6 months and 16 years. Yamane et al. [5] reported that neural disorders occured before 3 years in 70% of patients, and before 5 years in 87%. In our study, the ages of symptom appearance were as follows. Symptoms of cavus deformity ranged from 2 years to 17 years; 70% of patients were below 8 years, and 56% were 5- to 8-year-old patients. The spastic paralysis group ranged from 3 years to 10 years, and 60% of patients were from 5 years to 8 years old. The flaccid paralysis group ranged 6 years to 14 years, and 50% of patients were from 5 years to 8 years old.

We analyzed the factors causing every symptom. Cavus deformity occurs because of paralysis of the intrinsic muscles of the foot by traction or distortion of the spinal cord, and equinus is caused by muscle imbalance owing to spasticity of the triceps surae. These symptoms often appear in tethered cord syndrome. The causes of spastic paralysis are mainly a disturbance of the spinal cord. Our cases suggested that the main causative factors are tethering of the spinal cord, the growth of the patients, and syringomyelia. The factors causing flaccid paralysis are considered to be a disturbance of the nerve roots. Some definite causes are tethering of the film terminale, adhesion of a nerve, invasion of the lipoma, growth of the patient, ischemia of the filum terminale, and disturbance of the nerve roots.

Conclusion

Tethered cord syndrome is a major cause of decreased neurological function of the lower extremities. Almost all children with spina bifida have a tetherd cord at birth. As the patient grows, deformities and increasing paralysis of the lower extremities frequently occur. It has generally been considered that neurological disorders are related to growth spurts, but in our study, the symptoms appeared in the age range from 5 to 8 years in more than half of the patients. That is before the growth spurt. On the other hand, symptoms appeared after 11 years old in about 20% of patients. Various delayed neurological disorders of the lower extremities may occur in patients with spina bifida before and during the growth period. These data indicate that continuous observation of the neurological status is important for children with spina bifida.

References

1. Anderson FM (1975) Occult spinal dysraphism. A series of 73 cases. Pediatrics 55:826–835
2. James CCM (1962) Spinal dysraphism. The diagnosis and treatment of prognosis lesions in spina bifida occulta. J Bone Joint Surg 44-B:828–840
3. Lindseth RE (1990) Myelomeningocele. In: Morrissy RT (ed) Pediatric orthopaedics. JB Lippincott, Philadelphia, pp 507–538
4. Nakamura T (1984) Diagnosis and treatment of tethered spinal cord syndrome, based on experience of 77 cases. J Jpn Orthop Assoc 58:1237–1251
5. Yamane Y, Kamegaya M, Shinada Y (1991) Clinical aspects of over 10-year-old patients with spinal dysraphism. Rinsho Seikei Geka (Clinical Orthopaedic Surgery) 26:401–406

Results of Achilles Tenodesis and Posterior Transfer of the Tibialis Anterior Tendon for Residual Calcaneous Deformity of Spina Bifida

Yutaka Oketani, Toshio Fujii, Akihiko Takashima, Kazuyuki Takamura, and Syusaku Matsuda

Summary. We retrospectively evaluated nine children who had lower-lumbar-level spina bifida and who had undergone Achilles tenodesis and transfer of the tibialis anterior to the calcaneus. The power of plantar flexion after transfer of the tibialis anterior to the calcaneus improved within 2 years in all cases but one. However, some cases had a tendency to lose power for a short period just after surgery. The power of plantar flexion after Achilles tenodesis and transfer of the tibialis anterior to the calcaneus improved within 1–3 years in most cases. In these cases, there was no tendency to lose power for a short period just after surgery. In relation to brace usage and condition at last follow-up, there were cases who used lightweight plastic ankle–foot orthosis (AFO) and no braces in both groups. However, there were some cases who needed a solid, heavy AFO and knee–ankle–foot orthosis (KAFO) because of the development of a varus deformity of the foot.

Key words. Tendon transfer, Calcaneous deformity, Spina bifida, Achilles tenodesis

Introduction

Residual calcaneous deformity of spina bifida often makes the foot unstable when standing, meaning that such patients are at a disadvantage for walking. An ankle–foot orthosis improves the ability to walk, but weight and cosmetic problems occur with growth. To treat this surgically, we performed a posterior transfer of the tibialis anterior tendon and Achilles tenodesis to improve foot instability and decrease the weight of the orthosis. There follows a summary and report of our results.

Materials and Methods

We retrospectively evaluated nine children who had lower-lumbar-level spina bifida and who had undergone Achilles tenodesis and transfer of the tibialis anterior to the calcaneus. The mean age at the time of surgery was 9.5 years, and the patients were monitored for an average of 4 years. Two of the patients had L5 neurosegmental levels, and seven had sacral levels. Preoperatively, all of the patients were community ambulators, and all used ankle–foot or knee–ankle–foot orthoses.

Fukuoka Children's Hospital, 2-5-1 Toujin-machi, Chuou-ku, Fukuoka, Japan

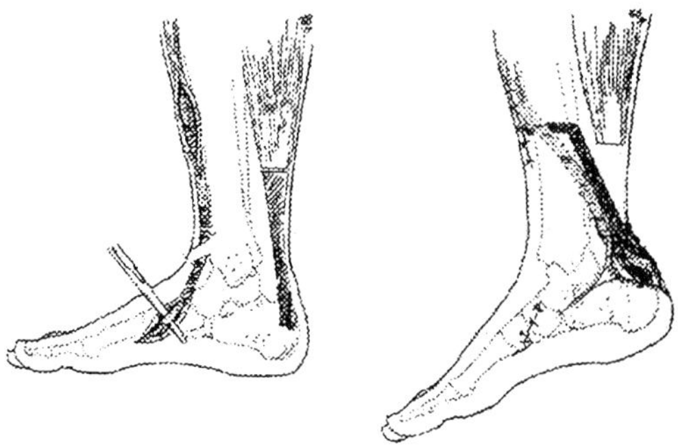

FIG. 1. A modification of the procedure described by Herndon et al. [1]

A modification of the procedure described by Herndon et al. [1] was used for the posterior transfer of the tibialis anterior muscle tendon. The tibialis anterior muscle was harvested at its insertion and passed through a window in the interosseous membrane to the posterior aspect of the calf. The tendon was then passed through a drilled hole in the calcaneus and secured with a suture of either wire or nonabsorbable multifilament nylon surgical strand tied over a button. Recently, we have occasionally used an anchoring device instead of this pull-through technique to transfer the tendon. We also cut the proximal end of the Achilles tendon and pulled the cut end through the drilled hole from the posterial to the anterial side of the tibia, and then sutured its end to the periosteum of the tibia (Fig. 1).

The indication for surgery was the presence of flexible calcaneal deformities of both feet. The preoperative tibialis anterior muscle strength was graded as level 4 or better in all cases using the manual muscle test (MMT). Depending on the power of their gastrocnemius–soleus complex, we selected one of two procedures, i.e. a posterior transfer of the tibialis anterior tendon, or a combination of a posterior transfer of the tibialis anterior tendon and Achilles tenodesis. Firstly, if the calf muscle was over MMT level 3, we undertook the posterior transfer of the tibialis anterior tendon only (group A). Secondly, if the calf muscle was under level 1, we performed the posterior transfer of the tibialis anterior tendon and Achilles tenodesis (group B).

Postoperative immobilization in a long-leg cast for 3 weeks was followed by a short-leg cast for an additional 3 weeks in the plantar flexion position. The patients were then fitted with a solid ankle–foot orthosis fixed at neutral, and encouraged to be mobile with full weight-bearing for 3–6 months. Six months after surgery, the patients, depending on their condition, used a soft, light-weight plastic ankle–foot orthosis fixed at neutral.

Observations and Results

Group A comprised 8 feet, and group B comprised 6 feet. The mean age at the time of surgery of group A was 9 years and 4 months, and that of group B was 8 years and 2 months. The average follow-up period for group A was 2 years and 9 months, and that for group B was 3 years and 9 months.

Group A had only one case who had a severe varus deformity of the foot, for which the medial release of the foot and triple arthrodesis was also necessary. However, for the other cases we only performed the posterior transfer of the tibialis anterior tendon and the additional plantar release of the foot (Steindler's operation) when necessary. The combined surgical procedures of group B had few cases which underwent the plantar release of the foot in addition to the posterior transfer of the tibialis anterior tendon and the Achilles tenodesis (Table 1).

TABLE 1. Additional operations of groups A and B

Group A								Group B						
Case	Level	Side	Age (years)	TA	Steindler	MR	Arthrodesis	Case	Level	Side	Age (years)	TA	AT	Steindler
Y.S.	L5	R	7	○	○			A.I.	L5	R	16.5	○	○	
		L	8	○	○			T.J.	L5	R	5.1	○	○	○
T.K.	L5	R	11.6	○	○					L	4.6	○	○	○
A.S.	L4	R	4.3	○	○									
A.H.	L5	L	16.6	○	○	○	○	Y.U.	L4	R	10.9	○	○	
T.N.	L5	R	12.4	○				H.N.	L5	R	6.1	○	○	○
		L	10.5	○	○					L	6.1	○	○	○
A.I.	L5	L	12.5	○										

TA, posterior transfer of the tibialis anterior tendon; AT, Achilles tenodesis; MR, medial release.

The power of plantar flexion of group A improved within 2 years after surgery in all cases but one. However, some cases had a tendency to lose power for a short period just after surgery. The power of plantar flexion of group B improved within 1–3 years in most cases. There was no tendency to lose power for a short period just after surgery (Fig. 2).

In relation to brace usage and condition at last follow-up, there were cases who used a lightweight plastic AFO and no braces in both groups. For example, one child managed to win a prize in an electric organ competition, and another child ran in a 1500-m race after treatment. However, there were some cases who needed a solid heavy AFO or KAFO because of the development of a varus deformity of the foot (Table 2).

Discussion and Conclusion

Patients with calcaneous deformities had some problems in walking. They walked with the knees in the flexion position and the ankle in the dorsiflexion position. Because they were unstable when standing on one foot, their stride length tended to be short. As their power to push off the floor was weak, their walking speed was slow.

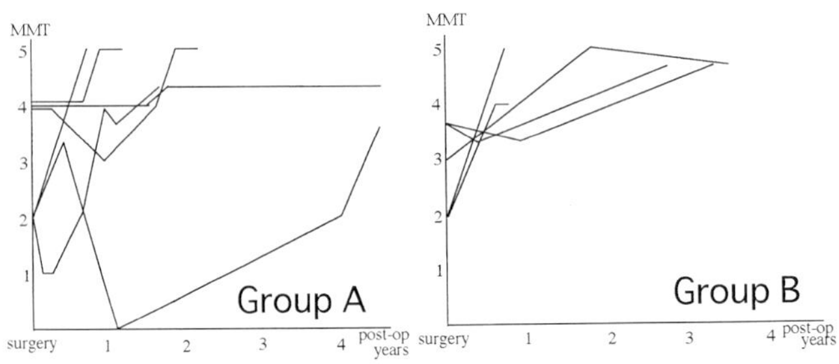

Fig. 2. Changes in plantar flexion muscle power. Group A improved within 2 years after surgery in all cases but one. Some cases had a tendency to lose power for a short period just after surgery. Group B improved within 1–3 years in most cases. There was no tendency to lose power for a short period just after surgery

Table 2. Condition at last follow-up

Case		Preop.	Postop.	Age (years)	Condition at last follow-up
A	Y.S.	Bil. KAFO	Bil. AFO	9	Running possible for 1.5 km
	A.S.	Bil. AFO	Free	7	Toe gait stable
	T.K.	Bil. AFO	Bil. HTS	14	Walking without orthosis
	A.H.	Bil. AFO	Bil. AFO	18	
	T.N.	Bil. AFO	Bil. AFO	15	Toe gait possible
	T.J.	Lt. AFO	Lt. AFO	8	
B	T.J.	Rt. AFO	Rt. HTS	8	
	A.I.	Bil. AFO	Lt. AFO Rt. AFO	17	Inside gait possible without orthosis
	H.N.	Bil. AFO	Rt. AFO	12	Varus deformity of right foot
	Y.U.	Bil. KAFO	Rt. AFO Lt. KAFO	11	Walking ability improved without orthosis

AFO, ankle–foot orthosis; KAFO, knee–ankle–foot orthosis; Bil., bitaleral; Lt., left; Rt., right.

Formerly, we performed surgical treatment using the posterior transfer of the tibialis anterior muscle tendon only for all patients who had problems walking. However, we noticed that in patients who had weaker plantar flexion power before the operation, there was a tendency for their plantar flexion power not to improve after surgery. To get more plantar flexion power and foot stability, we decided to perform the posterior transfer of the tibialis anterior tendon and Achilles tenodesis together. The reason for this is that in Japan shoes are not worn inside the house, which means that spina bifida patients are unable to wear braces indoors. It is therefore desirable to improve push-off power, if possible, so that the patients can function in bare feet indoors. We therefore selected a number of cases to undergo surgical treatment using these criteria. Consequently, they could use a lighter orthosis, and improve their standard of daily life indoors because of their foot stability.

The results of Achilles tenodesis and posterior transfer of the tibialis anterior tendon for residual calcaneous deformity of spina bifida are as follows.

1. There was no difference in MMT between the two groups.
2. The combined procedures of the posterior transfer of the tibialis anterior tendon and Achilles tenodesis improved plantar flexion power, and enabled the patients to use a lighter orthoses than with the posterior transfer of the tibialis anterior tendon alone.
3. In patients who underwent the posterior transfer of the tibialis anterior tendon and the Achilles tenodesis, foot stability improved when walking barefooted.

Reference

1. Herndon CH, Serong JM, Heyman CH (1956) Transposition of the tibialis anterior in the treatment of paralytic talipes calcaneus. J Bone Joint Surg 38A:751–760

Management of Ankle and Hindfoot Valgus in Spina Bifida

Luciano Dias

Valgus deformity of the ankle joint is commonly seen in the L4–L5-level spina bifida child. Valgus deformity can be a significant problem for brace fitting in the low-lumbar-level child. Clinically, these children consistently have a calcaneus foot with a valgus ankle associated with external tibial torsion. The gastrosoleus strength is 0, and excessive laxity of the Achilles tendon is seen, characterized by marked passive ankle dorsiflexion beyond 30°–40°. The deformity can be seen quite early, but it becomes more severe, leading to problems with orthotic fitting, and with medial malleolar pressure sores, around the ages of 4–6 years or older.

In the normal ankle joint, the fibula usually extends more distally than the tibia, and the relationship among the medial malleolus, the lateral malleolus, and the talus is important for the normal biomechanics of the ankle joint.

When growth at the lower tibial epiphysis is interrupted, a relative overgrowth of the fibula takes place which results in a varus deformity at the ankle. In the paralytic limb, abnormal shortening of the fibula and of the lateral malleolus result in valgus tilt of the talus, with subsequent valgus deformity at the ankle.

In 1981, we reported an extensive study on valgus deformity of the ankle joint in myelomeningocele and abnormal shortening of the fibula [4]. It was found that a relative shortening of the fibula was a quite common radiological finding, but that a clinically significant valgus deformity of the ankle does not occur so frequently, being seen mainly in the L4–L5-level child.

Roentgenographic Measurement of Fibular Shortening

No radiological criteria quantitates fibular length at the ankle level. In 1981, Dias devised a radiological method to quantitate the degree of fibular shortening [4].

The fibular growth plate is more sharply defined than the tip of the lateral malleolus in anteroposterior ankle roentgenographs. Therefore the relationship between the distal fibular growth plate and the dome of the talus can be used as a measure of fibular length. In a normal ankle, the distal fibular growth plate is located approximately 2–3 mm proximal to the dome of the talus during the first 4 years of life. After the age of 6, the distal fibular growth plate

Department of Orthopaedic Surgery, Northwestern University, 680 N. Lakeshorf Dr. Suite Chicago, IL 60611, USA will gradually become distal to the dome of the talus, and over the age of 8, the fibular growth plate is approximately 2–3 mm distal to the dome of the talus.

We studied 86 ankles in spina bifida children, which showed that the amount of shortening was related to the patient's age, with an average yearly progression of 1.3 mm.

We also noted that the paralysis of the soleus musculature had a direct relationship to the fibular length. In the group of patients in which the soleus was rated as poor-minus to poor, the average shortening was 7.2 mm (range 5–8 mm). In the group of patients in which the soleus was completely paralyzed, the average shortening was more than 10 mm. Therefore, in spina bifida, a shortening of the fibula seems to be secondary to soleus paralysis.

In the normal ankle joint, the tibial and talar articular surfaces are parallel. With the abnormal growth of the fibula and fibular shortening, the normal distribution of forces applied to the tibial articular surface is altered and this, according to the growth curve proposed by Frost [5a], leads to an abnormal growth of the epiphysis. The increased compression forces applied to the lateral portion of the tibial epiphysis inhibit cartilage growth, and a decrease in compression forces on the medial portion of the tibial epiphysis accelerates growth. Such an imbalance creates a valgus tilt of the tibial articular surface, which is directly related to the degree of fibular shortening. A moderate to severe degree of lateral wedging is seen in children when the amount of shortening exceeds 10 mm.

Treatment

Surgical treatment of a valgus ankle is indicated when the deformity causes problems with orthotic fitting and cannot be alleviated by orthotic changes. Three different methods of surgical treatment have been described. Tendo-Achilles tenodesis to the fibula was first described by Westin and Defiore [16] for patients with poliomyelitis. Dias, and more recently, Stevens and Toomey [14, 15], described the operation for patients with spina bifida. Our long-term follow-up after this procedure has shown unpredictable results. In about 30% of our cases we noticed stretching of the tenodesis, leading to minimal stimulation of the fibular growth. At present we do not advise this treatment. A hemiepiphysiodesis is indicated for mild deformities. Recently, Stevens (PM Stevens, personal communication) has presented his experience with this technique using a cannulated ankle orthosis (AO) screw. It is important to place the screw in the most medial position, and completely vertical. This procedure can be done in the outpatient department. In order to avoid a permanent closure of the physis, Stevens has advised removal of the screw within 2 years of its insertion. We have limited experience with this procedure at present. In the past, we have used the technique described by Burkus et al. [3] using staples or the Pfemister technique. We feel that the cannulated screw technique is easier, and we advise the use of this technique for the hemiepiphysiodesis. With the growth arrest of the medial aspect of the physis, and continued growth of the lateral aspect, there is a gradual correction of the lateral wedging of the tibial epiphysis, which corrects the valgus tilt. If overcorrection occurs, the epiphysiodesis should be completed laterally.

In a more severe valgus ankle deformity in an older child with no growth potential remaining, we suggest supramalleolar varus derotation osteotomy. Osteotomies of the distal tibia have a high incidence of complications such as delayed union, nonunion, wound infection, wound dehiscence, and loss of correction. To prevent some of these complications, multiple holes should be drilled and the osteotomy should be completed with an osteotome rather than with power instruments. If any rotational misalignment is present, which is commonly seen in external tibial torsion, then at the same time that the valgus deformity is corrected, a derotation of the distal fragment should be performed. We advise the use of a long-leg cast, nonweight-bearing, for 3 weeks followed by a short-leg weight-bearing cast for another 3 weeks, or until there is complete healing of the osteotomy.

Recently, Lubicky (J Lubicky, personal communication, 1996), from the Shriners Hospital in Chicago, presented his experience with a very low wedge osteotomy, very close to the tibial plafond, leading to an excellent correction of the valgus deformity.

When analyzing a valgus deformity, it is also important to recognize that frequently there may be an associated valgus hindfoot. In this situation, a medial sliding osteotomy of the os calcis is indicated. The supramalleolar varus osteotomy and the medial sliding osteotomy can be done at the same time.

Valgus Hindfoot

Excessive valgus hindhoot is often associated with a valgus deformity at the ankle joint, which exacerbates the valgus hindfoot. Initially, this deformity can be controlled with a well-fitting orthosis.

The indications for surgical treatment of a valgus deformity of the hindfoot is limited to patients with pressure sores, callosities, or problems with shoe wear or bracing. Among a number of procedures designed to correct valgus hindfoot deformity, medial displacement osteotomy of the os calcis appears to be a simple and effective procedure, with the correction based on the realignment of the os calcis and a new orientation for the action of the Achilles tendon. The concept of displacement osteotomy of the os calcis is not new, and was well described by Koutsogiannis [8a] in 1971 as a treatment for idiopathic flat foot. Koman et al. [8] also used the procedure to treat cerebral palsy and other neuromuscular diseases. We have been using this technique in spina bifida since 1981. We strongly advise against any subtalar joint fusion such as the Grice extraarticular arthrodesis, which has been described as the classic approach for valgus hindfoot.

Recently, Gallien [6] reported on experience with subtalar arthrodesis in children with spina bifida. Of the 14 cases, 61% were successful. Ross and Lyne [10a], however, reported 80% unsatisfactory results in spina bifida.

Medial displacement osteotomy has been reported by several authors as an effective means of correction for valgus hindfoot.

Postoperatively, the K-wire that is used for internal fixation is removed at 2 weeks, and then a short-leg walking cast is applied for another 4 weeks.

Torosian [15a], Dias, and Gabrieli reviewed their experiences with this procedure in 38 feet in 27 patients; they reported that 82% of patients had a satisfactory result. As part of the procedure, any associated soft tissue contractures should be corrected at the same time, such as peroneus tendon release or Achilles tendon release. Any rotational misalignment should also be addressed by an osteotomy of the tibia, with seven having been performed in this study.

The final goal of the treatment is a supple, plantigrade, and braceable foot, which is the reason why we feel that subtalar joint arthrodesis is contraindicated in spina bifida.

References

1. Banra JV, Sutherland DH, Wyatt M (1982) Anterior tibial transfer to the os calcis with Achilles tenodesis for calcaneal deformity in myelomeningocele. J Pediatr Orthop 1:125
2. Bliss HG, Menelaus MG (1986) The results of transfer of the tibialis anterior to the heel in patients who have a myelomeningocele. J Bone Joint Surg 68A:1258

3. Burkus JK, Moore DW, Raycroft JF (1983) Valgus deformity of the ankle in myelodysplastic patients: correction by stapling of the medial part of the distal phisis. J Bone Joint Surg 65A:1157
4. Dias LS (1981) Ankle valgus in children with myelomeningocele. Dev Med Child Neurol 20:627
5. Dias LS, Busch M, Tachdjian MO (1987) Surgical treatment of severe hindfoot valgus by medial displacement osteotomy of the os calcis. Orthop Trans 11:35
5a. Frost HM (1973) Bone modeling and skeletal modeling enoses. Thomas, Springfield (IL)
6. Gallien R, Morin F, Marquis F (1989) Subtalar arthrodesis in children. J Pediatr Orthop 9:59
7. Gross PM, Lyne D (1980) The Grice procedure: indications and evaluation of long-term results. Clin Orthop 153:193
8. Koman LA, Mooney JF, Goodman A (1993) Management of valgus hindfoot deformity in pediatric cerebral palsy patients by medial displacement osteotomy. J Pediatr Orthop 13:180–183
8a. Koutsogiannis E (1971) Treatment of mobile flatfoot by displacement osteotomy of the calcaneus. J Bone Joint Surg (Br) 53:96
9. Mahorta D, Puri R, Owen R (1984) Valgus deformity of the ankle in children with spina bifida aperta. J Bone Joint Surg 66B:381
10. Maskin M (1965) Tibiofibular relationship in paralysed limbs. J Bone Joint Surg 47B:500
10a. Ross PM, Lyne D (1980) The Grice procedure indications and evaluation of long-term results. Clin Orthop 153:195
11. Sanda JPS, Skinner SR, Banto PS (1984) Posterior transfer of the tibialis anterior in low level myelodysplasia. Dev Med Child Neurol 26:100
12. Schafer MF, Dias LS (1983) Myelomeningocele: orthopaedic treatment. Williams and Wilkins, Baltimore, p 160
13. Sharrard WJW, Webb J (1974) Supramalleolar wedge osteotomy of the tibia in children with myelomeningocele. J Bone Joint Surg 56B:458
14. Stevens PM (1987) Relative hypoplasia of fibula and associated ankle valgus. J Pediatr Orthop 7:605
15. Stevens PM, Toomey E (1988) Fibular achilles tenodesis for paralytic ankle valgus. J Pediatr Orthop 8:169
15a. Torosian C (1995) American Academy of Orthopedic Surgery. Orlando, February 20, 1995
16. Westin GW, Defiore RJ (1975) Tenodesis of the tendo-achilles to the fibula for a paralytic calcaneus deformity. J Bone Joint Surg 56-A:1541

Evaluation and Treatment of Pes Cavus in Spina Bifida

James G. Gamble

Summary. Cavus feet become a problem for patients with spina bifida as they enter school age and progress into adolescence. Cavus is an abnormally high-arched foot with associated soft tissue and skeletal changes. The types of cavus are cavovarus, calcaneocavus, and cavoplantaris. Mobility is graded as first degree for supple cavus feet, second degree for feet with some rigidity, and third degree for rigid cavus with contracture and articular deformity. Soft tissue releases are used for supple cavus, and osteotomies are required to correct bony deformity. For severely nonplantigrade, rigid pes cavus, a Hoke-type triple arthrodesis can restore a satisfactory plantigrade position.

Key words. Cavus foot, Cavovarus, Calcaneocavus, Spina bifida

Introduction

Foot deformity that requires surgical correction occurs in more than 90% of children with spina bifida [2, 3]. However, it is usually when children with spina bifida reach school age or adolescence that pes cavus becomes a problem. The purpose of this chapter is to discuss four questions concerning cavus feet in children with spina bifida: (1) What is pes cavus? (2) Why is it a serious problem? (3) How can we evaluate it? (4) How can we treat cavus feet in patients with spina bifida?

What is Pes Cavus?

Pes cavus is a foot that has an abnormally high arch, and pes cavus has some component of forefoot plantar flexion on the midfoot and is associated with other changes such as soft tissue contractures and bony deformities. The major soft tissue contractures in pes cavus involve the plantar fascia and clawing of the toes. The bony deformities include dorsiflexion and varus of the calcaneus, plus equinus and varus of the forefoot.

Guillaume Duchenne (1806–1875) investigated cavus feet in the nineteenth century using the newly discovered galvanic methods. He concluded that cavus is caused by an imbalance between the relatively strong extrinsic muscles and weaker intrinsic muscles of the foot. Since

Orthopaedic Surgery, Stanford University School of Medicine, Packard Children's Hospital, Palo Alto, CA 94304-5341, USA

Duchenne's contributions, our scientific understanding of the cause of cavus has not advanced very much.

However, we have advanced in our understanding of the varieties of cavus feet and in the subtleties associated with treatment. We understand that not all cavus feet are alike, and this recognition has led to a classification based on the type and severity of the deformities [6]. There are three general types of pes cavus. *Cavovarus* is a foot with the major deformity involving plantar flexion of the first ray and varus of the heel. *Calcaneocavus* is a foot where the primary deformity is dorsiflexion of the calcaneus coupled with plantar flexion of the forefoot. *Cavoplantaris* is a foot with minimal involvement of the calcaneus, but with the forefoot in severe plantar flexion at the first and fifth rays. The severity of cavus deformity is graded as *first degree* if the foot is supple and passively correctable, *second degree* if passive correction is limited by soft tissue contractures, and *third degree* if the foot is rigidly deformed due to articular, skeletal, and soft tissue changes.

Why is it a Problem?

Prior to school age, pes cavus is usually an incidental finding in patients with spina bifida. During school years and adolescence, a patient with spina bifida who has pes cavus feet that are rigid and insensate can have great difficulty with shoe fit, and can experience decreased standing balance and increased gait instability. These patients have a markedly uneven weight distribution, with more pressure being taken by the lateral border of the foot and the metatarsal heads. They develop plantar callosities which can progress to pressure ulceration, soft tissue infection, and even osteomyelitis.

Brinker et al. [1] reported a very high incidence of foot problems in sacral-level spina bifida. In 36 skeletally mature patients, 27 had skin breakdown on the foot, 23 had soft tissue infection, and 15 had developed osteomyelitis in at least one bone of the foot. Kinsman and Doehring [4] reviewed 98 hospital admissions of adult spina bifida patients and determined that 47% of their problems were due to preventable conditions such as renal calculi, urologic infection, and pressure ulceration, including foot ulceration. After evaluating clinical indicators of foot ulceration in ambulatory patients with spina bifida, Maynard et al. [5] found a correlation with foot rigidity, nonplantigrade position, and past performance of a surgical arthrodesis. We have found that the most serious problem for adolescents with rigid pes cavus is pressure ulceration along the lateral border of the foot or the metatarsal heads, and this is associated with the nonplantigrade position.

How is Pes Cavus Specifically Evaluated?

As with any foot problem, the evaluation begins with a visual inspection of the dorsal and plantar surfaces of the foot and toes. The range of movement is measured for the ankle, subtalar joint, metatarsal phalangeal, and proximal and distal interphalangeal joints. Clawing of the toes and the ability to passively correct the clawing is noted.

The first specific evaluation for cavus is to determine whether the foot is supple, and thus amenable to soft tissue release, or whether the foot is rigid, in which case it will be necessary to perform osteotomies as well as soft tissue releases to obtain a correction. One of the best ways to tell if a cavus foot is supple is to perform the Coleman block test [6]. To perform this test, the physician observes the heel as the patient places the lateral aspect of the foot on a 2-cm block of wood and bears their own weight with the medial aspect of the foot on the floor and the lateral aspect on the block. If the heel comes out of varus with weight bearing, the cavus is supple, and the foot can be corrected with soft tissue releases such as a plantar fasciiotomy.

The next specific evaluation for cavus relies on weight bearing radiographs to determine the relative position of the forefoot to the hindfoot and the midfoot. This is accomplished by measuring the calcaneal pitch angle, which is normally around 30°, and the angle of Meary, which is normally 0° [6].

How is Pes Cavus Treated in Patients with Spina Bifida?

The general rules of pes cavus treatment also hold true for spina bifida patients, except that particular care should be taken to achieve a plantigrade posture at the time of surgery. In the case of a supple cavovarus, satisfactory correction can be achieved with plantar fascia release coupled with flexor and/or extensor tenotomies and capsulectomies as needed. One possible tendon transfer in this situation is the Jones procedure for transfer of the extensor hallucis longus tendon to the neck of the first metatarsal, coupled with a fusion of the interphalangeal joint. For second-degree cavovarus feet which have some rigidity, a plantar fascia release may not be sufficient to correct the cavus, and it will be necessary to perform an osteotomy of the calcaneus or the first metatarsal.

For calcaneocavus, the operation of choice is a calcaneal osteotomy plus a plantar release. The osteotomy can be either a wedge or a crescent osteotomy, depending on the preference of the surgeon. For cavoplantaris, a midfoot osteotomy can achieve considerable correction, particularly when Chopart's joint is involved in the deformity. It will most likely be necessary to perform a plantar release and separately address the toe deformities.

The most difficult situation with pes cavus in spina bifida patients is the treatment of feet that have a rigid, nonplantigrade cavus due to skeletal and articular deformities coupled with soft tissue contractures. In these cases, the options are limited by the geometric changes in the bones and joints. Triple arthrodesis may be the only way to achieve a correction. However, triple arthrodesis has been held to be an unfavorable operation in patients with spina bifida owing to the risk of articular damage proximal and distal to the fused joints. Dias has stated that it is preferable to avoid arthrodesis in the feet of spina bifida patients if at all possible [2]. As previously mentioned, Maynard et al. [5] found a high incidence of foot problems in spina bifida patients if the foot was rigid, if the position was nonplantigrade, or if a previous arthrodesis had been performed. We prefer to consider these findings as an endorsement of the plantigrade position rather than a condemnation of arthrodesis, and our observations of triple arthrodesis as a salvage procedure for severe foot deformity in patients with spina bifida support this belief.

Between the years 1982 and 1996, we have followed 13 patients with spina bifida who underwent 16 triple arthrodeses. Three patients had bilateral procedures. Nine patients were community ambulators and 4 were household ambulators. The indications for arthrodesis were a nonplantigrade position in all 16 feet plus recurrent ulceration in 10 of the 16 feet. All of the community ambulators had been required to use crutches or a wheelchair to maintain nonweight-bearing mobility prior to the procedure.

All patients underwent a Hoke-type arthrodesis using intraoperative fixation with percutaneous pins and postoperative immobilization in a cast. Early complications included 2 superficial wound infections and 3 pin tract infections, which were all resolved with the use of oral antibiotics. All pins had been removed at an average of 8 weeks. All patients achieved union of the subtalar and midtarsal joints at an average time of 17 weeks. At the last follow-up, 15 of the 16 feet had remained plantigrade. One patient had experienced recurrent ulceration at the base of the fifth metatarsal due to over-supination, but this problem resolved with the use of customized soft orthotics and a wide shoe.

Our experience indicates that at early to intermediate follow-up, triple arthrodesis can produce a plantigrade foot in spina bifida patients with severe, rigid deformity. Ideally, it is preferable to maintain as much motion as possible in the feet of patients with spina bifida, but some patients will have such severe cavus deformity that all other measures, short of major skeletal surgery, are destined to fail. In this situation, triple arthrodesis, with the goal of obtaining a plantigrade position at the time of surgery, can greatly improve the foot posture.

References

1. Brinker MR, Rosenfeld SR, Feiwell E, Granger SP, Mitchell DC, Rice JC (1994) Myelomeningocele at the sacral level. Long-term outcomes in adults. J Bone Joint Surg 76A:1293–1300
2. Dias LS (1983) Foot. In: Shafer MF, Dias LS (eds) Myelomeningocele orthopaedic treatment. Williams and Wilkins, Baltimore, pp 179–213
3. Harris MB, Banta JV (1990) Cost of skin care in the myelomeningocele population. J Pediatr Orthop 10:355–361
4. Kinsman SL, Doering MC (1996) The cost of preventable conditions in adults with spina bifida. Eur J Pediatr Surg 1:17–20
5. Maynard MJ, Weiner LS, Burke SW (1992) Neuropathic foot ulceration in patients with myelomeningocele. J Pediatr Orthop 12:786–788
6. Wenger DR, Rang M (1993) The art and practice of children's orthopaedics. Raven, New York, pp 168–175

Abstract

The Surgical Treatment for Foot Deformity in Spina Bifida

Koji Noyori, Kikuo Kameshita, Shigeharu Okuzumi, Jun-ichiro Nakamura, and Yoshio Mukawa

The purpose of this study was to describe the results of the management of various combinations of deformity and paralysis in the feet of children with spina bifida, and to evaluate the principles of treatment.

One hundred and sixty-five feet of 118 patients, 62 boys and 55 girls, had at least one operation between 1970 and 1995. Most feet (80%, 131/165 feet) had low lumbar functional level (L4–L5). We operated on 39 equinovarus, 52 varus, 38 calcaneovarus, 8 equinus, 6 calcaneovalgus, 12 valgus, and 2 cavus deformities. Thirteen cavus, 13 claw toes, and 12 hammer toes were combined with other deformities. Since 1980, a combined operation has been used to correct deformities. This operation consists of posteromedial release, subtalar arthrodesis by cancellous grafts to obtain stability of the paralytic foot, arthrodesis of calcaneocuboid joints (Evans or reverse Evans), posterior tendon transfer of plantar flexors (tibialis posterior, flexor digitorum longus, flexor hallucis longus), and tenodesis of Achilles tendon in cases with a brace or zero triceps surae motor strength.

Satisfactory correction by this combined operation was obtained in most plantigrade feet. Very few decubitus and recurrence were seen.

Department of Orthopaedic Surgery, Kanagawa Children's Medical Center, Yokohama, Japan

Moderator's Comments on Sessions—Foot Pathology

Makoto Kamegaya

Seven papers were presented by five doctors from Japan and two from other countries. Dr. H. Yanagida and Dr. K. Yoh presented the incidences of foot deformities in spina bifida patients in Japan. Dr. Yanagida (Fukuoka, Japan) reported that 84% of 103 patients had some foot deformities, of which 45% had a varus or equinovarus foot. Dr. Yoh (Chiba, Japan) reported that the rate of foot surgery in all 90 operations which had been undertaken in the past 25 years was 61%. The patients with L4, L5, or S1 > motor level most frequently complained of foot problems. Foot surgery was very helpful to protect the feet from pressure sores and to make the walking pattern more stable, but it did not improve the ability of transfer to an upper level.

Dr. Ito (Aichi, Japan) presented a very interesting paper about the delayed onset of neurological disorders which were sometimes observed during the growth period, such as cavus deformity of the foot, and spastic or flaccid paralysis of the low extremities. He also reported that spasticity of the hamstring and adductor muscles was considerable in cases with lumbar lesion, and clonus tended to occur in cases with sacral lesion.

Dr. Noyori (Kanagawa, Japan) showed the results of the following combined operations: posteromedial release, subtalor arthrodesis, arthrodesis of the calcaneo-cuboid joint, posterior tendon transfer of plantar flexors, and tenodesis of the Achilles tendon. These were done for patients with various combinations of foot deformities. They were satisfactory for plantigrade foot and the prevention of foot pressure sores.

Dr. Oketani (Fukuoka, Japan) showed the surgical results of Achilles tenodesis and posterior transfer of the tibialis anterior tendon for residual calcaneus deformity. In a final review, he found improvements in foot stability and orthoses-free walking.

Dr. Dias (Chicago, USA) presented the management of ankle and hindfoot valgus in spina bifida. He first reported on how he developed a method for measuring fibular shortening on a plain radiograph. In the treatment, he recommends a surgical operation only when the deformity caused problems with orthotic fitting and cannot be alleviated with orthotic changes. Medial displacement osteotomy was recommended as the most effective procedure to get a plantigrade and braceable foot.

Finally, Dr. Gamble (Palo Alto, USA) reported on the treatment of cavus foot in spina bifida. His operative indication was soft tissue release for mild supple cavus deformity, and osteotomy or arthrodesis for rigid cavus in older patients.

Chiba Children's Hospital

Foot problems are really troublesome for community ambulators with spina bifida. Pressure sores often make a condition incurable, in spite of all kinds of treatment, and the deep infections which follow sometimes induce osteomyelitis of the metatarsals or phalanges bone. The treatment not only costs a lot, but it also takes a long time until the patient can go back to normal life. We orthopedic doctors must make an effort to protect patients from these problems with the modern concepts that were discussed in this session.

Urology

Neurogenic Bladder

Cellular Signaling in the Bladder: Implications for Treatment

LAURENCE S. BASKIN[1,3], SIMON W. HAYWARD[1,2], RONALD A. SUTHERLAND[1], MICHAEL S. DISANDRO[1], AXEL A. THOMSON[2], and GERALD R. CUNHA[1,2]

Mesenchymal–Epithelial Interactions

Embryologically, the urinary bladder is derived from undifferentiated mesenchyme and endoderm of the urogenital sinus and allantois. During development, the undifferentiated mesenchyme differentiates into bladder smooth muscle [1]. What are the signaling mechanisms that allow this process to occur? Previously, we have shown that epithelium is necessary for bladder smooth muscle differentiation [2] (Fig. 1). Using the rat as an experimental model, we first defined the ontogeny of both epithelial and smooth muscle differentiation using a panel of smooth muscle and epithelial proteins [1]. The smooth muscle proteins, α-actin, myosin, vinculin, desmin, laminin, and vimentin are sequentially expressed as a function of developmental stage. In the embryonic rat bladder at 14 days gestation, none of these markers were detected by immunostaining, whereas at 16 days gestation, when smooth muscle is first noted by histologic criteria, α-actin-staining cells are detected in the periphery of the bladder. Subsequently, these actin-positive cells sequentially acquire the remaining smooth muscle markers. We hypothesized that epithelial mesenchymal signaling is required for the smooth muscle differentiation to occur [2]. To test this hypothesis, 14-day embryonic rat bladders (prior to the differentiation of smooth muscle) were isolated and the epithelium was separated from the mesenchyme following tryptic digestion which degrades the epithelial basement membrane [3]. The isolated bladder mesenchyme, bladder mesenchyme recombined with urothelium, and intact embryonic bladders were then grown underneath the kidney capsule of syngeneic hosts. The intact 14-day embryonic bladders underwent normal differentiation, defined by the expression of smooth muscle proteins. In contrast, when isolated bladder mesenchyme was grown alone underneath the kidney capsule, the tissue survived, but the mesenchyme did not differentiate into smooth muscle. However, when bladder mesenchyme was recombined with bladder epithelium, smooth muscle differentiation occurred, although this was less organized than if the epithelium was left intact in its natural state.

The same experiments were repeated in vitro, where intact embryonic bladders prior to smooth muscle differentiation were grown on top of filter paper nourished by standard tissue culture medium. Compared with bladder mesenchyme cultured alone, again there was

[1] Department of Urology, [2] Department of Anatomy, and [3] Department of Pediatrics, University of California, San Francisco, UCSF Children's Medical Center, San Francisco, CA 94141, USA

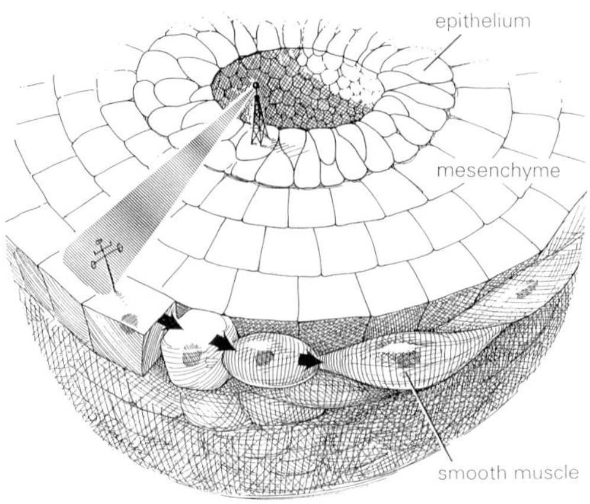

FIG. 1. Epithelium is required for bladder mesenchyme to differentiate into bladder smooth muscle. Signaling occurs via an unknown mechanism, possibly diffusable growth factors (From [10], with permission)

impressive growth of the intact organs. When epithelium was recombined with bladder mesenchyme, again the growth was greatly improved compared with the mesenchyme alone. Labeling of the organ culture experiments with ^{3}H-thymidine showed extensive cellular proliferation in the tissue recombinants composed of bladder mesenchyme plus bladder epithelium and in intact bladders, whereas in the mesenchyme alone, little growth occurred. Histologically, tissue recombinants of bladder mesenchyme plus epithelium structures revealed healthy cellular histology, whereas the bladder mesenchyme alone showed evidence of cellular degeneration.

A final experiment determined whether epithelium from a different species could induce bladder smooth muscle differentiation. This hypothesis was tested by performing a unilateral nephrectomy in nude mice [2]. Undifferentiated, 14-day rat bladder mesenchyme with the epithelium removed was then surgically attached to the severed mouse ureter. The bladder mesenchyme and mouse ureter were allowed to grow for 1 month in situ, with the idea that the ureteral epithelium would induce smooth muscle differentiation of the rat bladder mesenchyme. As expected, the mouse urothelium was able to induce smooth muscle differentiation in the rat bladder mesenchyme, resulting in the expression of smooth muscle differentiation markers. Species-specific probes confirmed that the epithelium was of mouse origin and the smooth muscle was from the rat. These experiments strongly support the concept that cellular signaling between the bladder epithelium and undifferentiated bladder mesenchyme is required for the induction of bladder smooth muscle.

A number of questions remain unanswered. Why does bladder smooth muscle initially form in the periphery of the bladder at the greatest distance from the signaling epithelium? Does signaling occur by diffusable factors (a hypothesis that we have subsequently been testing), or does it occur by cellular contact of mesenchymal cells with the epithelial basement membrane followed by signaling peripherally through the undifferentiated mesenchyme to the subserosal zone? These questions are the basis for further research.

Growth Factors

If diffusable growth factors play a role in smooth muscle differentiation, one would expect to see differences in their expression during development. We therefore utilized RNAse protection assays for a panel of growth factors at strategic times during bladder development and smooth muscle differentiation [4]. Specifically, we examined bladders at the embryonic stage before smooth muscle development (14 days gestation), at the time of first smooth muscle differentiation (16 days gestation), and then at 18 days gestation, newborn, 20 days postnatally, and in adulthood. We quantified growth factors that have known differentiation properties in other organ systems. Specifically, we assessed transcripts for KGF and the KGF receptor, TGF-α and EGF receptor, and the TGF-β family. We found that TGF-β-2 and -3 are regulated as a function of development, being expressed at a high level in early gestation and then decreasing as a function of time. TGF-α and KGF were expressed in the opposite fashion, being minimally expressed in the embryonic period with a greater expression in the mature bladder.

We then created a model of bladder outlet obstruction in the rodent in order to study the effect of obstruction on smooth muscle remodeling [5]. This resulted in a six-fold increase in bladder volume and a five-fold increase in bladder weight, as well as a doubling of smooth muscle cell diameter. The message for the growth factor TGF-β-2 increased two-fold, and TGF-β-3 increased five-fold. The message for TGF-α was elevated ten-fold. In contrast, the transcripts for KGF and the receptors for KGF and EGF did not exhibit any changes. TGF-β is known to affect extracellular matrix synthesis, and it may be that the changes in the bladder wall and increased matrix deposition resulted from the up-regulation of these growth factors.

Bladder Wound Healing

Further evidence for cellular signaling via growth factors has been shown with our model of bladder wound healing [6]. Again, using the rodent as a model, an incisional wound was created in the bladder and then sutured with primary closure. Histological analysis revealed that the bladder epithelium regrew over the defect within 24–48h. RNase protection assays of growth factors showed an eight-fold increase in the expression of KGF when compared with sham-operated and control animals. Interestingly, this increased expression occurred in the first 12–24h, corresponding to the period of intense epithelial proliferation noted histologically. At 5 and 7 days, when the epithelium had completely regrown, the expression of KGF had returned to normal.

Another interesting finding is that when the bladder wall was sampled at a distance from the injury, there was still an up-regulation compared with sham and nonoperated animals, suggesting that global signaling occurs throughout the bladder in response to injury, which facilitates epithelial repair. (Fig. 2) The impressive proliferative ability of the urothelial cell is amazing, since it is normally quiescent, with a turnover every 6 months to a year. However,

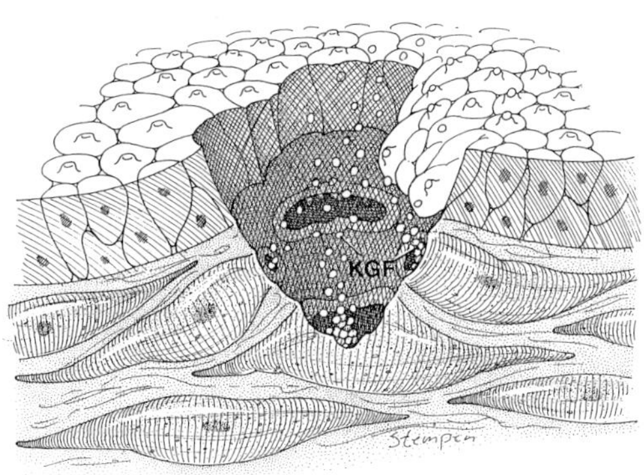

FIG. 2. Keratinocyte growth factor (*KGF*) is released from bladder stroma cells during bladder injury and directly acts through its urothelial located receptor to cause proliferation and regrowth of urothelial cells, mending the bladder injury (From [10], with permission)

following bladder epithelial injury, KGF released by the stroma elicits receptors on the epithelial surface to cause the urothelium to proliferate. Further support for the direct effect of KGF in the bladder was tested by experimentally injecting human recombinant KGF subcutaneously into neonatal mice. In comparison to saline controls, urothelial proliferation was greatly elevated as judged by thymidine labeling. Similar findings have been reported for the monkey bladder by Ye et al. [7].

One of the most clinically relevant areas of bladder signaling may occur at the border between the native bladder and augmented intestinal segments [8]. Here the bladder urothelium is put into an environment where it receives signals from the stroma of the native bladder as well as the stroma of the gastrointestinal graft. Although the incidence of tumors in augmented bladders is low, tumors tend to occur exactly at this surgical juncture. We hypothesize that the abnormal signaling at this site leads to aberrant communication, leading to this cellular atypia. Further work is underway using tissue recombinations to assess the effects of intestinal stroma on bladder urothelium, and vice versa.

Bladder Replacement

One of the most exciting areas of bladder research is the development of new methods of bladder augmentation which avoid the use of intestinal segments. We have created a model of bladder augmentation in which we use an acellular tissue matrix to elicit regeneration of bladder tissue (Fig. 3) [9]. In this model, the dome of the bladder is excised (again, this was first performed in the rodent model), and an acellular tissue matrix made from either the bladder or the stomach is sutured to the surgical defect. The acellular matrix is prepared by incubating the bladders or stomachs of adult rats in distilled water for 1 h to lyse the cells and to release the intracellular contents. The tissues are then suspended in 40 ml of 40% sodium deoxycholate (Sigma Chemical St. Louis, MO, USA), for 2–4 h, followed by treatment with 2000 kunitz units of deoxyribonuclease I (Sigma) in 1 M sodium chloride solution for 1–2 h. This process is repeated 1–3 times to extract all cellullar material. Histological confirmation shows an absence of cells. The preparation of the acellular matrix is designed to avoid complete removal of potentially important growth factors, as well as other extracellular matrix ligands. After suturing the acellular matrix patch in place, the animals were killed at serial time points to study the interface between the native bladder and the acellular matrix

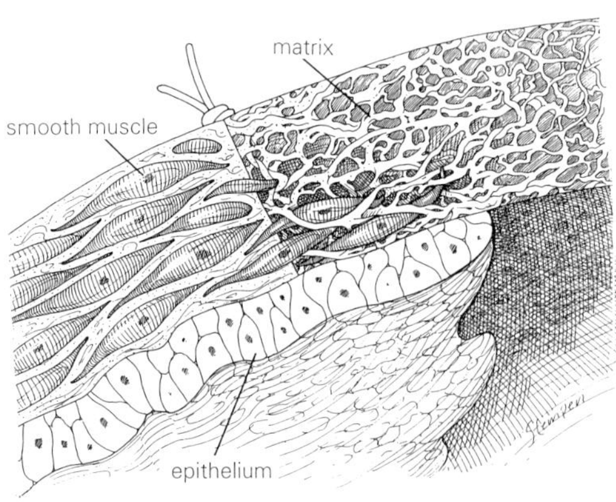

Fig. 3. A model of bladder regeneration with an acellular tissue matrix shows that urothelium, smooth muscle, and nerves can grow into the tissue matrix most likely to be under the influence of stromal–epithelial cellular communication (From [10], with permission)

tissue. Complete reepithelization with urothelial cells occurred by 4 days, and smooth muscle regenerated into the acellular matrix by 2 weeks postgrafting. Interestingly, the smooth muscle grew in juxtaposition to the epithelial surface, which matured into normal-size bundles by 26 weeks postgrafting.

Neovascularity was seen by 2 weeks, and neural elements from the native bladder formed around the developing bundles of smooth muscle as early as 4 weeks. These animals were able to function normally. Careful histological analysis showed that the acellular tissue matrix did not regenerate into a completely normal bladder, but over time smooth muscle bundles did organize into their appropriate positions in the periphery of the bladder, and the urothelium itself covered this matrix, presumably under the influence of KGF from the tissue injury [6]. This model has been very useful for studying the cellular signaling that occurs in the native bladder, especially in relation to potential bladder augmentation and bladder replacement.

Conclusions

In conclusion, cellular signaling plays an integral part in bladder development and the bladder's response to injury, such as obstruction and wound healing. A better understanding of these processes should allow for the strategic design of new therapies, especially in relation to bladder augmentation and bladder replacement.

Acknowledgments. Supported by NIH Grants K08 DK02397-01, CA 59831, DK51101, and DK 47517. This paper was previously published as Cellular Signaling in the Bladder, Frontiers in Bioscience, 2:592–595, December 1, 1997 (used with permission).

References

1. Baskin LS, Hayward SW, Young P et al. (1996) Ontogeny of the rat bladder: smooth muscle and epithelial differentiation. Acta Anat 155:163–171
2. Baskin LS, Hayward S, Young P et al. (1996) Role of mesenchymal–epithelial interactions in bladder development. J Urol 156:1820–1827
3. Baskin LS, Hayward SW, Sutherland RA et al. (1996) Mesenchymal–epithelial interactions in the bladder. World J Urol 14:301–309
4. Baskin LS, Sutherland RS, Thomson A et al. (1996) Growth factors and receptors in bladder development and obstruction. Lab Invest 75:157–166
5. Sutherland RS, Baskin LB, Elfman F et al. (1997) The role of type IV collagenases in rat bladder development and obstruction. Pediatr Res 41:430–434
6. Baskin L, Sutherland R, Thomson A et al. (1997) Growth factors in bladder wound healing. J Urol 157:2388–2395
7. Yi ES, Shabaik AS, Lacey DL et al. (1995) Keratinocyte growth factor causes proliferation of urothelium in vivo. J Urol 154:1566–1570
8. Barrington J, Fulford S, Griffiths D et al. (1997) Tumors in bladder remant after augmentation enterocystoplasty. J Urol 157:482–486
9. Sutherland RS, Baskin LB, Hayward SW et al. (1996) Regeneration of bladder urothelium, smooth muscle, blood vessels and nerves into an acellular tissue matrix. J Urol 156:571–577
10. Baskin LS (1997) The fate of the bladder in patients with congenital infravesical obstruction. Current opinions in urology. Rapid Science Publishers, London

Abstract

Uroneurology: The Mechanism of Neurogenic Bladder Disease

William E. Kaplan

The function of the lower urinary tract is to provide effective storage and voluntary emptying. Management goals are designed to either increase storage at low pressure or improve bladder emptying. The detrusor is made up of a mesh of smooth muscle fibers. These fibers coalesce at the bladder neck and proximal urethra. The bladder neck and proximal urethra work in concert to provide continence and probably to initiate bladder emptying. Smooth muscle fibers of the proximal urethra and bladder neck do provide the basis for the internal sphincter. Urethral resistance is dependent on smooth muscle tone in this region. The voluntary striated muscle of the external sphincter provides conscious urinary stream interruption. With a functional internal sphincter, the external sphincter will prevent stress urinary incontinence, but is not essential for routine urinary control. Unfortunately, many children with neuropathic bladders have poor to absent internal sphincter control.

The function of the lower urinary tract is affected by both autonomic and somatic innervation. The efferent innervation of the bladder and urethra are derived from the sympathetic and parasympathetic autonomic system, while the external sphincter responds to innervation from the somatic pudendal nerve. The response to parasympathetic stimulation is a sustained bladder contraction. Acetylcholine is the neurotransmitter for the parasympathetic system, both preganglionic and postganglionic. Acerylcholine is probably not the only parasympathetic neurohumoral transmitter. Numerous other substances have been cited as neurotransmitters for the parasympathetic system. The sympathetic system originates between cord segments T11-L2 and terminates as postganglionic fibers at the bladder and urethra as the hypogastric nerve. The neurohumoral transmitter for the sympathetic postganglionic innervation is norepinephrine. There are at least two different receptor types in the lower urinary tract responding to norepinephrine stimulation. The classic description are the alpha adrenergic receptors, responding by contraction, while the beta adrenergic receptors respond by relaxation. Experimentally, the sympathetic nervous system promotes urine storage by beta activation to increase bladder accommodation and by activation of the alpha receptors to increase outlet resistance. Utilization of the knowledge of receptors, and the pharmacotherapy directed at these receptor sites, results in a rational approach for modulation of bladder function. Unfortunately, the vast majority of children with spina bifida do not have pure lesions of the spinal cord and most patients have mixed lesions, resulting in either a failure to store or a failure to empty efficiently. When outlet resistance is low, the child is

Department of Urology, Northwestern University Medical School, Chicago, U.S.A., and Division of Urology, Children's Memorial Hospital, Chicago, IL, U.S.A.

usually at little risk of developing upper tract changes because of increased compliance; however, when outlet resistance is elevated, and intravesical pressure rises about 40 centimeters of water, there is risk of developing bladder trabeculation and reflux that could compromise upper tract function and drainage. The primary method of management of these patients is with catheterization and pharmacotherapy. The pharmacotherapy is directed towards the receptors in the bladder body and bladder neck. Anticholinergic therapy such as probanthine or oxybutynine hydrochloride is the mainstay for improving bladder volume and decreasing bladder pressure. Increasing outlet resistance by using pharmacotherapy is usually unrewarding; however, alpha receptor stimulation with medication such as ephedrine, or its derivatives can be tried. Voluntary voiding at low pressure may be helped by decreasing outlet resistance with alpha blockers or, occasionally, skeletal muscle relaxation may help in a very select group of patients. Again, the goal is to provide effective emptying, but not at the expense of bladder compliance.

Abstract

Indication of Surgical Interventions for Neurogenic Bladder

RICARDO GONZALEZ

This lecture will review the main surgical interventions often required to manage the urinary tract of children and young adults with spina bifida. Surgical procedures usually supplement but do not replace intermittent catheterization and pharmacologic agents.

Vesicostomy. Temporary diversion indicated in infants with high intravesical pressure who cannot be catheterized or do not respond to anticholinergic medications.

Ureteral reimplantation. Procedure to correct vesicoureteral reflux. Indicated when the sterility of the urine cannot be maintained or the reflux persists despite adequate bladder management. For a good result, it is essential to have good bladder capacity and compliance, therefore this operation is sometimes combined with bladder augmentation.

Bladder augmentation. Classically done by adding a segment of reconfigured bowel to the bladder. It is used to increase capacity and compliance when pharmacologic agents fall. The indications are to preserve the upper urinary tract and to enhance continence. New techniques for augmentation are discussed in another lecture.

Procedures to enhance bladder outlet resistance. These procedures are used to achieve continence in patients with sphincter incompetence. They are often combined with a bladder augmentation. Of the many procedures described, the author has the greatest experience and success with the artificial urinary sphincter.

Continent cutaneous appendico-vesicostomy (Mitrofanoff procedure). Is used in patients that for anatomical or other reasons cannot catheterize through the urethral meatus. It is often used to give patients greater independence.

Continent cutaneous appendico-cecostomy (Malone procedure). Achievement of fecal control is as essential as achievement of urinary continence. This procedure allows self-administration of antegrade enemas. It is indicated for patients with fecal incontinence who cannot self-administer rectal enemas.

Department of Urology, Children's Hospital of Michigan, Wayne State University, Detroit, Michigan, USA

Effects of Clean Intermittent Catheterization on Bladder Deformity in Spina Bifida Patients

Hitoshi Momose, Akihide Hirayama, Hiroki Kashiwai, Yoichi Kawata, Naoya Hirata, and Kaoru Yamada

Summary. A retrospective study was conducted to investigate the relationship between the age of starting clean intermittent catheterization (CIC) and its effects on urinary tract deterioration. One hundred and twelve spina bifida patients on CIC at evaluation, who had been followed up for longer than 10 years, were divided into 4 groups according to the age of starting CIC: Group 1 started CIC before 5 years old, Group 2 between 6 and 10 years, Group 3 between 11 and 15 years, and Group 4 after 16 years. Incidences of bladder deformity increased according to follow-up years in all groups. Incidence of improvement of vesicoureteral reflux (VUR) at 1 year after starting CIC was significantly higher in Group 1. It is concluded that some spina bifida patients are at risk of progressing bladder deformity which is refractory to CIC, and that the early introduction of CIC has a beneficial effect against VUR.

Key words. Spina bifida, Clean intermittent catheterization, Bladder deformity, Vesicoureteral reflux

Introduction

One of the most important goals in the urological management of patients with neurogenic bladder dysfunction is the preservation of renal function, and bladder deformity found radiographically is considered to be a potential risk factor for upper urinary tract deterioration which leads to renal damage [1].

Because of its low pressure conditions and high efficiency in urinary drainage, clean intermittent catheterization (CIC) is widely accepted as a standard method of urological management in patients with neurogenic bladder dysfunction, including those with spina bifida [2,3].

This retrospective study was conducted to investigate the effects of CIC on urinary tract deterioration, especially bladder deformity, with reference to the age of starting CIC.

Materials and Methods

Of 154 spina bifida patients who had undergone initial urological examination before 5 years old at Hoshigaoka Koseinenkin Hospital and had been followed up for longer than 10 years, 112 (41 males and 71 females) were on regular CIC at evaluation. The age at evaluation ranged

Department of Urology, Hoshigaoka Koseinenkin Hospital, 4-8-1 Hoshigaoka, Hirakata, Osaka 573-8511, Japan

from 10 to 24 years old (mean 15.9 years) and the follow-up period ranged from 10 to 20 years (mean 13.4 years). The patients had been on regular CIC for 8.0 years on average (range 2–15 years).

The patients were divided into 4 groups according to age at starting CIC: Group 1 ($n = 23$) started CIC before 5 years old (preschool age); Group 2 ($n = 55$) started between 6 and 10 years (younger school age); Group 3 ($n = 26$) started between 11 and 15 years (older school age); Group 4 ($n = 8$) started after 16 years.

Clinical records were reviewed, and the effects of CIC on the morbidity of urinary tract diseases were compared among groups.

Results

Sequential Changes in the Incidence of Urinary Tract Diseases in Initially Normal Patients

The incidences of bladder deformity, vesicoureteral reflux (VUR), and hydronephrosis during follow-up in patients who did not suffer from these lesions at the start of CIC are shown in Tables 1–3, respectively. As shown graphically in Fig. 1, the incidence of bladder deformity increased with age. The early introduction of CIC results in the delayed occurrence of new lesions, especially that of bladder deformity (Fig. 2).

TABLE 1. Incidence of bladder deformity during follow-up in patients who did not suffer from it when starting clean intermittent catheterization (CIC)

Group	Age at CIC introduction (years)	Years after introducing CIC		
		1	5	10
1	0–5	1/8[a]	3/8	3/5
2	6–10	3/23	12/20	2/4
3	11–15	0/11	3/9	2/3
4	≧16	0/1	0/1	–
Overall (%)		4/43 (9.3)	18/38 (47.4)	7/12 (58.3)

[a] No. of deformed bladders/No. of bladders evaluated.

TABLE 2. Incidence of vesicoureteral reflux (VUR) during follow-up in patients who did not suffer from it when starting CIC

Group	Age at CIC introduction (years)	Years after introducing CIC		
		1	5	10
1	0–5	1/32[a]	3/32	1/17
2	6–10	1/89	8/85	1/28
3	11–15	0/41	5/27	0/7
4	≧16	0/11	2/6	–
Overall (%)		2/173 (1.2)	18/150 (12.0)	2/52 (3.8)

[a] No. of ureters with VUR/No. of ureters evaluated.

TABLE 3. Incidence of hydronephrosis during follow-up in patients who did not suffer from it when starting CIC

Group	Age at CIC introduction (years)	Years after introducing CIC		
		1	5	10
1	0–5	0/35[a]	2/35	2/18
2	6–10	0/92	4/86	4/25
3	11–15	0/50	0/32	0/6
4	≧16	0/13	3/8	–
Overall (%)		0/190 (0)	9/161 (5.6)	6/49 (12.2)

[a] No. of renal units with hydronephrosis/No. of renal units evaluated.

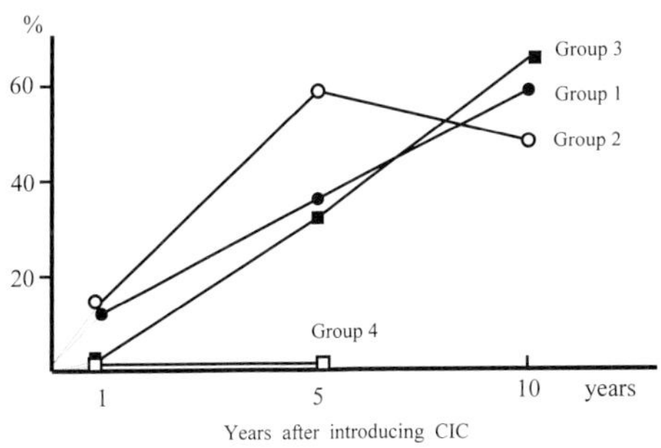

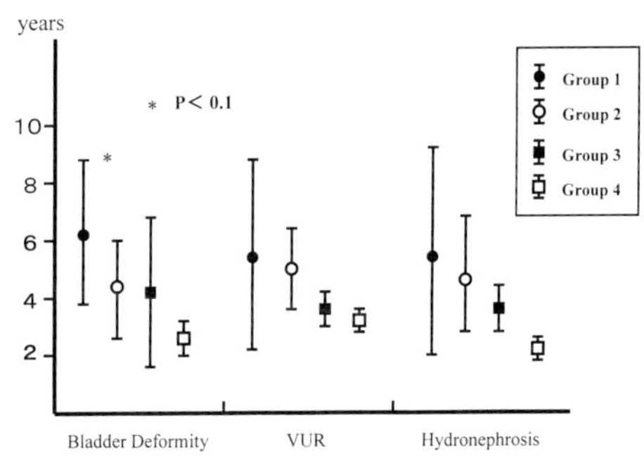

FIG. 1. Sequential changes in the incidence of bladder deformity in patients who did not suffer from it when starting clean intermittent catheterization (CIC)

FIG. 2. Time until the detection of urinary tract lesions after the introduction of CIC. VUR, vesicoureteral reflux

Improvement in Urinary Tract Lesions after the Introduction of CIC

The incidences of improvements in bladder deformity, VUR, and hydronephrosis after introducing CIC are shown in Tables 4–6, respectively. As shown graphically in Fig. 3, the incidence of an improvement in VUR in Group 1 1 year after starting CIC is significantly ($P < 0.05$) higher than the other groups.

Discussion

From the results of this retrospective study, it is evident that some groups of spina bifida patients are at risk of progressing bladder deformity for which CIC is not an effective preventative. Bladder deformity is considered to be attributable to high intravesical pressure and/or chronic bacterial infection of bladder mucosa, and it is well known that bladder deformity precedes upper urinary tract deterioration such as hydroureter or hydronephrosis. Theoretically, CIC performed in the correct way provides high-efficiency (i.e., no residual urine), low-pressure conditions for urinary drainage. Because of the retrospective nature of the analyses, it is difficult to draw any conclusion about the causes of progressing bladder deformity refractory to CIC from this set of data. CIC performed in an incorrect manner, or

TABLE 4. Incidence of improvements in bladder deformity

Group	Age at CIC introduction (years)	Years after introducing CIC 1	5	10
1	0–5	3/15[a]	2/15	1/8
2	6–10	2/32	4/32	0/14
3	11–15	2/16	1/9	0/1
4	≧16	0/6	0/3	–
Overall (%)		7/69 (10.1)	7/59 (11.9)	1/23 (4.3)

[a] No. of bladders improved/No. of bladders evaluated.

TABLE 5. Incidence of improvements in VUR

Group	Age at CIC introduction (years)	Years after introducing CIC 1	5	10
1	0–5	8/14[a]	8/14	3/9
2	6–10	6/21	7/19	1/8
3	11–15	0/12	2/8	0/1
4	≧16	0/3	0/2	–
Overall (%)		14/50 (28.0)	17/43 (39.5)	4/18 (22.2)

[a] No. of ureters improved/No. of ureters evaluated.

TABLE 6. Incidence of improvements in hydronephrosis

Group	Age at CIC introduction (years)	Years after introducing CIC 1	5	10
1	0–5	6/11[a]	6/11	2/8
2	6–10	5/18	5/18	3/11
3	11–15	1/3	1/3	1/2
4	≧16	0/1	–	–
Overall (%)		12/33 (36.4)	12/32 (37.5)	6/21 (28.6)

[a] No. of renal units improved/No. of renal units evaluated.

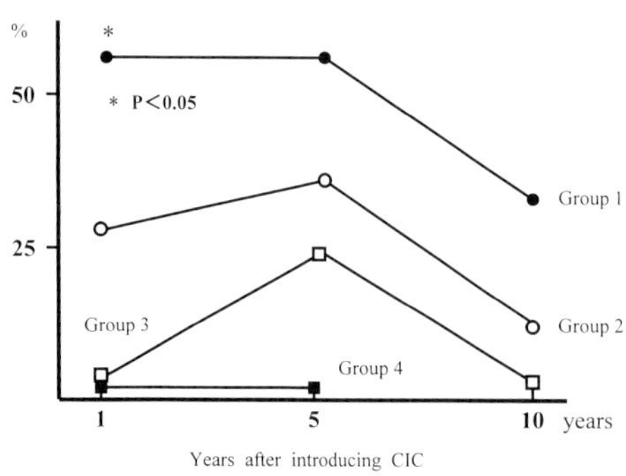

FIG. 3. Sequential changes in the incidence of improvements in VUR

high-pressure urinary storage due to detrusor hyperreflexia could be suspected of contributing to bladder deformity. A further prospective study is necessary to resolve this issue.

Another notable result is the significantly higher incidence of improvements in VUR in Group 1 than in the other groups. This means that the early introduction of CIC has a beneficial effect on improving VUR. Although no detailed data are available on the relationship between the grade of VUR and the incidence of its improvement in this study, it is reasonably expected that VURs of low grade will be better candidates for this benefit brought about by CIC. The currently available treatments for VUR of spina bifida patients include transurethral injection therapy [4] and ureteral reimplantation, often combined with augmentation cystoplasty [5, 6]. In cases of low-grade VURs, the first choice of treatment is CIC, and more invasive methods should be reserved only for refractory cases.

References

1. Anderson RU (1983) Urodynamic patterns after acute spinal cord injury. Association with bladder trabeculation in male patients. J Urol 129:777–779
2. Geraniotis E, Koff SA, Enrile B (1998) The prophylactic use of clean intermittent catheterization in the treatment of infants and young children with myelomeningocele and neurogenic bladder dysfunction. J Urol 139:85–86
3. Wu HY, Baskin LS, Kogan BA (1997) Neurogenic bladder dysfunction due to myelomeningocele. Neonatal versus childhood treatment. J Urol 157:2295–2297
4. Engel JD, Palmer LS, Cheng EY, Kaplan WE (1997) Surgical versus endoscopic correction of vesicoureteral reflux in children with neurogenic bladder dysfunction. J Urol 157:2291–2294
5. Mitchell ME, Piser JA (1987) Intestinocystoplasty and total bladder replacement in children and young adults. Followup in 129 cases. J Urol 138:579–584
6. Tsuji Y, Saito M, Kondo A, Narushima M, Otani T (1998) Vesicoureteral reflux and urinary tract incontinence in myelodysplastic patients. A comparison between those who had anti-reflux surgery alone and those who were treated by anti-reflux surgery combined with bladder augmentation with or without sling operation. Jpn J Urol 89:43–49

The Outcome of Management Based on Urethral Resistance in Myelodysplastic Children

Hiroshi Tanaka, Hidehiro Kakizaki, Shinya Kobayashi, Takashi Shibata, Kaname Ameda, and Tomohiko Koyanagi

Summary. The relevance of urethral resistance to upper tract deterioration (UTD) in myelodysplastic children and the outcome of conservative treatment based on urethral resistance were analyzed.

Fifty-four children were divided into two groups based on high (group 1) or low (group 2) urethral resistance, which was determined by leak-point pressure or maximum urethral closing pressure. Clean intermittent catheterization was instituted for all group 1 children and for group 2 children with UTD.

The incidence of UTD at presentation was 55% in group 1 and 13% in group 2 ($P < 0.01$). UTD was refractory to conservative management in 16% of group 1. The upper tract was normal in 84% of group 1 and 87% of group 2.

In conclusion, urethral resistance is relevant to UTD in untreated myelodysplastic children. Although UTD was refractory in a small fraction of children with high urethral resistance, the outcome of conservative treatment was generally satisfactory irrespective of urethral resistance.

Key words. Myelodysplasia, Upper tract deterioration, Urethral resistance

Introduction

Since the introduction of clean intermittent catheterization as a safe and reliable method of urinary management for vesicourethral dysfunction [11], the treatment of children with myelodysplasia has been significantly improved. Along with wide acceptance of intermittent catheterization, urodynamic studies have been performed on children with myelodysplasia to detect those who are at high risk from upper urinary tract deterioration. McGuire et al. [12] reported that in children with myelodysplasia there was a strong correlation between vesical leak-point pressure of more than 40 cm of water and upper tract deterioration. Kobayashi et al. [9] reported that maximum urethral closing pressure of more than 50 cm of water is a poor prognostic factor for reflux in children with myelodysplasia. In addition, Bauer et al. [1] recommended that intermittent catheterization should be instituted early for myelodysplastic infants with detrusor sphincter dyssynergia who are at high risk from upper

Department of Urology, Hokkaido University School of Medicine, North-15 West-7 Kita-Ku, Sapporo 060-8638, Japan

tract deterioration. Thus, prophylactic use of intermittent catheterization has been recommended to prevent upper urinary tract deterioration in children with myelodysplasia, in whom urodynamic studies demonstrated prognostically unfavorable patterns [5]. However, the optimal timing to initiate clean intermittent catheterization in children with myelodysplasia is controversial. Some have suggested that renal preservation can be accomplished equally without prophylactic use of intermittent catheterization by delaying treatment until the onset of upper tract deterioration [8, 13].

Our treatment strategy is to institute clean intermittent catheterization to prevent upper tract deterioration proactively in myelodysplastic children with high urethral resistance, or to treat upper tract deterioration as a primary therapy.

This retrospective study is aimed at clarifying the relevance of urethral resistance to upper urinary tract deterioration, and the outcome of urinary management based on urethral resistance in children with myelodysplasia.

Materials and Methods

We retrospectively reviewed the records of 54 children (29 boys and 25 girls) with vesicourethral dysfunction secondary to myelodysplasia who were less than 16 years old at initial evaluation and had a minimum follow-up of 12 months. Mean age at initial evaluation was 3.6 years (1 month to 16 years), and follow-up periods ranged from 12 months to 25 years (mean 9.2 years). Based on urethral resistance measured as leak-point pressure, or maximum urethral closing pressure at initial evaluation, they were divided into two groups. The high urethral resistance group (group 1) consisted of 31 children with leak-point pressure of more than 40 cm of water [12] or maximum urethral closing pressure of more than 50 cm of water [9]. The low urethral resistance group (group 2) consisted of 23 children with leak-point pressure of less than 40 cm of water or maximum urethral closing pressure of less than 50 cm of water.

The initial evaluation included excretory urography (IVP) or renal sonography and voiding cystourethrography. Urodynamic examination was also performed at initial evaluation, which included filling cystometry and urethral pressure profilometry. Filling-water cystometry was performed in all children to assess vesical compliance, the presence of detrusor hyperreflexia (phasic vesical pressure increase more than 15 cm of water), and leak-point pressure using an 8–10°F urethral catheter with a slow to medium filling rate (10–30 ml/min). Vesical compliance was calculated by dividing the volume change by the change in vesical pressure before a steep pressure increase occurred. Vesical pressure to overcome urethral resistance (leak-point pressure) was recorded during filling cystometry. Urethral pressure profilometry was also performed in some children to determine maximum urethral closing pressure with an empty bladder.

Periodic reassessment with imaging studies (IVP or renal ultrasound and, if necessary, voiding cystourethrography) as well as filling cystometry was performed every 6–12 months. After the clinical condition stabilized, the interval of evaluation was set longer than that initially adopted.

Our treatment strategy was basically a conservative one, a mainstay of which is to institute clean intermittent catheterization for all children with documented high urethral resistance (group 1), and for those with vesicourethral reflux or hydronephrosis in the low urethral resistance group (group 2) to prevent or normalize upper tract deterioration as a primary therapy. In addition, intermittent catheterization was instituted for children in group 2 with urinary incontinence requiring treatment after they reached school age. Thus, all children of group 1 and 16 children of group 2 were placed on clean intermittent catheterization. In group 2, the indication for clean intermittent catheterization was upper tract deterioration and/or conversion of urethral resistance from low to high during follow-up in five children, and to improve urinary incontinence in 11 children. Other conservative strategy included drug treatment with anticholinergics, which was prescribed for children with low vesical compliance or detrusor hyperreflexia, and was used in 20 children in group 1 and 10 children in group 2. Bladder augmentation was performed when upper tract deterioration was refractory to these conservative treatments.

The incidence of upper tract deterioration, including hydronephrosis or vesicoureteral reflux (VUR) at initial evaluation and during follow-up, and the final status of the upper tract were compared between the two groups.

Statistical significance was analyzed using contingency table analyses (χ^2 test) for categorical variables, and Mann–Whitney's *U* test for numerical variables.

Results

Initial Urodynamic Evaluation

The incidence of detrusor hyperreflexia was significantly higher in group 1 (52%) than in group 2 (33%). However, vesical capacity as well as compliance were not significantly different between the two groups (Table 1).

Incidence of Upper Tract Deterioration

The incidence of upper urinary tract deterioration in the form of VUR or hydronephrosis at initial evaluation was significantly different between the two groups (Table 2): 17 of 31 (55%) in group 1, and 3 of 23 (13%) in group 2 ($P = 0.0017$). During follow-up, de novo upper tract deterioration was detected in 5 children (3 in group 1 and 2 in group 2) at the ages of 1, 7, and 8 in group 1, and 7 and 8 in group 2. The incidence of de novo upper tract deterioration was 10% in group 1 and 9% in group 2, and there was no statistical difference (Table 2). In

TABLE 1. Results of initial urodynamic study

	Group 1	Group 2	*P* value
Bladder capacity (ml)[a]	147 ± 99	149 ± 85	Not significant
Vesical compliance (ml/cm water)[a]	8.3 ± 8.2	9.6 ± 5.3	Not significant
Detrusor hyperreflexia[b]	18/31 (58)	4/23 (17)	0.0026

[a] Mean ± S.D.
[b] No. of children/total (%).

TABLE 2. Upper tract condition at initial evaluation and throughout follow-up

Upper tract condition	Group 1	Group 2	*P* value
Upper tract deterioration at initial evaluation	17 (55%)	3 (13%)	0.0017
De novo upper tract deterioration during follow-up	3 (10%)	2 (9%)	Not significant
Normal throughout follow-up	11 (35%)	18 (78%)	0.0018

group 1, the underlying cause of de novo upper tract deterioration was persistent low vesical compliance in 1 child, gradually decreasing vesical compliance during follow-up in 1 child, and poor obedience to intermittent catheterization in 1 child, while in group 2, it was conversion of urethral resistance from low to high during followup in 1 child, and it was uncertain in the other. Normal upper tract was maintained from the initial to the follow-up evaluation in 11 children (35%) of group 1 and in 18 children (78%) of group 2 ($P = 0.0018$, Table 2). Of all the 25 children in whom upper urinary tract deterioration was detected at initial evaluation or developed during follow-up, significant hydroureteronephrosis without VUR occurred in only one child of group 1, while the other 24 children (19 of group 1 and 5 of group 2) had VUR with or without upper tract dilation. Reflux was bilateral in 7 of 19 (37%) in group 1 and in 3 of 5 (60%) in group 2. High-grade reflux (grade III or more) was noted in 12 of 19 (63%) in group 1 and in 4 of 5 (80%) in group 2. Thus, there was no obvious correlation between reflux grade or laterality and urethral resistance.

Outcome of Treatment for Upper Tract Deterioration

Of 19 children of group 1 with reflux, the reflux was resolved in 10 cases (53%), improved in 3 cases (16%), and stable in 2 cases (10%) following intermittent catheterization (Table 3). The other 4 children with reflux (21%) required bladder augmentation to preserve renal function. Overall, 69% of group 1 with reflux had resolution or improvement of VUR with conservative management. Of 5 children in group 2, reflux resolved in 2 cases (40%) and improved in 1 case (20%) with intermittent catheterization (Table 3). The response to conservative management was also compared between high- and low-grade reflux. The conservative approach led to resolution or improvement in 10 of 16 (63%) children with high-grade reflux, and in 6 of 8 (75%) children with low-grade reflux (Table 3). Thus, reflux grade at diagnosis did not affect the outcome of conservative treatment. Hydroureteronephrosis without reflux in one child in group 1 was refractory to conservative treatment.

Bladder Augmentation

Five children in group 1 (16%) in whom advanced upper tract deterioration and severely impaired vesical function had been documented at initial evaluation required bladder augmentation after bladder decompressive treatment with intermittent catheterization and anticholinergics for a mean period of 4.8 years (2–9 years). Four of 5 children had high-grade reflux, and the remainder had bilateral severe hydroureteronephrosis. Mean age at bladder

TABLE 3. The outcome of conservative treatment for reflux

	Group 1 ($n = 19$)	Group 2 ($n = 5$)	Total ($n = 24$)
Resolution	10 (53%)	2 (40%)	12 (50%)
Improvement	3 (16%)	1 (20%)	4 (17%)
Stable	2 (10%)	2 (40%)	4 (17%)
Refractory (augmentation)	4 (21%)	0	4 (17%)
	High-grade reflux (n = 16)		Low-grade reflux (n = 8)
Resolution	6 (38%)		6 (75%)
Improvement	4 (25%)		0
Stable	2 (12%)		2 (25%)
Refractory (augmentation)	4 (25%)		0

augmentation was 7.1 years. After bladder augmentation, all children obtained a normal upper tract and an adequate low-pressure, large-capacity bladder [10].

Upper Tract Status at Final Evaluation

At final evaluation, the upper tract was demonstrated to be normal in 26 children (84%), improved in 3 children, and stable in 2 children in group 1, while it was normal in 20 (87%), improved in 1, and stable in 2 in group 2.

Discussion

The present study revealed that urethral resistance is relevant to upper urinary tract deterioration in untreated myelodysplastic children, and that conservative treatment with intermittent catheterization is very effective for normalization or improvement of upper urinary tract deterioration in myelodysplastic children irrespective of urethral resistance.

Several urodynamic risk factors for upper urinary tract deterioration have been described in patients with myelodysplasia. McGuire et al. [12] introduced the concept of leak-point pressure, and proposed that high leak-point pressure (more than 40 cm of water) is a risk factor for upper urinary tract deterioration in myelodysplastic children. Kobayashi et al. [9] have shown that high maximum urethral closing pressure (more than 50 cm of water) is relevant to the occurrence of vesicoureteral reflux in patients with myelodysplasia. Because most patients with myelodysplasia are considered as having relatively fixed urethral resistance, which denotes that the urethral sphincter does not show dynamic behavior during bladder filling, leak-point pressure is assumed to be correlated with maximum urethral closing pressure [14]. Based on these earlier findings, urethral resistance in this study was determined by either leak-point pressure or maximum urethral closing pressure. This study showed that the incidence of upper urinary tract deterioration before treatment was significantly different between myelodysplastic children with high or low urethral resistance (55% versus 13%). Additionally, the present study indicated that there was no correlation between urethral resistance and reflux grade, which reflects a previous report [4].

The overall incidence of de novo upper tract deterioration during follow-up was not statistically different between group 1 and group 2 (10% versus 9%). The most plausible cause of de novo upper tract deterioration was sustained high bladder storage pressure due to persistent or worsened low vesical compliance, or poor compliance with the catheterization regimen in group 1 children, and conversion of urethral resistance from low to high in group 2 children. Age at occurrence of de novo upper tract deterioration was almost exclusively 7–8 years in this study. From these results, children with myelodysplasia, irrespective of urethral resistance, should be closely followed with imaging and urodynamic studies until at least school age to detect early signs of de novo upper tract deterioration.

In this study, conservative treatment by clean intermittent catheterization with or without anticholinergics accomplished resolution or improvement of reflux in 13 children (69%) with high urethral resistance and the outcome of conservative management was not significantly related to urethral resistance. Additionally, we found that there was no significant association between the grade of reflux at diagnosis and the final outcome of conservative management as reported by Cohen and Flood [2, 4]. Therefore we believe that conservative management should be considered primarily to treat myelodysplastic children with upper tract deterioration, even in those with high-grade reflux.

Recently some authors suggested that early intervention from infancy might prevent irreversible bladder dysfunction in children with myelodysplasia and reduce the need for bladder augmentation [3]. The reported incidence of bladder augmentation to resolve upper tract deterioration in myelodysplastic children with a poor prognostic factor who had been treated prophylactically from infancy is 4% by Kasabian et al. [6] and 11% by Wu et al. [15], while 28% of myelodysplastic children with upper tract deterioration who had been treated expectantly with radiological observation required bladder augmentation [7]. Although our treatment strategy was to institute clean intermittent catheterization in myelodysplastic children with high urethral resistance regardless of age or upper tract status, bladder augmentation was required in 16% of those with high urethral resistance. All the 5 children who underwent bladder augmentation were 3 years old or more when they were referred to our institution with advanced upper tract deterioration and severely damaged vesical function. Aggressive medication and intermittent catheterization did not have an impact on their established upper tract deterioration. Thus, early and appropriate monitoring from infancy is mandatory for successful conservative treatment.

Conclusions

Urethral resistance determined by leak-point pressure or maximum urethral closing pressure was relevant to upper urinary tract deterioration in untreated myelodysplastic children.

Clean intermittent catheterization with or without anticholinergics was instituted proactively as a primary therapy for myelodysplastic children with high urethral resistance and for those with upper urinary tract deterioration. The outcome of these conservative regimens was satisfactory, with preservation or normalization of upper tract status in the majority of children irrespective of urethral resistance. However, in a small fraction of children with high urethral resistance (16%) who presented with established upper tract deterioration, bladder augmentation was required. Thus, early and appropriate monitoring from infancy is essential in the management of children with myelodysplasia.

References

1. Bauer SB, Hallett M, Khoshbin S, Lebowitz RL, Winston KR, Gibson S, Colodny AH, Retik AB (1984) Predictive value of urodynamic evaluation in newborns with myelodysplasia. JAMA 252:650–652
2. Cohen RA, Rushton HG, Belman AB, Kass EJ, Majd M, Shaer C (1990) Renal scarring and vesicoureteral reflux in children with myelodysplasia. J Urol 144:541–544
3. Edelstein RA, Bauer SB, Kelly MD, Darbey MM, Peters CA, Atala A, Mandell J, Colodny AH, Retik AB (1995) The long-term urological response of neonates with myelodysplasia treated proactively with intermittent catheterization and anticholinergic therapy. J Urol 154:1500–1504
4. Flood HD, Ritchey ML, Bloom DA, Huang C, McGuire EJ (1994) Outcome of reflux in children with myelodysplasia managed by bladder pressure monitoring. J Urol 152:1574–1577
5. Geraniotis E, Koff SA, Enrile B (1988) The prophylactic use of clean intermittent catheterization in the treatment of infants and young children with meningocele and neurogenic bladder dysfunction. J Urol 139:85–86
6. Kasabian NG, Bauer SB, Dyro FM, Colodny AH, Mandell J, Retik AB (1992) The prophylactic value of clean intermittent catheterization and anticholinergic medication in newborns and infants with myelodysplasia at risk of developing urinary tract deterioration. Am J Dis Child 146:840–843
7. Kaufman AM, Ritchey ML, Roberts AC, Rudy DC, McGuire EJ (1996) Decreased bladder compliance in patients with myelomeningocele treated with radiological observation. J Urol 156:2031–2033

8. Klose AG, Sackett CK, Mesrobian HJ (1990) Management of children with myelodysplasia: urological alternatives. J Urol 144:1446–1449
9. Kobayashi S, Shinno Y, Kakizaki H, Matsumura K, Koyanagi T (1992) Relevance of detrusor hyperreflexia, vesical compliance and urethral pressure to the occurrence of vesicoureteral reflux in myelodysplastic patients. J Urol 147:413–415
10. Kobayashi S, Koyanagi T, Ameda K, Kakizaki H, Matsuura S, Shibata T, Sasaki Y (1996) Augmentation cystoplasty in children. Akt Urol 27:35 (Suppl)
11. Lapides J, Diokuno AC, Silber SJ, Lowe BS (1972) Clean intermittent self-catheterization in the treatment of urinary tract disease. J Urol 107:458–461
12. McGuire EJ, Woodside JR, Borden TA, Weiss RM (1981) Prognostic value of urodynamic testing in myelodysplastic patients. J Urol 126:205–209
13. Teichman JMH, Scherz HC, Kim KD, Cho DH, Packer MG, Kaplan GW (1994) An alternative approach to myelodysplasia management: aggressive observation and prompt intervention. J Urol 152:807–811
14. Wang SC, McGuire EJ, Bloom DA (1988) A bladder pressure management system for myelodysplasia—clinical outcome. J Urol 140:1499–1502
15. Wu HY, Baskin LS, Kogan BA (1997) Neurogenic bladder dysfunction due to myelomeningocele: neonatal versus childhood treatment. J Urol 157:2295–2297

A Case Study of Successful Self-Catheterization in an Adolescent with Spina Bifida, Mental Retardation, and Severe Motor Impairment

Eri Shinoki[1], Taiko Hirose[2], Kiyomi Yoshimura[2], Akemi Hamamatsu[2], Chizuko Horio[2], Masako Takamatsu[2], Masako Satohisa[2], and Yuko Hamada[1]

Summary. A description of nursing intervention to assist a female adolescent with spina bifida, mental retardation, and severe motor impairment so that she successfully completed a clean intermittent catheterization (CIC) program. The nursing intervention had three stages and took 13 months. This case study shows a way to intervene in a difficult case with an adolescent who did not fully meet the criteria to achieve self-catheterization. Important factors in completing the CIC program included self-motivation, appropriate nursing interventions, and the belief of the nurse that the patient could carry out the CIC program. In addition, the primary nurse was a competent coordinator who organized the health care professionals' skills to assist the patient and her family, who were also very supportive. Some problems and challenges encountered by this adolescent are highlighted.

Key words. Spina bifida, Adolescent, Mental retardation, CIC, Institution, Nursing

Introduction

Since the introduction of clean intermittent catheterization (CIC) in the United States during the 1970s, CIC has also been used in the care of children who have spina bifida in Japan [1, 2, 5]. CIC has improved not only the management of children with bladder dysfunction, but also of children with VUR, urinary tract infections, and urinary incontinence [7]. Many studies have reported successful teaching of self-catheterization skills to children with spina bifida [3, 6, 9, 10]. Steps in performing self-catheterization have been suggested by nurses and other clinical professionals, based upon studies and clinical experiences [4, 8]. Many have suggested the specific criteria necessary for success in accomplishing CIC, including physiological, developmental, and motivational components.

The female adolescent with spina bifida in this case study did not fully meet these suggested criteria. In addition to spina bifida, she had hydrocephalus, neurogenic bladder, Arnold–Chiari malformation, severe motor impairment, and mental retardation. The strongest motive for her performing self-catheterization seemed to be a wish to be independent from, and not a burden to, her mother. Her mother also wanted her to do self-catheterization and she knew this.

[1] School of Nursing and Social Services, Health Sciences University of Hokkaido, Ishikari-Tobetsu, Hokkaido 061-02, Japan
[2] Hokkaido Prefectural Rehabilitation Center for Handicapped Children, Sapporo, Hokkaido, Japan

The purpose of this case study is to report the nursing process by which this adolescent with multiple handicaps succeeded in learning self-catheterization.

Case Report

The subject was a 13-year-old girl who had a lumbar lesion, below L1 for perception, and below L4 for motor activity. She had resided in an institution for handicapped children in Hokkaido since she was 8 years old. She also had hydrocephalus, Arnold–Chiari malformation, mental retardation (IQ 41), and severe motor impairment. She did not fully meet the criteria suggested by Segal et al. [8] (Table 1). She had severe difficulty with motor activities; her pincer grasp was so premature that not only her index finger and thumb but also her middle finger involuntarily worked together when she grasped a catheter. In addition, her index finger and thumb did not have true opposition in pinching. Her hipjoint abduction was very narrow (an angle of 30° on one side and 20° on the other). To stay in an upright position by herself, she needed to be supported by special equipment surrounding her back and both sides. Thus it was hard for her to grasp the catheter or any held device while keeping in an upright position. She had worn diapers since birth, and nurses had managed intermittent urinary catheterization seven times per day. She was totally dependent on nurses in bladder management. Because of her mental retardation, she did not appear to have enough comprehension for appropriate bladder management. She could not tell time, and she did not fully understand numerical concepts, but she could count to 10. Nurses and physicians, as well as occupational and physical therapists at the institution, did not think she was ready to perform self-catheterization. She has been in a wheelchair, and with the exception of bladder and bowel management, she managed the activities of daily life almost independently, although such activities were time consuming; for example, she spent an hour dressing, 40 min feeding, and 30 min washing her face and brushing her teeth.

Her parents were devout adherents of a new religion, Mahikarikyo, and in order to avoid violating the precepts of their religion, they rejected surgery, medications, and using a pillow filled with ice. In spite of these limitations, the subject expressed a willingness to perform self-catheterization when she was 13 years old. Her family also wanted her to be independent

TABLE 1. Developmental components for a successful CIC program

Component
Toddler's drive for autonomy
Preschooler's drive for independence
Acquisition of self-recognition and self-identity
Emotional development to feel comfortable with manipulations necessary to self-catheterize
Ability to tell time or understand the concept of time
Ability to keep records
Ability to solve problems in unfamiliar settings
Fine motor and self-skills
Sufficient attention span
Manual dexterity
Ability to ignore distracting stimulus
Ability to imitate others
Ability of child to reach perineum and to balance self

Italics indicate components which this patient could not achieve.

in her bladder management. Her primary nurse decided to teach her to perform self-catheterization and to help her overcome various difficulties.

Nursing Process

Period I. Introducing CIC (April–July, 1995)

Assessment. Although she had strong motivation to perform catheterization, she did not understand the rationale for performing catheterization or the principles of the catheter procedure. She could not maintain a stable upright position. She did not understand why a clean catheter technique is needed, and did not have the skills to accomplish clean catheterization. In addition, it was hard for her to spread her labia and identify her urethral meatus because she could not stay upright and could not spread her legs far enough apart due to her motor impairment.

Objectives.

1. To identify reasons for performing catheterization and its steps with a clean procedure.
2. To maintain a stable upright position during catheterization.

Specific Content and Teaching Strategies

Because of her mental retardation, she did not understand the rationale for the CIC program. However, she was motivated by her mother's desire that she perform CIC and she wanted to be independent from her mother. The primary nurse thought it was the right time for her to learn self-catheterization. First, the nurse let her observe the nurses' proper procedure during CIC. The nurses explained what they did by using easy words and concrete concepts. Simultaneously, they showed her the urethral meatus by using a mirror. She could not watch the mirror as she manipulated the catheter due to her difficulty in keeping an upright position. Therefore, the primary nurse described the site of the urinary meatus as "Tsuru Tsuru" (Japanese meaning slippery tactility) and trained her to find the site of "Tsuru Tsuru" with her finger's tactile sense. Then the nurse took her hand and helped her insert a catheter into the urinary meatus. At this period the nurse instructed her using hand-on-hand instruction. She was provided with devices for catheterization by herself, and taught their uses. Procedural steps were written in a table and posted on the wall in the bathroom so that she and a nurse could follow them. Hand-washing and cleaning the catheter were specifically and intentionally trained. She needed repeated instructions and demonstrations to understand the steps of performing catheterization, and she sometimes forgot to provide some of the devices during the steps. The nurse read the steps each time, because she could not read some Japanese characters; by the end of period I, she had memorized all the steps. Nurses gave her positive feedback whenever she did well on these procedures and encouraged her progress in the CIC program. Further, the nurse taught her ways of observing urine in a urinal, and helped her identify the nebulous urine about which she needed to notify the nurses. Since her torso could not stay upright, an occupational therapist designed a device to support her back. However, the upright posture supported by this first device was not appropriate for catheterization, and she could not maintain a stable sitting posture. Next, she started muscle training to enhance her arm strength by handling a wheelchair weighted with a 5-kg sand bag for 500 m to 1 km a day. Although she had always worn trousers, the nurse asked her mother to make a skirt that would lessen the difficulties of her manipulation of the catheter. The mother was very cooperative and made the skirt quickly.

Period II. Mastering Skills for Self-Catheterization (August–December, 1995)

Assessment. She had gradually memorized the steps of the CIC program and understood the necessity of clean procedures. She could also identify nebulous urine, measure urine volume by guessing more or less than average, and report these findings to the nurses. She was still highly motivated to perform self-catheterization. She seemed ready to move forward in demonstrating self-catheterization. However, since the back support to keep her in an upright position did not work well, it first needed to be redesigned and remade. Her parents continued to be supportive of her performing self-catheterization.
Objectives.
1. To stay in an upright posture during the CIC program.
2. To acquire the skills for performing self-catheterization.

Specific Contents and Teaching Strategies

The support equipment was remodeled and another was made. The new arch-type equipment supported both her back and her sides. She could then easily maintain an upright position during the CIC procedure.

The primary nurse had her demonstrate CIC: washing hands, preparing equipment, washing the catheter, moving from her wheel chair to the toilet, positioning herself, removing her diaper, putting the urinal in front of her genitalia, cleaning her hands and labia with cleansing pads, spreading her labia, locating her urethral meatus, inserting the catheter, withdrawing the catheter, washing the catheter, replacing equipment, and washing her hands. After self-catheterization she put everything she used back in order. She went through this process repeatedly with the nurses' help. The nurses assisted her in finding her urinary meatus by grasping her index finger to help her locate it, and by holding her legs open. The nurses always told her to "look for Tsuru Tsuru," and they recorded the time spent locating it. She expressed happiness in her face when she could precisely locate her urinary meatus. These accumulated training sessions helped her succeed in finding it. Then she started to demonstrate self-catheterization with the nurse. As mentioned before, her manual dexterity was immature and poor. It was hard for her to insert the catheter. However, when she tried to insert a catheter by herself, she accidentally performed self-catheterization. She said, "Nurse Hamamatsu, I could do it" with a shyly delighted expression.

After this successful insertion, the primary nurse set the goal of having her demonstrate self-catheterization 4 times out of 7 times of catheterization in a day under nurses' monitoring. The nurse never forced her to do self-catheterization routinely. Sometimes the nurses helped with catheterization when she did not have enough time to do it alone. At the same time, the nurse asked her parents to encourage her to perform self-catheterization with the same steps and procedures at home when she went back home for a short stay.

Period III. Being Independent from Mother in CIC (January–April, 1996)

Assessment. She could perform self-catheterization, but it was time consuming. She needed help during the whole process of CIC, from preparing the devices, to self-catheterization, to putting the devices back in order and washing her hands. She still had trouble balancing in a sitting posture during the CIC procedure. She needed better balancing ability in order to return to an upright position.

Objective. To be able to complete the CIC program without a nurse's help.

Specific Contents and Teaching Strategies

First, the nurses encouraged her to carry out the whole CIC procedure by herself, and tried not assist her with their hands but just observe her demonstration. The nurses recorded in a table the time she spent from grasping to successfully inserting a catheter. The time decreased from 5–12 min at first to 15 s–2 min after 1.5 months (Fig. 1). She was encouraged and pleased by the table that documented her increased speed in self-catheterization.

She started muscle training, in which she raised her body from her wheelchair seat by her hands for 10 s 3 times before going to bed every night, so that she could balance her torso during the CIC program without a nurse's help. The effect of this exercise on her motor activity both improved her balance and helped her to spread her labia more easily. As a result, she was able to find her urinary meatus even sooner. Of course she sometimes mistakenly inserted the catheter into her vagina, but the nurses never criticized her when this occurred.

The primary nurse set the goal of having her complete CIC 6 times out of 7 times a day. She performed the CIC procedure by herself, without even a nurse's observation. She was asked to call a nurse after she was done. She could notice the time to perform CIC by associating it with daily events, even though she could not tell the time.

When she went to her parent's home for a short stay, she could perform the CIC procedure without her mother's help. She showed increased self-esteem and satisfaction with this success.

Discussion

This case study shows a successful CIC program for an adolescent with spina bifida when it had seemed impossible that she could complete the program. At the beginning, she could not meet half of the developmental components for successful CIC programs summarized by Segal et al. [8]. However, she and her primary nurse were determined to carry out the CIC program and they succeeded. This study suggests that there might need to be fewer components to achieve self-catheterization than those found before. The most important factor in this study was a strong motivation in the patient and the primary nurse. Once they decided to complete the CIC program, they never gave up. They continued their efforts until they suc-

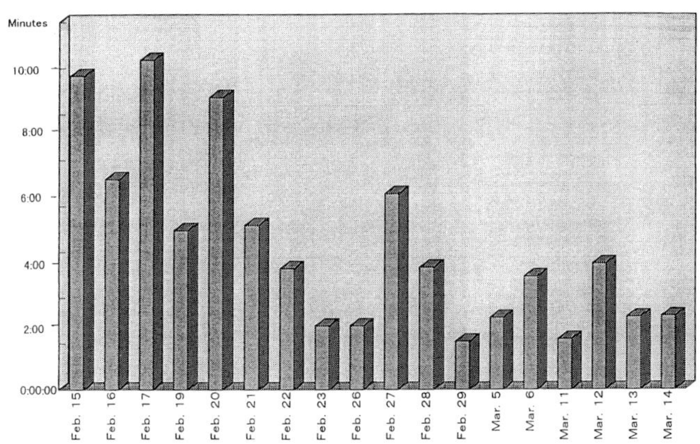

FIG. 1. Average time spent from grasping to inserting catheter

ceeded. This adolescent with spina bifida had an honest and earnest personality. She was gentle and obedient by nature, and was a hard worker. The primary nurse trusted in her potential to achieve the CIC program. The nurses had been very persistent, and instructed her over and over until she acquired the skills. The primary nurse coordinated the skills of the health care providers in the institution. The patient had their attention and creative efforts, and she made progress in the CIC program. Her parents were also very supportive, and wanted her to perform self-catheterization.

Now, in 1997, she consistently performs self-catheterization 4 times a day. She still needs help from nurses to remove her diaper, which has never been dry because her parents still refuse to allow her medication to make the diaper dry up because of their religious beliefs. In addition, she still does not have bowel management. She is 15 years old now, and wants to go to a high school for handicapped children and receive special education. It is hard to be accepted at the high school because they do not have a school nurse who can take care of her, nor facilities in which she can perform CIC. If she is able to do self-catheterization in a wheelchair by herself, it may be possible for her to attend the school. Now she and the primary nurse are working on this challenge so that she will be able to go to the high school.

References

1. Fukazawa K (1997) Bladder management in spina bifida children. Jpn Uro Nurs 2:18–24
2. Hannigan K (1988) Teaching catheterization to children. Urol Clin N Am 15:653–660
3. Iwakawa A, Senoh K, Nakajima M (1991) Some devices useful for teaching self-catheterization to children. Jpn Urol Surg 4:47–51
4. Kawabe K, Ogawa A, Sakaguchi R (1988) Indication for self-catheterization. Jpn Urol Surg 1:1025–1030
5. Momose H, Yamada K, Yamamoto M, Natsume O, Hirao Y, Okajima E (1996) Bladder management in spina bifida. Jpn Hainyo—Shougai Pract 4:151–155
6. Rickert VI, Edmond WA, Rickert CP, Thornsberry RG (1990) Behavioral method for teaching self-catheterization skills to anxious children with myelomeningocele. Arch Phys Med Rehabil 71:715–753
7. Sanematsu H, Nemoto R, Nakamura I (1994) Urinary management of patients with spina bifida. Jpn J Tottori Med Assoc 22:146–148
8. Segal ES, Deatrick JA, Hagelgans NA (1995) The determinants of successful self-catheterization programs in children with myelomeningoceles. J Pediatr Nurs 10:82–88
9. Shimizu N (1993) Clean intermittent catheterization (CIC) for spina bifida patients. Jpn Pediatr Surg 25:1137–1141
10. Takagi R (1988) Training: technique and result. Uro Surg 1:1031–1036

Augmentation Cystoplasty in Children with Spina Bifida

Hidehiro Kakizaki, Shinya Kobayashi, Kaname Ameda, Takashi Shibata, Hiroshi Tanaka, Katsuya Nonomura, and Tomohiko Koyanagi

Summary. During the last 9 years, 11 children with spina bifida (ages 3–14 years with a mean of 7.7 years; 6 girls and 5 boys) underwent augmentation cystoplasty (AC) for intractable neurogenic vesical dysfunction (NVD). The primary indication for AC was upper urinary tract deterioration in 7 and urinary incontinence in 4 that were refractory to a conservative regimen of clean intermittent catheterization and anticholinergics. A sling procedure using a free graft of anterior rectus fascia was simultaneously performed in 7 who had urethral sphincter incompetence. Postoperatively, the upper urinary tract was normalized or improved in all patients. Two of 4 children with severe incontinence became dry, while the other 2 experienced a dramatic improvement of incontinence. Bladder capacity and compliance were markedly increased after the operation. Long-term complications were not encountered, except for bladder stone in 2 cases. In spina bifida children with intractable NVD, augmentation cystoplasty can yield a highly satisfactory outcome.

Key words. Spina bifida, Augmentation cystoplasty, Incontinence, Neurogenic vesical dysfunction, Urodymanics

Introduction

The majority of children with spina bifida have neurogenic bladder despite early closure of the spinal defect. Neurogenic dysfunction of the bladder and urethra can cause upper urinary tract deterioration and urinay incontinence, which are major urological problems in the management of children with spina bifida.

Since the advent of clean intermittent catheterization as a safe method of bladder emptying for patients with vesicourethral dysfunction [15], urinary management of children with spina bifida has been dramatically improved. Conservative treatment using clean intermittent catheterization alone or in combination with anticholinergics has been successful in preserving the upper urinary tract and achieving urinary continence in many children with spina bifida [2, 7, 8, 12]. However, a small group of children have persistent ureteral reflux or urinary incontinence despite the maximal conservative treatment.

Persistent ureteral reflux or hydroureteronephrosis is usually caused by poor bladder compliance or detrusor hyperreflexia, while refractory urinary incontinence is caused by either

Department of Urology, Hokkaido University School of Medicine, North-15 West-7 Kita-Ku, Sapporo 060-8638, Japan

urethral sphincter incompetence or poor bladder storage function, or both. If conservative treatment with intermittent catheterization and anticholinergics is unsuccessful to improve bladder storage function, augmentation cystoplasty is a reasonable next step to resolve urological problems in children with spina bifida [14].

We describe our experience of augmentation cystoplasty in children with spina bifida to highlight surgical outcomes and long-term complications.

Patients and Methods

During the past 9 years, 11 children with spina bifida underwent augmentation cystoplasty in our hospital. Patients age ranged from 3 to 14 years, with a mean of 8 years. The indications for augmentation cystoplasty were upper urinary tract deterioration in 7 and urinary incontinence in 4, both of which were refractory to maximal conservative treatment with intermittent catheterization and anticholinergics. The upper urinary tract deterioration involved persistent high-grade reflux in 6 patients, and severe hydroureteronephrosis in 1. These upper tract changes were caused by poor bladder storage function (poor bladder compliance).

Preoperative evaluations of the lower urinary tract included cystography, cystometry, a urethral pressure profile (UPP), and electromyography of the external urethral sphincter (EUS-EMG). The methodological details of the urodynamic studies have been described previously [1, 13].

In all patients, the terminal ileum was used for augmentation cystoplasty. Goodwin's cup-patch technique was used in the first 5 patients, and Hautmann's method was performed in the other 6 patients. Basically, the bladder was opened widely by transverse oblique cystotomy, and an intestinal segment, which was fashioned into a U-shape (Goodwin) or a W-shape (Hautmann), was anastomosed to the bladder. Ureteral reimplantation was performed simultaneously in 4 patients, and fascial sling (Fig. 1) in 7 patients (5 boys and 2 girls). Fascial sling was indicated in patients with urethral sphincter incompetence, which was diagnosed as hypoactive sphincter on EUS-EMG, low urethral closure pressure (< 40 cm H_2O) on UPP, low detrusor leak point pressure (< 30 cm H_2O) on cystometry, or incompetent bladder neck on cystography [9].

Periodic reevaluations were performed postoperatively, including cystography and urodynamic studies. Laboratory data were also examined regularly to evaluate electrolyte disturbance and vitamin deficiency. If indicated, ultrasonography, excretory urography, or renal

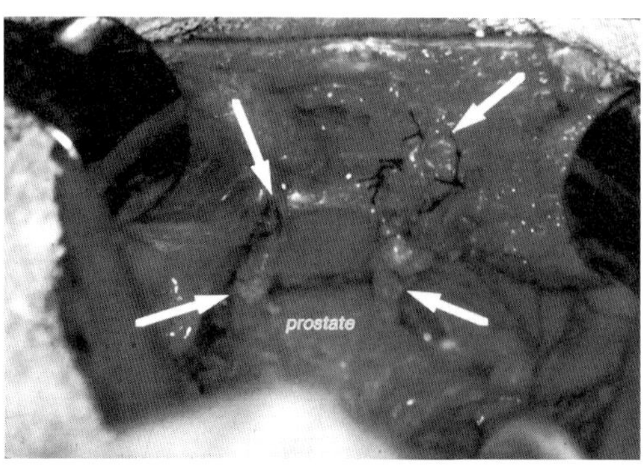

FIG. 1 A fascial sling, obtained from the rectus fascia, was placed around the prostatic apex in a male patient

scintigraphy with ^{99m}Tc-diethylene triamine pentaacetic acid (DTPA) or ^{99m}Tc -dimercapto-succinic acid (DMSA) were performed to assess the upper urinary tract.

Results

Augmentation cystoplasty was highly successful in all patients. After augmentation cystoplasty, reflux was resolved in all patients (Fig. 2) and hydroureteronephrosis was improved in 1 patient. Of 4 patients for whom the indication of augmentation cystoplasty was urinary incontinence, 2 became dry, while the other 2 experienced a dramatic improvement in their incontinence. Overall, 9 of 11 patients (82%) became dry after augmentation cystoplasty.

The characteristics of postoperative urodynamic studies were a significant increase in bladder capacity (from 119 ± 41 to 360 ± 99 ml) and compliance (from 4.9 ± 3.5 to 31 ± 13 ml/cm H_2O) (Fig. 3). No significant change in maximal urethral closure pressure on UPP was noted after fascial sling (from 40 ± 13 to 50 ± 19 cm H_2O).

During follow-up (from 3 to 9 years), 2 developed bladder stones (at 10 and 19 months after the operation, respectively), which were successfully managed by endourology. Diarrhea was worsened in 1 patient after the operation. Oral administration of cholestyramine is very effective in treating diarrhea in that patient. Other complications such as metabolic acidosis, vitamin B_{12} or folic acid deficiency, or bladder rupture were not encountered in any patients. As for the upper urinary tract, normal renal function is maintained in 10 patients. However, in the remaining patient who had presented with established renal damage, renal function gradually deteriorated, and she subsequently underwent successful renal transplantation.

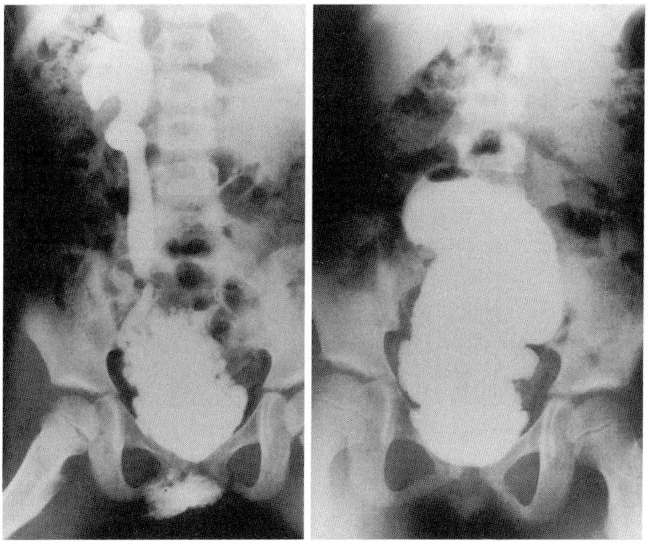

a Before operation

b After operation

FIG. 2 **a** Pre- and **b** postoperative cystography in a 5-year-old girl. High-grade ureteral reflux in the right side disappeared after augmentation cystoplasty without antireflux ureteral reimplantation

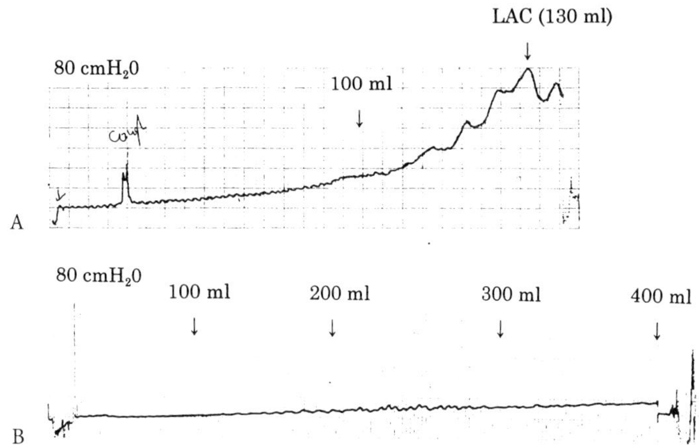

FIG. 3 **A** Pre- and **B** postoperative cystometrogram in a 12-year-old girl. Bladder capacity and compliance were markedly improved after augmentation cystoplasty

Discussion and Conclusions

The present study indicates that augmentation cystoplasty together with additional procedures can provide highly satisfactory outcomes for upper urinary tract preservation and urinary continence in patients with spina bifida. However, careful long-term follow-up is mandatory for urinary calculi and possible metabolic derangement.

Since the introduction of intermittent catheterization as a safe and reliable method of urinary management for vesicourethral dysfunction, the treatment of children with spina bifida has been significantly improved. Along with wide acceptance of intermittent catheterization, urodynamic studies have been performed in children with spina bifida to detect those who are at high risk of upper urinary tract deterioration. Vesical leak point pressure of more than 40 cm H_2O [16], maximal urethral closure pressure of more than 50 cm H_2O [13], and the presence of detrusor-sphincter dyssynergia (incoordination) [3] have been shown to be important risk factors for upper urinary tract deterioration in untreated children with spina bifida. Thus, prophylactic use of intermittent catheterization has been recommended to prevent upper urinary tract deterioration in children with spina bifida in whom urodynamic studies have demonstrated prognostically unfavorable patterns [6, 10]. This strategy has been adopted in our institute. However, the optimal timing to initiate intermittent catheterization in children with spina bifida is controversial. Some have indicated that preservation of the upper urinary tract can be accomplished equally without prophylactic use of intermittent catheterization, since the delayed use of intermittent catheterization can still normalize upper urinary tract deterioration if identified early and managed promptly [12, 18]. Despite these controversies regarding the optimal timing to initiate intermittent catheterization in children with spina bifida, its role in preserving the upper urinary tract, with or without anticholinergics, as well as achieving urinary continence is universally accepted. Recently, it has been suggested by some authors that early treatment from infancy with intermittent catheterization and anticholinergics might prevent irreversible bladder dysfunction in children with spina bifida and reduce the ultimate need for surgical intervention, especially bladder augmentation, which is the last resort for normalizing intractable high bladder-storage pressure

[5]. The reported incidence of bladder augmentation in children with spina bifida who had been treated from infancy with prophylactic intermittent catheterization because of poor prognostic factors is 4% [10] and 11% [19], while 28% of children with upper urinary tract deterioration required bladder augmentation if treated expectantly with radiological observation [4]. In our institute, bladder augmentation was performed in about 16% of children with spina bifida who had a urodynamic risk factor of high bladder-storage pressure.

In addition to upper urinary tract deterioration, which is refractory to conservative treatment, urinary incontinence is another indication for augmentation cystoplasty. In children with spina bifida, both bladder and urethral dysfunction could be responsible for urinary incontinence. We performed a fascial sling in several children simultaneously with bladder augmentation, particularly when the preoperative urodynamic studies suggested the presence of urethral sphincter incompetence, as defined previously [9]. In male patients, however, we failed to reveal significant urodynamic changes in stress urethral pressure profilometry, and it is not certain if the fascial sling provides a significant additive effect on continence in male patients [14]. However, of 11 children in this study, all of whom had been incontinent preoperatively, 9 (82%) became continent after bladder augmentation with or without fascial sling. The remaining 2 patients also experienced a dramatic improvement of urinary incontinence postoperatively. Taken together, excellent or fair results in urinary control were achieved in all of the patients following bladder augmentation with or without fascial sling.

Possible long-term complications of augmentation cystoplasty with intestine include urolithiasis, diarrhea, metabolic derangement, and bladder perforation [11]. In our study, the postoperative complication rate was relatively low except for bladder stone in 2 patients and worsened diarrhea in 1, and metabolic derangement was not encountered, although a longer follow-up period is required. The reported incidence of urolithiasis after augmentation cystoplasty ranged from 6% to 30%, including bladder and upper urinary tract stones [17]. The development of bladder stone might be associated with persistent bacteriuria or retention of mucus, and thus strict adherence to frequent catheterization and bladder irrigation with saline might be recommended to prevent recurrent bladder stone [17].

In one patient who had presented with established renal damage due to intractable bladder dysfunction, successful augmentation cystoplasty did not have an impact on the prognosis of renal function. When bladder dysfunction is refractory to maximum conservative treatment, bladder augmentation should be considered without undue delay before the establishment of significant renal damage. Even if end-stage renal failure develops, restoration of lower urinary tract function by bladder augmentation is a prerequisite for successful renal transplantation in patients with intractable bladder dysfunction.

In conclusion, augmentation cystoplasty, with or without additional procedures such as ureteral reimplantation or fascial sling, can provide highly satisfactory outcomes for upper urinary tract preservation and urinary continence in patients with spina bifida. However, careful long-term follow-up is mandatory for urinary calculi and possible metabolic derangement.

References

1. Ameda K, Kakizaki H, Yamashita T, Nonomura K, Shinno Y, Kemmotsu O, Koyanagi T (1997) Feasibility of urodynamic study (combined cystometry and electromyography of the external urethral sphincter) under general anesthesia in children. Int J Urol 4:32–39
2. Baskin LS, Kogan BA, Benard F (1990) Treatment of infants with neurogenic bladder dysfunction using anticholinergic drugs and intermittent catheterisation. Br J Urol 66:532–534

3. Bauer SB, Hallett M, Khoshbin S, Lebowitz RL, Winston KR, Gibson S, Colodny AH, Retik AB (1984) Predictive value of urodynamic evaluation in newborns with myelodysplasia. JAMA 252:650–652
4. Bloom DA, Knechtel JM, McGuire EJ (1990) Urethral dilation improves bladder compliance in children with myelomeningocele and high leak point pressure. J Urol 144:430–433
5. Edelstein RA, Bauer SB, Kelly MD, Darbey MM, Peters CA, Atala A, Mandell J, Colodny AH, Retik AB (1995) The long-term urological response of neonates with myelodysplasia treated proactively with intermittent catheterization and anticholinergic therapy. J Urol 154: 1500–1505
6. Geraniotis E, Koff SA, Enrile B (1988) The prophylactic use of clean intermittent catheterization in the treatment of infants and young children with myelomeningocele and neurogenic bladder dysfunction. J Urol 139:85–86
7. Hernandez RD, Hurwitz RS, Foote JE, Zimmern PE, Leach GE (1994) Nonsurgical management of threatened upper urinary tracts and incontinence in children with myelomeningocele. J Urol 152:1582–1585
8. Joseph DB, Bauer SB, Colodny AH, Mandell J, Retik SB (1989) Clean, intermittent catheterization of infants with neurogenic bladder. Pediatrics 84:78–82
9. Kakizaki H, Shibata T, Shinno Y, Kobayashi S, Matsumura K, Koyanagi T (1995) Fascial sling for the management of urinary incontinence due to sphincter incompetence. J Urol 153: 644–647
10. Kasabian NG, Bauer SB, Dyro FM, Colodny AH, Mandell J, Retik AB (1992) The prophylactic value of clean intermittent catheterization and anticholinergic medication in newborns and infants with myelodysplasia at risk of developing urinary tract deterioration. Am J Dis Child 146:840–843
11. Khoury JM, Timmons SL, Corbel L, Webster GD (1992) Complications of enterocystoplasty. Urology 40:9–14
12. Klose AG, Sackett CK, Mesrobian HG (1990) Management of children with myelodysplasia: urological alternatives. J Urol 144:1446–1449
13. Kobayashi S, Shinno Y, Kakizaki H, Matsumura K, Koyanagi T (1992) Relevance of detrusor hyperreflexia, vesical compliance and urethral pressure to the occurrence of vesicoureteral reflux in myelodysplastic patients. J Urol 147:413–415
14. Kobayashi S, Koyanagi T, Ameda K, Kakizaki H, Matsuura S, Shibata T, Sasaki Y (1996) Augmentation cystoplasty in children. Akt Urol 27 (suppl.):35–37
15. Lapides J, Diokno AC, Silber SJ, Lowe BS (1972) Clean, intermittent self-catheterization in the treatment of urinary tract disease. J Urol 107:458–461
16. McGuire EJ, Woodside JR, Borden TA, Weiss RM (1981) Prognostic value of urodynamic testing in myelodysplastic patients. J Urol 126:205–209
17. Shinojima H, Kakizaki H, Nonomura K, Yamashita T, Kanagawa K, Koyanagi T, Nantani M, Matsuno T (1994) Bladder calculus after augmentation ileocystoplasty in children. Jpn J Urol 85:1374–1379
18. Teichman JMH, Scherz HC, Kim KD, Cho DH, Packer MG, Kaplan GW (1994) An alternative approach to myelodysplasia management: aggressive observation and prompt intervention. J Urol 152:807–811
19. Wu HY, Baskin LS, Kogan BA (1997) Neurogenic bladder dysfunction due to myelomeningocele: neonatal versus childhood treatment. J Urol 157:2295–2297

Vesicoureteric Reflux and Urinary Incontinence in Myelodysplastic Patients: A Comparison Between Those who Underwent Antireflux Surgery Alone and Those who were Treated by Antireflux Surgery and Bladder Augmentation, With or Without Sling Operation

Atsuo Kondo[1], Masahiko Saito, and Yoshikazu Tsuji[2]

Introduction

Recent information about surgical intervention to correct such problems as vesicoureteric reflux and urinary incontinence associated with myelodysplasia has not made much impression on urologists or patients. Therefore, conservative treatment such as clean intermittent catheterization, with or without anticholinergics, has persistently been used for in some patients despite being of little clinical effectiveness. We feel that when these conservative modalities fail, surgical treatments should be taken into consideration.

We started to treat myelodysplastic patients in 1972. During the first 10 years we treated children mainly with conservative strategies, and did not feel justified in treating urological pathologies with surgery. However, it gradually became clear that clinical symptomatologies could not always be properly controlled by conservative means, and patients needed surgical intervention for incontinence, reflux, and a low compliance bladder. It is known that reflux and incontinence are the major causes of morbidity in myelodysplasia, and they are present in 30% and 90% of patients, respectively. We have treated patients with reflux by a crossover method reported in 1982 [4] and later by Orikasa's method [6]. For urinary incontinence, we initially used artificial sphincters [7], but stopped because of frequent mechanical failures. A sling operation with rectus fascia was our subsequent choice of treatment [5]. When bladder augmentation is required for low compliance and/or small bladder capacity, clam's operation [1] or Goodwin's ileal cup-patch method [3] have been used. The aim of this study is to compare the surgical outcomes between two groups of myelodysplastic patients; one group underwent antireflux surgery alone, and the other group was treated with antireflux surgery and bladder augmentation, with or without a sling operation.

Patients and Methods

Two groups of myelodysplastic patients were analyzed. Group A comprised 17 patients, 3 males and 14 females, whose ages varied from 3 to 18 years, with a mean of 9.5 years. They underwent surgery for correction of reflux, with a mean follow-up period of 11.7 years. Group

[1] Department of Urology, Komaki Shimin Hospital, Komaki 485-8520, Japan
[2] Nagoya University Hospital, Nagoya 466-8550, Japan

B consisted of 21 patients, 8 males and 13 females, with a mean age of 10.1 years (3–21 years). They were operated on not only for reflux but also for other pathologies, with a mean follow-up period of 3.7 years. Patients in group A were operated on for reflux by the crossover method [4]. For those in group B, Orikasa's method [6] was used for reflux surgery, and a detubularized ileum [1, 3] was used for bladder augmentation. Furthermore, 11 of the 21 patients simultaneously had a sling operation using rectus fascia.

Clinical parameters were assessed by fluoroscopic urodynamic studies, sonography, radioisotope studies, urinalysis, and blood chemistry. In 1996, postal questionnaires were sent to obtain the latest subjective assessments of the patients about the surgery they underwent.

Results

Surgical outcomes are given in Table 1. Reflux disappeared in 79% of group A (19/24 renal units) and 86% of group B (25/29 renal units) patients, and there was no statistical difference between them. Although an increase in both bladder capacity and bladder compliance is statistically significant in the two groups, group B did show an obvious superiority over group A. Subjective assessments of the operation are summarized in Table 2. There was no statistical difference between the two groups regarding patient satisfaction (analyzed by means of a visual analogue scale, with 100 being the highest satisfaction score and 0 the lowest), degree of continence, and numbers of clean intermittent catheterizations per day. However, after surgery the number of urinary tract infections was significantly lower in group B than in group A.

TABLE 1. Surgical outcomes in groups A and B

	Preoperation	Postoperation	*P* values
Group A			
Reflux corrected		79% (19/24)[a]	
Bladder capacity	158 ml	220 ml	<0.05
Bladder compliance	6.0	9.6	<0.01
Group B			
Reflux corrected		86% (25/29)[a]	
Bladder capacity	157 ml	326 ml	<0.01
Bladder compliance	5.1	32.1	<0.01

[a] Not significantly different ($P > 0.05$).

TABLE 2. Subjective assessments based on postal questionnaires

	Group A	Group B	*P* values
Satisfaction (VAS[a])	81	77	>0.05
Continence (patients[b])	86%	90%	>0.05
No. of CIC per day	5.7	4.8	>0.05
Absence of UTI (patients)	79%	100%	<0.05

[a] Visual analogue scale.
[b] Patients having complete continence or slight incontinence.
CIC, clean intermittent catheterization; UTI, urinary tract infection.

Renal insufficiency following antireflux surgery developed in one girl in group A, which was the worst complication we experienced. Several complications developed with bladder augmentation, in particular malfunctions of the ventriculoperitoneal (VP) shunt tube developed in 4 patients, and these subsequently required 14 surgical revisions. Incomplete ileus, bladder stone, contralateral reflux, and persistent diarrhea have also developed in a few patients.

Discussion

We found that video-urodynamic studies were extremely important to investigate the lower urinary tract prior to operation, and to follow up patients. Recently, Wang et al. [8] confirmed that a leak-point pressure of more than 40 cm of water indicated the imminent danger of upper urinary tract problems. In our series, the surgical outcomes of the two different techniques used for reflux were the same in both groups.

Although enterocystoplasty greatly increased bladder capacity and bladder compliance in patients in group B, its adverse effects, such as incomplete ileus, VP shunt malfunctions, acidosis, and possible bladder malignancy in the long term, cannot be neglected. The detubularized ileum could theoretically be replaced by an autoaugmentation procedure [2] which does not require incorporating the ileum and subsequently reduces the number of intraabdominal complications, but the latter cannot always guarantee an increase in bladder capacity, and is therefore a significant drawback of this surgery.

Conclusion

Surgical intervention for reflux was of clinical effect. Although adverse effects of surgery occurred more often in patients in group B, these patients enjoyed a significant improvement in bladder capacity and bladder compliance. We conclude that when conservative therapy fails to cure or improve vesicoureteric reflux and urinary incontinence, surgical intervention should be taken into consideration.

References

1. Bramble FJ (1982) The treatment of adult enuresis and urge incontinence by enterocystoplasty. Br J Urol 54:693–696
2. Cartwright PC, Snow BW (1989) Bladder autoaugmentation: early clinical experience. J Urol 142:505–508
3. Goodwin WE, Winter CC, Barher WF (1959) "Cup-patch" technique of ileocystoplasty for bladder enlargement or partial substitution. Surg Gynecol Obstet 108:370–372
4. Kondo A, Otani T (1987) Correction of reflux with the ureteric crossover method: clinical experience in 50 patients. Br J Urol 60:36–38
5. McGuire EJ, Lytton B (1978) Pubovaginal sling procedure for stress incontinence. J Urol 119:85–84
6. Orikasa S (1990) A new antireflux operation. Eur Urol 17:330–332
7. Scott FB, Bradley WE, Timm GW (1974) Treatment of urinary incontinence by an implantable prosthetic urinary sphincter. J Urol 112:75–80
8. Wang SC, McGuire EJ, Bloom DA (1988) A bladder pressure management system for myelodysplasia—clinical outcome. J Urol 140:1499–1502

Sensory Skin-Fascial Flap Application to Nonsensitive Perianal Region in Patients with Sacral Myelomeningocele: Report of Two Cases

Shun-ichi Makino, Akira Nishi, Hiroaki Komuro, Takafumi Kusaka, Kazuki Ueda, and Kyotaro Kanazawa

Summary. It is known that an inferior gluteal thigh flap (IGTF) is suitable for the reconstruction of pelvic sites. ITGF is sentient, thick, and available for remote areas from the posterior thigh. We applied an ITGF to recover a sense of their skin on the perianal region in two patients with sacral myelomeningocele of S2 and S3 segments. We report our surgical techniques and results. The IGTF was prepared from the right lower leg in both cases. It was deeply implanted into the anus after a two-thirds circumference excision of the anal verge and pecten. Nonsensitive perianal skin was also excised. The IGTF is supplied by the descending branch of the inferior gluteal artery (DBIGA), and is innervated by the posterior femoral cutaneous nerve (PFCN) originating in the S1 and S2 segments. In both cases the flap survived and maintained a pain and touch sense postoperatively. Patients became perceptive of stools during bowel movements. The management of anal incontinence is gradually improving.

Key words. Inferior gluteal thigh flap, Meningocele, Anal incontinence

Introduction

An inferior gluteal thigh flap (IGTF) was first applied in the reconstruction of pelvic lesions by Hurwitz in 1980 [1]. An IGTF is a flap from the posterior thigh. It is sentient, has a rich fat layer, and is available to remote areas as a long flap. An IGTF is often used as a sensory skin flap to treat sacral and ischiadic pressure sores in plastic surgery [2].

It is known that patients with sacral myelomeningocele have anal and urinary incontinence due to congenital damage to the spinal cord. In addition, they have nonsensitive skin in the perineum and perianal region.

For the recovery of nonsensitive skin lesions, we used an IGTF in two patients with sacral myelomeningocele in S2 and S3 segments. These patients were suffering from poor management of incontinence. We report on these two cases and our surgical procedures in the ITGF application.

Division of Pediatric Surgery and Plastic Surgery, Department of Surgery, Jichi Medical School, Tochigi 329-04, Japan.

Case Reports

Case 1

A 5-year-old male was admitted to Jichi Medical School Hospital (JHSH) after poor management of anal incontinence. At 1 day after birth, he had a skin covering operation for a myelomeningocele. Postoperatively, diminished anal muscle contraction and constipation were noted. There were no symptoms or signs of urinary bladder dysfunction or of hydrocephalus. At 1 year of age, he developed tethered cord syndrome accompanied by occasional urinary infections and loss of dry time. In MRCT investigations, an elongation of the spinal cord and an adhesion at the second sacral vertebra (S2) were observed. In spite of a fine untethering operation using Dacron sheet, there was no improvement. Postoperatively, he had a nonsensitive area in the perineum and perianal region, which are segments S3–S5 of the dermatome. He had no awareness of bowel movements, and had frequent staining. The patient was mentally normal, and had a normal gait. Although he wanted to attend ordinary primary school, his parents insisted that his condition should improve first.

Case 2

A male child aged 2 years and 10 months was admitted to JMSH owing to anal incontinence. Previously, he had undergone two operations. The first operation was a dura and skin plasty for sacral myelomeningocele in the S3 segment performed 42 h after birth. The second was a Ramstedt operation for pyloric stenosis performed at 38 days of age. Pre- and postoperatively after the first operation he had total urinary and anal incontinence, diminished anal muscle contraction, and constipation. He had a nonsensitive area in the perineum and perianal region. As he wore a diaper, his perianal site became easily erosive due to occasional diarrhea. His parents insisted that his condition be improved.

Surgical Procedure

The patient was placed in the jackknife position. Prior to the actual operation, we used X-marks to indicate the right greater trochanter and the ischium, and drew lines toward the popliteal fossa to prepare for a parabolic skin fascial flap (Fig. 1). Between the two X-marks were the posterior femoral cutaneous nerve (PFCN), a descending branch of the inferior gluteal artery (DBIGA), and coexisting veins (Figs. 2 and 3). The PFCN is a pure sensory nerve and covers dermatomes S1 and S2 of the posterior thigh (Fig. 4). The DBIGA is the last branch of the internal pelvic artery. The flap was 8 cm wide and 20 cm long. A skin incision was made from the lower end of the parabola near the popliteal fossa. We extended the incision and exfoliated the skin flap toward the gluteus maximus muscle. The flap contained a thick fat layer and the posterior fascia lata just over the fascia of the muscles of the posterior thigh. The PFCN and DBIGA had perforating branches directed toward the biceps femoris muscle and the semimembranous muscle. Using a nerve stimulater, we distingushed the main PFCN from the perforating branches, and cut the perforating branches. The main PFCN and DBIGA were observed on the side of the flap. Exfoliation was completed at the lower end of the gluteus maximus muscle and reached to a line between the X-marks (Fig. 5). The flap was sufficiently long and was rotated easily toward the perianal region. We made another skin incision in the direction of the anus from the medial X-mark. In addition, we incised the perianal region, anal verge, and pecten. We incised about two-thirds of the circumference. The

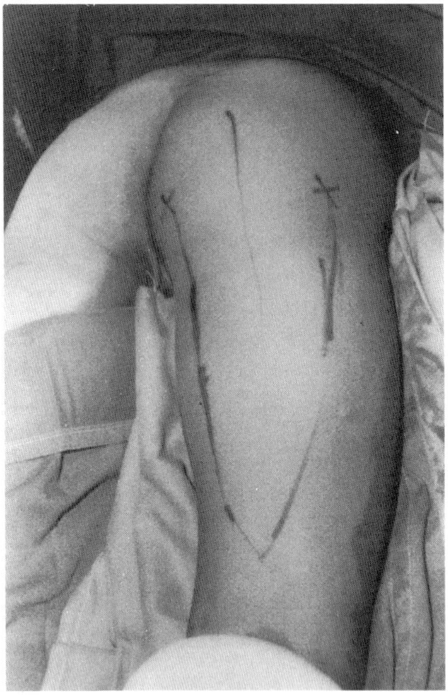

FIG. 1. X-marks were used to indicate the greater trochanter and ischium. A parabolic line for an inferior gluteal thigh flap (IGTF) was drawn (Case 1)

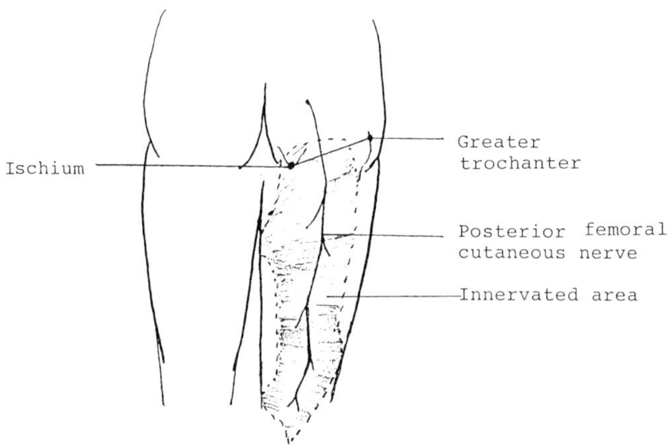

FIG. 2. The posterior femoral cutaneous nerve (PFCN) runs midway between the two X-marks and innervates the IGTF

flap was rotated about 90° inter-nally. For flap application to the anus, we employed the lateral edge of dermatome S1 to the rim of the anus. The dermatome S1 segment should be more sensitized than the S2 segment. Anastomosis with anal mucosa was carried out by 3-0 vicryl. Penrose drains and a portex drain were placed into the subcutaneous space. The skin was closed by 3-0 nylon (Fig. 6). The operating time was about 4h and the blood loss was about 50ml in both cases.

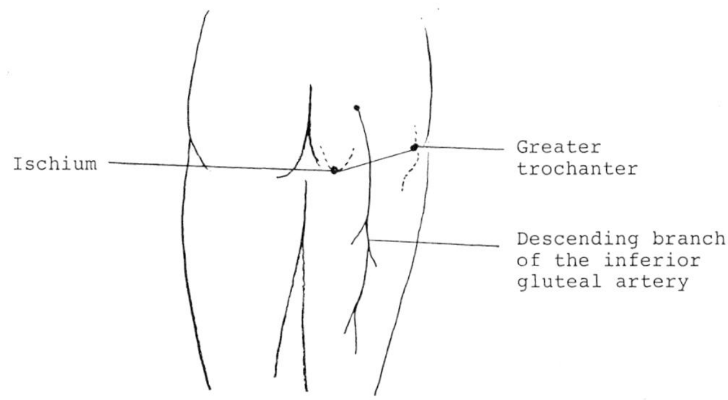

FIG. 3. A descending branch of the inferior gluteal artery (DBIGA) runs near the PFCN and supplies the ITGF

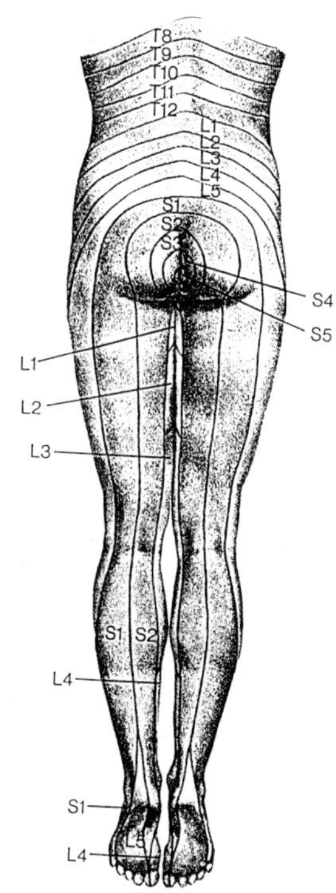

FIG. 4. The dermatome of the lumbosacral region and the posterior thigh. The S1 and S2 segments were innervated by the PCFN. The PCFN was implanted to segments S3, S4, and S5

Operative Results

After 13 months in one patient and 8 months in the other, the flaps are sentient and the appearance is acceptable (Fig. 7 and 8). We urged both patients to pay attention to bowel movements, and suggested that the perianal region should be kept clean and dry. Currently,

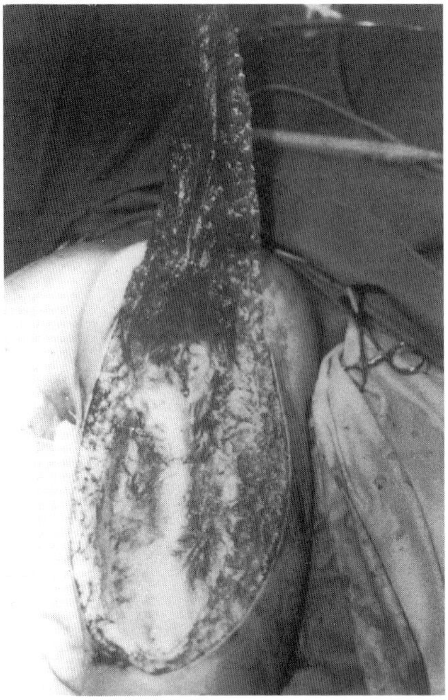

Fig. 5. The flap is prepared. The main PCFN, DBIGA, and fascia lata are contained in the flap (Case 1)

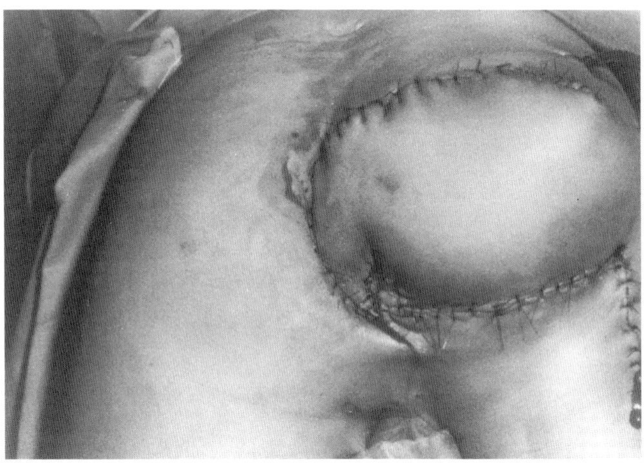

Fig. 6. The application of the flap to the perianal region is completed (Case 1)

although both patients complain of pain from the posterior thigh, they have gradually become aware of bowel movements after evacuation. We also noted that management was improving.

However, these operations revealed certain problems: (1) it is difficult to have sensitivity in the early postoperative period; (2) it is difficult to evacuate large hard stools because of

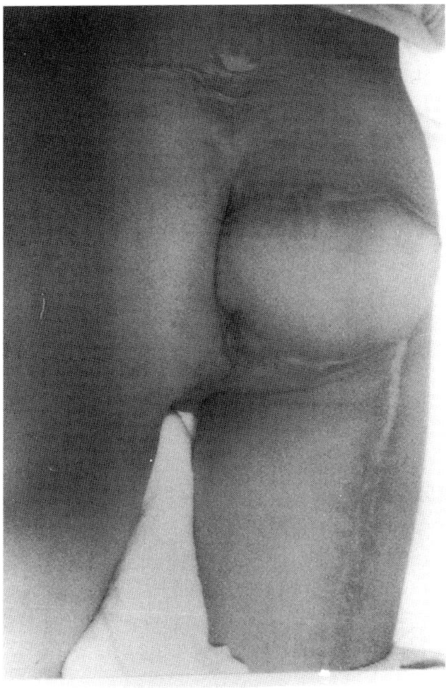

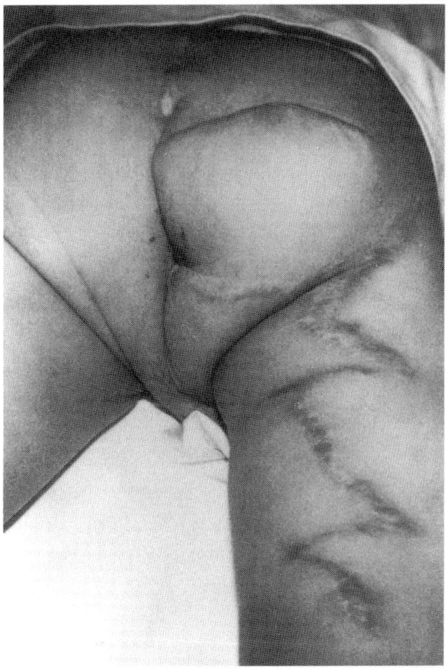

FIG. 7. The appearance of the flap 13 months into the postoperative period in Case 1
FIG. 8. The appearance of the flap 8 months into the postoperative period in Case 2

the scar; (3) it is difficult to maintain the same sitting position for long periods because of numbness of the right leg.

Discussion

It is known that patients with a sacral myelomeningocele have frequent anal and urinary incontinence. They also have a nonsensitive skin region in the perineum and the anus. The present patients passed cubic, inspisated, viscous stools because of paralyses of the colon and rectum. Onuf's nucleus in the spinal cord was congenitally damaged. The patients noticed a bowel movement when stools touched remote skin areas or by its unpleasant smell. They usually had a delay in its management. In spite of having a normal mentality and gait, incontinence was a serious handicap in kindergarten or primary school. It was not suprising that their parents wished to improve this condition. In compliance with their wishes, we performed the operation.

Our operative indications are now described. (1) Ethical problems have to be resolved. Both parents or a person in parental authority must consent to the results of the operation. The operation uses new surgical techniques and is focused only on an improvement in the management of bowel movements after evacuation. There is no change in urinary and anal incontinence. Patients have a long scar on the back of the leg after the operation. (2) Patients should be of normal mentality and have almost normal gait. They should also have the ability to attend kindergarten or an ordinary school. We also insist that patients have no hydrocephalus and no V-P shunt in order to avoid multiple surgery. (3) Patients must have intact dermatomes of segments S1 and S2, which is of prime importance. We checked this repeatedly by needle stabbing before the operation. Dermatomes S1 and S2 are innervated by the PFCN, which derives from the upper part of the damaged spinal cord. We could use an IGTF in both cases.

Case 1 had spina bifida in the S2 segment, but fortunately his dermatome S2 was intact. Case 2 had spina bifida in the S3 segment, and was suitable to undergo surgery. We excised two-thirds of the circumference of the anal verge and pecten because we had noted that total excision caused anal constriction due to scarring. For the implantion of the flap, the edge of the dermatome S1 side was facing the anus to maintain a reliable sensation.

There have been no published reports of an IGTF application for recovering sensitivity around the perianal region of patients with myelomeningocele. We consider that these symptoms have been ignored for too long, as they are the result of intractable congenital damage. However, plastic surgeons often treat pressure sores in the sacral area using an IGTF. Recently, the application of an IGTF in patients with myelomeningocele were reported by Rosen et al. [3]. They treated pressure sores in two cases. One was a 15-year-old male, and the other was an adult. They used an IGTF in both cases as an island flap. They also described an IGTF application for a imperforated anus in which a vagina was constructed. The results were not documented. It is very interesting that Rosen et al. reported that they applied an IGTF in a patient with spina bifida of segments L3-S1. In one of their two cases, they observed sensitivity in the flap postoperatively. The patient should not have had sensitivity in the IGTF.

There is a similar method in use to treat pressure sores. Dibbell et al. [4] reported the application of a tensor fascia latae (TFL) myocutaneous flap in two patients with myelomeningocele. The flap was innervated by the lateral femoral cutaneous nerve (LFCN), which originates in segments L1, L2, and L3. They recommended the use of TFL in patients with myelomeningocele which occurs in higher segments. However, these patients had a poor blood supply to the legs. Their legs were anoxic and cold, and we hesitate to take even an IV root. We believe that TEL is not ideal for the reconstruction of sensitivity around the perianal region.

Former operative techniques for anal incontinence were evaluated. The results of Picrell's operation and derivatives which use skeletal voluntary muscle have not been satisfactory so far. If other innovative methods are developed, we should not neglect insensitive skin lesions of the perineum and perianus in patients with myelomeningocele.

In the two cases described here, the flap survived completely and is gradually functioning as a sensory flap. Our operative results revealed the problems mentioned above, but the overall results seem to be acceptable to the patients.

References

1. Hurwitz DJ (1980) Closure of a large defect of the pelvic cavity by an extended compound flap based on the inferior gluteal artery. Br J Plast Surg 33:256
2. Walton R (1982) Inferior gluteal thigh flap. In: Mathe S, Nahai F (eds) Clinical applications for muscle and musculocutaneous flaps. Mosby, St. Louis, pp 490–505

3. Rosen JM, Mo ST, Liu A (1990) Experience with the island inferior thigh flap compared with other local flaps for the reconstruction of the pelvic area. Ann Plast Surg 24:498–509
4. Dibbell DG, MaCraw JB, Edstrom LE (1976) Providing useful and protective sensibility to the sitting areas in patients with meningocele. Plast Reconstr Surg 64:796

Surgical Management of the Neurogenic Bladder

Laurence S. Baskin

Patients with myelomeningocele or neurogenic bladder include many different types, ranging from the obvious back deformities, to patients who have a small spinal dimple. The incidence of spina bifida is about 1:1000 newborn infants. Presently, the urological aspects of spina bifida can be effectively treated [1]. A contemporary goal is to eliminate the diagnosis of myelomeningocele from the list of patients requiring renal transplantation.

There are three goals of urological treatment of myelomeningocele, with the primary goal being preservation of renal function. The second goal, at an appropriate time, is the achievement of urinary and fecal continence. The final goal is to facilitate independence, self-esteem, and a healthy sexual function for our patients [1].

Surgical treatment of patients with myelomeningocele starts in the newborn period [2, 3], because it is necessary to define which type of bladder these patients have when they are born. Prior to hospital discharge, the status of the bladder is defined urodynamically. The bladder is declared to be hostile or friendly, and therapy is instituted based on these preliminary findings. These findings are then correlated with renal bladder sonography.

All of our urodynamic studies are done by simple observation of the pressures involved in the cyclical filling and emptying of the bladder. Simultaneous fluoroscopy, perineal myography, and cystometrics can be monitored. We attempt to document the nature of the baby's voiding. Is the bladder contracting and emptying? Is the bladder normal? Is there vesicoureteral reflux? Is the bladder smooth-walled? What is the condition of the sphincter and the posterior urethra? More simply, does the infant void, and is this a coordinated void? In the newborn period it is possible to document severe trabeculation, massive reflux, and dyssynergia (with the dilated posterior urethra and the abrupt cutoff at the external sphincter). This suggests that the damage to the urinary tract is occurring well before birth.

Electromyography (EMG) tells us if the sphincter is relaxing while the bladder is contracting. When we measure EMG activity, we use electrocardiography (ECG) pads. We do not use needles or a rectal probe in an attempt to simplify our studies and to make them more acceptable to the children and their families.

As mentioned, the goal of newborn urodynamics is to document whether the bladder is hostile and needs intervention, or friendly and acceptable for observation. This will be determined by what is happening to the urethra. In this example from a newborn baby (Fig. 1), the neurologic defect has been closed. The urodynamics show that the urethra has minimal

Department of Urology, University of California, U575, 533 Parnassus Ave., San Francisco, CA 94143-0738, USA

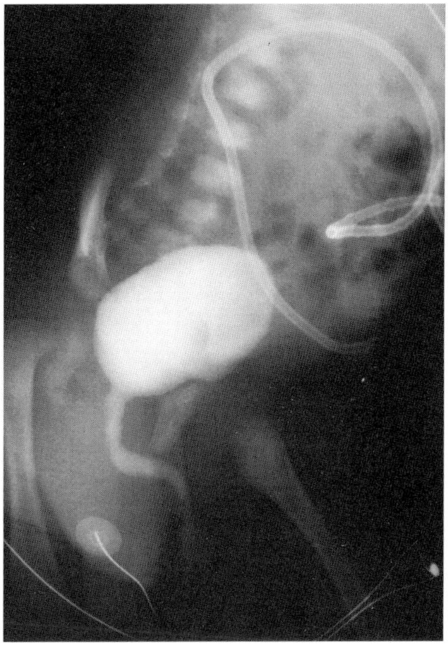

FIG. 1. Cystogram of a neonate with weak urethral resistance or a poor sphincter. Note the smooth bladder wall without vesicoureteral reflux. This patient is not at risk from upper tract damage or urinary tract infections

resistance. This is a patient we would put into a safe observation category. We are not going to start intermittent catheterization because there is little pressure in the bladder due to the minimal resistance offered by the urethra. While this is great for the family early on, it becomes a continence issue when they are 4 or 5 years old. This is a two-edge sword. We do not have to worry about the patient immediately, but as yet we do not have a perfect operation to correct urinary incontinence. However, there are many operations which will ensure an improvement. We would monitor this patient by ultrasound. If the patient had a urinary tract infection, we would repeat the urodynamics, because these lesions can change, especially as the child grows. Also, the cord can tether, and new problems can occur. We recommend embarking on a continence procedure before they enter kindergarten.

At the opposite end of the scale is the patients with a hostile bladder in the neonatal period (Fig. 2). Urodynamics show that there are clearly major problems. The dyssynergic sphincter can be seen, where the bladder contracts without urethral relaxation, and compliance is very poor with massive reflux. Such a patient has high risk of trouble, and we would start them on intermittent catheterization immediately. We use 0.1 mg/kg of anticholinergic oxybutynin divided into three doses. We would also monitor these patients by ultrasound in order to see stabilization of the upper tracts.

We have found this treatment to be very effective for patients with high-pressure bladders. In a study from UCSF, we confirmed the classic findings of Stuart Bauer from Boston. Urodynamic testing is carried out in newborn babies between 9 and 30 days of age. They are then classified as patients with hostile bladders, or those with bladders that will give little trouble [2, 3]. About 25% will have a little sphincter activity, and they can simply be observed. The other group, of approximately 65% of the patients, will have a hypertonic spastic bladder with a dyssynergic sphincter. These patients are the ones who are at the highest risk. Then there is the last group, about 10% of patients, who will have a flaccid bladder and a reasonable sphincter. This is really the most hopeful category because there is an excellent chance

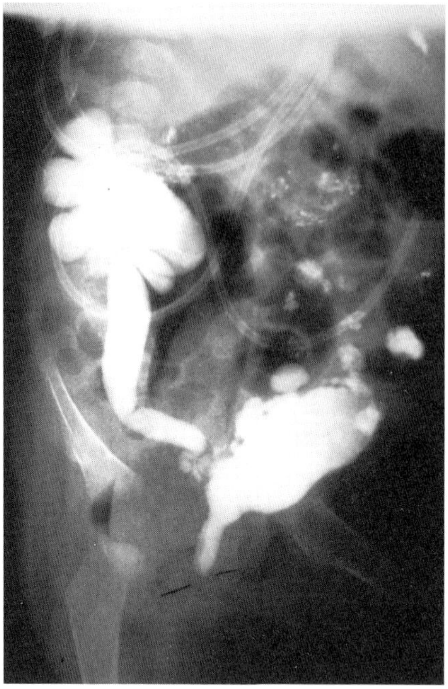

FIG. 2. Cystogram of a patient with a hostile bladder showing dyssynergic voiding with a closed sphincter, trabeculated bladder, and vesicoureteral reflux. This patient is at risk from upper tract damage and recurrent urinary tract infections, and was managed with anticholinergic medication and intermittent catheterization

of continence later on. These findings are correlated with renal bladder sonography, and both groups will receive treatment. It is possible that bladder function may change, and patients can move between one category and the other. Sometimes we are very uncertain which category they should be in, because urodynamic studies on babies is not an exact science. They scream, and are not happy. It is very difficult to measure pressures in the newborn using a 5 French tube, and sometimes it is not clear what is going on. We always try to assess the whole picture. In other words, if the ultrasound is perfect (normal kidneys and no bladder-wall thickening), it is unlikely that the baby has a problem bladder. However, if the ultrasound shows massive hydronephrosis, and the cystogram part of the urodynamics shows reflux and trabeculation, it is very worrying. If the diagnosis is uncertain, the patient is recalled and the urodynamic tests are repeated in about 2 months, or earlier if they have a urinary tract infection. It is necessary to be flexible in these studies. Even when the most up-to-date equipment is available, the results need to be interpreted, and interpretation is the real job of the physician.

Presently, we have well over 100 patients who were first treated in the newborn period. Our original group of 35 patients did very well with an initial treatment of intermittent catheterization and anticholinergic medication [2]. Two patients were withdrawn from the study because they required vesicostomy, one because we could not control upper tract changes and infection, and the other because of urethral trauma. However, a vesicostomy to keep pressures down and the baby infection-free is very rare. With intermittent catheterization and anticholinergic medication, the majority of patients (95%) will have stable upper tracts. This group has tolerated the intermittent catheterization perfectly and remains without infection, and about three-quarters of them actually became dry, which is the second goal for patients with spina bifida [2].

We were also able to conclude from our original study that oxybutynin, which had not been approved by the pharmaceutical companies for use in neonates, was safe and effective in newborns [2]. We also found that spinal shock after back closure is a real phenomenon, so these bladders can change and need to be followed up. Our results have agreed reasonably well with those of Bauer. We found that with intermittent catheterization and anticholinergic treatment, only 8% of patients had any trouble. Without treatment, we found that about 50% of them had upper tract complications. Therefore, our approach is now early aggressive preventive therapy. I am not an advocate of watchful waiting until trouble happens. I think we can prevent problems. I use the analogy of hypertension. You do not wait for a stroke, you treat early on when the patient is asymptomatic.

To test the hypothesis that intermittent catheterization will prevent future problems, we did a retrospective study on 50 neonates who were treated at birth [4]. We compared this group with 50 patients who were referred or treated after 4 years of age to see whether early intervention meant fewer upper tract problems and fewer infections. These patients were followed up for between 5 and 12 years, and we found that the renal outcome was equivalent in both groups. However, we also found that patients who first had treatment in the newborn period had fewer bladder augmentations over the course of the study. We concluded from this that if we treat patients early, and keep their bladder pressures low, we will preserve bladder function and they will have a better chance of not requiring major surgery later in life.

We also believe that there is a psychological benefit in early intervention. I have generally found that it is difficult to start intermittent catheterization when patients are older. The families do not accept it and it becomes more of a radical therapeutic option, whereas a mother will do anything for her newborn baby. Therefore we prefer to start catheterization in the neonatal period. Sometimes it is no longer needed after a year or two because the urethral resistance becomes less and the patient is easy to monitor. However, if catheterization is started at birth, and reconstruction becomes necessary at 5 or 6 years old, it is no problem for the parents to restart temporary catheterization. We advocate starting almost every patient on intermittent catheterization until we can prove urodynamically that their sphincter is so weak that they do not need it.

Many new patients are ambulatory myelomeningocele patients who have not been diagnosed. One example was a 9-year-old girl who was a champion skier from Lake Tahoe. She was having recurrent urinary tract infections and she also wet herself (Fig. 3). Examination by X-ray showed a very scrambled spine, and she actually had a closed lipomyelomeningocele that had been undiagnosed. Urodynamic tests revealed a trabeculated bladder, poor compliance, severe vesicoureteral reflux, and a relatively poor kidney. We treated her with intermittent catheterization and oxybutynin, and the results were spectacular. She is now completely dry and her infections have cleared up. As with any teenager, the treatment consisted of more than just filling out a prescription. She required a lot of teaching, and a lot of support when the initial diagnosis was confirmed.

I will now consider vesicoureteral reflux associated with spina bifida. We know that reflux in these patients corresponds to high bladder pressures. We believe that if the pressure can be brought under control, the reflux will be cured in the majority of cases. I believe that the literature will also support this view.

As we started to treat a larger group of ambulatory patients with myelomeningocele, we wanted to know if walking meant that they were urinating satisfactorily. In other words, if the motor function to the lower extremities is well preserved, is the bladder function preserved as well. The answer is no. If you are an ambulatory patient with myelomeningocele, you have the same chance of having a neurogenic bladder as a myelomeningocele patient

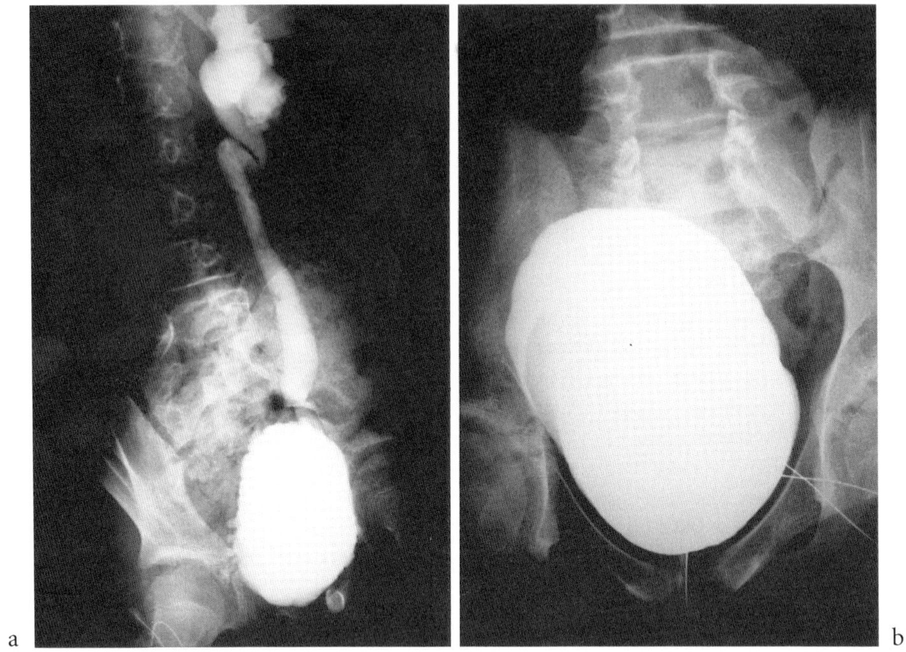

FIG. 3. **a** Cystogram of an adolescent with a neurogenic bladder prior to treatment with intermittent catheterization and anticholinergic medication. Note the trabeculated bladder and vesicoureteral reflux. **b** Cystogram after treatment with intermittent catheterization and anticholinergic medication. Note the smooth-walled bladder and the resolution of the reflux

who has had some type of gait abnormality. In fact, in our group of 45 ambulatory myelomeningocele patients, only three had normal urodynamics documenting normal voiding [5]. So walking does not necessarily mean satisfactory urination. Therefore ambulatory patients must have the same kind of urological evaluation as patients with ambulation deficiencies.

It is rare for intermittent catheterization and anticholinergic medication not to work in the newborn period. Such unusual patients will have recurrent infections or increasing hydronephrosis. In this type of patient, we would recommend vesicostomy, which is a very effective form of treatment for a minority of patients with neurogenic bladders. The best location for the vesicostomy is between the umbilicus and the pubic bone. The concept is that the bladder will now cycle but under low pressure with the pop-off from the vesicostomy. Before kindergarten, reconstruction with closure of the vesicostomy and augmentation cystoplasty will be performed.

In patients with neurogenic bladders that require augmentation, the choice of bowel segment depends on many factors [1]. Classically, ileum was used, with sigmoid colon also being a suitable segment. In selected patients with neurogenic bladders and no urethral sensation, we have recently used gastric segments. We have performed over 45 gastrocystoplasties, and Ueoka and Tanikaze from Kobe have performed 15 [6]. Both centers have had excellent long-term results. Technically, when performing a gastrocystoplasty it is important to preserve the blood supply. Most commonly, we base the gastric segment on the right gastroepiploic artery (Fig. 4). The stomach is thick like the bladder, and quite acceptable for

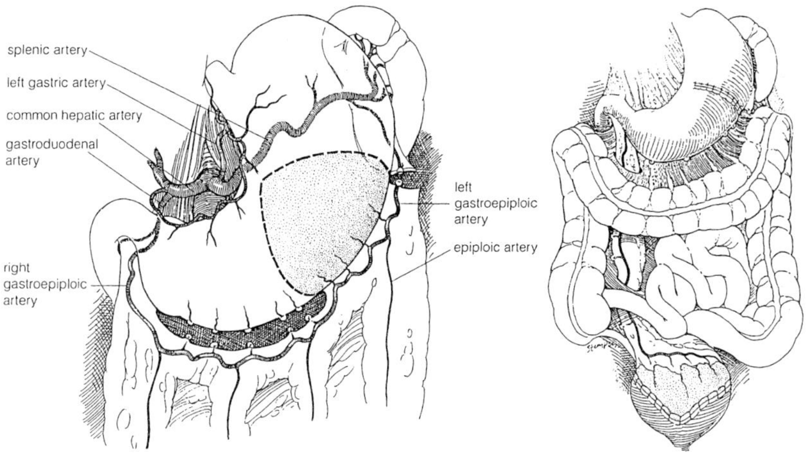

FIG. 4. Schematic diagram of a gastric segment with anatomical landmarks used in the gastrocystoplasty operation

reimplantation of ureters or to accept an appendical Mitrofanoff. The only problem that patients have when a stomach segment is used is that they cannot eat as much after the surgery. We encourage them to spread their meals out over their day until their stomach expands.

At this institution, Kogan has pioneered physiological studies on what happens to the stomach segment when it is put into the bladder [7]. The answer is, once a stomach, always a stomach. If the patient is in a restaurant where, for example, they serve incredible Kobe beef, when they see that beef, their bladder is going to start excreting acid. When they see a meal or eat a meal, as their stomach expands, gastrins are excreted. When that gastrin circulates through the blood system, it causes acid secretion from the stomach patch. It acts just like a stomach, even though it has been removed from its initial environment. When the patient has a meal, the titratable acid increases and the pH decreases. Therefore, once a stomach, always a stomach. The only trouble we had, which should not be a major problem in Japan or the United States, is that if a patient gets flu, they sometimes have trouble with dehydration or losing salt. We recommend supplementation with salt, which is not hard to find in developed countries. These patients are a little more susceptible to electrolyte abnormalities when they dehydrate. We always warn the parents, and we have not had any major clinical problems. Ease of catheterization for these patients is perfect, and again I emphasize that because they have been through this process at an early age, it is not a serious problem to start again after their reconstruction.

In terms of complications, the stomach has many of the same problems as any form of surgical treatment [6]. The most serious complication would be augmentation perforation. That has not occurred in this institution for many years. We have been selective about offering reconstruction to patients and families with stable social environments. The stomach has advantages which do not apply to metabolic abnormalities of acidosis because of the acid secretions, but there can be obvious alkalosis-type problems, especially with dehydration. One patient had to have another operation because she did not catheterize as well as we would have liked, and let her bladder fill to over 1000 cc. That patient was eventually treated with a composite ileal gastric augmentation.

Over the last 10 years we have recorded the progress of 45 patients [6]. In this group, as stated above, there was one reoperation for an electrolyte abnormality, and another as the result of a surgical error. The second patient had a gastric ileal fistula 6 months later that needed surgical repair. Because we selected only patients with neurogenic bladders and no urethral sensation, we have had not major problems with hematuria dysuria syndrome. I emphasize again that patient selection is critical. We have not used gastric cystoplasty for patients with posterior urethral valves or exstrophy because of the risk of hematuria dysuria syndrome.

To summarize, we have three goals in our treatment of spina bifida patients: preserving renal function, achieving urinary and fecal continence, and self-esteem and autonomy [1]. We have been working hard, especially with the older patients, both male and female, on their sexuality, and issues of possible fertility. We have also been using the antegrade continence enema (ACE) Malone on a few patients, when indicated, to control fecal incontinence.

References

1. Sutherland RS, Mevorach RA, Baskin LS, Kogan BA (1995) Spinal dysraphism in children: an overview and an approach to prevent complications. Urology 46:294–304
2. Baskin LS, Kogan BA, Benard F (1990) Treatment of infants with neurogenic bladder dysfunction using anticholinergic drugs and intermittent catheterisation. Br J Urol 66:532–534
3. Bauer SB, Hallett M, Khoshbin S, Lebowitz RL, Winston KR, Gibson S, Colodny AH, Retik AB (1984) Predictive value of urodynamic evaluation in newborns with myelodysplasia. JAMA 252:650–652
4. Wu HY, Baskin LS, Kogan BA (1997) Neurogenic bladder dysfunction due to myelomeningocele: neonatal versus childhood treatment. J Urol 157:2295–2297
5. Mevorach RA, Bogaert GA, Baskin LS, Lazzaretti CC, Edwards MS, Kogan BA (1996) Lower urinary tract function in ambulatory children with spina bifida. Br J Urol 77:593
6. Kurzrock E, Baskin L, Kogan B (1998) Gastrocystoplasty: is there a consensus. World J Urol 16:242–250
7. Bogaert GA, Mevorach RA, Kim J et al. (1995) The physiology of gastrocystoplasty: once a stomach, always a stomach. J Urol 153:1977–1980

Electromyographic and Manometric Anorectal Evaluation in Children Affected by Meningomyelocele

R. Del Gado, D. Brescia, G. Del Gado, D. Del Gaizo, G. Polidori, A. Tamburro, and F. Ausiello

Summary. Fecal incontinence is often undervalued in children affected by spina bifida. We conducted an electromanometric evaluation of the anorectal tract (at rest and under stimulation) in 83 children affected by meningomyelocele to evaluate the degree of functional damage and so provide appropriate treatment; 37 of these children also underwent surface electromyography. Recording perfusion catheters (0.1 ml/s) were placed at rectal and anal level.

Overall sphincter pressure was reduced in all patients (15–25 mm Hg; n.v. 25 ± 25 mm Hg) and the anal canal functional length was shorter (1–1.8 cm) compared with age-matched controls. Inhibitory anal- and rectal-sphincteric reflexes were normal in all patients, but amplitude, duration, and sensitivity were not constant. Recordings of rectal-sigmoid motility revealed sudden, fast, and high-pressure waves of peristaltic progression followed by prolonged pauses. Treatment consisted of daily emptying of the rectum to avoid fecal retention. Fifteen patients with prolapse and sphincteric hypotonia (<10 mm Hg) underwent cerclage with sustained good results. Further studies are required to establish an appropriate diagnostic–therapeutic protocol for such cases.

Key words. Electromyography, Manometry, Fecal incontinence, Meningomyelocele

Introduction

Children affected by spina bifida frequently present anorectal motility disorders that clinically appear as fecal incontinence with or without persistent constipation. Medullar lesions in meningomyelocele (MMC) patients are asymmetric and can result in defects at different levels: bladder, rectum, pelvic floor, and the lower limbs. In almost all patients, lesions in the anorectal region cause slowing of rectal and/or rectal-sigmoid motility secondary to pregangliar cholinergic neuron alterations, loss of anal canal and pelvic floor sensitivity, deranged external anal sphincter function, altered motility of the anal levator muscles, and preservation of the internal anal sphincter reflex but loss of motor coordination by sacral neurons, so that MMC patients do not have a regular peristalsis.

These anorectal motility disorders induce persistent constipation with or without fecal incontinence, and differ from other intestinal disorders such as Hirschsprung-like disease,

---

Dipartimento di Pediatria, Università degli Studi di Napoli, Via S. Andrea delle Dame, 4, 80138 Naples, Italy

functional constipation, and traumatic lesions. In patients affected by spina bifida, fecal stasis is caused by slowing of motility and loss of anal canal sensitivity [1].

Electromyographic and electromanometric anorectal evaluations in these children show slightly reduced levels of basal rectal pressure, slightly increased rectal compliance compared with normal values, an external anal sphincter defect with lack of, or very decreased, reflexes, and an apparently normal basal anal canal pressure, but voluntary contraction does not lead to a rise in basal pressure.

The absence of rectal-sphincteric coordination induces a vicious circle that, starting from the slack progression or nonprogression of the feces, leads to fecal dehydration: the feces increase in size and become solid, thereby slowing transit even further, and local irritation causes anomalous contractions.

Treatment in MMC consists of avoiding excessive fecal retention in an attempt to prevent a further reduction of the already poor rectal-sigmoid motility and to take advantage of any eventual residual rectal sensitivity. In older and collaborating children, the treatment of choice is to increase abdominal pressure with an abdominal press, to administer a "scoriae"-enriched diet in order to obtain feces of a normal consistency, and a weekly continence enema. If intestinal function becomes regular, patients can control fecal incontinence and soiling. In young and noncollaborating children, daily emptying of the rectum is obtained with the administration of hypertonic lactulosium solution and enema [2–4].

While evaluation parameters of the neuropathic bladder are well standardized, as to both values and treatment guidelines, data on the neuropathic rectum are scarce and contradictory. Moreover, the results of functional examination are not always an aid to treatment strategy. The aim of this study was to try to establish the degree of functional damage, based on electromyography and manometry of the anorectal tract, in a group of children affected by MMC, and thus to provide the most appropriate treatment.

Materials and Methods

Eighty-three children affected by MMC underwent anorectal manometry. Thirty-three of these children also underwent surface electromyography. We thus evaluated the overall sphincter pressure, the inhibitory anal reflex, the rectal-sphincteric reflex, and rectal motility during stimulation and at rest. We used a manometric apparatus that consisted of two pressure probes: one placed at a point corresponding to the internal sphincter, and the other placed at the level of the rectal ampulla. Two n.6 catheters linked to 0.5-ml perfusion pressure tranductors were introduced for 2 min. To assess the degree of functionality, we used a catheter with an inflatable ball at one end, placed at rectal ampulla level, to induce inhibitory anal- and rectal-sphincteric reflexes by applying decreasing stimulations (i.e., 60, 50, 40, 30, 20, 15, 10, and 5 cc sufflations).

Results

Overall sphincter pressure was reduced in all patients (15–25 mm Hg), and the functional length of the anal canal (the continence rectal zone) was reduced compared with age-matched controls (1–1.8 cm vs. 2–2.5 cm). The inhibitory anal reflex was normal in all patients, although its amplitude, duration, and sensitivity were reduced compared with normal values. In other words, in these patients, the rectum had the characteristics typical of a neuropathic rectum: the inhibitory anal reflex was not constant, i.e., sometimes a different response was obtained by stimulating the same patient at exactly the same level. The rectal-sphincteric response was also very inconstant, and the peristaltic activity of the anal canal was increased, i.e., an enhanced number of slow and low pressure waves.

The MMC patients affected by fecal incontinence underwent daily emptying of the rectum so as to avoid the retention of solid fecal pellets, and consequent internal sphincteric relaxation. External sphincteric hypotonia exacerbates the situation because it does not relieve the incontinence. In no case did we perform the Maloney appendix-cutaneous-stomia. Fifteen patients who presented prolapse and sphincteric hypotonia (<10 mm Hg) underwent cerclage with 2/0 prolene, which resulted in an improvement in the overall sphincter tone. There was a partial expulsion of the thread in two patients, so the cerclage was removed.

Conclusions

This study using electromyographic and manometric techniques to evaluate the degree of functional anorectal damage in children affected by MMC and fecal incontinence shows that these patients had a neuropathic rectum. The paucity of data on the condition and the lack of treatment guidelines have lead to empiric treatment of fecal incontinence, each center using different therapeutic procedures. In addition, the urologic situation of patients with a neuropathic rectum is often considered more important than fecal incontinence, which consequently can be undervalued and incorrectly treated. There is a need for further studies to establish an appropriate diagnostic protocol and treatment guidelines for patients affected by a neuropathic rectum.

References

1. Arhan P, Faverdin C, Devroede G, Pierre Kahn A, Scott H, Pelierin D (1984) Anorectal motility after surgery for spina bifida. Dis Colon Rectum 27(3):159–163
2. Loening-Baucke V, Desch L, Wolraich M (1988) Biofeedback training in patients with meningomyelocele and fecal incontinence. Dev Med Child Neurol 30(6):781–790
3. Wald A (1981) Use of biofeedback in treatment of fecal incontinence with meningomyelocele. Pediatrics 68(1):45–49
4. Whithead WE, Parker LH, Masek BJ, Cataldo MF, Freeman JH (1981) Biofeedback treatment of fecal incontinence in patients with myelomeningocele. Dev Med Child Neurol 23(3):313–322

Nitrofurantoin Prophylaxis for Bacteriuria and Urinary Tract Infection in Children with Neurogenic Bladder on Intermittent Catheterization

Theresa A. Schlager, Susan Anderson, Julie Trudell, and J. Owen Hendley

Summary. The objective of this work was to determine the effect of nitrofurantoin prophylaxis on the rates of bacteriuria and symptomatic urinary tract infection in children with chronic neurogenic bladder on clean intermittent catheterization. We exsamined whether the frequency of resistant organisms rose on prophylaxis, and if so whether this increase in resistant organisms would lead to an increase in the number of urinary tract infections.

The study was designed as a double-blind, placebo-controlled, cross-over trial of nitrofurantoin versus a look-alike placebo. Each child was studied for 11 months. They received one of the study drugs for 5 months, then no drug (wash-out) for 1 month, then the alternate study drug for 5 months. Weekly home visits were made during the study period. During each visit a sample of bladder urine was obtained by intermittent catheterization, all signs and symptoms of urinary tract infection were recorded, and all medications were recorded as well as a capsule count of the study drug.

Fifteen children each completed 11 months of study. During nitrofurantoin use, the frequency of bacteriuria remained high. Cultures of 74% (203/274) of the 274 samples taken when on placebo were positive for a pathogen ($\geq 10^4$ colony-forming units per milliliter) compared with 65% (165/252) of the 252 samples taken when on nitrofurantoin. However, the bacterial species responsible for bacteriuria were altered: *E. coli*, the most common pathogen isolated while taking placebo, was replaced by resistant *Klebsiella* spp. and *Pseudomonas* spp. while taking nitrofurantoin. The carriage of these resistant organisms tripled while taking nitrofurantoin. Symptomatic infection dropped by half with nitrofurantoin, but this decline was due solely to infections caused by *E. coli*. Despite an increased frequency of resistant organisms with nitrofurantoin prophylaxis, an increase in urinary tract infections due to these resistant organisms did not occur.

We concluded that routine use of nitrofurantoin prophylaxis in an attempt to eradicate bacteriuria in patients with chronic neurogenic bladder is not effective. Thus prophylaxis is not recommended for bacteriuria. The findings of this study do not allow us to make a general recommendation regarding prophylaxis for symptomatic infections.

Department of Pediatrics and Emergency Medicine, University of Virginia, PO Box 10014, Charlottesville, VA 22906-0014, USA

Introduction

Bladder emptying is a life-long problem in patients with neurogenic bladder due to myelomeningocele or spinal cord injury. Clean intermittent catheterization (CIC) performed several times a day is the standard technique for emptying the bladder in patients with neurogenic bladder [1]. A disadvantage of CIC is that inoculation of bacteria into the bladder urine is inevitable in the course of repeated catheterization of the bladder. In previous work, we found that bacteriuria was present in 75% of urine samples collected from children with neurogenic bladder on CIC who were followed for 6 months [2]. In addition, pyuria was associated with bacteriuria two-thirds of the time. Bacteriuria, even with pyuria, did not predict the presence of symptomatic urinary tract infection (UTI) and was not associated with deterioration of the upper urinary tract during the 6-month period of study. Antimicrobial prophylaxis is commonly used in patients with chronic neurogenic bladder on CIC in an attempt to prevent bacteriuria and symptomatic infection, but the effectiveness of this strategy has not been established. A problem in investigating the efficacy of prophylaxis is differentiation between bacteriuria and symptomatic infection. In addition, concerns about the long-term use of prophylactic antibiotics in patients with neurogenic bladder include not only drug toxicity, but also the emergence of more resistant bacterial species to cause bacteriuria and infection [3].

In this study, we examined the effect of nitrofurantoin prophylaxis on rates of bacteriuria and UTI in children with chronic neurogenic bladder on CIC using a double-blind, placebo-controlled, cross-over design. Infection was differentiated from bacteriuria [2]. Nitrofurantoin was chosen rather than TMP–SMX because of its minimal effect on fecal and periurethral flora [4], low rate of development of resistant bacteria, and minimal adverse side effects [5, 6].

Methods

Population

Children (2–18 years of age) with neurogenic bladder who were voiding by CIC four times a day were enrolled if they lived at home and had a normal upper urinary tract by renal ultrasonography and voiding cystourethrogram. All children continued to receive medical care from their primary physician during the study; no therapies were withheld or altered except that children who had been on antimicrobial prophylaxis discontinued their prophylaxis 2 weeks prior to entry into this study. The urine cultures obtained for the study did not influence the child's care, since the results were kept on file by the research technologist in the pediatric microbiology laboratory and were not available to either the child's physician or the investigator during the study. The protocol was approved by the University of Virginia Human Investigation Committee.

Fifteen of the 16 children enrolled completed the study. One child was removed from the study owing to a 4-week hospitalization for torsion of an ovarian cyst. Ten of the 15 participants were girls; five children were 2–5 years of age, and the remaining ten were 6–18 years of age. Fourteen children had neurogenic bladder caused by myelomeningocele; for one child with neurogenic bladder secondary to traumatic spinal cord injury, the study began 1 year after injury.

Design

Each child served as his/her own control in this double-blind, placebo-controlled, cross-over trial of nitrofurantoin versus a look-alike placebo. Children were enrolled in a staggered fashion according to geographical location from March 1993 to July 1996. Each child was studied for 11 months; for 5 months (330 total patient weeks) they received one of the study drugs, then for 4 weeks they had no drug (wash-out), and then for 5 more months (330 total weeks) they had the alternate study drug. A "wash-out" period was provided in order to prevent a carryover effect of nitrofurantoin into the placebo period in the children who received the placebo second. Eight children were randomly assigned by the research pharmacist to receive the placebo for the first 5 months, and seven children were assigned to receive nitrofurantoin for the first 5 months. The placebo or nitrofurantoin were taken once a day at bedtime, 7 days a week.

Nitrofurantoin was dispensed in capsule form by the pharmacist in two strengths; 25 mg for children less than 25 kg in weight, and 50 mg for children heavier than 25 kg. The placebo was also dispensed as a capsule, identical in size and color to the nitrofurantoin capsule. The study drug was discontinued if a child received an antibiotic from his/her physician. After the antibiotic course was completed, the study drug was restarted.

Each child was visited weekly for 11 months in his or her home by the investigator (TAS) or study nurse. At each visit, a capsule count of the study medication was performed (compliance), and symptoms and signs of UTI, and all medications were recorded. In addition, a sample of bladder urine that had been collected during routine CIC on the day of the home visit was picked up. Urine obtained during CIC was placed in a sterile cup, immediately refrigerated, and then plated within 10 h after collection. Organisms were identified by standard methods [7].

Definitions

The appropriate definition of significant bacteriuria in terms of species and number of organisms per milliliter of urine is unclear in this population. For this study, a positive urine culture result (bacteriuria) was defined as greater than $\geq 10^4$ colony-forming units of a bacteria per milliliter of urine obtained by bladder catheterization [8]. Symptomatic infection (UTI) was defined as bacteriuria *with* fever, abdominal pain, change in continence pattern, or change in color or odor of urine. This definition of symptomatic UTI is in accordance with guidelines developed at the Round Table Discussion of Symptoms of UTI in Neurogenic Bladder at the October 1990 meeting of the American Academy for Cerebral Palsy and Developmental Medicine in Orlando, Florida [2]. The distinction between urinary tract pathogens and nonpathogens in a patient with neurogenic bladder has also not been established. For this study the Enterobacteriaceae, *Enterococcus* spp., *S. aureus*, *S. saprophyticus*, and group B streptococci were designated as "usual pathogens"; coagulase-negative staphylococci, alphahemolytic streptococci or nonhemolytic streptococci, and *Corynebacterium* spp. were designated as "commensal" organisms.

Analysis

Acquisition of bacteriuria was defined as the detection of a bacterial species that had not been isolated in the previous 2 weeks. Bacterial carriage was defined as the number of consecutive weeks that a species was present after acquisition. Statistical analysis was done with the Fisher exact test (two-tailed).

Results

Effect of Nitrofurantoin on Bacteriuria and Symptomatic Infection

Two hundred and seventy-four urine samples were collected during 330 patient weeks on the placebo (range 12–20 samples per child), and 252 samples were collected during 330 patient

TABLE 1. Frequency of bacteriuria and symptomatic infection during an 11-month study in eight children on placebo first (Group 1) and seven children on nitrofurantoin first (Group 2)

	Group 1	Group 2
Months 1–5	Placebo	Nitrofurantoin
Positive/total	130/155 (84%)	81/112 (72%)
UTI	11	5
Month 6 (washout)	No drug	No drug
Positive/Total	16/24 (67%)	19/24 (79%)
UTI	2	0
E. coli	11/24 (46%)	8/24 (33%)
Months 7–11	Nitrofurantoin	Placebo
Positive/total	87/140 (62%)	84/119 (71%)
UTI	4	8

weeks on nitrofurantoin (range 12–19 samples per child) (Table 1). The discrepancy between the numbers of urine samples and patient weeks relates to patient compliance. Each week an attempt was made to collect a urine sample. Two hundred and three (74%) of the 274 samples on the placebo were positive for a pathogen compared with 165 (65%) of 252 samples on nitrofurantoin (203/274 vs. 165/252, $P = 0.04$). A commensal species was detected in 43 of the samples during the placebo period, and in 13 of the samples during the nitrofurantoin period. Typically, commensals were isolated along with a pathogen; commensals alone were detected in 12 samples during the placebo period and in four samples during the nitrofurantoin period.

Nineteen symptomatic infections occurred in 11 children (1–4 UTI/child) while on the placebo compared with nine infections in eight children (1–2 UTI/child) on nitrofurantoin (19 UTI/330 weeks vs. 9 UTI/330 weeks, $P = 0.048$). Children with UTI were seen by their physician and were treated with an oral antibiotic for 7 days. All did well; none was hospitalized for UTI. Four children (two on the placebo and two on nitrofurantoin) were treated for a diagnosis other than UTI (sinusitis, bronchitis, pharyngitis, skin boil) with a course of oral antibiotic for 7–10 days.

We examined for evidence of a carryover effect of nitrofurantoin into the placebo period in the seven children who received the placebo second (Table 1). For this we compared the frequency of bacteriuria during the washout period in the children who received the placebo first (Group I) with the frequency during the washout period in the children who received nitrofurantoin first (Group II). Sixteen (67%) of 24 samples collected during the washout period in Group I were positive for bacteria compared with 19 (79%) of 24 samples collected during the washout period in Group II ($P = 0.05$). Thus there was no evidence of a carryover of nitrofurantoin into the washout period. Consequently, the two placebo periods were combined for analysis. Note that the two UTI that occurred during the washout period were not counted.

Effect of Nitrofurantoin on Carriage of Bacterial Species

E. coli was the most common pathogen detected during the placebo period (Table 2), followed by *Klebsiella* spp. and *Pseudomonas* spp. The frequency of acquisition and the duration of carriage of *Klebsiella* spp. and *Pseudomonas* spp. were similar. *Klebsiella* spp. were carried for 15 weeks and *Pseudomonas* spp. were carried for 24 weeks, so these two species

TABLE 2. Results. Bacterial carriage and symptomatic urinary tract infections during 330 patient weeks on a placebo and 330 patient weeks on nitrofurantoin

Bacteria	Placebo		Nitrofurantoin	
	Weeks of carriage	No. of UTI	Weeks of carriage	No. of UTI
E. coli	149	13	35	2
Klebsiella/ Pseudomonas	43	2	140	2
Other pathogens[a]	64	4	71	5
Commensals	53	0	24	0

[a] *Proteus* spp., *Enterobacter* spp., *Serratia* spp., *Citrobacter* spp., *Acinetobacter* spp.

were combined for analysis. A variety of other pathogens (*Proteus* spp., *Enterobacter* spp., *Serratia* spp., *Citrobacter* spp., *Acinetobacter* spp.) followed *E. coli*, *Klebsiella* spp., or *Pseudomonas* spp. in frequency. The carriage of *E. coli* was considerably reduced by the use of nitrofurantoin (Table 2). *E. coli* was carried for 149 weeks out of the 330 weeks on placebo compared with only 35 weeks during 330 weeks on nitrofurantoin ($P = 0.00001$). In contrast, the carriage of *Klebsiella/Pseudomonas* increased from 43 weeks on the placebo to 140 weeks on nitrofurantoin (43/330 vs. 140/330, $P = 0.00001$). This balancing of the reduction in *E. coli* by the increase in *Klebsiella/Pseudomonas* resulted in only a modest overall reduction in the frequency of bacteriuria during use of nitrofurantoin (Table 1). Carriage of other pathogens was not different on nitrofurantoin (64/330 vs. 71/330, $P = 0.5$); carriage of commensal organisms decreased on nitrofurantoin (53/330 vs. 24/330, $P = 0.00004$).

The number of symptomatic UTIs was reduced by 47% on nitrofurantoin, from 19 on the placebo to 9 (Table 2). This overall reduction was due to a reduction in infections due to *E. coli* from 13 during 330 placebo weeks to two in 330 nitrofurantoin weeks ($P = 0.01$). UTI due to *E. coli* occurred in seven children (1–3 UTI/child) on the placebo. In contrast, only two children (1 UTI/child) had a UTI due to *E. coli* while on nitrofurantoin. The reduction in *E. coli* infections paralleled the reduction in *E. coli* carriage (Table 2). In contrast, the number of UTIs due to *Klebsiella/Pseudomonas* remained constant (two on the placebo and two on nitrofurantoin) despite a tripling in the number of weeks of carriage. The number of UTIs due to other pathogens was similar on both placebo and nitrofurantoin. There were no UTIs associated with commensal organisms.

Effect of Nitrofurantoin on Acquisition of Bacteria

The effect of nitrofurantoin was examined in more detail by investigating the acquisition and carriage of bacteria in individual patients (Table 3). Twelve patients (Nos. 1, 2, 4–6, 9–15) acquired and carried *E. coli* for 1–21 weeks during the placebo period (Table 3). The use of nitrofurantoin was associated with elimination of the acquisition of *E. coli* in four of these patients (Nos. 5, 9, 11, 15) and a decrease in the length of carriage in the remaining eight patients (Nos. 1, 2, 4, 6, 10, 12–14). The pattern of acquisition and carriage of *Klebsiella/Pseudomonas* was the mirror image of *E. coli*. While on the placebo, eight patients (Nos. 1, 3, 4, 6, 8, 12, 13, 15) acquired and carried *Klebsiella/Pseudomonas*. While on nitrofurantoin, four patients (Nos. 2, 5, 10, 11) acquired *Klebsiella/Pseudomonas* and carriage was

TABLE 3. Results. Number of weeks in each episode[a] of bacterial carriage during the placebo and nitrofurantion periods

	E. coli		*Klebsiella* spp./or *Pseudomonas* spp.		Other pathogens		Commensals	
Patient No.	Placebo	Nitro.	Placebo	Nitro.	Placebo	Nitro.	Placebo	Nitro.
1	16	1,9	1,5	1,3,10	1,1	1,6	1,2,5	
2	1,1,2,4[a]	1,1		1,1,2,2,3		1,1,1,2,3	1,1,1,5	1,1,1
3			1,1	4	1,2,3,4	3,5,5	1,1,2,6,9	1,9
4	1,17	1	1	15		3		
5	1,1,2			5,11				
6	1,7	1,2	1,15	5,8			1,1,1,7	3,1
7					1,1	1,1,7		
8			5,8		1,3,15	1,18		
9	1,1,1				1,1			
10	19	3,4,8		2	5	2		
11	21			2,3,6,13				1,1,1
12	12	1,1	3	1,1			7	1,1
13	19	1	1	3	1,3,4	2,3,5		
14	19	1						1,1
15	1,1		1	3,15,15	16		1	
Total weeks of carriage	149	35	43	140	64	71	53	24

[a] Every number represents one episode of carriage which may have lasted either 2 week or as long as 19 weeks.
Nitro, nitrofurantoin.
Other pathogens: *Proteus* spp.; *Enterobacter* spp.; *Serratia* spp.; *Citrobacter* spp.; *Acinetobacter* spp.
Commensals: Coagulase-negative staphylococci; *Corynebacterium* spp.; Alpha-or-non-hemolytic streptococci

usually longer. The pattern of carriage of other pathogens was no different on placebo or nitrofurantoin. Carriage of commensals was sometimes longer during on the placebo.

Discussion

Bacteriuria appears to be common and inevitable in patients with chronic neurogenic bladder on CIC for bladder emptying [2, 9]. The periurethra of patients with neurogenic bladder is colonized with enteric organisms presumed to have originated from the gastrointestinal tract [10]. Intermittent catheterization performed several times a day may facilitate the inoculation of periurethral bacteria into the bladder urine [11]. Of the species which colonize the periurethra, *E. coli* is the most frequently isolated from the urine [10]. An explanation for the dominance of *E. coli* in bacteriuria in patients with neurogenic bladder is suggested by the work of Anderson et al. [12]. They utilized an in vitro model to examine the outcome of mixed infections of urine in the presence of voiding. These investigators inoculated sterile urine into a bladder model with *E. coli* and either *Klebsiella* spp. or *Pseudomonas* spp. so as to provide a concentration of 10^5 cfu/ml of both organisms. Simulated voiding was performed every 4h, and quantitative cultures of the bladder urine were done at 2-h intervals over 24h. *E. coli* outgrew both *Klebsiella* spp. and *Pseudomonas* spp. in a mixed culture. At 24h, *E. coli* represented greater than or equal to 99% of the viable counts obtained from culture of the urine in the bladder model. Anderson et al. concluded that the rapid growth rate of *E. coli* will result in dominance of this organism in a mixed culture.

Our findings in vivo are in accord with the in vitro work of Anderson et al. [12]. In our patients with chronic neurogenic bladder, it seems likely that organisms other than *E. coli* are simultaneously inoculated with *E. coli* into the bladder urine during CIC. Without antibiotic pressure, *E. coli* bacteriuria was detected in 40% of the samples collected, and *Klebsiella/Pseudomonas* was present in 10%. When we applied antimicrobial pressure with prophylactic nitrofurantoin, the frequency of *E. coli* bacteriuria dropped to 14% of samples, and that of *Klebsiella/Pseudomonas* bacteriuria rose to 20% of samples. Thus, when *E. coli* and *Klebsiella/Pseudomonas* were present in the urine, *E. coli* outgrew everything else. When *E. coli* was inhibited by nitrofurantoin, *Klebsiella/Pseudomonas* was able to grow without competition. As a consequence, the use of nitrofurantoin resulted in a change in the organisms, but the frequency of bacteriuria was altered very little.

Since the rate of bacteriuria with pathogenic bacteria was similar with both placebo and nitrofurantoin, it would be expected that the number of symptomatic infections would be the same if the presence of organisms in high titer in bladder urine was sufficient to cause symptomatic illness. In fact, a potential drawback to the use of prophylaxic antibiotics is the risk of infections with resistant organisms [3, 13]. In our study, although carriage of *Klebsiella/Pseudomonas* tripled during nitrofurantoin, the number of infections did not increase. The lack of symptomatic illness despite 10 000 to 100 000 cfu *Klebsiella/Pseudomonas* per milliliter of urine suggests that numbers of bacteria are not sufficient on their own to cause UTI in this population. Importantly, our fear that an increased frequency of resistant organisms would lead to an increase in the number of UTI was not realized.

The reason that infections due to *Klebsiella/Pseudomonas* did not rise is unclear. Virulence factors appear to be more common in *E. coli* isolated from symptomatic urinary tract infections compared with *E. coli* isolated from asymptomatic bacteriuria [14]. Little is known about the role of virulence factors in infection due to *Klebsiella* spp. or *Pseudomonas* spp. Podschun et al. [15] examined isolates of *Klebsiella* spp. (*K. pneumoniae* and *K. oxytoca*) from symptomatic infections and asymptomatic bacteriuria in patients with normal bladders. They found that K2 capsular type accounted for most infections due to *Klebsiella* spp. Type I fimbriae and serum resistance were more commonly found in isolates of *Klebsiella* spp. from symptomatic infections compared with those from asymptomatic bacteriuria. A variety of virulence factors have been identified for *P. aeruginosa* (adhesins, protease, hemolysin, phospholipase C, pyoverdin), but their role in the pathogenesis of UTI is unclear [16]. It would of interest to examine virulence factor expression in strains of *Klebsiella* spp. and *Pseudomonas* spp. in our population, as most strains of *Klebsiella/Pseudomonas* did not cause symptomatic infection. The implication is that these strains would not express virulence factors.

Previous work on antimicrobial prophylaxis in chronic neurogenic bladder is difficult to interpret since bacteriuria is usually not differentiated from infection [17–19], and patients on different bladder-emptying methods (abdominal pressure, suprapubic aspiration, intermittent catheterization) may be combined for analysis [20]. Our findings of a modest decrease in symptomatic infection with little change in the rate of bacteriuria are similar to work by Mohler et al. [21]; bacteriuria was unchanged on prophylaxis and symptomatic infections occurred with a frequency of 1.86 per 100 patient days on the placebo and 1.11 per 100 patient days while on TMP–SMX. Unfortunately, the bacterial species detected on the placebo and on TMP–SMX prophylaxis were not stated, so we were unable to observe whether a change in organisms occurred as in our study.

In patients with neurogenic bladder, bacteriuria and symptomatic infection must be considered as separate entities. Nitrofurantoin prophylaxis will alter the species of organism isolated from bacteriuria, and will halve the number of infections due to nitrofurantoin's inhibition of *E. coli*. Whether nitrofurantoin prophylaxis is beneficial to a patient must be decided on an individual basis in view of our results. Routine use of nitrofurantoin prophylaxis in an attempt to eradicate bacteriuria in this patient population is not effective. In view of the fact that persistent bacteriuria was not associated with a deterioration of the upper urinary tract (renal ultrasound and voiding cystourethrogram) in children followed for 6 months [2], we feel that attempts to eradicate bacteriuria with antimicrobial prophylaxis are not justified. The findings of this study do not allow a general recommendation to be made regarding prophylaxis for symptomatic infections.

Acknowledgments. Supported by the Pendleton Pediatric Infectious Disease Research Laboratory, and by a grant from the March of Dimes Birth Defects Foundation.

References

1. Lapides J, Kiokno AC, Silber SJ, Lowe BS (1972) Clean intermittent self-catheterization in the treatment of urinary tract disease. J Urol 107:458–461
2. Schlager TA, Dilks S, Trudell J, Whittam TS, Hendley JO (1995) Bacteriuria in children with neurogenic bladder treated with intermittent catheterization: natural history. J Pediatr 126: 490–496
3. Boyarsky S, Labay P, Hanick P, Abramson AS, Boyarsky R (1974) Care of the patient with neurogenic bladder. Little, Brown, Boston, pp 145–158
4. Stamey TA, Condy M, Mihara G (1977) Prophylactic efficacy of nitrofurantoin macrocrystals and trimethoprim-sulfamethoxazole in urinary infections. N Engl J Med 296:780–783
5. Waisbren BA, Crowley W (1955) Nitrofurantoin: clinical and laboratory evaluation. Arch Int Med 95:653
6. Marshall Jr M, Johnson III SH (1959) Use of nitrofurantoin in chronic and recurrent urinary tract infection in children. JAMA 169:919–922
7. Baron ET, Finegold SM (eds) (1990) Methods for identification of etiologic agents of infectious disease. In: Bailey and Scott's diagnostic microbiology, 8th edn. Mosby, St Louis, pp 323–519
8. Hellerstein S (1982) Recurrent urinary tract infections in children. Pediatr Infect Dis J 1:271–279
9. Stover SL, Lloyd LK, Waites KB, Jackson AB (1991) Neurogenic urinary tract infection. In: Woolsey RM, Young RR (eds) Neurological clinics: disorders of the spinal cord. Harcourt Brace Jovanovich, Philadelphia, pp 741–755
10. Schlager TA, Simon VA, Hendley JO, Whittam TS (1995) Clonal diversity of *Escherichia coli* causing baceriuria in patients with neurogenic bladder (abstract). 35th Interscience Conference on Antimicrobial Agents and Chemotherapy, September
11. Horton TM, Stamm WE (1996) The vaginal flora in urinary tract infections. In: Mobley HLT, Warren JW (eds) Urinary tract infections. ASM Press, Washington, pp 67–94
12. Anderson JD, Eftekhar F, Aird MY, Hammond J (1979) Role of bacterial growth rates in the epidemiology and pathogenesis of urinary infections in women. J Clin Microbiol 10:766–771
13. Johnson JR (1996) Treatment and prevention of urinary tract infections. In: Mobley HLT, Warren JW (eds) Urinary tract infections. ASM Press, Washington, pp 95–118
14. Eden CS, de Man P (1987) Bacterial virulence in urinary tract infection. Infect Dis Clin N Am 1:731–749
15. Podschun R, Sievers D, Fischer A, Ullmann U (1993) Serotypes, hemagglutinins, siderophore synthesis, and serum resistance of *Klebsiella* isolates causing human urinary tract infections. J Infect Dis 168:1415–1421
16. Woods DE, Vasil ML (1994) Pathogenesis of *Pseudomonas aeruginosa* infections. In: Baltih A, Smith RP (eds) *Pseudomonas aeruginosa* infections and treatment. Dekker, New York, pp 21–50
17. Anderson RU (1979) Non-sterile intermittent catheterization with antibiotic prophylaxis in the acute spinal cord injured male patient. J Urol 124:392–394

18. Kuhlemeier KV, Stover SL, Lloyd LK (1985) Prophylactic antibacterial therapy for preventing urinary tract infections in spinal cord injury patients. J Urol 134:514–517
19. Johnson HW, Anderson JD, Chambers GK, Arnold WJD, Irwin BJ, Brinton JR (1994) A short-term study of nitrofurantoin prophylaxis in children managed with clean intermittent catheterization. Pediatrics 93:752–755
20. Biering-Sorensen F, Hoiby N, Nordenbo A, Ravnborg M, Bruun B, Rahm V (1994) Ciprofloxacin as prophylaxis for urinary tract infection: prospective, randomized, cross-over, placebo controlled study in patients with spinal cord lesion. J Urol 151:105–108
21. Mohler JL, Cowen DL, Flanigan RC (1987) Suppression and treatment of urinary tract infection in patients with an intermittently catheterized neurogenic bladder. J Urol 138:336–340

Abstract

Spina Bifida and the Urinary Excretion of Glycosaminoglycans

D. Antuzzi[1], M. Scanu[2], L. Venuti[1], P. Ferrara[1], R. Ricci[1], and E. Salvaggio[1]

Neurogenic bladder caused by spina bifida (SB) is frequently affected by recurrent bacterial infections. The neurological impairment produces alterations to the bladder's internal surface and, as a consequence, a distrophy of the bladder mucosa. Glycosaminoglycans (GAG) or acid mucopolysaccharides are linear polymers of a uronic acid and a hexosamine, and are a fundamental part of the bladder wall structure. A small quantity of GAG is excreted in the urine either as a result of glomerular filtration, or from a leak of the upper urinary tract.

The aim of this study was to investigate a possible correlation between the excretion of GAG and bladder wall degeneration. GAG expressed as μg/mg creatinine was measured according to the modified method described in Hesse et al. (1986). The Na tetraborate-carbazole method was employed to measure the total GAG. The excretion of GAG in 39 patients affected by SB and 36 healthy controls matched by age is shown in Table 1. Subjects and controls, aged 0–8 years, were divided into four age groups since GAG excretion presents a large variability during the early years.

Computation of the median and of the Wilcoxon test statistic at a 5% level suggests that GAG excretion in SB subjects 0–5 years old is similar to that of normal controls. GAG excretion in older SB subjects (over 5 years) is significantly higher than in normal controls.

In conclusion, SB subjects present an increased excretion of GAG after the age of 5 years. These values are an important parameter in the evaluation of the physiopathological condi-

Table 1. Excretion of GAG in 39 SD patients and 36 controls

	Spina bifida		Controls		
Age (years)	Median	Int. range	Median	Int. range	WTSL
0–1	93.07	24.67–156.81	79.50	59.83–119.29	n.s.
1–3	73.76	48.36–108.17	71.30	60.86–115.21	n.s.
3–5	58.47	21.52–82.05	31.38	28.94–37.86	n.s.
5–8	33.75	22.60–48.70	22.72	12.92–24.28	0.0469

WTSL, Wilcoxon test significance level $P = 0.05$; n.s., not significant.

[1] Department of Pediatric Clinics, Catholic University of the Sacred Heart, Rome, Italy.
[2] Department of Statistics, University "La Sapienza", Rome, Italy.

tion of the bladder wall, and hence may be considered a good marker for the beginning of bladder mucosa distrophy and for monitoring the clinical course of the disease.

References

1. Di Ferrante NM (1967) The measurement of urinary mucopolysaccharides. Annal Biochem 21:98–106
2. Hesse A, Wuzel H, Wahlensieck W (1986) The excretion of glycosaminoglycans in the urine of calcium-oxalate stone patients and healthy persons. Urol Int 41:81–87
3. Dische Z (1947) A new specific colour reaction of hexuronic acids. J Biol Chem 167:189–192

Management of Bowel Problems in the Patient with Spina Bifida

MASAHIKO SAITO[1] and ATSUO KONDO[2]

Summary. Most patients with spina bifida and/or their parents face fecal incontinence and/or intractable constipation. One hundred and twenty-five questionnaires relating to bowel control were sent to patients with spina bifida who lived in the Tokai area in Japan. Ninety-four (43 male and 51 female) were returned. Seventy-three patients (78%) were suffering from bowel symptoms, including intractable constipation, fecal incontinence, stinks, and genital dermatitis. Sixty-one patients used a diaper or pad for fecal incontinence or soiling. There were no significant differences in the results of the questionnaires between male and female. When the results were compared between children (<16 years old) and adults (≥16 years old), adult patients had less frequent evacuation of feces and less frequent fecal incontinence, and consequently more patients were satisfied with their present defecation methods.

The bowel problems of 16 patients were satisfactorily managed by a large-volume water enema. However, 8 patients stopped using this method because of persistent soiling following the enema. To control chronic constipation and frequent soiling, appendicocutaneostomy (Malone's antegrade continence enema: ACE) was performed for two patients. In both cases the bowel is well managed by an antegrade enema through the abdominal stoma twice a week. This procedure might be beneficial for bowel problems in patients with spina bifida.

Key words. Spina bifida, Fecal control, Neurogenic bladder

Introduction

The surgical treatment of spina bifida and associated hydrocephalus ensures long-term survival in most patients selected for treatment. Bowel problems are one of the major problems affecting their quality of life and producing dependence on others [2]. Recently, major advances have been made in the nonoperative and operative management of fecal incontinence and/or intractable constipation [1,3–5]. These specialist centers report excellent results [3–5], but it seems that only a minority of patients have access to this treatment, and most continue to suffer the socially isolating stigma of bowel problems. In this study we attempted to clear the bowel problems of patients with spina bifida based on the results of questionnaires.

[1] Daido Steel Hoshizaki Clinic, 2-30 Daido-cho, Minami-ku, Nagoya 457-8545, Japan
[2] Department of Urology, Komaki Municipal Hospital, Komaki, Japan

Patients and Method

Questionnaires were sent to 125 patients with spina bifida who lived in the Tokai area in Japan. The questionnaires addressed details of methods and results of bowel management. Wherever possible, the questionnaires were completed by the patients themselves, but if this was not possible, by their mother or father.

Ninety-four of the 125 (75%) questionnaires were returned. The mean age was 15.1 years (range 1–47 years), with 51 females and 43 males. Their mean height and mean body weight were 131.6cm and 37.5kg, respectively. Fifty-two patients could walk by themselves, 16 walked on crutches, and the other 22 used a wheelchair regularly. Eighteen patients had undergone bowel surgery: this was enterocystoplasty using the end of the ileum in 16, and surgery for ileus of unknown origin in 2 patients.

Results

Seventy-three (78%) patients suffer from bowel problems such as intractable constipation (50), soiling (44), stink of feces (17), and genital dermatitis (11). The general condition of the feces was constipation in 48 patients, repeat of constipation followed by diarrhea in 21, and frequent fecal incontinence in 5. Sixty-one used a diaper or pad regularly for fecal incontinence. Only 11 patients defecated naturally. Other patients used adjuvant treatment for fecal evacuation. Thirty-four practiced manual evacuation, 17 used a large-volume water enema, 16 regularly used laxatives, and 13 used a glycerin enema. Frequency of defecation was once or more on every day in 33 patients, every other day in 27, twice a week in 22, and once a week in 11. Frequency of fecal incontinence was once or more on every day in 16 patients, every other day in 11, twice a week in 9, once a week in 33, and very rare or none in 20. Sixty-four patients were satisfied with their present defecation method and had no major problems. The other 30 wanted to try to find a better method of bowel control.

There were no differences in the results between male and female. There was no significant difference between the method for movement. No significant results were observed in the patients with bowel surgery. In contrast, when we compared results between adults (over 16 years old) and children (less than 16 years old), adult patients were less embarrassed by fecal problems and fewer used a diaper for soiling. The frequencies of defecation and fecal incontinence were rarer in the adult group. This finding suggested that in the adult group, bowel control and feces are well managed when compared with those of children.

Seventeen patients used a large-volume water enema for control of constipation, and 14 of them were satisfied. However, 8 patients stopped using this method mainly because of persistent soiling following the enema. They complained of it taking a long time to complete, and of suffering sometimes from postenema diarrhea.

Two of our patients had undergone Malone's antegrade continence enema (ACE), which was done in combination with enterocystoplasty or autoaugmentation. In both cases constipation and diarrhea are well managed by an antegrade continence enema twice a week.

Discussion

Patients with spina bifida have many problems which require a multidisciplinary approach to their management, i.e., access to pediatricians, neurosurgeons, urologists, and orthopedicians. In spite of recent progress in the management of patients with spina bifida by careful coordination of these services, many patients still suffer from bowel problems [2]. Even with adjuvant treatment such as manual evacuation, laxatives, and/or enemas, 62% of patients in this study use a diaper or pad because of soiling. This indicates the inadequency of current treatments. This study showed that fecal problems were well managed in adult patients when compared with children. We had speculated that problems of fecal incontinence should become greater as patient gets older, and patients or their parents make efforts to control feces by themselves.

Shadling and Gilmour [4] described the use of the enema continence catheter in 112 patients with spina bifida, and all were clean. We also recommended a large-volume water enema, which similar to that of Shadling and Gilmour, for patients with severe constipation, and 74% of users were satisfied. However, the length of time it takes to complete and the prolonged soiling which follows this procedure are major problems.

An operation has been developed in which the appendix is used to provide continent catheterizable access to the cecum, through which an ACE procedure can be administered; the results are excellent in patients with spina bifida [3, 5]. Although an operation is required, this technique is less cumbersome and easier to use than the large-volume water enema. If patients are to be offered the best chance of being clean, these newer methods of treatment should always be considered as an option.

References

1. Malone PS (1995) The management of bowel problems in children with urological disease. Br J Urol 76:220–223
2. Malone PS, Wheeler RA, Williams JE (1994) Continence in patients with spina bifida: long-term results. Arch Dis Childhood 70:107–110
3. Roberts JP, Moon S, Malone PS (1995) Treatment of neuropathic urinary and faecal incontinence with synchronous bladder reconstruction and the antegrade continence enema procedure. Br J Urol 75:386–389
4. Shandling B, Gilmour RF (1987) The enema continence catheter in spina bifida: successful bowel management. J Pediatr Surg 22:271–273
5. Squire R, Kiely EM, Carr B, Ransley PG, Duffy PG (1993) The clinical application of the Malone antegrade colonic enema. J Pediatr Surg 28:1012–1015

Pediatric Neurology

Seventeen-Year Experience with Children with Meningomyelocele Born by Cesarean Section Prior to Rupture of Amniotic Membranes

DAVID B. SHURTLEFF[1], SHARON DUGUAY[1], JOHN LOESER[2], and RICHARD ELLENBOGEN[3]

Summary. We examined 17 years of experience with 238 patients with meningomyelocele without kyphosis or cephalopelvic disproportion as an indication of cesarean section delivery. Sixty-four of 84 (64/84) patients born by cesarean section before rupture of the amniotic membranes, with or without labor, exceeded the proportion of similar, minimally paralyzed patients born by cesarean section after rupture of the amniotic membranes (20/38; $X^2 = 5.7$, df = 1, $P = 0.02$) and after vaginal birth (65/115; $X^2 = 7.8$, df = 1, $P = 0.005$). From 1982 to 1987, the incidence of newborns born with meningomyelocele (25–48 per year) exceeded the numbers born from 1988 to 1996 (7–20; $T = 6.2$, df = 13, $P = 0.00003$). Cesarean section delivery before rupture of the amniotic membranes apparently indicates a more favorable outcome for infants diagnosed with meningomyelocele and movement of their legs in utero. However, more study is required to further define the degree of protrusion of nerves, placode, and meningomyelocele sac beyond the dorsal plane of the back, and whether breech presentation or spinal cord hypoplasia adversely affect infant outcome despite cesarean section delivery before rupture of the amniotic membranes.

Key words. Spina bifida aperta, Meningomyelocele, Prenatal diagnosis, Cesarean section, Rupture of amniotic membranes

Stark and Drummond in 1970 [19], Ralis in 1975 [12], and Hutchins et al. in 1996 [6] described spinal cord injury in humans with meningomyelocele "consistent with occurrence during delivery." Until prenatal diagnostic techniques such as maternal serum alpha-fetoprotein screening [9] and ultrasound [11], the avoidance of birth trauma could not be achieved.

In 1986, Chervenak et al. [2] and Shurtleff et al. [14] reported small, statistically insignificant series of prenatally diagnosed infants with meningomyelocele born after prelabor cesarean section. These studies appeared to support the hypothesis that avoidance of perinatal trauma to the meningomyelocele may decrease secondarily acquired paralysis. Subsequently, Bensen et al., in 1988 [1], and Sakala and Andree, in 1990 [13], published larger, retrospective studies of infants born by cesarean section and reported no benefit as compared with groups born vaginally. Hogge et al. [5] reported that 14 infants

[1] Division of Congenital Defects, Department of Pediatrics, [2] Department of Neurological Surgery, [3] Division of Pediatric Neurosurgery and Department of Neurological Surgery, University of Washington and Children's Hospital and Regional Medical Center, PO Box 5371, Seattle, WA 98105, USA

diagnosed prenatally were brought to term, delivered by cesarean section, and given a good prognosis.

Luthy et al. [8] in 1991, reported on a prospective study of 47 infants delivered by cesarean section before labor began, 35 after labor began, and 78 delivered vaginally, over an 11-year period. Those infants born before onset of labor by cesarean section had a motor level of 3.3 (±3.0) spinal segments below their proximal anatomic level, measured by plain radiographs of the spine. Those with labor and cesarean section or born vaginally had 0.9 (±4.1) and 1.1 (±2.3) spinal segments below their anatomic level, respectively, which was a significantly favorable difference ($P < 0.001$ for both comparisons). However, Cochrane et al. [3] reported in the same year that cesarean section did not favorably affect the ambulatory status of their patients born by this method.

In 1994, Hill and Beattie [4] reported on a prospective study of 25 infants, of which 10 were delivered by prelabor cesarean section and 15 by other methods. They left unanswered the question of whether cesarean section delivery improved the neuromuscular potential of fetuses identified as having open spina bifida aperta.

Also in 1994, in the same journal, Shurtleff et al. [16] reported on 14 years' experience with infants born vaginally and by prelabor cesarean section with intact amniotic membranes, or by other methods after amniotic membrane rupture. They compared neuromotor levels to anatomic levels defined by plain radiographs, and concluded that rupture of the amniotic membranes, not the duration of labor, in the presence of dorsally protruding neural elements and movements of knee and ankle are the three criteria for selecting cesarean section for fetuses with meningomyelocele to improve pregnancy outcome for the fetus.

This 17-year follow-up of the cohort in Seattle is to address the following hypothesis. Neuromotor levels over time are preserved sufficiently to warrant cesarean section birth if the following prenatal criteria are met: (a) ultrasound demonstrates movement of the lower leg and ankle; (b) amniotic membranes are intact at the time of cesarean section delivery by the method of Chervenak et al. [2]; (c) there is absence of kyphosis.

Methods

All children with a diagnosis of meningomyelocele seen in the University of Washington Birth Defects Clinic and born since January 1, 1979, were reviewed. When each child is registered for an initial visit, an interview with the parents and a review of the medical records establish the method of delivery, duration of labor, time interval between rupture of the amniotic membranes and delivery, and the indication for cesarean section, if pertinent. Serial evaluations of neuromotor levels were determined at 6-month intervals from birth to 2 years of age, and yearly thereafter, according to McDonald et al.'s [10] modification of Sharrard's classification. Data were entered into a Patient Data Management System (PDMS/fx) [15].

Neuromotor level was determined by physical therapists who did not know about the method of delivery. Fetuses with no leg movement noted at knee or ankle in utero and an indication of cephalopelvic disproportion for cesarean section, and those infants with congenital kyphosis, were excluded from this study. Those infants with rupture of the amniotic membranes, with or without perceived labor, were considered as a separate group from those born vaginally or by cesarean section before rupture of the amniotic membranes. Infants born by cesarean section with intact amniotic membranes, with or without labor, were hypothesized as the group who would benefit most from nontraumatic birth. This update is modified from an analysis of prelabor cesarean section to cesarean section before rupture of the amniotic membranes, based on our observations reported in 1994 [16, 17].

Results

Table 1 shows that the proportion of patients with the lowest levels of paralysis (low lumbar [L4–5], sacral, and no loss classifications) in the cesarean section group before rupture of the amniotic membranes, with or without labor (64/84), was greater than that in the cesarean section group delivered after rupture of the amniotic membranes (20/38; $X^2 = 5.7$, df = 1, $P = 0.02$, odds ratio = 2.88, 95% confidence limits 1.2–7.0), and also greater than that in the vaginally delivered group (65/116 or 56%; $X^2 = 7.8$, df = 1, $P = 0.005$, odds ratio = 0.4, 95% confidence limits 0.2 and 0.8). The groups for comparison were chosen as midlumbar and above versus low lumbar, sacral, and no loss, because there is general agreement in the literature that high lumbar and thoracic-level lesion patients are not usually permanent ambulators, and patients with low lumbar and sacral-level lesions or no loss remain ambulators.

Table 2 demonstrates a significant reduction in births per year after the introduction of prenatal diagnosis and elective termination of pregnancy for patients other than those with Spanish surnames ($T = 6.2$, df = 13, $P = 0.00003$). There was no decrease in the number of births amongst those with Spanish surnames ($T = 0$, df = 13, $P = 1$).

Discussion

Neuromotor levels were chosen as the outcome measures in this study rather than ambulatory status as reported by Cochrane et al. [3] because of the difference in emphasis placed on ambulation and use of wheelchairs by different centers [7]. Most authors writing about mobility of patients with meningomyelocele agree that the least paralyzed are most likely to ambulate throughout life. This study was undertaken to test the observation of Cochrane et al. [3] that cesarean section did not influence long-term ambulatory ability.

Our study differs in that we did not practice selection of high-level lesion patients for less than optimal care, as did Cochrane et al. [3] for some time during their retrospective study. We have used specific prenatal diagnostic criteria for selection of patients, and we are conducting an ongoing, prospective study. Bensen et al. [1], Cochrane et al. [3], and Sakala and

TABLE 1. Neuromotor levels in three groups of patients with meningomyelocele born by different methods

Neuromotor level	C/S with RAM	C/S without RAM	Vaginal delivery
T	11	7	23
L1–2	4	6	13
L3	3	7	15
L4–5	8	27	2
Sacral	12	31	58
No loss	0	6	5
Total	38	84	116

C/S, cesarean section delivery; RAM, ruptured amniotic membranes.
See text for statistical significance.

TABLE 2. Number of patients born per year in The University of Washington Birth Defects Clinic

Year	Spanish surname	Nonhispanic	Total
1982	3	38	41
1983	4	44	48
1984	1	24	25
1985	2	31	33
1986	4	22	26
1987	0	31	31
1988	3	15	18
1989	4	16	20
1990	1	16	17
1991	2	16	18
1992	2	11	13
1993	5	9	14
1994	1	12	13
1995	2	11	13
1996	1	6	7

See text for statistical significance.

Andree [13] also did not provide information about fetal indications for and against cesarean section for improved fetal outcome. Both these studies are also retrospective and, like that of Cochrane et al. [3], do not mention the status of amniotic membranes at the time of delivery, or the presence of kyphosis.

Our second set of data (Table 2) extends by 2 years our original observations in 1994 [16] that prenatal diagnosis is significantly reducing the number of children being born with meningomyelocele in our population. Patients with Spanish surnames were identified as a separate group because they are primarily antiabortion, Roman Catholics, who refuse prenatal diagnosis if they understand that the only alternatives are abortion of an affected fetus or routine delivery. The complexities of meningomyelocele, such as hydromyelia, kyphosis, spinal cord tethering, and cord hypoplasia, discussed previously [16, 17] and elsewhere in this symposium [18], require carefully planned, long-term follow-up and large enough study populations to correctly sort out influences that significantly alter the outcome. Our change in emphasis from prelabor cesarean section to cesarean section before rupture of the amniotic membranes took 15 years and a sufficient number of patients to establish features such as kyphosis that mitigate against an improved outcome [14–16].

Technology [9, 11] has provided us with prenatal diagnostic abilities that have allowed us to test the theories of Stark and Drumond [19] and Ralis [12] about secondary injury at birth superimposed on meningomyelocele lesions. However, several questions remain about the use of cesarean section delivery before rupture of the amniotic membranes to improve fetal outcome. Will imaging techniques allow us to identify spinal cord hypoplasia, a condition that leads to a nonambulatory status probably not altered by method of delivery? Can sufficient prospective data be collected about the degree of protrusion of the meningomyelocele sac beyond the dorsal plane of the back to provide guidance as to which patients cannot be improved by cesarean section as opposed to which may? We agree with Hill and Beattie [4]. Better coordination within programs between obstetricians, ultrasonographers, and teams treating children with meningomyelocele needs to be developed. Multiple-center studies using a common computerized database would greatly accelerate the rate at which we can answer questions about the management of children with meningomyelocele. The need for multiple-center studies is becoming more urgent as frequency of meningomyelocele at birth diminishes (Table 2).

Acknowledgments. This study was supported by the Department of Neurological Surgery, University of Washington, the National Foundation for the March of Dimes, and gifts to the Birth Defects Clinic, University of Washington.

References

1. Bensen JT, Dillard RG, Burton BK (1988) Open spina bifida: does cesarean section improve prognosis? Obstet Gynecol 71:532–534
2. Chervenak FA, Duncan L, Ment LR (1984) Perinatal management of meningomyelocele. Obstet Gynecol 63:376–380
3. Cochrane D, Aaroynk K, Sawatsky B, Wilson D, Steinbok P (1991) The effects of labour and delivery on spinal cord function and ambulation in patients with meningomyelocele. Child's Nerv Syst 7:312–315
4. Hill AE, Beattie F (1994) Does cesarean section delivery improve neurological outcome in open spina bifida? Eur J Pediatr Surg Suppl I, 4:32–34
5. Hogge WA, Dungan JS, Broobs MP, Dilks SA, Abbitt PA, Thiaqardjahs, Ferguson JE (1990) Diagnosis and management of prenatally detected myelomeningocele: a preliminary report. Am J Obstet Gynecol 163:1061–1065
6. Hutchins GM, Meuli M, Meuli-Simmen C, Jordan MA, Heffez DS, Blakemore KJ (1996) Acquired spinal cord injury in human fetuses with myelomeningocele. Pediatr Path Lab Med 16:701–712
7. Liptak G, Shurtleff DB, Bloss JW, Baltus-Hebert E, Manitta P (1992) Mobility aids for children with high-level myelomeningocele: parapodium vs. wheelchair. Dev Med Child Neurol 33:473–481
8. Luthy DA, Wardinsky T, Shurtleff DB, Hollenbach KA, Hickok DE, Hyberg DA, Benedetti T (1991) Cesarean section before the onset of labor and subsequent motor function in infants with meningomyelocele diagnosed antenatally. New Engl J Med 324:662–666
9. Main DM, Mennuti MT (1986) Neural tube defects: issues in prenatal diagnosis and counseling. Obstet Gynecol 67:1–16
10. McDonald CM, Jaffe KM, Shurtleff DB, Menelaus MB (1991) Modifications to the traditional description of neurosegmental innervation in myelomeningocele. Dev Med Child Neurol 33:473–481
11. Nicolaides KH, Campbell S, Gabbe SG, Guidetti R (1986) Ultrasound screening for spina bifida: cranial and cerebellar signs. Lancet 2:71–74
12. Ralis ZA (1974) The role of mechanical intrauterine pressure in the pathogenesis of paralytic limb deformities. J Bone Joint Surg [Br] 56:383–389
13. Sakala EP, Andree I (1990) Optimal route of delivery for meningomyelocele. Obstet Gynecol Survey 45:209–212
14. Shurtleff DB (1986) Selection process for the care of congenitally malformed infants. In: Shurtleff DB (ed) Myelodysplasias and exstrophies. Grune & Stratton, Orlando, pp 89–116
15. Shurtleff DB (1991) Computer data bases for pediatric disability. Phys Med Rehabil Clin NA 2:665–687
16. Shurtleff DB, Luthy DA, Nyberg DA, Mack LA (1994) The outcome of fetal myelomeningocele brought to term. Eur J Pediatr Surg 4, Suppl I:25–28
17. Shurtleff DB, Luthy DA, Nyberg DA, Benedetti TJ, Mack LA (1994) Meningomyelocele: management in utero and postnatum in neural tube defects. Wiley, Chichester (CIBA Foundation Symposium 181), pp 270–286
18. Shurtleff DB, Moskowitz D, Weinberger E, Duguay S, Loeser J (1997) Anatomy of the spinal cord with meningomyelocele. International Symposium on Spina Bifida, Part II of III, Kobe, Japan
19. Stark G, Drummond M (1970) Spina bifida as an obstetric problem. Dev Med Child Neurol (Suppl) 22:157–160

Long-Term Prognosis of the Mental Activities of Hydrocephalus Associated with Spina Bifida

Masaya Segawa

Summary. The long-term prognosis of mental activity with hydrocephalus associated with spina bifida was evaluated in 10 patients by correlating their IQ/DQ with neurological and clinical electroneurophysiological findings. It was revealed that the development of the circadian sleep–wake (S–W) cycle and normal crawling before 12 months correlated to high IQ/DQ levels, and that co-occurrence of epilepsy, leakage of atonia of REM stage into NREM stages (atonic NREM), and asynchronism of sleep spindles correlated to reduced IQ/DQ levels. The latter was particularly noted for hydrocephalus associated with spina bifida in cases of congenital hydrocephalus. The co-occurrence of other dysraphic malformation and perinatal asphyxia affected IQ/DQ levels, but early shunting showed no apparent relation to mental activities. Delay in the development of the circadian S–W cycle was related to delay in the determination of hand dominance or left-handedness, and in a few patients to autistic behavior, but the latter was not marked compared with hydrocephalus due to aqueductal stenosis. An association with epilepsy affected IQ/DQ levels of all patients with congenital hydrocephalus whatever the cause. Co-occurrence of sleep-related correlates, particularly of atonic NREM, was related to a decrease in IQ/DQ levels with age. The circadian S–W cycle and atonic NREM are modulated by the aminergic neurons of the brainstem, which have important roles in the functional maturation of the brain. Sleep spindles are modulated by the structures of the rostral brainstem. Thus, co-occurrence of a particular lesion in the rostral portion of the brainstem may relate to mental activities and their prognosis for hydrocephalus associated with spina bifida. Epilepsy may cause turbulence in the immature brain under insufficient modulation of the aminergic neurons.

Key words. Hydrocephalus associated with spina bifida, IQ/DQ, Sleep–wake cycle, Atonic NREM, Asynchronism in sleep spindle, Hand dominance, Aminergic neurons

Introduction

Hydrocephalus is a fairly frequent associated disorder of spina bifida. Although this association often causes mental disability, its prognosis and pathophysiology have not been clarified. In this study, we evaluated the long-term prognosis of mental activities

Segawa Neurological Clinic for Children, 2-8 Surugadai Kanda, Chiyoda-ku, Tokyo 101-0062, Japan

for hydrocephalus associated with spina bifida, and investigated its pathophysiology by correlating the levels of mental activity with neurological and clinical-electroneurophysiological findings.

Materials and Methods

Ten patients with hydrocephalus associated with spina bifida were the subjects of this study. There were 4 males and 6 females, who had been referred to our clinic for neurological evaluation at ages ranging from 2 months to 13 years 6 months. Ages at last examination ranged from 5 years 3 months to 20 years 4 months. Ventriculoperitoneal (V-P) shunts were performed in all children at ages ranging from 10 days to 5 years: 4 cases before 1 month, 2 in the 1st month, 1 each in the 2nd and 4th months, and the other 2 after 1 year, 3 years 7 months, and 5 years. Only two patients showed shunt-malfunction; one of these was associated with Chiari malformation type II and agenesis of the corpus callosum.

As well as the routine evaluation of motor and psychomental abilities, the development of the circadian sleep–wakefulness (S–W) cycle, the age (months or years) when first crawling, and the age when hand dominance was determined and the side of that dominance were investigated. If hand dominance was not determined by 3 years of age, that child was assessed as ambidextrous. In the neurological examination, the pattern of locomotion in crawling or walking was carefully evaluated. We also examined whether the children could close their eyes on command and do pronation/supination movements of their arms by the age of 5 years or older. Psychobehavioral analysis was performed according to our personal check list for the clinical evaluation of behavior typical of infantile autism in reference to the activities of the brain stem aminergic neurons (Table 1). For clinical neurophysiological examinations, routine EEG with simultaneous recording of the mentalis muscle EMG and an electrooculogram were performed. With the recording of the surface EMG of the mentalis muscle, leakage of axial atonia of REM stage (sREM) into NREM stage, that is, atonic NREM, was evaluated.

The results of these clinical and laboratory examinations and the ages at which V-P shunt was performed were correlated with the levels of IQ/DQ assessed at or just before their last visit. Their IQ levels were evaluated by Tanaka–Binet or WISC-R tests. For patients with severe mental disability, the DQ levels were assessed by other tests.

TABLE 1. Check list for psychobehavioral function

A. Impairment in accommodation to novel environments
   Extreme rote memory
   Insistence on sameness
   Lack of social relatedness
B. Hyperkinesia
   Stereotyped movement
   Abnormal dependence
   Aggressiveness
   Self-mutilation
C. Failure in eye-to-eye contact
   Inability in finger pointing
   Echolalia
   Pronominal reverse

Results

As shown in Fig. 1, the levels of IQ/DQ against the ages when V-P shunt was performed were lower in patients operated on before they were 1 month old.

Among the 4 patients operated on before they were 1 month old, one with an IQ of 58 and one with a DQ of 14 also had other anomalies of the brain, i.e., Arnold–Chiari malformation type II and meningomyelocele, respectively. The former patient also had agenesis of the corpus callosum, and the latter had myoclonic seizure from infancy. Patients operated on after 1 month of age had a higher IQ than those operated on before, except for two patients: one operated on at 1 month had had perinatal asphyxia, and the other operated on at 3 years 7 months had had fever-induced convulsions at 1 year of age, which was later diagnosed as partial epilepsy. In the others there were no neurological complications, except for the one operated on at 2 months who had had severe neonatal jaundice which needed ultraviolet phototherapy.

The results of correlative studies between IQ/DQ levels and clinical symptoms are shown in Fig. 2.

As shown in the left-hand column, an IQ higher than 90 was observed only in patients who had developed the circadian S–W cycle before 12 months of age. Also, 4 of the 5 patients had an IQ/DQ of over 80, except for the one who had Arnold–Chiari malformation.

The center column of Fig. 2 demonstrates comparative IQ/DQ levels between patients who began to crawl before or after 12 months of age.

Four patients began to crawl before 12 months, 3 of them could crawl with a normal pattern, and 2 showed IQ levels higher than 100. The other one, who had the lowest IQ level in this group, showed an abnormal pattern of crawling with total flexor posture and was unable to do the pronation/supination movements of the arm. On the other hand, of the 6 patients who could not crawl before 12 months, 4 showed an abnormal pattern of crawling. Among them, the one who had the lowest IQ (14) could not crawl. One patient who crawled

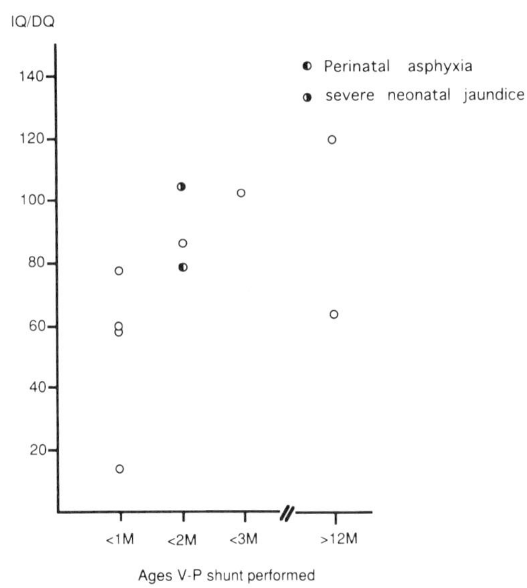

FIG. 1. Final IQ levels and ages at V-P shunt in congenital hydrocephalus with spina bifida

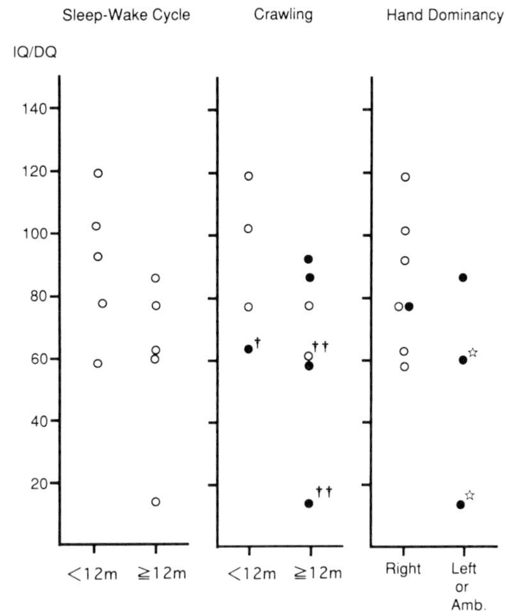

FIG. 2. Correlation of IQ/DQ levels and the development of neurological correlates. The *left column* shows the correlation of IQ/DQ levels between patients who developed a circadian sleep–wake cycle before and after 12 months of age. The *center column* shows the results of the same study on the development of crawling. *Closed circles*, abnormalities in posture and pattern of crawling; *single dagger*, inability in pronation/supination movment of the arms; *double dagger*, inability in pronation/supination movement and closing eyes on command. The *right column* shows the side of hand dominance assessed at age 5 years and the correlation with IQ/DQ levels. *Right*, right-handed; *left* or *amb*, left-handed or ambidextrous; *closed circles*, patients with a delay in the development of a circadian sleep–wakefulness cycle; *star*, patients with abnormal psychobehavior, as shown in Table 1

with a normal pattern but had an IQ of 60 was shown to have difficulties in closing the eyes on command and in the pronation/supination movements of the arms. The other 3 patients who began to crawl after 1 year of age had IQs of 77, 85, and 93, respectively. Among them there was no apparent difference in IQ/DQ levels whether the pattern of crawling was normal or not.

The right-hand column of Fig. 2 shows a comparison of IQ/DQ levels between right-handed patients and those who were left-handed or ambidextrous.

Of the 10 patients, 7 were right-handed, 2 were left-handed and 1 was ambidextrous. Two of 7 right-handed patients and all 3 left-handed or ambidextrous patients (shown by a closed circle in this figure) had delay in development of the circadian S–W cycle. Among the 7 right-handed patients, 3 had IQs higher than 93, while the other 4 showed IQ levels lower than 80. These 4 had neurological complications and/or one or more clinical electroneurophysiological abnormalities (see below). Two non-right-handed patients (marked by a star in Fig. 2) showed abnormalities in the analysis of psychobehavioral function shown in Table 1. One ambidextrous patient with meningomyelocele had poor accommodation to novel environments, and insistence on sameness, the abnormal behaviors shown in category A, all items of category B, and echolalia and pronominal reverse from category C. The other patient with left-handedness showed hyperkinesia, stereotyped movements, and abnormal dependence from category B, and echolalia and pronominal reverse from category C, while he had no symptoms from category A. These IQ levels were 14 and 60, respectively. Patients who had none of the psychobehavioral abnormalities listed in Table 1 had IQs higher than 60, except for the one with Chiari malformation type II and agenesis of the corpus callosum who had an IQ level of 58.

Figure 3 demonstrates the results of correlative studies between IQ/DQ levels and the presence or absence of clinical epileptic seizures and two clinical electroneurophysiological correlates, atonic NREM and asynchronism in sleep spindles. As shown in this figure, the

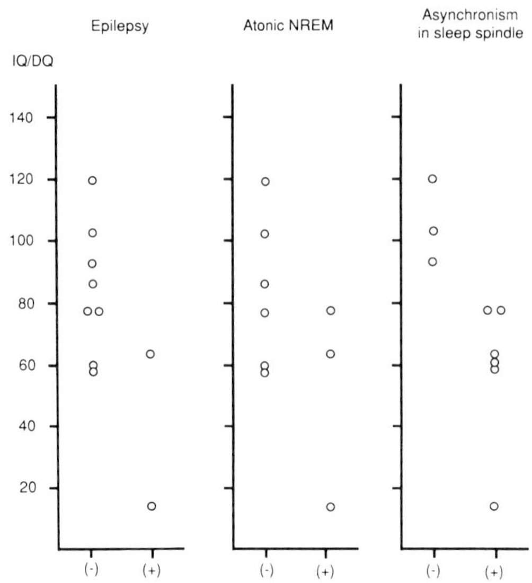

FIG. 3. Correlation of IQ/DQ levels and co-occurrence of epilepsy and the existence of clinical electroneurophysiological correlates. *Plus*, co-occurrence or existence of these clinical or clinical electroneurophysiological parameters; *minus*, patients who did not have these parameters

presence of these clinical and laboratory findings had an apparent correlation with the lower levels of IQ/DQ. No patient who had at least one of these clinical or clinical neurophysiological findings had an IQ/DQ higher than 80.

Age variations of IQ/DQ levels are shown in Fig. 4. As shown in this figure, the IQ/DQ levels tended to reduce with age. This tendency was observed from late childhood and in those who had one or more of the following signs and symptoms, i.e., delay in development of the circadian S–W rhythm, atonic NREM, and asynchronism in sleep spindles. This was more marked in patients with atonic NREM (shown by closed circles in the figure). One patient showed a marked decrease in IQ level with the development of atonic NREM in the course of an illness.

Discussion

The levels and prognosis of mental activity for hydrocephalus associated with spina bifida were dependent on co-occurrence of other dysraphic malformations, abnormalities of the central nervous system, or particular neurological, neuropsychological, and clinical electroneurophysiological findings.

There was no correlation between the age of shunting and IQ/DQ levels. The lower IQ levels in patients operated on before 1 month of age, compared with those operated on in later months, were considered to be due to association with other dysraphic malformations, i.e., meningoencephalocele and Arnold–Chiari malformation. Perinatal asphyxia and association with epileptic convulsions might cause a lowering of IQ levels, although these complications did not cause an early shunt operation. On the other hand, neonatal jaundice seemed to have no apparent influence in lowering the levels of IQ/DQ.

Although there is a report suggesting early shunting for better IQ levels (presented by T. Tomosugi et al. at the ISSB, 1997), mental retardation of patients with hydrocephalus associated with spina bifida was largely dependent on its association with other anomalies or complications (presented by M. Choux at the ISSB, 1997) and had no correlation with age of initial

Fig. 4. Age variation of IQ and atonic NREM in congenital hydrocephalus with spina bifida

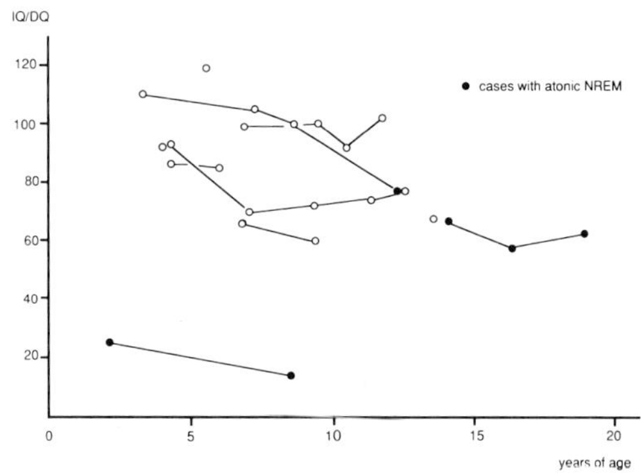

neurosurgical treatment (presented by Y. Nakagawa et al. at the ISSB, 1997). The present study confirmed these results.

On the other hand, the present study revealed the presence of certain neurological and clinical electroneurophysiological symptoms or signs correlated with the levels and prognosis of mentality. The former included the development of the circadian S–W cycle, crawling in infancy, determination of hand dominance to the right by early childhood, and association with epileptic convulsions. In the latter there was the presence or absence of atonic NREM and asynchronism of sleep spindles. As well as these, the co-occurrence of epilepsy, which has particular psychobehavioral and neurological symptoms, seemed to relate to low IQ/DQ levels.

Delay in the development of the circadian S–W cycle and in crawling, and the presence of atonic NREM are also observed in infantile autism and Down syndrome, and they are shown to relate to their mental dysfunction and psychobehavioral abnormalities [1–3].

Studies on infantile autism revealed that abnormality in development of the circadian S–W cycle relates to the behavioral disorders shown in Category A of Table 1, and also to delay in determination of hand dominance, i.e., delay in the development of functional lateralization, but does not relate to levels of IQ/DQ [1]. On the other hand, abnormalities in locomotion correlated to low IQ/DQ levels [4].

In Down syndrome, early development of the circadian sleep–wake cycle is related to an increase in IQ/DQ levels [3], but IQ/DQ levels are significantly higher in patients who began to crawl and walk early and in whom atonic NREM disappeared early [3].

In infantile autism, the age of being able to step with normal interlimb coordination are shown to correlate to the age of being able to close their eyes on command and, to those able to do so, the pronation/supination movements of the arm [4]. As difficulties in closing the eyes on command and in the pronation/supination movements of the arm in infantile autism are signs of possible orofacial apraxia and limbkinetic apraxia, abnormalities in the development of locomotion suggest impairment in the development of functional specialization of the cortex in this disorder [4].

In both diseases, hypofunction or abnormality in the aminergic neurons of the brainstem are considered as pathognomonic.

The S–W cycle is modulated by the suprachiasmatic nuclei, but for its synchronization to the 24-h day–night cycle, the serotonin (5HT) neurons have an important role. During development, the 24-h day–night cycle of the S–W cycle develops by the end of the 4th month. For normal functioning of this aminergic neuron, adequate daytime stimulation is necessary.

Disturbance in the development of the S–W cycle in very early infancy by endogenous and/or exogenous causes results in behavioral disorders similar to infantile autism.

Locomotion is promoted by the propriospinal circuit between the brachial and the lumbosacral stepping generators, which are executed by tonic innervation from the supraspinal locomotion center [5]. This center, the midbrain locomotion region or the pedunculopontine nuclei, is modulated by the brainstem aminergic neurons [6].

In this study, delay in the development of the S–W cycle was correlated with delay in the development of hand dominance and the particular language disturbances of echolalia and pronominal reverse. However, there was no apparent correlation between the development of the S–W cycle and IQ/DQ levels, although high IQ levels were observed only in patients who had developed the S–W cycle in infancy and were right-handed.

In hydrocephalus associated with spina bifida, starting to crawl in infancy with a normal pattern was related to high IQ levels. On the other hand, delay in crawling with an abnormal posture showed low IQ/DQ levels and also signs of developmental orofacial and/or limb-kinetic apraxia, suggesting delay in the development of functional specialization of the cortex. However, there was no apparent correlation between the age of starting to crawl and IQ/DQ levels as observed in autism and Down syndrome.

In infantile autism as well as Down syndrome, the abnormal locomotion is entirely due to the hypofunction of the serotonin (5HT) neurons, which reduces the tonic innervation to the lumbosacral stepping generator. The same pathophysiology may occur in some patients with spina bifida, but the dysraphic abnormality of the spinal cord may develop lesions in the lumbosacral stepping generator which could cause abnormal locomotion without any relation to the suprasegmental neurons. In animal experiments, these aminergic neurons, i.e., the 5HT neurons and the noradrenergic (NA) neurons, are known to have important roles in the synaptogenesis of the cortex in the neonatal period [7, 8], which corresponds to the first one or two years in humans.

Early lesions in the 5HT neurons cause abnormalities in cognitive function after maturation [9] and behavioral disorders similar to social isolation [10]. Lesions in the NA neurons cause stagnation of head growth [11], and lesions of the dorsal bundle of these neurons result in failure in the extinction of memorized behavior, called dorsal bundle extinction effects [12], which simulates extreme rote memory and the insistence on sameness observed in infantile autism [2]. On the other hand, combined lesions of 5HT and NA neurons with dopamine (DA) neurons cause friendliness in comfortable situations, but aggressiveness in isolation, which is called muricide [13].

By referring to the results of animal experiments, the psychomental abnormalities shown in category A of Table 1 are shown to be due to the dysfunction of the 5HT or NA neurons [2, 12]. For the abnormalities in category B, supersensitized dopamine receptors are shown to be involved, which occur secondarily following early dysfunction of the DA neurons. However, for abnormal dependence, aggressiveness, and selfmutilation or panic states, dysfunction of the 5HT and NA neurons are also thought to be involved, as in "friendliness" and "muricide" in animal experiments [13]. Echolalia and pronominal reverse, shown in category C, are signs of the language of the nondominant hemisphere, or a failure in the development of the functional lateralization of the cortex [2]. Poor eye-to-eye contact and failure in finger-pointing are signs of a lack of communication, or failure in the development of the functional specialization of the cortex.

The psychobehavioral abnormalities shown in Table 1 were observed in infantile autism. These were not common in hydrocephalus associated with spina bifida, and those in categories A and B were only observed in severely affected patients.

It is noteworthy that the presence of atonic NREM and/or asynchronism in sleep spindles was correlated to low IQ/DQ levels, and both, particularly the presence of atonic NREM, were related to a decrease in these levels with age. Atonic NREM is a sign of leakage of axial atonia of the REM stage into the NREM stage, and suggests hypofunction of the dorsal raphe serotonergic (5HTergic) neurons and/or the locus ceruleus noradrenergic (NAergic) neurons. Moreover, the neural pathway executing atonia in the REM stage is the same pathway which develops postural atonia and prevents locomotion. Atonic NREM is observed in normal infants in the first 4 months, but after 6 months, atonia is only observed in the REM stage. Thus, in hydrocephalus associated with spina bifida, the presence of atonic NREM implies a dysfunction of the brainstem, which causes postural atonia and failure in locomotion. Asynchronism of sleep spindles is a common feature in infancy, but the presence of it in childhood suggests certain abnormalities in the interhemispheric connections, or dysfunction of the rostral portion of the brainstem.

Experimental studies on the pathogenesis of myeloschisis in Splotch-delayed mice with exogenous lectin showed glial infiltration on the dorsal surface of the neural placode, the primitive floor of the 4th ventricle (presented by K. Takahashi, H. Tanaka, S. Nakahara et al. at the ISSB, 1997). However, the agent primarily affects the sensory neurons of the primitive brainstem, but not the motor neurons. So in the dysraphic state, spina bifida might have a lesion of the aminergic neuron of the brainstem located on its dorsal surface. This strongly suggests the involvement of the aminergic neurons of the brainstem, which develop atonic NREM in those patients with hydrocephalus associated with spina bifida.

We have also performed an evaluation on congenital hydrocephalus caused by aqueductal stenosis or meningitis of neonates or young infants. The results of this evaluation are shown in Table 2, together with those of the present study. As shown in this table, the clinical neurological and clinical electroneurophysiological findings correlated with IQ/DQ were different depending on the causes of the hydrocephalus. Among them, ambidexterity or left-handedness and asynchronism in sleep spindles were particularly correlated with hydrocephalus associated with spina bifida. Atonic NREM was also a causative factor in hydrocephalus due to aqueductal stenosis, and epilepsy related to low IQ/DQ in all hydrocephalus cases. In hydrocephalus due to aqueductal stenosis, psychobehavioral abnormalities, such as autism, are often observed, suggesting early 5HTergic hypofunction. However, these features were observed in only 2 of 10 patients with hydrocephalus associated with spinal bifida, who were the subjects of this study.

Thus, in hydrocephalus associated with spina bifida, there exists a particular pathophysiology for lower IQ/DQ levels which is different from those caused by other etiologies. It might be dysfunction of particular brainstem aminergic neurons, probably the 5HTergic neurons, which cause abnormalities in the development of the circadian S–W cycle and leakage of axial atonia of the REM stage into the NREM stage. However, in contrast to congenital

TABLE 2. Parameters of clinical neurology and clinical electroneurophysiology correlated with low intelligence in congenital hydrocephalus

	S—W cycle	Crawling	Hand dominance	Atonic NREM	Synchronism in spindles	Epilepsy
SB	+	−	±	+	+	+
AS	+	+	−	+	−	+
PM	−	−	−	−	−	+

S—W cycle, sleep—wakefulness cycle; SB, spina bifida; AS, aqueductus stenosis; PM, post-meningitis.

hydrocephalus due to aqueductal stenosis, brainstem aminergic neurons related to autistic behavior might be preserved or only slightly affected. The increase in the number of ambidexterous patients in this study may partly be due to the delay in the development of the S–W cycle. Alternatively, this might be caused by abnormal interhemispheric connections due to associated dysraphic anomalies of the brain. This abnormality may also relate to the asynchronism of sleep spindles.

The pathophysiology of epilepsy as a causative factor for low IQ/DQ levels is not known. However, in hydrocephalus associated with spina bifida, as well as that caused by aqueductal stenosis, the epileptic pathophysiology might cause turbulence in the maturation of the cortex, which would disturb or delay the development of functional lateralization and specialization.

Evaluation of the function of the aminergic neurons in hydrocephalus associated with spina bifida is important, not only for arriving at a prognosis, but also for preventing brainstem dysfunction by improving or strengthening the environment in early infancy, as the functions of these aminergic neurons are influenced by environmental stimulation.

References

1. Segawa M, Katoh M, Katoh J, Nomura Y (1992) Early modulation of sleep parameters and its importance in later behavior. Brain Dysfunction 5:211–223
2. Segawa M (1989) A neurological model of early infantile autism. No-To-Hattatsu 21:170–180
3. Segawa M (1993) Pathophysiology of Down syndrome: considerations from clinical neurology. Neuropathology 13:301–303
4. Segawa M (1998) A neurological model of early infantile autism. Brain Science (Tokyo) 20:169–175
5. Miller S, van der Burg J (1973) The function of long propriospinal pathways in the coordination of quadrupedal stepping in the cat. In: Stein RB, Pearson KG, Smith RS, Redford JB (eds) Control of posture and locomotion. Advances in behavioral biology, vol 7. Plenum Press, New York, London, pp 561–577
6. Mori S, Matsuyama K, Kohyama J, Kobayashi Y, Takakusaki K (1992) Neuronal constituents of postural and locomotor control systems and their interactions in cats. Brian Dev 14(suppl):S109–S120
7. Koh T, Nakazawa M, Kani K, Maeda T (1991) Investigation of origin of serotonergic projection to developing rat visual cortex: a combined retrograde tracing and immunohistochemical study. Brain Res Bull 27:675–684
8. Lewitt P, Harvey JA, Friedman E, Simansky K, Murphy H (1997) New evidence for neurotransmitter influences on brain development. Trends Neurosci 20:269–274
9. Mazer C, Muneyyirci J, Taheny K, Raio N, Borella A, Whitaker-Azmitia P (1997) Serotonin depletion during synaptogenesis leads to decreased synaptic density and learning deficits in the adult rat: a possible model of neurodevelopment disorders with cognitive deficits. Brain Res 760:68–73
10. Valzelle L (1978) Affective behavior and serotonin. In: Essman WB (ed) Serotonin in health and disease, vol 3. The central nervous system. Spectrum, New York, London, pp 145–201
11. Brenner E, Mirmiran M, Uylings HBM, Van Der Gugten J (1983) Impaired growth of the cerebral cortex of rats treated neonatally with 6-hydroxydopamine under different environmental conditions. Neurosci Lett 42:13–17
12. Tanaka S, Miyagawa F, Imai H, Hidano T (1987) Effects on learning of the lesion on the dorsal noradrenergic bundle. Juntendo Med J (Tokyo) 33:271–272
13. Valzelli L, Garattini S (1972) Biochemical and behavioural changes induced by isolation in rats. Neuropharmacology 11:17–22

Abstract

Outcome of Spina Bifida and Present Attitude Towards Prenatal Diagnosis in Europe

PIERRE GRESSENS, P. LEBARBIER, I. HUSSON, P. COLLIN, C. BONNIER, G. PENNECOT, and P. EVRARD

The frequency of new cases of spina bifida (SB) has largely decreased in the last 10 years in several countries of western Europe. The emergence of widespread prenatal diagnosis is probably the main cause of this reduced incidence of SB, at least in France and Belgium. However, knowledge of the outcome of SB remains important in western Europe for at least three reasons: (i) the follow-up of the large cohort of SB children born before the generalization of prenatal diagnosis; (ii) the follow-up of patients who have escaped the prenatal diagnosis or where abortion was refused by the parents; (iii) to provide appropriate and complete information to parents who have an affected fetus. We have reviewed the outcome (between the ages of 5 and 20 years) of 39 SB cases followed in a Belgian center and of 98 French cases. Three major aspects were evaluated: (i) frequency and types of surgery and their benefits; (ii) sociopsychological adaptation; (iii) educational level and learning disabilities. An average of 5.6 surgical interventions were performed for each affected child, and 78% of the hospitalizations were linked to surgical procedures. In the Belgian population, 54% of surgical cases were orthopedic in nature and 28% were performed by urologists; modifications of CSF derivation accounted for 17% of surgical procedures. Common urological interventions included cystostomy (24%), intermittent clean catheterization (38%), and bladder augmentation (21%). Despite surgical and medical treatments, 79% and 62% of children were reported to have remained chronically incontinent for urine and feces, respectively. The French study was focused on orthopedic treatments and performances. Follow-up showed that 39% were able to walk, 19% walked with help, and 42% were in a wheelchair. We also found that 40% of children had hip interventions, and 26% of these had good results. Half of the patients had surgical corrections to their feet (with multiple interventions in most cases); the results were considered to be good in 37% of cases. Among 31 cases with spinal balance problems (mostly lumber scoliosis and severe kyphosis), 16 were operated on, with mixed results. To evaluate the cognitive performance and sociopsychological problems of these patients, Belgian parents and affected children were submitted to a phone questionnaire. The results showed that 66% of families described the disease as a major social handicap, and each child had an average of 2.6 sessions of reeducation (speech or motor) per week. Also, 58% of children had experienced high levels of anxiety and/or depression (mostly

Pediatric Neurology and Orthopedic Surgery Services, Robert-Debre Hospital, Paris, France, and Pediatric Neurology Service, St-Luc Hospital, Brussels, Belgium; Centre P. Dottin, ASEI, Ramonville-St-Agne

between 12 and 15 years old), although none of the patients was currently followed by a psychologist/psychiatrist. Of the children affected, 76% (mostly under the age of 10 years) considered their existence to be enjoyable, although only half of their parents had the same feeling. In terms of education, 45% of the children were in special schools (mostly for cerebral palsy patients), while 56% of the children in the normal educational system were at least 1 year behind for their age. Although the size of the sample was limited, 54% of the children with school problems, and who were older than 10 years, had a history of CSF derivation dysfunction, while none of the children who were at the right school level for their age had had this complication during the study period.

Abstract

A Study of Physical Development in Patients with Myelomeningocele

Kuniko Shirane[1], Kazunari Yoshida[1], Tsutomu Iwaya[1], Reizo Shirane[2], Akira Morone[3], and Nobuhiko Haga[4]

The neurological paralysis of patients with myelomeningocele results in motor disabilities, particularly in ambulation. The deterioration in ambulation is often caused by an increase in body weight during the developmental period. This study was undertaken to clarify the pattern of physical development of children with myelomeningocele.

The subjects were 85 children with myelomeningocele, whose clinical details were clear since birth. Investigations of height, weight, neurosegmental level, and clinical status were performed longitudinally.

After the age of 1 year, body height was smaller than normal and the differences in body height between patients with myelomeningocele and normal children became significant with age. The children with neurological involvement above L4 level were smaller in height than those with neurological involvement below L5 level.

As for body weight, differences from normal children were small at preschool age, and in adolescence the differences became even smaller. The body weights of children with hydrocephalus were higher than of those without hydrocephalus. In adolescence, the heights were smaller and the weights were greater in patients with myelomeningocele who had a history of meningitis.

[1] Section of Rehabilitation Medicine for the Physically Disabled, Tohoku University Graduate School of Medicine, Sendai, Japan

[2] Department of Neurosurgery, Tohoku University School of Medicine, Sendai, Japan

[3] Department of Orthopaedics, Takuto Rehabilitation Center for Physically Handicapped Children, Sendai, Japan

[4] Department of Pediatric Orthopaedics, Shizuoka Prefectural Children's Hospital, Shizuoka, Japan

Abstract

Obesity and Overweight in a Group of Patients with Myelomeningocele

Roberto Del Gado, Donatella Del Gaizo, Daniela Brescia, Giuseppina Polidori, and Angela Tamburro

The nutritional status of patients with myelomeningocele needs careful attention because of its potential impact on skeletal development and the risk of cardiovascular disease. A.A. found a high prevalence of obesity and short stature in myelomeningocele (MMC) children. The purpose of this study was to report on the nutritional status of our patients with MMC. Nutritional status was evaluated in 32 children with MMC (14 boys and 18 girls between the ages of 2.3 and 12.7 years; mean ± SD = 7.1 ± 3.2 years). Nineteen out of the 32 subjects who entered the study were ambulatory (13 without any support and 6 with splints) and 13 were nonambulatory. During the period of the study, anthropometry and dietary recall were also performed in a control group of 30 healthy children, 15 boys and 15 girls, aged 2–15.2 years (mean ± SD = 5.9 ± 3.1 years). Body weight was measured by a counterweight scale. The subjects were weighed in their inner clothes. Stature was obtained by a Harpenden wall-mounted stadiometer, carefully measured in order to obtain the maximum elongation of the rachis. Triceps and subscapular skinfolds were measured with a Lange skinfold caliper; mid-arm muscle circumference was measured using a tape. Weight-for-height index (WHI), Quetelets' body mass index (BMI), arm muscle area (AMA), and fat area index (FAI) were calculated from the measured indices following Frisancho. On the morning of anthropometric assessment, a blood sample was taken from MMC patients. The sample was worked up for hemoglobin (Hb), hematocrit (Ht), serum protein (Prot), albumin (Alb), and transferrin (TRF) by standard methods. Serum calcium (Ca), phosphorus (P), and alkaline phosphatase (ALP) were evaluated by colorimetric methods. Intact parathyroid hormone (PTH) concentrations were measured using a kit for immunoradiometric assay (IRMA). A 24-h dietary intake recall was provided by all subjects at the start of the study with a visual memory system. Intakes were assessed with a computer code based on available data (Dietosystem). Nutrient intake was espressed as a percentage of recommended dietary allowances according to the age of the subject. Patients had significantly lower stature than controls, and 11 out of 32 had a stature score less than −2 Z. BMI and subscapular skinfolds were significantly higher in patients than in controls, and 10 out of 32 patients had BMI and subscapular skinfold scores greater than 2 Z. There were no significant differences between patients and controls with respect to WHI, AMA, or FAI. Three patients had Hb and Ht levels below, and TRF levels above, the normal range for age. Above normal values were found for P and PTH in 2 patients and for ALP in 8 patients. Prot, Alb, Ca, and P values were normal in all the MMC patients.

Department of Pediatrics, II University of Naples, Naples, Italy

The primary findings of our study were that the MMC patients had significantly lower stature and higher weights, and greater fat deposits in the trunk but not peripherally (arms). Thirty-four percent of the children had stature scores less than −2 Z, and 31% had BMI and subscapular skinfold scores greater than 2 Z. In our patients, subscapular skinfolds but not triceps skinfolds were significantly higher than in controls. This indicates that subcutaneous fat accumulates mainly in the trunk. In this respect it is worth noting that subscapular skinfolds are better associated with cardiovascular disease risk factors than are triceps skinfolds. MMC children appear to be of short stature and at risk of low bone mass a well as of cardiovascular disease secondary to the excess of stored fats. These risk factors seem to depend on reduced mobility rather than on excessive energy or low calcium intake.

Moderator's Comments on Sessions—Pediatric Neurology

Pierre Gressens and Shigehiko Kamoshita

This child neurology session was composed of five talks addressing different aspects of spina bifida, including prenatal diagnosis with primary and secondary prevention, optimal mode of delivery, postnatal growth and development with the impact of obesity, and consequences of hydrocephalus on neurophysiological parameters.

Dr. Pierre Gressens reminded us that attitude of physicians towards prenatal diagnosis of spina bifida is very defferent between cultures, countries, and even among practitioners of a given country. Based on the retrospective analysis of a French–Belgian cohort of children with spina bifida, he underlined some important aspects in the management of spina bifida: (i) the optimal care of these patients requires a multidisciplinary approach; (ii) a large proportion of these children will undergo multiple surgery during a large part of their infancy and adolscence; (iii) psychological support for these patients might be critical; (iv) cerebrospinal fluid derivation dysfunction could negatively impact on cognitive functions.

Dr. David Shurtleff summarized some crucial studies showing the benefits of cesareans vs. vaginal delivery for the motor outcome of children with spina bifida. He further underlined the deleterious influence of ruptured membranes on motor outcome. He also raised the critical issue of the primary prevention of spina bifida by folic acid, suggesting that antioxydant therapeutics could be more efficient because his colleagues had observed free radical scavenger deficiencies in their population of spina bifida patients. In terms of prenatal evaluation of prognosis, Dr. Shurtleff underlined two criteria of poor motor and cognitive outcome: severe kyphosis and spinal cord hypoplasia. Finally, he also reminded us of the differences existing in the attitude towards prenatal diagnosis of spina bifida among different "subpopulations" in the United States.

Dr. Kuniko Shirane addressed the physical development of patients with spina bifida. Although body height was normal at birth, they showed a progressive slowing down of growth rate with age. The severity of the short stature was determined, at least in females, by the neurosegmental level of the spinal cord defect. The authors had also studied the potential effects of hydrocephalus and meningitis on body height.

Dr. Masaya Segawa's presentation was focused on the long-term prognosis of ten patients with spina bifida and hydrocephalus. This study aimed to look for a correlation between cognitive outcome and EEG, polygraphy, time of crawling, hand dominance, or epilepsy occurrence. The authors showed abnormal EEG basal activity and atonic non-REM sleep in these patients, with the polygraphic abnormality being associated with lower cognitive function. Interestingly, time of crawling was not predictive of cognitive level, suggesting that delay in crawling in these patients was mainly due to spinal cord defects.

Dr. Roberto Del Gado addressed the issue of the negative impact of obesity. Their anthropometric study and bone mineral content measurements revealed that children with spina bifida were overweight, and had a short stature, a bone-mineral deficiency, and an increased scapular skinfold measurement. Furthermore, they had a normal caloric and nutrient intake, suggesting a vicious circle: skeletal deformities will induce short stature and will discourage physical exercise, inducing overweight and bone demineralization, which will aggravate skeletal deformities. Based on these data, the authors recommended developing specific programs of physical activity for children with spina bifida.

Nursing

Nursing Care of Mothers with a Newborn with Spina Bifida Child

Michiko Ebina

Summary. This chapter focuses on the early psychological care of the mother after a baby is born with spina bifida. There are five moments when intervention is necessary. The first is at the time of diagnosis, before the birth of the baby. The second is at an "encounter" between medical professionals and the family of the baby. The third moment is when the situation is explained, and it is important to consider from whom the explanation should come. In Japan, the explanation is generally, first given to the father and others, not to the mother. The fourth is when the mother has received an explanation about the diseased state of her newborn from the attending physician, and is upset. The fifth time is when the family is prepared for discharge. At that time, a nurse mitigates the family's tensions, urges the family to ask the physician questions, and questions the physician instead of the family having to do so.

Key words. Nursing care, Mother, Spina bifida, Newborn, Explanation

This chapter focuses on the psychological care of the mother after a baby is born with spina bifida. It will cover the period from birth to 1 month of age, and will include the period during which the infant with spina bifida is born, surgery is performed, the wound has healed, and the mother has been given guidance on infant care in preparation for discharge from the hospital. According to Drotar et al. [1], this period is the time when the parents adapt to the birth of a baby with a congenital malformation, i.e. it is a time of shock, then of denial, and then of mixed emotions of both sorrow and anger.

At the end of this chapter, I express my own point of view on a few of the problems which a mother has to face after the discharge of her child from the hospital.

The severity of spina bifida differs greatly, depending on whether it is the occulta type or aperta type, and also what level of the spine is affected [2–4]. The occulta type is generally mild, while the aperta type is quite severe. All of the babies described in my examples had spina bifida aperta. After discharge, the infant will need to visit the hospital frequently. Although details will depend on the system of the hospital concerned and the attending physician, the mother and baby will need to visit the urological section for follow-up of urinary disturbances [5, 6], the orthopedic section for gait disturbances [7], and the rehabilitation section for early assessment and therapy [8]. Therefore, it is not unusual for the mother and infant to visit the outpatient clinic 2 or 3 times per week.

Department of Child-Maternal Health Care Nursing, Kobe City College of Nursing, 3-4 Gakuen-nishimachi, Nishi-ku, Kobe 651-2103, Japan

There are five main aspects of the psychological care of the mother when a baby is born with spina bifida aperta.

The first need for psychological care comes at the time of diagnosis, before the birth of the baby. At present, with the advancement of medical technology, the diagnosis of a fetus with spina bifida before birth is possible by measuring the α-fetoprotein in the amniotic fluid using ultrasound or magnetic resonance imaging (MRI) [9]. In general, there are two problems associated with diagnosis before the birth of the baby.

One is the reliability of the diagnosis. The second is to check how well the physician in charge and the nurse understand this disease and its implications. I will not discuss diagnosis before birth in this chapter, but I wish to emphasize that 90% of the children with spina bifida live a long time, 80% have normal intelligence, and 85% can walk [10–12].

The second psychological aspect of care concerns the "encounter" between the medical professionals and the family of the baby [13]. By encounter, I do not mean just a routine meeting, but a deep communication between them which touches their souls and arouses profound respect for this other human being. In other words, we must ensure the correct attitude of the medical professionals at the time of the explanation to the family. When spina bifida and its long-term prognosis is explained to the parents, they are initially in shock and do not remember the theoretical explanation very clearly. What they do remember is the attitude of the physician and the nurse at the time of the explanation, and especially their nonverbal communication. The physician and nurse need to inform the parents of the facts of the disease objectively, without distortion, with the understanding that the parents can overcome the mental shock. Moreover, they should convey to the parents what potential the child has, what kind of care should be provided to the baby in order not to limit such potential, and what support services that are available to both the baby and the parents. It is important for the physician and nurse to convey how eager they are to cooperate with and support the parents. Regarding nursing care, nurses are required to update their knowledge about this disease and its treatment. If they have not kept up-to-date, they will be obliged to follow the physician's values when contacting the family.

Generally, the family is skeptical, even if the medical professional gives an explanation incorporating a forward-looking message. Nurses should search for good points about the child and convey them to the family. If they praise the child by saying such things as "she will become a beauty as she has a high nose," or "he has clever-looking eyes," the family will be encouraged for a long time while they are raising the child.

The third critical time in the psychological care of the mother is when the explanation is given and from whom the explanation comes [14, 15]. In Japan, the explanation is generally first given to the father, the grandfather or the grandmother, not to the mother. This is primarily owing to the long-standing belief that immediately after delivery of the baby, the mother is in a mental state which is not totally normal and may be unstable, and she will respond to matters concerning her child so sensitively that she cannot accept the condition of her child accurately. Unfortunately, most obstetricians and other medical staff members still believe this.

Often, a mother feels immediately after the delivery of her baby that there is something abnormal in her child, probably when she does not hear the words, "Congratulations!", "your baby has a perfect body," which she is unconsciously expecting after delivery. It is said that the atmosphere in the delivery room turns from one of enthusiasm to one of unusual quietness. Even if the mother asks, "How is my baby"? the physician or nurse merely replies by saying that the baby is alright.

In Japan, the earliest time at which the mother learns of the condition of her newborn baby may be 2 or 3 days after delivery, when the information is given to the mother by a medical professional. There have been cases in which a mother heard the information from the family more than a week after the delivery. In local regions, there are a number of cases in which the attending physician explained spina bifida to the mother 21 days after the birth.

How would the mother feel if she was left without information for as long as 3 weeks?

Reactions differ among individuals. Some received the delayed information positively as consideration on the part of the husband and the attending physician not to cause her anxiety. Other mothers became angry, saying that they were very worried about what had happened to the child, and felt as if they were going mad. A few specific cases are described below.

Mrs. B was not given any explanation by the attending physician or nurse during her week of hospitalization after delivery. The day of her discharge, while waiting for a ride, her grandmother awkwardly revealed the condition of the newborn baby, saying "The nurse told me that the baby will not live until 6 years of age."

Mrs. C received only fragmentary information from her husband after repeated questioning, although he visited the hospital every day to meet the baby and to take her frozen breast milk. Twenty-one days after birth, the mother drove alone to the hospital. The young mother first saw her baby lying in the prone position receiving a drip infusion, with its legs bandaged. Upon seeing this, she was thrown into a panic! This was a shocking situation, which she had never imagined possible.

Immediately after the birth of her baby, Mrs. D was shown the bifida lesion on the lower back of her newborn. The physician explained the necessity of the newborn being transferred to another hospital for an immediate operation. During the 1 week hospitalization period, she received a clear explanation of the condition of the newborn, with photos, as well as answers to her questions from physicians and nurses. She said, "Such an explanation was useful for me to accept the disorder of my child."

It is important that the nurse should not necessarily side with the physician concerning the mental state of the mother immediately after delivery. Instead, the nurse should gather data and discuss with the physician the feelings of the mother. The nurse will be closest to the mother, and in the best position to influence the physician, who will probably tend to hold to more traditional beliefs and behavior.

The fourth psychological aspect of care concerns the distress of the mother after receiving the explanation about the diseased state of her newborn from the attending physician [14, 15]. This distress consists of two stages. One is a state of shock immediately after hearing the explanation. Some mothers will not come to the hospital to see their newborn. Sometimes, the nurse wonders whether to wait and how long to wait. If there is no contact from the mother or the father, the nurse should contact the family by telephone. The nurse should express concern about the mother, and enquire when she is next scheduled to visit the hospital. The nurse must be careful to talk to the mother persuasively, not threateningly.

When the mother comes to the hospital, the nurse should speak kind words to her and lovingly tend the newborn in front of her. The nurse then positively conveys to the mother how the newborn behaves, with such phrases as, "the baby sucks milk well," "the baby cries at appropriate times," or "the baby belches loudly." All of these are good signs of a healthy baby. After hearing of the newborn's responsiveness in detail from the nurse, the mother tends to become more open and familiar, and more accepting of the newborn. The nurse should arrange opportunities for the mother to touch her child, and request her to help care for the child so that she will have the actual feeling of mothering her child. In spite of the nurse's attempts, and the mother may never touch her child, and she may even require some assistance. In such cases, the nurse should collect a wide range of information related to the mother's home life, such as her relationship with her husband and the response of other relatives. Depending on necessity, the nurse may propose various measures to the physician.

Affter the initial state of shock, the next stage begins. This is when the mother recollects the physician's words fragmentarily and asks the nurse a few irregular questions to confirm the doctor's words. This confirmation work takes the form of the mother speaking to the nurse while she gives the child milk or changes a diaper. The nurse thus plays a critical role in supplementing the physician's explanation. For instance, this condition is related to the central nervous system, and family members may be worried about the "intelligence" of the child. The family may also express fears that the child may be unable to walk. However, they seem to overcome this fear after an explanation that the ability to walk differs among individuals.

When providing such explanations, the nurse is required to respond in a timely manner to the mother's words, always keeping in mind that there is hope for the child.

The fifth vital time for the mother is when she and the family are preparing for the baby to be discharged [15, 16]. At that time, the nurse mitigates the family's tensions, urges the family to ask the physician questions, puts some questions to the physician instead of leaving it to the family, and contributes to the formation of a relaxed atmosphere where the family feels that "any question is alright." Sometimes, during the conversation, the family may become distraught or begin crying. On such occasions, the nurse should arrange for a quiet place to attend to the family.

Unfortunately, actual nursing care in Japan does not socially permit the ideal behavior just described. Even if nurses feel the necessity to be with the family, they must pretend that they did not see their need, offer apologies, and say they have lots of other work to do. However, I strongly believe that it is very important for nurses to create the opportunity to sit down and discuss health issues with the patient's family sincerely and wholeheartedly. This behavior will guarantee a high standard of nursing care, promote the patient's understanding, and enhance the nurse's feelings of job satisfaction.

I also think that it is important for nursing management or the head nurse to rearrange the nursing staff's work responsibilities so as to address patient teaching. Then the attitude of "I will attend to the mother, because I was the nurse present when she gave birth," becomes a common, accepted practice. If the nurse can make contact with the mother in the ways described above, both of them can share a significant time, and deepen their mutual understanding and shared values about the situation. The nurse can thereby provide an effective, high level of psychological care to the mother.

Finally, I would like to propose two systems of support for mothers after discharge from the hospital. I recently talked with a group of 10 mothers in Ibaragi Prefecture, Japan, who had infants with spina bifida. These proposals were put forward at that meeting. The first proposal is a system of 24-h telephone consultation and/or a nurse visiting the family during the daytime. Although the mothers were taught how to care for the child after discharge, they realized that they had many questions about "minute things" when they returned home and began caring for their child alone. They could not judge whether these minute things were trifles or were very important. The mothers unanimously said that for 1 month after leaving the hospital, they were anxious every day about whether their care was correct or not. They often felt as if they were going mad! Mothers often said that it takes at least a year before they become confident and feel that they can provide adequate care for their child.

The second proposal is the presence of nurseries for the family visiting the hospital. In the current situation, where the family tends to be split into small units, the installation of a nursery in the outpatient clinic of the hospital is essential to creating an environment in which the mothers can visit the hospital without concern about their other children. One possibility for realizing this proposal widely is to evaluate hospitals with outpatient nurseries using a scoring system to be added to the health insurance system.

Acknowledgments. I wish to express my appreciation to Prof. Haruo Ohkawa and Assistant Prof. Mayumi Iwakawa, Pediatric Surgery Department of Tsukuba University, for their advice, and to the mothers of the group of patients with spina bifida in Ibaragi Prefecture for their response to my interview.

References

1. Drotar D, Baskiewicz A, Irvin N, Kennell JH, Klaus MH (1975) The adaptation of parents to the birth of an infant with a congenital malformation: a hypothetical model. Pediatrics 56:710–717
2. Inukai K (1996) Spina bifida. Perinatal Med 26:1263–1266
3. Morone A (1996) Rihabilitation of the patiant with spina bifida-the latest trend-. Jnp J Rihabil Med 33(3)
4. Takei F, Oi S (1996) Embryology of spina bifida. Jnp J Pediatric Surg 28:12–24
5. Tanaka K, Ishidoh T (1996) Long-term prognosis of patients with spina bifida. Jnp J Pediatric Surg 28:102–106
6. Miyano T, Morioka A, Horikoshi T, et al. (1996) Perinatal Med., Neurogenic bladder dysfunction and Spina Bifida. 26(6), 1996-6
7. Kimizuka M (1996) Orthopedic Management of Spina Bifida. Jnp J Pediatric Surg 28:85–91
8. Morone A (1996) Rihabilitation of the Patiant with Spina Bifida. Jnp J Pediatric Srg 28:92–97
9. Morioka A, Miyano T, Horikoshi T (1997) Prenatal Diagnosis and Prevention of Spina Bifida. Jnp J Pediatric Surg 28:25–29
10. Iwasaki Y (1996) Primary Management of Spina Bifida. Jnp J Pediatric Surg 28:30–35
11. Tamaki N, Kurata H (1996) Treatment of Hydrocephalus Associated with Spina Bifida. Jnp J Pediatric Surg 28:36–39
12. Iwaya T, Yoshida K (1996) The Physical Growth and Social Skill of Myelomeningocele Children. Sogo Rehabilitation 24(10)
13. Klaus MH, Kennell JH/Translation: Takeuchi T, Kashiwagi T, Yokoo K (1990) Parent-Infant Bonding "Care of Mother with Congenital Malformation" pp 327–373
14. Kabe K, Tamai M (1944) Teno Hirano Inochi "The Life in the Palm of Mother's hand", Yumiru Shuppan, Tokyo
15. Nobe A (1993) Mahoo no Te no Kodomotachi-Senten Ijou wo Ikiru "Children with Magic Hands", TaroJirosha, Tokyo
16. Porepore Kurabu (1995) Imadoki Shogaiji no Hahaoya Monogatari "Now, A Story of Mother with Handicapped Children", Budosha, Tokyo

Continuing Care of Children with Spina Bifida at an Outpatient Clinic

MIHO NARAMA

Summary. Children with spina bifida accompanied by chronic conditions acquire the activities of daily life and adapt to social life individually. The purposes of this study were (1) to examine the characteristics of independent activities in daily life in young Japanese children with spina bifida, (2) to identify the relationship between their independent activities in daily life and home care by their mothers, and (3) to identify the relationship between their independent activities in daily life and the stress of their mothers. The subjects were 19 pairs of Japanese mothers and their young children with spina bifida. It was found that the quality of home care by mothers influenced the activities of daily life of their children. Furthermore, it was found that problems related to the mobility of the children were the main stressors of their mothers. These findings suggested that nursing interventions in the outpatient clinic need to focus not only on illness-related risk reductions, but also on the progression of developmental tasks.

Key words. Young children, Activities of daily living, Home care, Stress of mothers

Introduction

Characteristics of Health Problems of Children with Spina Bifida and their Families in Japan

Illness Management of Children with Spina Bifida

Most children with spina bifida have various disabilities, and they continuously need some specific daily care. In Japan, most children with spina bifida perform intermittent self-catheterization. Most parents of young children are burdened with this specific daily care, because they assume responsibility for these tasks. There is a gradual transition of these responsibilities and self-care task performance from parents to school-age children [5]. In the process of transition, there may be various problems related to the physical conditions of children with spina bifida. It is necessary to consider these developmental factors in order to improve illness management at home.

School of Nursing, Hamamatsu University, 3600 Handa-cho, Hamamatsu, Shizuoka 431-31, Japan

Developmental Tasks of Children with Spina Bifida

Healthy children are able to acquire the activities of daily life and adapt to social life through their developmental processes. Most children with spina bifida have bowel and urinary control problems and disabled mobility, and their developmental processes may be different from those of healthy children. Factors contributing to the independent activities in daily life of children with spina bifida include not only developmental level, but also the severity of their disabilities as well as the quality of illness management and lifestyle help. Therefore it may be especially important for children with spina bifida to improve their health status and lifestyle in infancy, so that they will be able to accomplish developmental tasks.

Stress of Children with Spina Bifida and their Families

In Japan, many researchers have focused on stress in children with health problems and in their parents [4]. In other countries, it has been found that the stress levels of parents of children with spina bifida were higher than those of parents of healthy children [2]. I have done a study to ascertain the relationship between illness management and stress in mothers of children with anorectal malformation who had disabled bowel control [3]. The findings indicated that the existence of several health problems in these children increased the stress level of their mothers. Thus, the stress of parents of children with spina bifida may be an important factor influencing the quality of parenting, the health status, and the developmental level of their children.

Therefore, it is necessary to assess illness and developmental factors in children with spina bifida and the stress of their parents comprehensively.

The Independence of Activities in Daily Life of Young Japanese Children with Spina Bifida and Its Relations to Illness Management, Improvement of Lifestyle by their Mothers, and Mother's Stress

The purposes of this study were (1) to examine the characteristics of the independent activities in daily life in young Japanese children with spina bifida, (2) to identify the relationship between these activities and home care by their mothers, and (3) to identify the relationship between the activities and stress in their mothers.

Methods

The subjects were 19 pairs of Japanese mothers and their young children (aged from 1 to 6 years) with spina bifida who were recruited from the outpatient clinic of a children's hospital in Shizuoka City, Japan. Most children needed some specific daily care, such as intermittent catheterization. Ten children also had hydrocephalus. Two types of questionnaire were used for data collection: a Japanese translated Parenting Stress Index (PIS) [1], and a self-developed questionnaire relating to home care by mothers and independent activities in daily life, e.g., eating, sleeping, dressing and undressing, hygiene, elimination, and mobility. The questionnaires were handed to mothers, who were asked to return them on the same day or by mail.

The PSI scores of mothers of healthy children were quoted from an earlier report as a comparison [4].

Results

Characteristics of Independent Activities in Daily Life

The accomplishment rates for the items related to eating, "using chopsticks to eat" and "eating most of the meal by oneself," increased with age and reached 100% by 4 years old. Most children performed the tasks "putting on socks by oneself" and "taking off outerwear by oneself," after 4 years old. The accomplishment rates of the items related to sleeping, "getting up at a regular time" and "going to bed at a regular time," reached over 60%, but 47.4% of children with spina bifida usually go to bed after 10 p.m. The accomplishment rates of the items related to hygiene, "washing one's hands before each meals and snacks" and "washing one's hands at the time of getting home," increased with age and reached 100% by 4 years old. The accomplishment rates of most items related to elimination and mobility were less than 50%. There are few children who accomplished "giving notice about defecation" and "giving notice about urination."

Most children with spina bifida used diapers. It was found that the accomplishments of "standing by oneself" and "walking by oneself" were influenced by the severity of the disabilities.

Relationships Among Independent Activities in Daily Life, Illness Management, and Improvement of Lifestyle by Helpful Mothers

Sixteen mothers performed intermittent catheterization of their children. The frequency of this care ranged from 3 to 8 times a day. Eight mothers performed intermittent catheterization with help from the fathers and grandmothers of the children. Furthermore, some mothers felt anxiety about the social disadvantages of children who needed intermittent catheterization. Four mothers performed bowel management of their children. Because some mothers could not understand what were good conditions for their children, they required information related to the method of bowel management. Six mothers performed rehabilitation training of their children to keep in a standing posture and to walk.

The accomplishments of three items of the independent activities in daily life were related to the frequency of intermittent catheterization. This means that there was a relationship between the regular and frequent performance of intermittent catheterization and the independence of the activities in daily life.

The total scores of improvement of lifestyle by mothers were related to the accomplishment of independence of dressing and undressing in two of the items.

Relationship Between Independent Activities in Daily Life and Mothers' Stress

The mean scores of PSI of mothers of children with spina bifida tended to be higher than those of mothers of healthy children. The score of a subcategory of PSI "perception of problematic issues related to child" were significantly higher in mothers of children who could not stand and walk by themselves than in mothers of children who could.

Discussion

Nursing Care to Promote Illness Management and Progress in Developmental Tasks

The research findings indicated that the accomplishment rates of independent activities in daily life related to eating and dressing and undressing increased slowly with age.

Furthermore, it found that the quality of improvement of daily health practice by mothers were related to whether children could dress or undress independently. Therefore, nurses need to focus on improving the daily health practice of children with spina bifida, and encourage parents to support children in mastering self-help tasks. In addition, nursing intervention should set individual goals relating to the severity of disability in the areas of elimination and mobility, because independence in these areas is directly influenced by disabilities.

Another important role when nursing children with spina bifida is promoting illness management at home. Although mothers were responsible for bowel management of their children, most of them were not satisfied with the defecating conditions of the children. Therefore, nursing intervention should include helping mothers to identify individual goals for the defecating conditions of their children, and providing information about the relationship between diet and constipation and the effective use of enemas. It was interesting that the illness management of adequate intermittent catheterization influenced the independent activities in daily life of children with spina bifida. These findings suggest that nursing intervention in the outpatient clinic needs to focus not only on illness-related risk reductions, but also on the progression of developmental tasks.

Nursing Care to Decrease Stress in Mothers

The findings suggest that problems related to the mobility of their children were the main stressors of mothers. Independence of mobility influenced the social life of children and the burden of parents. Therefore it may be important for nursing intervention to help mothers to understand these characteristics of their stress, and to provide information related to the prospects in this area and useful social resources.

Most mothers feel anxious about the influences of elimination problems on children's social life. Because children with spina bifida usually receive treatment at various medical units depending on their physical problems, it will be difficult to provide holistic care for elimination problems. Nurses need to fulfil a unique role as a coordinator and as a specialist, so that daily problems may be solved and mothers' stress may decrease.

References

1. Abidin RR (1990) Parenting stress index, 3rd edn. Charlottesville Pediatric Psychology Press
2. Kazak AE, Marvin RS (1984) Differences, difficulties, and adaptation: stress and social networks in families with a handicapped child. Fam Relat 33:1–11
3. Miho N (1997) The relationships among acquirement of defecation control of children with anorectal malformation after surgery, parenting and parenting stress of their mothers. J Chiba Acad Nurs Sci 3:24–31
4. Mitsue M, Yuriko K, Miho N, Yoshiko K, Junko T (1997) Determinants of stress experienced by mothers of young chronically ill children: the comparison with healthy children. J School Nurs Chiba Univ 19:45–51
5. Peterson PM, Rauen KK, Brown J, Cole J (1994) Spina bifida: the transition into adulthood begins in infancy. Rehabil Nurs 19:229–238

Nursing Care for School-Aged Children with Spina Bifida in an Institution

Taiko Hirose[1], Akemi Hamamatsu[2], and Kiyomi Yoshimura[2]

Summary. This chaptes focuses on nursing care for school-aged children with spina bifida residing in an institution. First, developmental issues in the school-age period are described. Second, nursing care to school-age children with spina bifida is discussed, and three cases of children with spina bifida who had nursing care in an institution in Hokkaido are given as examples. Finally, the article outlines the implications for nursing care of school-aged children with spina bifida in institutions and in the community in Japan. School age was defined as the period from elementary school to middle school, that is, 6–15 years old.

Key words. Spina bifida, Adolescent, CIC, Institution, Handicapped children

Introduction

Today at least 85% of the children born with myelomeningocele, the most severe form of spina bifida, can be expected to reach adulthood [4]. In order for these children to effectively make the transition to adulthood, school age is an important developmental stage [7]. School age is defined as the period from elementary to middle school, that is, 6–15 years old. The school-age child uses knowledge and experience to increase self-control in all aspects of care. The internal self, the social self, and the socially comparative self become more prominent at this stage. Self-esteem, group identity, and Erikson's stage of industry versus inferiority are also important dimensions of self in this period. The child also spends considerably more time with peers, both at school and outside of school. Egocentric thinking is weakened, and altruism appears [6].

For children with spina bifida, nurses need to facilitate the school-age child's independence in personal care and help prevent secondary disability, as well as foster continued growth and development, independent mobility, and educational success [1, 3, 5, 7]. Nurses may also help the child develop self-esteem, a positive self-image, and optimal social skills with peers [2].

How are these goals accomplished? An example of such care can be seen in the nursing care provided in an institution for handicapped children in Hokkaido, Japan. The institution has four units, where about a hundred children with physical and mental disabilities reside. There are usually 2–3 children with spina bifida. One unit has 30–35 inpatients, and 16 nurses

[1] School of Nursing and Social Services, Health Sciences University of Hokkaido, Ishikari-Tobetsu, Hokkaido 061-02, Japan

[2] Hokkaido Prefectual Rehabilitation Center for Handicapped Children, Sapporo, Hokkaido, Japan

take care of them. A nurse is assigned as the primary nurse for 2–3 children, usually for about 2 years; the primary nurse makes nursing plans and evaluates nursing interventions for her patients. A nursing plan lasts from 1 to 6 months. Nurses work with physicians, physical therapists, occupational therapists, speech therapists, nannies, medical social workers, nutritionists, and teachers in the school attached to the institution. The primary nurse coordinates effective care by organizing the health professionals' care for the children. Nurses care for the children 24 hours a day with a three-shift system: day, evening, and night shift.

The disabilities of children with spina bifida who are institutionalized are often so severe that they cannot stay at home; some are there because there is no school for handicapped children near their home. They go to the school for handicapped children that is attached to the institution, and have rehabilitation training during the day. After coming back to their unit in the evening, they have free time before going to bed. They go home to visit their families for short stays during weekends and school breaks. There are many events and activities throughout the year, such as picnics, sports day, sea-bathing, a fireworks display, and various parties.

Nurses help the children perform personal care as independently as possible and help them remain free of secondary disability where possible. They also help them to acquire appropriate growth and development, maintain independent mobility, and have an appropriate education.

There follow three case studies of children with spina bifida who have resided at the institution. Because bladder and bowel management are two of the main issues for school-age children with spina bifida, these three studies focus on nursing care to achieve or improve bladder and bowel management.

Case Study A

Case study A is a 14-year-old boy who has resided at the institution since he was 6 years old. He has myelomeningocele (lesion at L5 motor level), neurogenic bladder, hydrocephalus, a hip dislocation, and mental retardation (IQ 70). He attends the school attached to the institution. He is independent in dressing, eating, hygiene, and bladder management, but not in bowel management. He uses a wheelchair. He started clean intermittent catheterization training (CIC) at 8 years old. He took 2 years to complete the training. He has such good manual dexterity that he is independent in bladder management at both school and in the institution. However, he still has problems with bowel management. He did not care when there was a strong fecal smell in his diaper, even at school, and he did not return to his unit to change the diaper and clean himself.

After he began participating in the wheelchair marathon team, he began paying attention to bowel management. An experience of rectal incontinence in the middle of a marathon gave him a strong drive to manage elimination during school time. His primary nurse recognized that it was the right time to start a bowel management program, especially since he had become independent in CIC. First, the nurse had him recognize the stain of stool on his buttocks by using a mirror. In this picture, the nurse is planning to apply a cleansing enema.

Case Study B

Case study B is a 12-year-old girl who resided at the institution for 2 years, from age 6 to age 8. Now she attends a special education class in a regular school in Hokkaido. She has myelomeningocele (lesion level: L1 motor level), neurogenic bladder, Arnold–Chiari malformation, epilepsy, and mental retardation (IQ 66). She is independent in dressing, eating, and hygiene, as well as bladder and bowel management. She too uses a wheelchair. Right after she entered the institution, she started the CIC program training, and took 1 year to complete it. She needed an additional year of training to successfully perform CIC in a wheelchair. When she was 8 years old, she was discharged from the institution, and she now performs CIC at school. She does not even need to wear diapers.

Case Study C

Case study C is a 15-year-old girl who has a lumbar lesion: below L1 for perception and below L4 for motor activity. She has neurogenic bladder, Arnold–Chiari malformation, hydrocephalus, and mental retardation (IQ 41). She has resided in the institution since she was 8 years old. Her manual dexterity was very poor and she had severe motor impairment. She needs a special support around her back and sides to stay in an upright position. In addition, even a nurse had difficulty finding her urinary meatus because of mild malformation. Her parents were devout adherents in a new religion, Mahikarikyo. In order to uphold the precepts of their religion, they rejected surgery, medication, and using a pillow filled with ice. None of the different health care professionals at the institution thought she was ready to perform self-catheterization.

However, when she was 13, she expressed a willingness to perform self-catheterization, and her family supported her. Nurses, especially her primary nurse, decided to teach her to perform self-catheterization and to help her overcome various difficulties to accomplish this. It took her a year and a month to complete the CIC program. At first, the nurse took her hand and helped her insert a catheter into the urinary meatus. After much effort, she was able to perform CIC by herself. She was eventually able to perform CIC successfully without help both at school and at her home. She still wears a diaper because she does not have independent bowel management, and she does not stay dry long. Next year, the plan is for her to be discharged from the institution to attend a high school for handicapped children. It is hard to be admitted to the high school because it does not have a school nurse who can take care of her and facilities where she can perform CIC. If she is able to do self-catheterization in a wheel chair by herself, it may be possible to attend the school. Now she and her primary nurse are working on this next challenge, so that she can participate in high school.

Discussion

Cases A, B, and C were all children with severe problems related to spina bifida; however, they all successfully completed the CIC program. It seems that their developmental stage contributed to their success in CIC, and the nurses did not miss important chances to start a CIC program. Case A could master the CIC technique quickly, but could not adjust to a regular schedule. He sometimes forgot, or skipped CIC. He did not change his diaper after stooling because he did not want to miss time playing with peers. Due to sensory dysfunction, he sometimes neglected bladder and bowl management. However, after he joined the wheelchair marathon he realized he should not annoy his peers with his fecal smell. He now has a strong drive to begin bowel management. Peer relationships and social activities are important to school-age children, and help them to develop firmer self-control.

Case B was fortunate in that she could enter the regular school in her community. It can be hard for a child with spina bifida to attend a regular school, because there is usually no private bathroom. Even if the school had a bathroom, a child's mother would have to visit the school 2–3 times a day to perform CIC. With independent bladder management, it has become easier for a child with spina bifida to go to a regular school. The school nurse becomes the key person to help.

The last case was the most severe, but she had the strongest motive to complete the CIC program: not wanting to be a burden to her mother. She knew how much her mother wanted her to be independent in bladder management. It is characteristic that a school-age child develops altruism.

Based upon the developmental characteristics of school-aged children, there are opportunities for nurses to assist school-aged children with spina bifida to achieve self-care independence. As shown in these three cases, inpatients in the institution are often multiply and severely disabled. They require care provided not only by nurses, but by many other health professionals in the institution.

Nurses primarily offer care in daily living, and coordinate the services the children need. For example, case C's primary nurse asked for assistance from an occupational therapist to make a device to hold her back upright, gave the information that she was able to do CIC at school to the teacher, and solicited the cooperation of the family in the CIC program. Not only did she address these issues, but she also took the family to the unit, and let them learn how to support case C in CIC. The primary nurse was C's main instructor in the CIC program and an advocate for C's success.

There is another nursing issue: home-based care for children with spina bifida. Nurses in an institution should also take responsibility for home care for the child in the community. We do not have a clinical nurse specialist in pediatric care yet, but there needs to be home-based care for handicapped children in Japan. A member of a support group for parents of children with spina bifida said she taught her daughter how to perform CIC at home, just before she entered a public school. She said that most nurses or physicians in general hospitals did not know about spina bifida, and that the support group members were her best consultants. Nurses in the institution have enough experience, knowledge, and human resources to care for families. If these nurses expand their work into the community, many children with spina bifida and their families will have higher quality care. The nurses could also work with support groups and school teachers, to give better care. The institution could be a center of nursing care for children with spina bifida.

Conclusion

In conclusion, we suggest that nurses in the institution expand their care into the community by encouraging children to return to the community, and by shortening the children's length of stay in the institution. We believe that nursing care for school-aged children with spina bifida in the twenty-first century in Japan should enable the children to live with their families and peers in the community.

References

1. Fukazawa K (1997) Bladder management in spina bifida children. Jpn Uro Nurs 2:18–24
2. Gray M (1993) Nursing planning, intervention, and evaluation for altered urinary function. In: Jackson DB, Saunders RB (eds) Child health nursing. Lippincott, Philadelphia, pp 1243–1317
3. Hafeman CA (1989) Teaching the younger patient. J Enterostom Ther 16:52–57
4. Kaufman-Rauen K (1992) A bright future for adults who have myelomeningocele. One form of spina bifida. Orthopaed Nurs 11(3):16–25

5. Murphy-Peterson P, Kaufman-Rauen K, Brown J, Cole J (1994) Spina bifida: the transition into adulthood begins in infancy. Rehabil Nurs 19:229–238
6. Santrock JW (1997) Life span development. Brown and Benchmark, Madison
7. Smith KA (1991) Bowel and bladder management of the child with myelomeningocele in the school setting. J Enterostom Ther 18:6–10

Nursing Care of Children with Spina Bifida in the United States

Joy Santiago Ito

Summary. The role of the nurse in the care of the child with spina bifida is a very important one. As nurses, we are in an enviable position in being able to affect the care of these children and their families. We need to continue to work closely with the spina bifida team and the children and their families to provide the best care possible.

Nursing is a key component in the management of children with spina bifida. The role of the nurse in the care of the child with spina bifida varies depending upon where one decides to find employment and the specialty one decides to pursue. Inpatient hospital nursing is by far the most well known. Yet, today, outpatient or ambulatory nursing has emerged as an integral part of the care of the child with spina bifida. Inpatient hospital stays have decreased dramatically over the past decade, and the number of outpatient procedures performed has increased. The combination of these two factors has had a dramatic impact on the role of the outpatient nurse and produced a shift in how and where care is provided.

Inpatient hospital nurses care for patients who are admitted to the hospital for observation, surgery, and disease management. The inpatient nurse is responsible for thorough assessment, evaluation, and management of patients during their entire hospitalization. It is expected that if a child with spina bifida is admitted to an inpatient floor, questions regarding neurological status, urology status, pediatric care, school status, transitioning issues and orthopedic care are addressed. Furthermore, it is important to recognize that the family plays a vital role in the well being of the child; therefore, family dynamics and problems are incorporated in the assessment and care of the child with spina bifida. The outpatient nurse holds a key position within the spina bifida team. At the Children's Memorial Hospital, we have nurses who are specialists in neurosurgery, urology, and orthopaedics, and a coordinator of the spina bifida team who provide direct patient care to the child with spina bifida. Key nursing roles and responsibilities in the management of the child with spina bifida are described below.

Children's Memorial Hospital, 2300 Children's Plaza, No. 28, Chicago, IL 60614, USA

Assessment, Evaluation and Direct Patient Care

The nurse has a responsibility to do a thorough assessment of the child to be able to provide comprehensive care. Evaluations include not only obtaining a good health history of the child, but also encompass every aspect of the child's development and spina bifida care. Direct patient care (medication administration, wound care, skin care, bowel and bladder management, range of motion, etc.) is provided by nurses in both the inpatient and outpatient settings. As an outpatient nurse, there are numerous opportunities to do phone assessments in between scheduled visits. The nurse, especially in the outpatient or ambulatory setting, acts as a triage nurse to identify and prioritize problems. Because of shortened inpatient stays, outpatient follow-up becomes crucial in assessing patients' health status, compliance with prescribed treatment, and overall management. Follow-up relating to treatment regimen is usually handled by phone and/or outpatient visits to the spina bifida center.

Patient and Family Teaching

A major component of the nurses's role in caring for the child with spina bifida is patient and family teaching. For new parents, nurses are instrumental in explaining, teaching, and providing as much information as possible about spina bifida. Before a newborn is discharged, it is our protocol that teaching is completed and families are knowledgeable about the care of their newborn as well as about spina bifida. The information provided includes an explanation of spina bifida, hydrocephalus, shunts, shunt malfunction, Chiari II, bowel and bladder management, urology test results, handling and developmental exercises, feeding and nutrition, and well-baby care. Teaching is then reinforced when the family comes to the clinic for the first time and/or in subsequent phone calls. As the child gets older, self bowel and bladder management is usually initiated in the outpatient area by the urology nurses and a urologist. When a child is an inpatient and requires CIC, inpatient nurses will do CIC teaching and at times consult with outpatient spina bifida nurses who may already have a rapport with the child and the family. Learning CIC and self-CIC is done as an outpatient. Follow-up is usually done by phone. Other patient education topics include shunt malfunction, tethered cord symptoms, hydromyelia, Chiari II, fractures, skin care management, brace wear, brace fit, brace care, exercise, and latex allergy. Explanations of testing procedures, hospital procedures, and protocols are also provided by the nurse. Often, for various reasons, the family will approach the nurse to request re-explanation or clarification of test results and the plan of care. The nurse must be aware of the treatment plan to be able to provide information to the family. Accurate and timely information provided to the family gives them confidence in the care their child is receiving, as well as providing an environment where the physician, nurses, and families communicate openly. Teaching and reinforcement of previous information is an ongoing process in both inpatient and outpatient settings. Parents and patients are encouraged to call with problems or questions at any time.

Coordination of Care

The nurse is in a position to coordinate care and services for the child with spina bifida, not only within the hospital, setting, but also with outside agencies. Referral to services outside the hospital, such as early intervention programs, therapy programs, school, respite, recreation, fitness, and family support are commonly considered. Coordination within team members and other hospital departments can also fall upon the nurse.

Collaborator

As nurses we offer ideas and innovations to assist with the care of our patients. The nurse acts as a collaborator with physicians, therapists, social workers, school staff, and other professionals to provide a comprehensive plan of care. Not only does the nurse collect information about the patient, but (s)he also seeks solutions to problems and concerns that have been identified. The nurse also evaluates whether current treatment plan is being implemented and whether it is still effective, and then makes revisions if necessary in collaboration with the team members and the patient and the family. The nurse acts as a liaison with the child/family and various physicians, hospital departments, and outside agencies, and provides the necessary feedback on how the child is doing. The nurse also acts as an advocate for the child and the family.

Support Person

The birth of a baby with a congenital defect is a highly charged emotional time for families. Hospitalizations, surgery, and dealing with the disability associated with spina bifida are also challenging. It is critical that the nurse be available to provide support to the children and their families during difficult times. We need to allow our families the space and opportunity to verbalize their thoughts, feelings, and emotions openly. Referral to support groups and to mental health care providers, when necessary, should always be an option.

Resource Person

The nurse acts as a resource not only to the child and the family, but also to other professionals within the hospital and the outside community. Nurses, along with the spina bifida team present at meetings, publish articles and research papers to provide updated and timely information.

Abstract

Children with Spina Bifida I Met in the School for Physically Handicapped Children: 1978–Today

Yoshiko Furuya

I have met several children who have spina bifida at the school for physically handicapped children where I work. The ages of the children with spina bifida range from 6 years (the elementary school) to 18 years (the high school education department), and the challenges they have been faced with are very varied.

I. Daily care at school.

1. Prevention of urinary tract infection.

(1) In my early years of service, starting from 1978, there were three ways that were used to help children's urination: urethrostomy (which we called "artificial bladders"); CREDE urination; intermittent self-catheterization. In those days, we were kept busy preventing urinary tract infection, but a great deal of effort was also made to solve such physical problems as how to help children put on artificial bladders and reduce foul odors from cloth diapers.

(2) In my later years of service, specifically from 1986, the majority of children were provided with intermittent self-catheterization, but some were using the CREDE urination method.

2. Lower body exercise, paralysis: detection of injuries, prevention of bed sores.

3. Hydrocephalus: observation of shunt troubles, coping with epilepsy.

4. Improvement and maintenance of motor functions (prevention of deformation, walking, etc.).

II. Preparation for self-management and independent life in society (including the sharing of problems that our school's graduates encountered).

III. Cooperation with parents and medical facilities.

We listened to what the parents of our children had to say, exchanged various information, including the results of health observations, and worked with the medial facilities. (For example, we discussed what instructions were given by a child's doctor, what kind of advice was provided by nurses, and what were the results of regular check-ups, etc.)

IV. Future challenges.

Kanagawa Prefectural Kamakura School for Handicapped Children, Kamakura, Japan

• Review the assumption of "Urethral catheterization = Medical practice". It is acceptable to have nonmedical personnel carry out urethral catheterization for a patient if self-catheterization is not available?
• The problem of a gap between ordinary schools and schools for the disabled children. Parents are in a dilemma as to which kind of school they are going to send their children to.

Moderator's Comments on Sessions—Nursing

Kayoko Yoshitake

Although I understood that this international symposium focused on school-age children and adolescents. I still wanted to cover all stages of development of children in this nursing session.

Especially when a child is young, the mother is the most important, key person for a growing child. I want to discuss how to help mothers adapt to a child with spina bifida, even while they are still on the delivery table, and then giving support to that mother while bringing up her child at home. I believe that nursing care of children with spina bifida should start right after the baby is born, or even before the moment of birth.

While a child is growing, the type of nursing intervention changes gradually with the developmental stage of the child: newborn, infant, toddler, preschooler, school-age child, and adolescent.

There are various places where nursing care is offered to these children, and places where each individual can get the most suitable service depending on their developmental stage and condition. This starts from a maternity ward where the baby is born, an intensive care unit after surgery, an outpatient department for children requiring continuous care at home, a 24-h care institution for children requiring long-term, institutionalized care, and special school for the handicapped for school-age children.

There are various places where nurses work for children with spina bifida. A nurse usually does not follow one child throughout his or her whole childhood, but stays in one place to take care of one category of children. For instance, some nurses work in a pediatric outpatient department, and some work in an institution for the handicapped.

We nurses must try to understand the total needs of each individual child on a long-term basis, even though we work in one place without following each individual child, in order to give better nursing care to all children with spina bifida.

I strongly desire that this symposium will give all nurses a good chance to appreciate the total nursing care of children with spina bifida through the presentations by five nurses speaking from five different standpoints.

All of those five nurses are working in the field of child nursing. The first nurse spoke about helping mothers and babies right after the baby is born; the second nurse spoke about helping young children and their families when they are brought up at home. The third nurse focused on the care of school-age children in institutions who need 24-h care, and the fourth nurse spoke about school life and care in a special school for the handicapped. She is a school nurse, and she also told us that many unique problems came from the very special Japanese school system. The fifth and last nurse came from the

United States. She told us about nursing care of children with spina bifida in the States.

I believe that this symposium could be a wonderful chance to appreciate the importance of the role of nurses who are working for children with spina bifida, and all of the nurses at this session clearly recognized our common desire to give better nursing care to all children.

Spina Bifida: An International Perspective

Children with Meningomyelocele in Hokkaido, Japan: From a Passive to an Active Approach

Yoshio Takahashi

Introduction

The serious problems affecting children suffering from meningomyelocele (MMC) include intellectual disorders associated with hydrocephalus, paralysis of both lower limbs associated with spinal anomaly, marked impairment of sensation in both lower limbs, and neurogenic bladder or bowel. We report the results of recent active physiotherapy, which consisted not only of the standard, conventional government-controlled systems, but also of physiotherapy in swimming pools and outdoors, and group education with normal children or other handicapped children.

Children and Methods

The subjects were 58 children suffering from MMC, with serious disorders from the time of birth, who underwent an evaluation of IQ, mobility, and bladder and bowel function when they were between 5 and 6 years of age. They were then divided into two groups. Group A consisted of 30 children who received conventional government-controlled physiotherapy involving functional assistance with braces, etc., and attended school. Group B consisted of 28 children who received physiotherapy in swimming pools and outdoors, as well as group education from an early stage in addition to conventional functional training. The IQ, mobility, and bladder and bowel function were compared between the two groups. The main aims of physiotherapy in swimming pools and outdoors, as well as music therapy, were relaxation, improved body balance, enhanced muscle power in the upper limbs, and improved communication. The main aims of group education were to achieve independence, cooperation, and socialization.

Case Reports

Case 1

The patient was a girl who is 10 years of age at present. She underwent an operation for MMC, mainly at the L4 level, and a shunt operation one day after birth. Deformity of both lower limbs was prominent.

Department of Pediatric Neurosurgery, Hokkaido Children's Hospital and Medical Center, 1-10-1 Zenibako, Otaru, Hokkaido 047-02, Japan

Physiotherapy in a swimming pool started from 2 years of age, mainly to achieve body balance, enhance muscle power in the upper limbs, and improve communication. At home, she played with toys and the upper limbs were strengthened by hanging from a strap, etc.

From 3 years of age, group education was started and the patient could walk independently using a brace. She participated in athletic meetings with the aid of braces and played outdoors, moving mainly with her upper limbs.

From 4 years of age, independent walking without the aid of a brace became possible.

At 6 years of age, she attended school regularly with the assistance of friends.

At 8 years of age, she underwent an operation on her lower limbs, and at 9 years of age, she could stand for long periods. She could walk and go anywhere without assistance. Her grades were better than those in some physically healthy children.

Case 2

The patient was a girl, who is 12 years of age at present.

She had MMC mainly at the L2 level. She underwent an operation for MMC and a shunt operation one day after birth. Deformity of both lower limbs was present.

From 1 year of age, she used a brace and was admitted to hospital with her mother for functional training, which continued until 2 years of age, but her balance was still poor.

Physiotherapy in a swimming pool started at 3 years of age to achieve better balance and upper limb training. From 3 years of age, emphasis was placed on functional improvement of the lower limbs. The degree of mobility training and functional training of the lower limbs was later reduced and group training began. Her behavior was the same as that of a normal child, and socialization improved as the upper half of her body became stronger.

At 5 years of age, she gained better mobility of her upper limbs by strengthening the limbs through such actions as rice-cake making, and she could walk with a cane. She attended school, could move without problems using a wheelchair, and participated in various events, such as class days and sports. Her life is the same as that of a normal child, except for the fact that she mainly moves about in a wheelchair. Intellectually, she is better than average.

Case 3

The patient was a boy, who is 7 years of age at present. He had MMC mainly at the L3 level.

He underwent an operation for MMC and a shunt operation on the day of birth. Deformity of both lower limbs was prominent.

Because he lived in the country, the physiotherapy at his central facility was inadequate, and there was no system by which he could receive group training.

From 3 years of age, he started physiotherapy in a swimming pool to achieve better balance. He strengthened the upper half of his body by actions such as climbing trees and participated in various events to achieve independence.

Although the system for educating such children was inadequate, he was forced to go to school and was treated the same as the normal children, except for mobility. His intellect is superior to some physically healthy children.

Case 4

The patient was a 12-year-old boy with an MMC mainly at the L4 level. He underwent an operation for MMC and a shunt operation on the second day after birth. Deformity of both lower limbs was marked. Because he lived in the country, training at a central facility was impossible. Because of the marked deformity of his lower limbs, he concentrated on mobility from an early stage, mainly by strengthening the upper half of his body. At present, he moves outdoors in a wheelchair and indoors using his upper limbs. He was placed 10th in a wheelchair marathon with adults participating.

Although he dislikes studying, he is intellectually superior to some physically healthy children. He shows excellent socialization, since he has liked sports from an early age and participates in sports meetings.

Result

Since adequate centralized training is impossible because Hokkaido covers a large area and is mainly rural and without any transport, and also because of prejudice, it is difficult to bring out a handicapped child's potential by conventional methods. Figures 1 and 2 show a comparison between physiotherapy in a swimming pool and outdoors, and group training with the conventional government central training method. Intellectual development at 6 years old was 83 ± 16 in group A and 96 ± 12 in group B: group B was significantly better. Independent walking without a brace was possible for 10 patients in group A (33%) and 18 in group B (64%). Independent movement for at least 10 m was possible for 14 patients (47%) in group A and 24 (89%) in group B. Mobility was significantly better in group B. Neurogenic bladder and bowel disorders were the same in groups A and B. In groups A, seven out of 30 patients (23%) attended school normally, while 27 patients (96%) in group B went to school regularly and continue to do so.

Discussion

MMC no longer requires emergency surgery, and the disorders can at least be reduced by physiotherapy in appropriate facilities (centers) with considerable experience. However, at the stable stage after the critical stage has passed, the abilities of the children can be enhanced further by physiotherapy in a swimming pool as outdoors, and music and group therapy in local groups, as seen in our patients.

The training provided at a center can be regionally standardized, but we believe that children can acquire the necessary skills under more pleasant conditions at a local level. It is

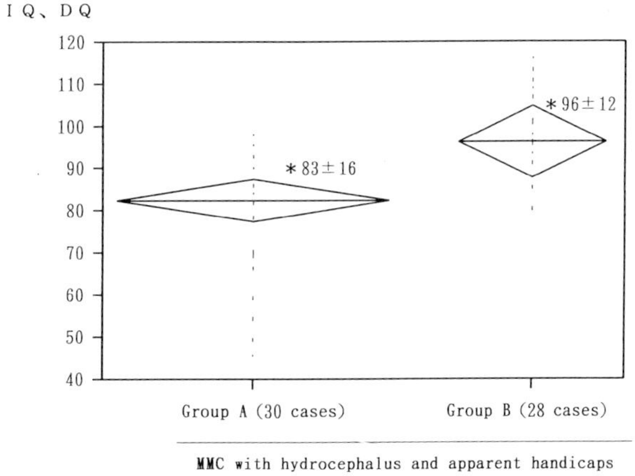

FIG. 1. Intellectual outcome (IQ or DQ) after 5–6 years for Group A and B who had meningomyelocele (MMC) with apparent handicaps. Group A: 30 children who received regular conventional government physiotherapy without other training. Group B: 28 children who received physiotherapy in swimming pools and outdoors, as well as group education from an early stage in addition to conventional training

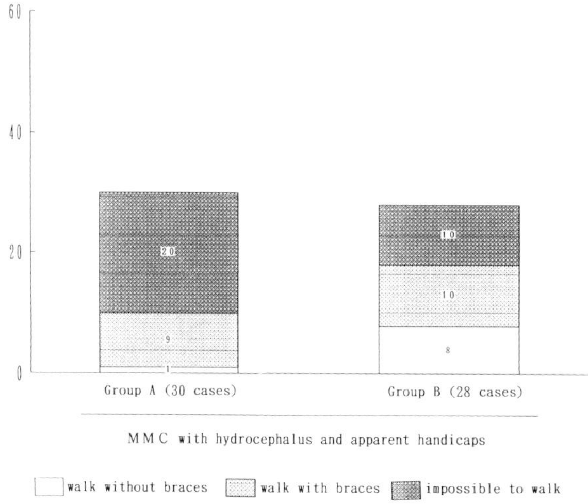

FIG. 2. Motor outcome after 5 ~ 6 years for Group A and B who had MMC with apparent handicaps

necessary to return children with MMC to their familiar area after the acute stage has passed and to make efforts to help them establish their roots in that area. In this way, space can be prepared in each area to bring out the children's abilities in normal life. The use of training methods which promote skills and methods which make the patients move on their own, based on flexible thinking, will be a plus for these children in the future. In other words, the abilities of the children cannot be sufficiently developed by the existing government-controlled training system.

Training which is concentrated at government centers after the critical stage has passed has actually caused children to drop out of society. If active training is carried out disorders in children with MMC will be reduced and it will be difficult to categorize such children handicapped in today's society.

MMC can now be diagnosed before birth. Therefore, the time has come when it is possible for children with MMC and their parents to meet before birth and create appropriate conditions in each area so that capable children can be raised based on a better understanding of the disease itself. The aim is not to make the children exactly the same as healthy children by acquiring all of their skills, but to concentrate on enhancing the function of the upper limbs and body balance. In this way, they can acquire the skills required for living.

Conclusion

The serious problems of children with MMC after their initial critical treatment are movement disorders, intellectual problems, and neurogenic bladder and bowel.

When emphasis is placed on the special nature of such children, it leads to a restriction of their living environment and often causes them to drop out of society.

To improve movement disorders and mental delay, it is important to create a living environment where the children can move actively at an early stage after treatment. Physiotherapy in a swimming pool and outdoors, group therapy, etc., appear to be more important than passive functional training at governmental facilities.

The abilities of children with MMC cannot be adequately nurtured by government systems, and new dynamic methods are required. To achieve this, it is necessary to change the way of thinking of parents, physicians, and other caretakers.

MTHFR 677C-T and Neural Tube Defects: An Evaluation in a Population from Southern Italy

A. Iolascon[1], B. Coppola[1], E. Miraglia Del Giudice[2], R. Carbone[1], D. Del Gaizo[2], M.T. Carbone[2], G. Aceto[1], M.F. Faienza[1], G. Del Gado[2], and R. Del Gado[2]

Summary. The risk of neural tube defects (NTDs) varies widely according to genetic background and diet. Clinical trials demonstrated that up to 70% of NTD can be prevented by folic acid supplementation in early pregnancy, and that mothers of children with NTD had higher homocysteine levels. Frosst et al. (1995) identified a common 677C-T mutation in the MTHFR gene, which results in decreased activity, increased thermolability of the enzyme, and raised plasma homocysteine concentrations. The frequency of this polymorphism varies among different populations. De Franchis et al. (1995) found that the prevalence of homozygotes for 677C-T mutation was 16.3% among 289 controls of Italian origin, which is more than three times higher than in the Netherlands. The aim of our study was to verify the frequency of the 677C-T mutation in a population of subjects affected by spina bifida and healthy controls from southern Italy. Although our population is too small for a complete statistical analysis, our results show that the prevalence of the 677C-T mutation is higher in southern Italy than in the Dutch population.

Key words. MHTFR, Spina bifida, NTDs, 677C-T mutation

Introduction

Neural tube defects (NTDs) are very complex embryological anomalies that arise during the development of the central nervous system, with a multifactorial transmission. They are caused by an alternate differentiation and fusion of the cranio-encephalic and dorsal medial structures, such as skin, muscles, rachis, meninx, neural tube, and nerve roots. Despite considerable progress in understanding these malformations, the etiology of most cases remains unknown [5]. The hypothesis that during human embryogenesis there is multisite closure of the neural tube, with regionally distinct genetic control, is possible in the light of the NTD occurring in trisomy 13, 18, and triploidy [9].

Many teratogenic factors, such as valproic acid, folic acid, alcohol, and maternal diabetes, have been involved in the pathogenesis of NTDs. Folic acid is a cofactor in the purine and

[1] Department of Pediatric Biomedicine, University of Bari, Policlinico, Clinica Pediatrica I, Piazza Giulio Cesare 11, 70124 Bari, Italy
[2] Department of Pediatrics, II University of Naples, Naples, Italy

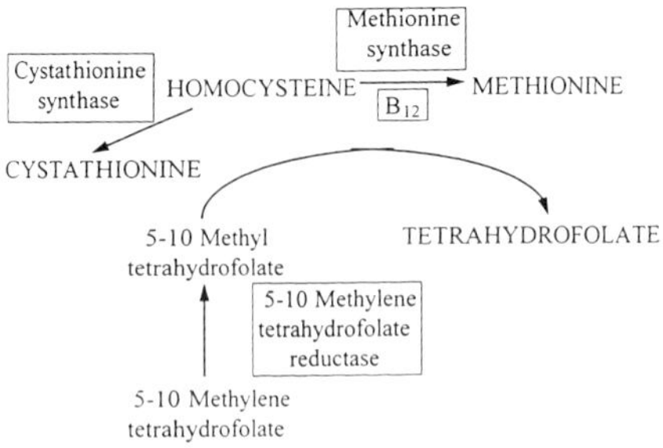

FIG. 1. Metabolic pathway of homocysteine remethylation

pirimidine biosynthesis, and is involved in the methylation pathway that goes from methionine to homocysteine, supplying the methyl groups. The methylation process is important for many proteins, and it appears to be essential for the integrity of myelin in vitamin B_{12} deficiency. The discovery that high levels of homocysteine are related to an increased risk of the development of arteriosclerosis and vascular disease has promoted interest in the study of the enzymes and cofactors involved in homocysteine metabolism [4].

During the last 5 years, attention has been focused on the enzymes related to the metabolism of the sulphorate aminoacids, particularly methylenetetrahydrofolate reductase (MTHFR). This enzyme catalyzes the synthesis of 5-methyltetrahydrofolate, a methyl donor, in the reduction of homocysteine to methionine (Fig. 1) [3, 7].

The human MTHFR gene has been localized to chromosome 1p36.3. The cDNA for MTHFR has been isolated, and nine rare mutations in patients with severe MTHFR deficiency have been identified [4]. The identification of each mutation in only one or two families shows the high degree of heterogeneity in this gene [4].

In 1995, Frosst et al. [3] identified a common 677C-T mutation in the MTHFR gene which results in decreased activity of the enzyme, increased thermolability, and raised plasma homocysteine concentration. Low serum folate concentration has been described in some, but not all, subjects homozygous for the thermolabile variant. In 1997, Molloy et al. [6] showed that in women homozygous for the MTHFR variant there were significantly lower concentrations of red cell folate. Plasma folate concentration is not a good indicator of folate status, particularly after sporadic vitamin supplementation. Therefore the analysis of red cell folate is necessary to obtain a true indication of tissue status.

The aim of our study was to verified the frequency of the 677C-T mutation in a population of subjects affected by spina bifida and their parents and healthy controls coming from southern Italy.

Materials and Methods

Patients

The study group consisted of 28 patients affected by spina bifida, 15 mothers, and 14 fathers. A control group of 67 subjects was recruited for this study. Genomic DNA was obtained by standard methods from peripheral blood leucocytes [8].

Methods

The presence of the 677C-T mutation was investigated by PCR of genomic DNA and restriction enzyme digestion with HinfI. The amplified fragment of the MTHFR gene spanned 198 bp. 677C-T substitution creates a HinfI recognition sequence which digests the PCR

TABLE 1. Prevalence of mutation in the subjects investigated

	677C/677C	C677/C677	C677T/C677T
Controls	18 (27%)	38 (57%)	11 (16%)
Patients	4 (14%)	14 (50%)	10 (36%)
Mothers	9 (33%)	13 (46%)	6 (20%)
Fathers	4 (14%)	12 (43%)	12 (43%)

product into 175 and 23 bp fragments, as shown on 10% silver-stained polyacrylamide gel. The prevalence of the 677C-T mutation in the subjects investigated is given in Table 1.

Results

The homozygous mutation was found in 10/28 (36%) of the patients affected by spina bifida, and in 3/15 (20%) and 6/14 (43%) of the mothers and fathers, respectively. In the control group, the 677C-T homozygous mutation was demonstrated in only 11/67 (16%) of the subjects examined.

Discussion

MTHFR deficiency is an autosomal recessive disorder [2]. Patients with severe MTHFR deficiency and residual enzyme activity of 0–20% present severe mental retardation and neurovegetative disorders which appear in the neonatal or adoloscent period [3].

The product of the MTHFR reaction, 5-methyltetrahydrofolate, is the predominant form of folate in plasma, whereas other folate derivatives, such as the enzyme substrate methylenetetrahydrofolate, are found mainly within cells. The effect of decreased MTHFR activity on folate metabolism is reflected by increased red cells and decreased plasma folate concentration in individuals homozygous for the mutations. Raised plasma homocysteine can be explained by the reduced availability of 5-methyltetrahydrofolate homozygous mutations.

The 677C-T mutation is the first identified genetic risk factor for spina bifida. The frequency of homozygous MTHFR polymorphism was two or three times greater among mothers, fathers, and patients with NTD. The study by van der Put et al. [11] confirms these findings in the Dutch population: 5% of 207 controls were homozygous for the 677C-T mutation compared with 16% of mothers, 10% of fathers, and 13% of patients with NTD. Thus the identification of this common mutation serves to illustate the concept of genetic predisposition to a disorder mediated by a specific environmental factor, in this case low folate intake. It is now clearly established that preconceptional folate supplementation prevents about 70% of all neural tube defects [10].

The frequency of this polymorphism varies among different populations, e.g., Japanese 2%, Brazilian 4%, and Irish 9%–12%. In 1995, De Franchis et al. [1] found that the prevalence of homozygotes for 677C-T mutation was 16.3% among 289 controls of Italian origin, which is more than three times higher than in The Netherlands. The reasons for the discrepancy between Italians and other white populations are unclear. Other common genetic variants, or probably environmental and dietary factors, could have a role in 677C-T mutation. The high folate intake that results from a Mediterranean diet (vegetables, fruit, and whole grains) might counterbalance the potentially negative effects of the high incidence of the mutation and explain the low incidence of neural tube defects.

Although our test population is too small for a complete statistical analysis, our results do allow several observations. The prevalence of the 677C-T polymorphism is higher in southern Italy than in the Dutch population. The frequency of the 677C-T mutation was very high in patients with NTD, and it should be regarded as a genetic risk factor.

In conclusion, NTDs represent a paradigmatic example of a genetic disease that can be greatly influenced by environmental elements.

References

1. De Franchis R, Sebastio G, Mandato C, Andria G, Mastroiacovo P (1995) Spina bifida, 677C-T mutation, and role of folate (letter). Lancet 346:1703
2. Goyette P, Sammer JS, Milos R, Duncan AMV, Rosenblatt D, Matthews RG, Rozen R (1994) Human methylenetetrahydrofolate reductase: isolation of cDNA, mapping and mutation identification. Nat Genet 7:195–198
3. Goyette P, Frosst P, Rosenblatt D, Rozen R (1995) Seven novel mutations in the methylenetetrahydrofolate reductase gene and genotype/phenotype correlations in severe methylenetetrahydrofolate reductase deficiency. Am J Med Genet 56:1052–1059
4. Goyette P, Christensen B, Rosenblatt DS, Rozen R (1996) Severe and mild mutations in cis for the methylenetetrahydrofolate reductase (MTHFR) gene, and description of five novel mutations in MTHFR. Am J Hum Genet 59:1268–1275
5. Hunter AG, Cleveland RH, Blickman JG, Holmes LB (1996) A study of level of lesion, associated malformations and sib occurence risks in spina bifida. Teratology 54:213–218
6. Molloy AM, Daly S, Mils JL, Kirke PN, Whitehead AS, Ramsbottom D, Conley MR, Weir D (1997) Thermolabile variant of 5,10-methylenetetrahydrofolate reductase associated with low red cell folates: implications for folate intake recommendations. Lancet 349:1591–1593
7. Ou CY, Stevenson RE, Brown VK, Schwartz CE, Allen WP, Khoury MJ (1996) Methylenetetrahydrofolate reductase genetic polymorphism as a risk factor for neural tube defect. Am J Med Genet 63:610–614
8. Sambrook J, Fritsch EF, Maniatis T (1989) Molecular cloning: a laboratory manual. 2nd edn. Cold Spring Harbor Laboratory Press, New York
9. Seller MJ (1995) Neural tube defects, chromosome abnormalities and multiple closure sites for the human neural tube. Clin Dysmorphol 4:202–207
10. Smithells RW, Sheppard S, Schorah CJ (1980) Possible prevention of neural tube defects by periconceptional vitamin supplementation. Lancet:339–340
11. Van der Put NM, Steegers-Theunissen RP, Frosst P, Trijbells FJ, Eskes TK, van den Heuvel LP (1995) Mutated methylenetetrahydrofolate reductase as a risk factor for spina bifida (comment). Lancet 346:1070–1071

The Situation of People with Hydrocephalus and Spina Bifida in Developing Countries

Pierre Mertens

As president of the International Federation for Hydrocephalus and Spina Bifida, known as "*if*," I am reporting on the world-wide solidarity between parents and people with hydrocephalus and spina bifida. I am grateful that there is now widespread recognition of the value of the input of "*if*'s" member organizations in improving the life of people with these disabilities.

While national organizations have to focus on service delivery in their own countries, "*if*" looks across borders and facilitates the creation of organizations in those countries where services are still poor or completely lacking.

This paper will tell you more about the situation of people with hydrocephalus and spina bifida in developing countries, and about the activities "*if*" is starting in East Africa. This information will show that the approach we propose in developing countries can be useful for rethinking the provision of care world-wide.

"*if*" started workshops on hydrocephalus and spina bifida in some developing countries to create awareness, and to hear from the participants about their present situation. We were surprised to find how many cases there are in developing countries, and we were astonished by their situation and living conditions.

Most of the children I met in Africa had not been operated upon. The head was very large, many children became blind and had no head control, and nearly all of them had cerebral palsy. They were more disabled than at birth, but they survived.

Early detection and treatment are essential to avoid additional disabilities. Organized treatment is not evident in Africa. It is very rare for everything to be available at one time: the patient, the surgeon, the anesthetist, the nurse, the drugs, the shunt . . . Even when everything is available, it is not certain that anything will happen. In poor countries you need money for everything that needs to be done. No money, no shunt, no anesthetist, no nurse, etc.

In many parts of Africa, national care is decreasing and the private sector works at European and American prices only for the elite who can afford to pay. We see the same situation in the ex-Soviet countries. One of the first problems we find is the shunt. In Kenya, Tanzania, and Ethiopia, patients themselves have to buy a shunt in Nairobi at the price of 4–5 months salary. Most hospitals have no shunts available. In an emergency, as is often the case with hydrocephalus, this is a very bad situation. No shunt, no operation.

Marialei 27, B2900 Schoten, Belgium

What is the Prevalence and Incidence of Hydrocephalus and Spina Bifida in Developing Countries?

Available statistics and other literature provide little information on the prevalence in Developing countries. Exact figures are not available because of a lack of registration. There are several reasons to believe that there are more cases of spina bifida in developing countries than in others. Pregnancies are unplanned, and two in ten children are malnourished and so are the mothers. Spina bifida is frequently the result of a lack of absorption of folic acid. As we know, the quality of food can have an influence on this. Without prevention campaigns, the incidence of spina bifida is now approximately 1–2 in 1000 live births.

The prevalence of hydrocephalus is higher than in the developed countries because:

- malnutrition during pregnancy can cause premature birth;
- prematurely born babies have higher risks of bleeding in the brain;
- birth trauma is high due to bad conditions of delivery.

Meningitis can result from many different infections: TB, syphilis, malaria, accidents/trauma, e.g., war, traffic accidents, etc.

Through our contacts, we know that Kenyatta National Hospital in Nairobi and the Mulago hospital in Kampala both have approximately 400–500 children with hydrocephalus and/or spina bifida every year. Most of the patients are sent back home without any help. These children have been brought to the hospital spontaneously, since there is no program of early detection. Often they come too late, as the head has already grown and secondary disabilities have appeared. As we know, the result of late or nontreatment of hydrocephalus can be death, blindness, enlarged head, cerebral palsy, epilepsy, or learning difficulties.

There are many reasons for late or nontreatment.

1. Lack of awareness of hydrocephalus and spina bifida.
2. Cultural influences. Many parents feel guilty, hide their child, and do not look for help.
3. Lack of information on treatment possibilities result in fieldworkers, traditional doctors, and MLRW not sending patients to specialized hospitals in time for treatment.
4. The medical system in most African countries has collapsed. National health care does not take care of these patients, and private care is too expensive.
5. The treatment is only carried out in the capitals of the countries.
6. Because of great distances, the patients have many transport problems, the children do not reach the national hospitals, or arrive too late to prevent damage.
7. Corruption and lack of formal management in the hospitals.
8. Lack of neurosurgeons. Most surgeons leave the country once they are trained to benefit from a better salary.

The Ugandan family described below is typical of very many throughout Africa. The child with hydrocephalus is 11 years old. Without no husband, her mother cares for the three children of her brother and sister-in-law who both died from AIDS, plus her own five children and the little son of her oldest daughter. She lives in a small house which is 1 day's travel from the hospital. She has no salary and lives from the food she can cultivate around the hut. It is a desperate struggle to survive, and every day she has to find food and water for ten people. Her daughter can not sit up because her head is too heavy for her little neck. She never leaves the hut, and has been lying there for 11 years. In the beginning her mother took her to the hospital once. She found a person to take care of the other children and a relative paid for the transport fee. She waited 2 days in the corridors of the hospital before a doctor looked only briefly at her daughter. He sent her away with the message "come back in 6 months." The child's head became larger and larger, and 6 monther later the mother had neither the energy nor the money to leave her family alone and to make the same long journey to the hospital. She no longer believed that this doctor would help her child, so she stayed at home and survived day by day.

Children with hydrocephalus and spina bifida are often hidden like the little Ugandan girl. Hidden and far from all statistics. It is not totally correct to say that nothing has been done for children with disabilities in developing countries. This child lives, has received food during the last 11 years, and has survived because of the care of her mother. The little girl speaks and laughs; she is part of the family.

In developing countries the mothers take care of their children. They are doing the major job. If we want to support children with disabilities, we also have to support the parents. This is the case all over the world. Mothers, fathers, brothers, and sisters are the basis of a full life for every child. Many developing countries have started community-based rehabilitation (CBR) projects where, considering the situation and the small funds available, the maximum possible is being done. The main strategy for our projects is also based on this CBR approach, which tries to make optimal use of all the human, material, financial, and other resources available to the community in its response to the problems of people with disabilities (PWDs).

In this approach, the training, monitoring, evaluation, and upgrading of local community rehabilitation workers are part of the strategy. They play an essential role in early detection, prevention, and timely referral, and in providing training and other services and support to persons with hydrocephalus and spina bifida within their homes and communities.

Our federation is building up expertise and is working on a positive scheme for offering help that can be applied in other parts of the world too. From the reports of our experts, we concluded that the success of future affordable activities will depend on collaboration between hospitals, surgeons, and community-based grassroots organizations working with disabled people within the communities. Such activities will only be viable if they make maximum use of the human, material, infrastructure, and financial resources available locally.

We therefore we work with existing surgeons, hospitals, and other programs. Our input is training, management, control, and financial help for the extra costs for treatment such as the shunt and the operation. We sign memoranda of understanding with all partners specifying each one's role, contribution, and responsibility.

In Dar Es Salaam, we have a functioning program that could be the model for other countries and regions. A CBR programme called CCBRT is doing the detection and rehabilitation. Every Saturday is operation day, and the surgeon is available in emergencies. In Dar Es Salaam, we can organize detection, treatment, and follow-up for a cost of only 200 US dollars per child. In the current economic situation, it is impossible for developing countries to meet the costs required for the basic care of children with hydrocephalus and spina bifida. In Uganda, the national health budget is 2 US dollars per person per year, and since they are facing problems such as AIDS, civil wars, malaria, etc., you can imagine that this is not realistic.

As President of "*if*," I travel around the world and look at it through a hole in the back of children. I visit families and hospitals. This gives me an idea of how a nation copes with health care, and with children and adults with severe disabilities. From my wide experience, I believe that good community-based rehabilitation (CBR) projects, such as already exist in some developing countries, could be the ideal rehabilitation system if combined with the material and financial possibilities of the developed countries.

It would take too long to explain in detail the whole CBR approach, but one very important aspect is that therapy should be as much a part of daily life as possible. Children should not be isolated from their friends in the neighborhood and their family. Ideal therapy is integrated in daily activities such as going to school, sitting in the classroom, eating, sleeping, etc. In developed countries also, therapists are moving into the community more and more to coach parents and children at home, and teachers at school. This recent evolution has been the method in developing countries for many years. In CBR programs, people with disabilities and their families are fully involved in deciding what steps should be taken, and are not regarded as passive receivers. The parents are also being trained, and are expected to coach the child.

CBR has many good elements which should be considered as we rethink treatment and therapy in the developed countries. Medical care should be part of a bigger, more holistic strategy, where medical action is reduced to the absolute minimum. We hope that our projects in developing countries will give us a chance to assess this approach, and that in the near future we can fully evaluate it.

Treatment and Care of Spina Bifida in Taiwan

T.-T. Wong[1], Tsui-Fen Yang[2], Wei-Perng Chen[3], and Alex Tong-Long Lin[4]

Summary. In the past 10 years, most of the patients with spina bifida in Taiwan have been referred to the Veterans General Hospital–Taipei for care and management. In this chapter, we retrospectively review our experience in 36 cases of myelomeningocele and 43 cases of lipomyelomeningocele. A total of 77.2% of myelomeningoceles were repaired in the first month of life, including 28.6% on the first day, 28.6% between 2 and 7 days old, and 20% from the second week to 1 month. There were 77.7% of lesions located in the lumbosacral or sacral regions. Hydrocephalus occurred in 66.7% patients. The clinical outcomes of the clinical group were normal intelligence in 76.2%, and various degrees of motor deficits in 81.6%. Only 5.6% of patients had normal voiding, and 25% of patients had normal or independent ambulation. A total of 50.8% of lipomyelomeningoceles were repaired within the first year of life. There were 95.3% of patients with lesions located in the lumbosacral or sacral regions. The neurological outcomes were different between the group with lesions repaired within the first year of life (group A) and the group who were older than 1 year (group B). In group A, 66.7% of patients had normal motor function and 50% had normal voiding. In group B, only 26.3% of patients had normal motor function, and 26.3% had normal voiding.

Key words. Myelomeningocele, Lipomyelomeningocele, Taiwan

Introduction

In Taiwan, the specialty of pediatric neurosurgery was first established at the Veterans General Hospital–Taipei in 1981. Before 1981, most of the infants with myelomeningocele or lipomyelomeningocele were managed by general pediatric surgeons. At present, we have five neurosurgeons who have received subspecialty training in pediatric neurosurgery in North America. Nowadays, most of the newborn infants with spinal dysraphism in Taiwan are cared

[1] Division of Pediatric Neurosurgery, Neurological Institute, Veterans General Hospital–Taipei and School of Medicine, National Yang-Ming University, No. 210, Shih-Pai, Taipei, Taiwan 11217, ROC

[2] Department of Physical Therapy, School of Medicine, National Yang-Ming Medical University, 155, Section 2, Lih-Nong Street, Taipei, Taiwan, ROC

[3] Division of Nephrology, Department of Pediatrics, Division of Urology, Department of Surgery, Veterans General Hospital–Taipei and School of Medicine, National Yang-Ming University, Taiwan, ROC

for and managed by them. However, the only spina bifida clinic was set up at the Veterans General Hospital–Taipei in 1994. In order to evaluate the care, management, and outcome of these patients, we retrospectively reviewed our experience at this hospital.

Patients and Methods

Thirty-six patients with myelomeningocele who were treated from 1986 to 1997, and 43 patients with lipomyelomeningocele who were treated from 1984 to 1997 were retrospectively reviewed. The parents' satisfaction with the operations and with Medicare in Taiwan was assessed by a questionnaire. For patients with myelomeningocele, data including age of repair, level of lesion, hydrocephalus, intelligence, and neurological outcome (motor deficit, voiding deficit, and ambulatory status) were collected and analyzed. For patients with lipomyelomeningocele, age of repair, level of lesion, and neurological outcome were reviewed. The differences in neurological status between the two groups of patients who had an operation before or after 1 year old were compared.

Results

Myelomeningocele

At the Veterans General Hospital–Taipei, patients were referred from different districts in Taiwan. Among 36 cases of myelomeningocele, 28.6% were operated on in the first day, 57.2% within the first week, and 76.2% in the first month after birth (Table 1). The locations of this congenital anomaly included the sacral (50%), lumbosacral (27.7%), midlumbar (8.3%), and high lumbar (13.9%) regions (Table 2). Twenty-four of the 36 patients (64%) had hydrocephalus, and 22 of them received a ventriculo-peritoneal shunt operation. There were two shunt infections. Two neonates developed symptomatic Arnold–Chiari malformations, and were surgically decompressed. Including a few cases operated on in other hospitals, 37 cases

TABLE 1. Age of operation for myelomeningocele and lipomyelomeningocele at the Veterans General Hospital–Taipei

Age of operation	Number of patients	%
Myelomeningocele		
1st day	10	28.6
2–7 days	10	28.6
2nd week–1 month	7	20.0
2–5 months	8	22.9
18 years	1	2.9
Lipomyelomeningocele		
1st month	11	25.6
2nd month–1 year	13	30.2
2–5 years	11	25.6
6–10 years	4	9.3
15–28 years	4	9.3

Location of lesions, anatomical locations of myelomeningocele and lipomyelomeningocele. Number of patients, number of patients with myelomeningocele and lipomyelomeningocele in different locations. %, percentage of patients with myelomeningocele and lipomyelomeningocele in different locations.

TABLE 2. Locations of myelomeningocele and lipomyelomeningocele

Location of lesions	Number of patients	%
Myelomeningocele		
Sacral	18	50
Lumbosacral	10	27.7
Midlumbar	3	8.3
High lumbar	5	13.9
Lipomyelomeningocele		
Sacral	10	23.3
Lumbosacral	31	72.1
Midlumbar	2	4.6

Age of operation, age of patient at time of repair. Number of patient, number of patient in different age group of repair. %, percentage of patients repaired in different age group.

TABLE 3. Intelligence of children with myelomeningocele

Age	Number of cases	Range of intellegence	Mean
>3 years	21	57–129	93
<3 years	16		75
Degree of mental retardation	%		
Normal	76.2		
Borderline	14.3		
Mild	9.5		

TABLE 4. Motor deficits of myelomeningocele and lipomyelomeningocele patients in postoperative follow-up

Motor deficits	Group 1 (%)	Group 2 (%)	Group 3 (%)
Normal	19.4	66.7	26.3
Sacral	27.8	4.2	15.8
Lumbosacral	27.8	29.2	52.6
Midlumbar	11.1		5.3
High lumbar	13.4		

Group 1, patients with myelomeningocele. Group 2, patients with lipomyelomeningocele with operation before 1 year old. Group 3, patients with lipomyelomeningocele with operation after 1 year old.

were involved in follow-up studies for intelligence, with 76.2% having normal intelligence, 14.3% borderline mental retardation, and 9.5% mild mental retardation. In 21 cases, the final intelligence studies were performed after 3 years of age. Their range of intelligence coefficients was between 57 and 129 (mean 93). In 16 cases, the final intelligence evaluations were made before 3 years of age, and the mean intelligence coefficient was 75 (Table 3). The majority of patients had abnormal neurological status relating to the spinal cord malformation. Motor function and deficits of the lower limbs were correlated with the spinal level of the placode. The motor function of the lower limbs was normal in only 19.4% of patients (Table 4). Voiding was normal in only 5.6% of patients (Table 5). Twenty-five percent of

TABLE 5. Voiding deficits of myelomeningocele and lipomyelomeningocele patients in postoperative follow-up

Voiding deficits	Group 1 (%)	Group 2 (%)	Group 3 (%)
Normal	5.6	50	26.3
Abnormal but continent	16.7	8.3	31.6
Stress incontinent		4.2	5.3
Incontinent	13.9	20.8	31.6
No record	13.9	16.7	5.3

Group 1, patients with myelomeningocele. Group 2, patients with lipomyelomeningocele with operation before 1 year old. Group 3, patients with lipomyelomeningocele with operation after 1 year old.

TABLE 6. Ambulatory status of myelomeningocele and lipomyelomeningocele patients in postoperative follow-up

Ambulatory status	Group 1 (%)	Group 2 (%)	Group 3 (%)
Normal/independent	25	75	63.2
Abnormal/independent	44.5	20.8	31.6
Walker	8.3		
Nonambulatory	44.4	4.2[a]	5.3

Group 1, patients with myelomeningocele. Group 2, patients with lipomyelomeningocele with operation before 1 year old. Group 3, patients with lipomyelomeningocele with operation after 1 year old. [a]A case of lipomyelomeningocele, transitional type, lumbosacral level, with progressive paraparesis 7 years after the first operation.

TABLE 7. Parent's satifaction with the operation and Medicare for myelomeningocele patients in the Veterans General Hospital—Taipei spina bifida clinic

	Satisfied with operation (%)	Satisfied with Medicare (%)
Satisfied	86.1	72.2
Unsatisfied		2.6
No answer	13.9	25

patients ambulated normally or independently (Table 6). In response to outpatient questionnaires, 86.1% of parents were satisfied with the management and 72.2% of parents were satisfied with the Medicare environment for myelomeningocele (Table 7).

Lipomyelomeningocele

Among 43 cases of lipomyelomeningocele, 25.6% were operated on in the first month after birth, and 55.8% within the first year (Table 1). The locations of this congenital anomaly included the sacral (23.3%), lumbosacral (72.1%), and lumbar (4.6%) regions (Table 2). Motor function of the lower limbs, gait and ambulatory status, and voiding were correlated with time of lipomyelomeningocele repair. More than 2/3 patients with repair within 1 year of birth had normal motor function of the lower limbs and were normal/independent ambulators. Voiding was normal in 50% of these patients. In those patients with lipomyelomeningocele repair after 1 year of age, about 1/4 of them had lower limb motor deficits, and 3/4 of them had voiding deficits (Tables 4–6).

Discussion

Myelomeningocele in newborn infants is devastating to the family. In Taiwan, as in other countries, parents worry about the intellectual and functional outcome of these infants. In our experience, some parents refused myelomeningocele repair because they learned that the disease might be associated with hydrocephalus, symptomatic Arnold–Chiari malformation, hydrosyringomyelia, weakness and atrophy of the lower limbs, and voiding and bowel movement problems. Changes in spinal curvature and late progressive neurological deterioration could occurr a few years after repair.

From experience of 36 myelomeningocele repairs and various operations for associated problems, it is encouraging that 86.1% of parents were satisfied with the management, and 72.2% of parents were satisfied with the environment of Medicare, for myelomeningocele.

All of the myelomeningocele defects in this series were small enough that soft tissue closure was achieved by simple undermining of the skin edges and approximation in the midline. If the infant was referred 24 h after birth, the defect was disinfected with diluted aqueous betadine for 3 days before repair. If hydrocephalus existed as the myelomeningocele was repaired, a ventriculo-peritoneal shunt was inserted simultaneously. Local complications and CSF leakage were rare. Twenty-two cases with hydrocephalus were shunted with only two infections. In our experience, simultaneous shunting was not a contributing factor to shunt infection [3, 8]. The intellectual outcome of these patients was promising, with 76.2% normal intelligence, 14.3% borderline mental retardation, and 9.5% mild mental retardation. The average of the intelligent coefficients was higher and more reliable in the group studied after 3 years of age (mean 93) than in the group studied only until 3 years old (mean 75). Thus, in this series, repair of defect, shunting of hydrocephalus, and intellectual outcome were not factors hindering the care and management. The most difficult issues were still the problems of voiding deficits, incontinence, lower limb weakness and atrophy, skeletal deformities, and long-term follow-up and detection of urinary and neurological deterioration for retethering and other treatable causes [2, 4, 6, 7, 9, 11]. We set up a multidisciplinary spina bifida clinic for this purpose. However, many of the parents were reluctant to use this facility if they feel there is no obvious neurological deterioration.

In a reported series of 14 infants and children in Taiwan, only 25% had intact neurological function on initial examination in comparison with the other reported series which had 37% [5, 12]. There is controversy in some quarters about untethering and repair of patients with lipomyelomeningocele [10, 13]. In the past few years, we have operated on infants with or without neurological symptoms, but not on stable teenagers and adults. Surgery performed during the first year of life has been reported as quite safe [1] when performed by an experienced pediatric neurosurgeon. In our experience, the neurological status was much better in the group operated on within 1 year of birth than in the group operated on after 1 year old. However, the review was not extensive and comprehensive enough to support a recommendation for the prophylactic repair of lipomyelomeningocele in asymptomatic infants. Surgery is usually easy and safe when performed for lipomas of the filum and lipomas of the conus (dorsal type). Operations for lipomas of the conus (caudal type and transitional type) are relatively difficult and hazardous because of the risk of injuring the lumbosacral roots. In lipomas of the conus after more than 5 years of follow-up, it was reported that only 53.1% of patients were still free of symptoms [10]. In this series, lipomas of the filum were excluded; all operations were for lipomas of the conus, including dorsal, transitional, and caudal type.

These patients should be followed up regularly at a spina bifida clinic for the possibility of retethering symptoms and a need for reoperation [4].

References

1. Byrne RW, Hayes EA, George TM, McLone DG (1995) Operative resection of 100 spinal lipomas in infants less than 1 year of age. Pediatr Neurosurg 23:182–186; discussion pp 186–187
2. Caldarelli M, Di Rocco C, Colosimo C Jr, Fariello G, Di Gennaro M (1995) Surgical treatment of late neurological deterioration in children with myelodysplasia. Acta Neurochir (Wien) 137:199–206
3. Gamache FW Jr (1995) Treatment of hydrocephalus in patients with meningomyelocele or encephalocele: a recent series. Childs Nerv Syst 11:487–488
4. Herman JM, McLone DG, Storrs BB, Dauser RC (1993) Analysis of 153 patients with myelomeningocele or spinal lipoma reoperated upon for a tethered cord. Presentation, management and outcome. Pediatr Neurosurg 19:243–249
5. Kanev PM, Bierbrauer KS (1995) Reflections on the natural history of lipomyelomeningocele. Pediatr Neurosurg 22:137–140
6. Laies A, Kasabian NG, Dyro FM, Scott RM, Kelly MD, Bauer SB (1993) The neurosurgical implications of continuous neurourological surveillance of children with myelodysplasia. J Urol 150:1879–1883
7. Lintner SA, Lindseth RE (1994) Kyphotic deformity in patients who have a myelomeningocele. Operative treatment and long-term follow-up. J Bone Joint Surg Am 76:1293–1300
8. Miller PD, Pollack IF, Pang D, Albright AL (1996) Comparison of simultaneous versus delayed ventriculoperitoneal shunt insertion in children undergoing myelomeningocele repair. J Child Neurol 11:370–372
9. Namima T, Uchi K, Nakagawa H, Aizawa M, Orikasa S (1996) Urological assessment for tethered cord syndrome of delayed onset following repair of meningomyelocele. Nippon Hinyokika Gakkai Zasshi (Japanese Journal of Urology) 87:1158–1166
10. Pierre-Kahn A, Zerah M, Renier D, Cinalli G, Sainte-Rose C, Lellouch-Tubiana A, Brunelle F, Le Merrer M, Giudicelli Y, Pichon J, Kleinknecht B, Nataf F (1997) Congenital lumbosacral lipomas. Childs Nerv Syst 13:298–334; discussion p 335
11. Reigel DH, Tchernoukha K, Bazmi B, Kortyna R, Rotenstein D (1994) Change in spinal curvature following release of tethered spinal cord associated with spina bifida. Pediatr Neurosurg 20:30–42
12. Shian WJ, Chi CS, Wong TT (1994) Lipomyelomeningocele: a 9-year review. Acta Pediatr Sin 35:57–62
13. Sutton LN (1995) Lipomyelomeningocele. Neurosurg Clin N Am 6:325–338

Management of Spina Bifida in India

Sanat N. Bhagwati

No epidemiological study of the incidence of spina bifida in India is available, although at Jerbai Wadia Hospital for Women, Mumbai, there was one case in 1432 births between 1993 and 1997.

As only a few spina bifida centers exist in the country, most of the patients who need organized rehabilitation and control of their incontinence are left to fend for themselves. Lack of institutional care and the want of proper guidance often results in the parents wandering from place to place seeking advice and medical help to make their children ambulatory, continent, and acceptable to society.

Spina Bifida Occulta

If spina bifida occulta is found on X-ray, it is left alone. However, if it is associated with cutaneous stigmata, nocturnal eneuresis, or urinary sphincter impairment, it is investigated further. Myelogram, computed tomography myelo, or magnetic resonance imaging are done to visualize the tethering of the cord. Even when asymptomatic, detethering of the cord is undertaken prophylactically these days by most neurosurgeons.

Spina Bifida Aperta

Meningocele is repaired as early as possible after birth, especially if there has been a leakage of CSF or if the covering skin is very thin. With only 650 neurosurgeons in the country, most of the cases are tackled by general surgeons or pediatric surgeons except in large metropolitan cities.

Myelomeningocele with Partial Neurological Deficit

Repair is undertaken early if there has been a leakage of CSF or if there is a threatened rupture of the sac. Otherwise it is delayed for 2–3 months to allow the child to grow a little to stand surgery better. Very often it is done by general surgeons or pediatric surgeons, who may not

Department of Neurosurgery, Bombay Hospital Institute of Medical Sciences, 12 Marine Lines, Bombay 400020, India

worry much about the placode or retethering. The milder foot deformities are then attended to by orthopedic surgeons.

Myelomeningocele with Complete Paraplegia and Sphincter Involvement

If not leaking CSF, patients are observed and referred to larger centers where they are operated upon by either general surgeons or pediatric surgeons immediately. Neurosurgeons often try to talk the parents out of surgery, especially when the socio-economic condition of the parents would not permit them to look after the crippled child for the rest of its life. When informed about the irreversibility of paraplegia, the parents often want the child to be left alone, hoping that the child might develop CSF leak, meningitis, or intercurrent infection and die.

When they do survive, such children remain totally paraplegic, with sphincter impairment, and develop urinary infection and back-pressure phenomena. They tend to develop sacral bed sores and trophic ulcers on the feet, with a foul-smelling purulent discharge, and the parents go from place to place seeking a cure. The mothers become attached to these children, neglecting the rest of the family. Not having the wherewithal to look after them, the family ends up in misery.

Unfortunately there are no institutions where these children can be housed or rehabilitated. In the few spina bifida centers that exist in the country, only outpatient counselling and physiotherapy are given.

Associated Hydrocephalus

If hydrocephalus is detected early, preoperative shunting is resorted to in most centers. The shunt works well if CSF is not infected, and often makes the sac of the myelomeningocele quite slack. If hydrocephalus develops after repair of the myelomeningocele, or if a CSF leak develops at the site of repair, a ventriculo-peritoneal shunt is inserted postoperatively.

Orthopedic Procedures

Kyphectomy or correction of scoliosis is not undertaken with the initial repair of myelomeningocele. It is undertaken only if the myelomeningocele becomes progressive.

Various procedures are undertaken with the aim of making the child more ambulatory.

1. Operative procedures undertaken for the hip joint.
   — For dislocated / subluxated joints:
      open reduction;
      femoral osteotomy;
      pelvic osteotomy.
   — Release of contractures.
   — Muscle tendon transfers.
2. Operative procedures undertaken for the knee.
   — Femoral osteotomy.
   — Release of contractures.
   — Muscle tendon transfers.

3. Operative procedures undertaken for the foot.
   — Correction of foot deformity.
   — Tendon transfers.
   — Triple arthrodesis or other fusion procedures for flaccid foot.

Management of Urinary Involvement

Urinary incontinence is a very common manifestation. It may be true incontinence with a small spastic dysreflexic bladder, or retention with overflow.

One should always do urodynamomatric studies to learn the state of the bladder and the sphincter so that appropriate therapy can be instituted. All children of 6 months of age and above should have these studies.

The aim of therapy would be to have the child "dry." The child is considered dry if the day-time dry interval is 4 h or more. The renal function of the child is judged by serial serum creatinine measurements.

Incomplete emptying of the bladder may be due to acontractible detrusor, bladder neck dyssynergia, or striated sphincter dyssynergia. For acontractile detrusor, Urecholine is administered. Phenoxybenzamine, Prazopress, or Terazosin are given for bladder neck dyssynergia, and Baclofen, Lioresal, or Diazepam for striated sphincter dyssynergia.

When there is incontinence or leakage of urine due to a spastic bladder, Probanthin, Oxybutinin, or Imipramine are given to lower the intravesical pressure. To increase the resistance in the urethral smooth muscle, Ephedrine, Actifed, or Imipramine are given.

When there is a large postvoid residue of urine in acontractile bladder or hyperreflexia with dyssynergia, clean intermittent catheterization 3–4 times a day is advised.

Artificial sphincter implantation may be attempted where there is a persisting leaking bladder due to a true lower motor neurone lesion. Teflon injection into the sphincter may be attempted to increase the urethral pressure. Urethral plugs may be used for females and penile clamps for males.

In the Spina Bifida Clinic at Jerbai Wadia Hospital for Children, about 100 children have been followed up over the last 5 years. As is common for urinary incontinence (after urodynamometric studies), they are given anticholinergic drugs such as Probanthine and Oxybutinin, or advised about clean intermittent catheterization. In 12 children, bladder neck tightening has been carried out, to increase the outlet resistance. In 10 children, bladder augmentation with ileoplasty or coloplasty has been carried out, and in 5 children, continence diversion was carried out to create a new continence catheterization channel.

Differences in Patient Populations Cared for in Various Areas of the World

David B. Shurtleff[1], Gregorio Arendar[2], Luciano Dias[3], Gerard Duguay[1], Sharon Duguay[1], and Malcolm Menelaus[4]

Summary. Computerized patient clinical abstracts for 3196 subjects from a total of 3616 were studied. All patients from each of four centers (National Children's Hospital in Buenos Aires, Children's Memorial Hospital of Chicago, Royal Children's Hospital in Melbourne, and Children's Hospital in Seattle), born between 1965 and 1996, were included. Significant differences in the number of patients in each center were found according to type of spina bifida, age, level of lesion, type of birth, and ability to walk. Despite large numbers of patients, restriction of analyses for proportion able to walk by age, and level of lesion yielded such small numbers in each cell as to render analyses questionable. The authors recommend that a larger number of centers should join an International Myelodysplasia Study Group, begin a collection of data according to common definitions, utilize the computerized Patient Data Management System, and initiate prospective collaborative studies.

Key words. Spina bifida, Spina bifida aperta, Meningomyelocele, Myelodysplasia, Ambulation, Walk, Epidemiology, Cesarean section, Multiple center studies, Collaborative studies

Introduction

Since studies of the treatment of patients with meningomyelocele in the late 19th century [2], there have been series of published cases with varying outcomes for different systems' function. These studies are too numerous to cite. Most also neither provide the reader with knowledge about the degree of initial impairment, nor provide a comparison of like cases. Most also contain no assessment of statistical significance. Recently, reports have begun to appear either combining data from several centers [3, 15], or comparing two or more centers' series [4, 6, 7].

The purpose of this paper is to report the variances among groups of patients with meningomyelocele being cared for in four different centers on three continents and in two hemispheres.

[1] Division of Congenital Defects, Department of Pediatrics, University of Washington and Children's Hospital and Regional Medical Center, PO Box 5371, Seattle, WA 98105, USA
[2] National Pediatric Hospital, Combate de los Pozos 1881, 1245 Buenos Aires, Argentina
[3] Children's Memorial Hospital, Department of Orthopedics, 680 N. Lakeshore Dr., Chicago, IL 60611, USA
[4] Royal Children's Hospital, 25 Victoria Parade, Collingwood, Vic. 3066, Australia

Materials and Methods

All patients have had clinical data entered into an IBM-compatible computer Patient Data Management System (PDMS), created over a 37-year period [13], using definitions developed by international advisory committees consisting of participants in an informal International Myelodysplasia Study Group (IMSG).

Definitions

Levels of lesion were defined as neuromotor levels according to Sharrard [11] as follows: thoracic and high lumbar (T/HL) = T1–T12, L1, L2, L1–2, L1–3; middle lumbar (mid-L) = L3, L2–4, L3–4; low lumbar (LL) = L4, L5, L4–5; sacral and no loss (Sacral NL) = S1, S2 and below, S1–3, S2–3, L5–S, and no loss. Hyphenated numbers indicated mixed lesions. With asymmetry, the stronger side was used for classification. Patients with other, more complex, patterns were eliminated from the analysis.

Ambulatory status has been defined as the usual means of locomotion as follows: nonambulatory means is carried, scoots or crawls at home and uses a stroller or wheelchair outside, or wheelchair use regardless of whether totally dependent, independent at home, or independent in the community; partially ambulatory means learning to walk, cruises or takes a few steps, scoots and crawls at home but ambulates with aids outdoors, or is a household ambulator with wheelchair use outdoors; ambulatory (walks) means ambulates with or without braces and/or crutches and no wheelchair is required.

Information was recorded using clinical data collection forms developed and modified by the IMSG over the past 20 years. Data were then entered into the PDMS database at each center, most prospectively at each visit, and some retrospectively from hospital or clinic records, either during retrospective studies or when patients were transferred into one of the centers. Data were transferred to the Division of Congenital Defects, University of Washington, Coordinators for PDMS and IMSG (authors GD and SD and DBS) in Seattle, Washington, USA, by data collection forms (from Melbourne initially), and later from Buenos Aires and Chicago on computer disk or tapes as well. Data were then merged and analyzed using PDMS/fx, the new version of PDMS developed by GD and SD on the FoxPro platform. Results were exported from PDMS/fx into files which were then translated into charts and graphs using Microsoft Excel.

Data were analyzed by using χ^2 and Fisher's exact for comparison of proportions.

Observations and Results

The numbers of patients included in this review compared with the total number of patients in each center's database are as follows: Buenos Aires, 370 of 383 (97%); Chicago, 1144 of 1184 (97%); Melbourne, 551 of 551 (100%); Seattle, 1131 of 1498 (76%). The years that data collection began were: Buenos Aires, 1975; Chicago, 1965; Melbourne and Seattle, 1955. Differences between the total number of patients and patients included in each analysis are accounted for in all series by missing, unknown, or questionable data, and patients born prior to 1955.

Frequency of Diagnosis: Meningomyelocele

The Buenos Aires population contained 293 patients with a diagnosis of meningomyelocele (MM) (79%), 13 with another diagnosis (4%), and 64 with no data (17%). The following figures are for the same three categories: Chicago, MM = 904/1144 (79%), other = 229/1144

(20%), unknown = 11/1144 (1%); Melbourne, MM = 369/551 (67%), other = 49/555 (9%), unknown = 133/155 (24%); Seattle, MM = 885/1131 (78%), other = 204/1131 (18%), unknown = 42/1131 (4%).

PDMS/fx allows the user to identify patients by many different diagnoses. The majority of IMSG participants use PDMS to record clinical data about children with various spinal cord or congenital musculoskeletal disorders.

Age of Patients

The ages of the patients vary significantly amongst the four centers, with those beginning to collect data and entering into PDMS more recently having the higher proportion of younger patients (Table 1).

The multiple-cell χ^2 analyses for all data in Table 1, as well as for population ages between Buenos Aires and the other three centers and Chicago and Seattle, were significant at the $P < 0.000001$ level. The age of patients in the database for Melbourne differed significantly from those in Chicago ($P = 0.004$) and Seattle ($P = 0.000004$).

Levels of Lesion

Differences between levels of lesions for populations in the four centers were calculated using only the data for which specific levels could be assigned. The multiple-cell χ^2 analyses for the four centers combined in Table 2, as well as population levels of lesion between Chicago and the other three centers, were significant ($P < 0.000001$). The levels of lesion of the populations in Buenos Aires differed from those in Melbourne ($P = 0.003$) and Seattle ($P = 0.000006$). There was no difference between the levels of lesion in Melbourne and Seattle ($P = 0.98$).

Ambulatory Status

Table 3 demonstrates that, despite grouping thoracic (T) and high-level lumbar (HL) levels, and ages 18 months to 8 years and those over 8 years of age, there are too few numbers in each cell for χ^2 analysis of ambulatory status when age and level of lesion are considered.

TABLE 1. Age of patients by decade of birth

Location	Number	1955–1965	1965–1975	1975–1985	1985–1995
Buenos Aires	370	–	–	53 (14%)	370 (86%)
Chicago	1144	–	162 (14%)	580 (51%)	402 (35%)
Melbourne	551	48 (9%)	104 (19%)	239 (43%)	160 (29%)
Seattle	1131	156 (14%)	305 (27%)	392 (35%)	278 (24%)

1975–1995			
All	$X^2 =$	df = 5	$P < 0.000001$ $P = < 10$
CH/Mel	$X^2 = 11$	df = 2	$P = 0.004$
Mel/Sea	$X^2 = 29$	df = 3	$P = 0.000004$ $P < 10^{-6}$

CH, Chicago; Mel, Melbourne; Sea, Seattle.

TABLE 2. Levels of lesion

Location	Number	T + H/L	Mid-L	LL	S and NL	Mixed or no data
Buenos Aires	370	85 (23%)	41 (11%)	107 (29%)	111 (30%)	26 (7%)
Chicago	1144	297 (26%)	57 (5%)	195 (17%)	526 (46%)	69 (6%)
Melbourne	551	138 (25%)	44 (8%)	83 (15%)	132 (24%)	154 (28%)
Seattle	1131	351 (31%)	125 (11%)	203 (18%)	350 (31%)	26 (7%)

x^2 without mixed or no data and sacral and no loss combined

	X^2	df	P
B.A./CH	54	3	$P < 10^{-6}$
B.A./Mel	14	3	$P = 0.003$
B.A./Sea	22	3	$P = 0.00006$
CH/Mel	36	3	$P < 10^{-6}$
CH/Sea	64	3	$P < 10^{-6}$
Mel/Sea	0.6	3	$P = 0.98$
Summary, all columns	48.4	6	$P < 10^{-6}$

B.A., Buenos Aires; CH, Chicago; Mel, Melbourne; Sea, Seattle.

TABLE 3. Ambulatory status

Location	T + H/L	Mid-L	LL	S and NL
Age 18 months to 8 years				
Buenos Aires	2/36	1/12	13/42	28/56
Chicago	14/116 (12%)	9/26	48/91	116/219 (53%)
Melbourne	6/25	3/10	12/20	38/45
Seattle	4/74	11/46	16/66	71/81
Over 8 years of age				
Buenos Aires	1/3	1/3	5/6	5/6
Chicago	21/55	4/5	16/19	69/70
Melbourne	2/19	3/7	8/10	34/35
Seattle	0/118 (0%)	5/25	30/49	127/128 (99%)

Fisher's exact analyses of proportions demonstrate significant differences between Chicago and Melbourne in only two age and lesion-level groups: T + HL over age 8 years ($P = 0.02$), and S + NL for 18 months to 8 years ($P = 0.0005$).

The Chicago populations differ significantly from the Seattle populations for those over age 8 years in the T + HL ($P < 0.00000001$), mid-L ($P = 0.02$), and LL ($P = 0.004$) groups. The Chicago LL and S + NL group amongst the 18-month to 8-year olds were also significantly different ($P = 0.0003$ and $P < 0.00000001$, respectively) from their peers in the Seattle population. The Melbourne population differs significantly from the Seattle population in the two T + HL age groups (both $P = 0.02$), and in the LL age 18 months to 8 years group ($P = 0.004$).

Type of Delivery

Data in Table 4 demonstrate the increase in recording delivery information for the three centers (Buenos Aires, Melbourne, and Seattle—no data available from Chicago) from 36/45 of cases in 1975–1985 to 92% in 1985–1995 in Buenos Aires, from 68% to 98% in Melbourne for the same two decades, and from 28% in 1965–1975 to 95% in 1985–1995 in Seattle (Buenos

TABLE 4. Type of delivery

	1965–1975	1975–1985	1985–1995
Buenos aires			
No data	–	9 (9/45)	21 (8%)
C/S	–	7 (7/45) (7/36)	15 (47%) (51%)
Vaginal	–	29 (29/45) (29/36)	112 (45%) (49%)
Total	–	45	248
Melbourne			
No data	–	61 (32%)	3 (2%)
C/S	–	39 (21%) (30%)	32 (24%) (25%)
Vaginal	–	89 (47%) (70%)	97 (74%) (75%)
Total	–	189	132
Seattle			
No data	181 (72%)	67 (22%)	10 (5%)
C/S	5 (2%) (5/69)	76 (25%) (32%)	103 (53%) (55%)
Vaginal	64 (26%) (64/69)	159 (53%) (68%)	83 (42%) (45%)
Total	250	302	196

Numbers in parentheses: 1st number, percentage or fraction of entire column; 2nd number, percentage or fraction of known methods of delivery.

Aires, X^2 $P = 0.04$ and $P < 0.000001$ for Melbourne and Seattle). The increases from 7/36 to 51% for cesarean section birth in the 1975–1985 to 1985–1995 decades in Buenos Aires and from 5/69 to 55% in the 1965–1975, 1975–1985, and 1985–1995 decades in Seattle for all known methods of delivery are significant (X^2 $P = 0.0009$ and $P = 0.000004$, respectively).

Discussion

We have purposely defined the ability to walk strictly as biped ambulation, with or without aids, in order to avoid controversies that have been reported elsewhere citing the advantages of biped ambulation and standing as opposed to use of wheelchairs [6, 7]. These case comparison studies involve too few patients and do not consider long-term evaluation of outcome [6] or the result of comparable programs. The Mazur et al. study [7] included wheelchair patients who had, as younger children, failed to achieve an upright ambulatory program [12]. The environment in Melbourne, with full-time schools for the disabled, provided more opportunity for physiotherapy than was available in Seattle and is no longer available in Melbourne.

A second conscious decision was to select the definition of level of neuromotor lesion according to Sharrard [11] and collapse the thoracic and high lumbar groups despite our understanding of the importance of the iliopsoas muscle to ambulation [10]. To use the more accurate neurophysiological classification of McDonald et al. [9] would have required a breakdown of the neuromotor levels to six or more, rendering analysis impossible because of the small numbers in each cell.

A third decision was to limit the analysis of age and ambulation to provide a comparison between younger and older patients, using 8 years of age as the limit (Table 3). A more extensive study looking at the patients by the age at which each was seen is planned, in order to determine the effects of the teenage years on the type of mobility in adulthood. Preliminary analysis by LD suggests that older patients in Chicago and Seattle have similar mobility outcomes despite different approaches in childhood.

The differences in these four populations as documented in the text (differences in frequency of diagnoses), and in Table 1 (differences in ages) and Table 2 (levels of lesion) illustrate the differences in populations due to many possible causes. Some of these causes may be the severity of lesions born into the cohort, differences in referral practices to the centers, selection criteria used by the centers and, possibly, methods of management.

Temporal changes in these aspects of the problem preclude applying, in the 21st century, long-term observations of the outcome of a cohort surviving after treatment 20–30 years ago [5]. Changes that we know have altered the cohorts in these four centers are listed below.

1. Prenatal diagnosis, as discussed elsewhere in this symposium, is decreasing the number (Tables 1 and 4) and the severity of patients born with meningomyelocele [14].
2. Selection of the more severely paralyzed; less aggressive care is practiced in Melbourne.
3. Referral to both Buenos Aires and Chicago is dependent on local health professionals, who have many possible reasons for selecting patients. In Buenos Aires, it may be consideration of how these technically complicated children can receive appropriate follow-up care if they live in impoverished or rural neighborhoods. In Chicago and Seattle, obstetricians and geneticists, some of whom may be influenced by managed care to seek the least expensive alternative, are increasingly the primary providers of information (frequently, in one author's (DBS) experience, deficient) to parents of a fetus with meningomyelocele.

This paper has included only a few of the known input variables that affect outcome. They have been chosen in order to illustrate the complexity of evaluating outcome for a multiple-system disorder such as meningomyelocele. We believe that with the declining number of cases and the complexity of problems presented by patients, that multicenter, collaborative studies should be organized.

First, participating centers should agree on definitions and collaborate to establish accuracy, reproducibility, and stability of measurements over time [1, 8]. Comprehensive, computer-based data should then be collected [13]. Prospective studies and the natural history of various components of the problems presented by patients with meningomyelocele can then be addressed [3, 4, 6, 7, 15]. Should any participants in the International Symposium on Spina Bifida: The Child, Part II of III want to join the International Myelodysplasia Study Group, we welcome them.

References

1. Bartlett MD, Wolf LS, Shurtleff DB, Staheli LT (1985) Hip flexion contractures: a comparison of measurement methods. Arch Phys Med Rehabil 66:620–625
2. Bayer C (1897) Ztchr f Heille Berl Vor der Operation der Spina Bifida and Encephalocele. Z Herlkronen Berlin 18:405–416
3. Broughton NS, Menelaus MB, Cole WG, Shurtleff DB (1993) The natural history of hip deformity in myelomeningocele. J Bone Joint Surg 75-B:760–763
4. Cuddeford TJ, Freeling RP, Thomas SS, Aiona MD, Rex D, Sirolli H, Elliott J, Magnusson M (1997) Energy consumption in children with myelomeningocele: a comparison between reciprocating gait orthosis and hip-knee-ankle-foot orthosis ambulators. Dev Med Child Neurol 39:239–242
5. Hunt GM (1990) Open spina bifida: outcome for a complete cohort treated unselectively and followed into adulthood. Dev Med Child Neurol 32:108–118
6. Liptak G, Shurtleff DB, Bloss JW, Baltus-Hebert E, Manitta P (1992) Mobility aids for children with high-level myelomeningocele: parapodium versus wheelchair. Dev Med Child Neurol 34:787–796

7. Mazur JM, Shurtleff D, Menelaus M, Colliver J (1989) Orthopaedic management of high-level spina bifida early walking compared with early use of a wheelchair. J Bone Joint Surg 71-A(1):56–61
8. McDonald CM, Jaffe KM, Shurtleff DB (1986) Assessment of muscle strength in children with meningomyelocele: accuracy and stability of measurements over time. Arch Phys Med Rehabil 67:855–861
9. McDonald CM, Jaffe KM, Mosca VS, Shurtleff DB (1991) Modifications to the traditional description of neurosegmental innervation in myelomeningocele. Dev Med Child Neurol 33:473–481
10. McDonald CM, Jaffe KM, Mosca VS, Shurtleff DB (1991) Ambulatory outcome of children with myelomeningocele: effect of lower extremity muscle strength. Dev Med Child Neurol 33:482–490
11. Sharrard WJW (1964) The segmented innervation of the lower limb muscles in man. Ann R Coll Surg Engl 35:106–112
12. Shurtleff DB (1965) Timing of learning: meningomyelocele patients. J Am Phys Therapy Assoc 46:135–148
13. Shurtleff DB (1991) Computer data bases for pediatric disability: clinical and research applications. Phys Med Rehabil Clin N Am 2(4)
14. Shurtleff DB, Duguay S, Luthy DA, Ellenbogen R, Loeser J (1997) Seventeen year follow-up of children born by pre-amniotic membrane rupture cesarean section. International Symposium on Spina Bifida: Part II of III, Kobe, Japan, September
15. Wright JG, Menelaus MB, Broughton NS, Shurtleff DB (1991) Natural history of knee contractures in myelomeningocele. J Pediatr Orthop 11(6):725–730

Ethics, Social Welfare, and Psychosocial Adjustment

Ethical Considerations in Care, Treatment, and Management

Bernard M. Dickens

Summary. This chapter briefly outlines contrasts between different orientations to ethics and addresses principles common to these different orientations.

Distributive justice requires nondiscrimination where differences in ability are morally immaterial. Spina bifida patients are accordingly entitled to medical care, access to public buildings, education, and, for instance, entertainment and recreation opportunities. They have no right, for example, to futile treatment or disproportionate assistance such as in mobility.

The principle of beneficence reinforces the ethical claims of spina bifida patients to education, recreation, entertainment, group activities with non-spina bifida adolescents, and, for instance, training for employment. Nonmaleficence requires that the activities of spina bifida patients to assist themselves should not be obstructed or frustrated, for instance by unreasonable conditions for patients' protection. The principle of autonomy requires that the wishes of children and adolescents be taken seriously, such as for companionship and opportunities, and the protective principle requires their protection against physical, psychological, sexual, and other abuse.

Key words. Ethics, Nondiscrimination, Justice, Education, Recreation, Employment, Training

Introduction

Some analysts and commentators approach ethics in terms of philosophical or religious absolute values, distinguishing right conduct from wrong conduct and ethical behavior from unethical behavior. They reject ethical pluralism and ethical relativity. However, modern bioethics, particularly when approached from an international perspective, recognize that different ethical approaches may be taken to an issue, and that it may be analysed at different levels of abstraction. Accordingly, an ethical assessment or conclusion may appear appropriate or inappropriate, but inappropriate conclusions are not necessarily unethical. They may simply be the results of different ethical orientations, of different prioritizations of ethical principles, or of different levels of ethical analysis.

Faculty of Law, Faculty of Medicine and Joint Centre for Bioethics, University of Toronto, 84 Queen's Park Crescent, Toronto, Ontario M5S 2C5, Canada

Ethical analysis helps to identify the issues that are involved in proposed forms of health care, social treatment, and personal management of children and adolescents who have spina bifida. Analysis in itself may not lead to self-evident conclusions, but it allows care-givers, family members, the children and adolescents themselves, and interested members of society in general to explain their preferences, and to compare and contrast the preferences of others. Ethics provide a common language of explanation and criticism, and allow those who prefer different approaches and conclusions to understand each other on the basis of mutual respect for their differences in approach, and to escape condemnation as being unethical when their ethical analyses result in conclusions with which others disagree.

Duty-Based Ethics

Orientations to ethical analysis may be based on perceptions of duty. The influential German philosopher Immanuel Kant advanced important ethical duties, notably that human beings should not be used only as instruments or as mere means to other people's ends, but should always be treated as ends in themselves, with respect for their human dignity, individuality, and personality. Further, every principle in accordance with which individuals are treated should be generalizable to all other individuals. Decisions in particular cases should not be approached as exceptions to rules of conduct in human behavior, but should be made in accordance with rules that the actors would be willing to have applied to themselves. By this test, rules applied to children and adolescents with spina bifida need special justification if they differ from rules applied to people of other ages, or to people who do not have spina bifida. Accommodation of a disability may justify different rules, but no disadvantage may be permitted on this basis.

The Kantian orientation is not religious, but religious texts also impose the duty that people "should do unto others as they would have others do unto them." Duty-based ethics often have a religious basis. All of the world's religions have ethical orientations, expressed through their recognized authorities. The Roman Catholic Church is most easily understood because, unlike religions such as Islam and Judaism, and other denominations of Christianity, that Church has a single highest authority, in the person of the Pope. He is entitled to speak on behalf of the church in terms that the Church considers to be infallible revelations of divine will. The Roman Catholic Church believes itself to be the one true faith that all members of the human race should hold, and it rejects ethical pluralism and relativity. It condemns as wrong and unethical views that differ from its own on such controversial issues as voluntary sterilization and abortion of fetuses affected with spina bifida, and suicide, including medically assisted suicide, by those who find their life and suffering unendurable.

Consequence-Based Ethics

Ethics based on duties claimed to come from nature or divine will relieve those who consciously observe them from responsibility for the consequences that result from obedience. In contrast are consequence-based ethics, or utilitarian ethics. These link causes and effects and hold that conduct is ethical that produces socially useful or beneficial results, and is unethical if it produces harmful consequences for society. Accordingly, conduct that produces social unhappiness is unethical, and conduct that produces "the greatest happiness for the greatest number" in a given society is ethical. Conduct is judged in its social results and setting, and conduct can be ethical in one society or in circumstances at one time that is unethical in another society or at another time.

Feminist Ethics

Several other orientations to bioethics exist beyond duty-based and consequentialist ethics, such as particular case-based ethics, described as casuistry. Of growing significance are feminist ethics. These react to the fact that traditional religious, academic, political, and professional institutions that have been sources of ethical analysis have not included women, and some, particularly more fundamentalist religious institutions, continue to exclude women from positions of authority. Feminist ethics introduce the impact of rules on women and how women are able to enjoy their lives, and question whether rules made by persons unaware of how the female half of humanity experiences life can truly be ethical. Feminist ethics address the discriminations women suffer on grounds of sex and gender, and require sexual and gender equality as a condition of ethical conduct. They raise the issue of whether children and adolescents with spina bifida are medically cared for, treated socially, or managed personally differently on the basis of their sex.

Ethical Principles

Because ethical orientations are different, and may produce different practical results, attempts have been made to identify common principles on which proponents of different ethical orientations agree, even if for different and perhaps incompatible reasons. Principles have been found that different ethical orientations accept, although, because they were identified before the rise of feminist ethics, feminist analysts criticize them as being not necessarily wrong in themselves, but incomplete. These principles are

1. respect for persons, which includes
   - autonomy for those competent for decision-making, meaning able to bear responsibility for their decisions, and
   - protection of those incapable of autonomy.
2. beneficence, meaning the duty to do good, which some interpret to include
3. nonmaleficence, meaning the duty to do no harm, and
4. justice, the ethical duty that the law claims to serve.

These principles will be elaborated below in the context of children and adolescents with spina bifida.

Levels of Ethical Analysis

Ethical principles can be applied at different levels of ethical analysis. Traditional, religious, or conscience-based ethics are applied in relations between individuals. Person-to-person ethics are often described as *microethics*. In contrast are social ethics, or *macroethics*, which address ethical conduct among human groups and between a group and an individual, whether a group member or an outsider. In addition are *mesoethics*, which are administrative or bureaucratic ethics, largely concerned with resource-allocation ethics, and *megaethics*, concerned with relations that transcend national boundaries and address such issues as environmental protection and immigration. Megaethics address, for instance, whether countries should allow immigration of families whose members include a child or adolescent with spina bifida. Many countries prohibit immigration of disabled persons who will burden the health care system, which a spina bifida patient may be considered to do.

Further analysis will address the different ethical principles that have been widely, although not universally, agreed. These principles have been proposed without clarification of how to resolve which principles have priority over others. They are therefore taken in an arbitrary or convenient sequence, not because the first is necessarily more important than the others. Each ethical analyst who addresses an issue must justify the heavier significance of any principle over any other.

Distributive Justice

Distributive justice addresses equitable allocation of risks and benefits, and of scarce resources. It requires that like cases be treated alike, which is the basis of the law's concern with precedents, and that different cases be treated in ways that recognize the differences, since it is unjust to disregard material or significant differences. Distributive justice also requires nondiscrimination in treatment of those whose differences from others are immaterial.

The issue must therefore be addressed of the extent to which children and adolescents with spina bifida are like others without that condition, and should be treated like they are and not be discriminated against on the basis of their condition, and the extent to which they are different and may justly require treatment that those without that condition do not need. Activities that children and adolescents can usually undertake unaided may be unavailable to those with spina bifida, unless perhaps they are afforded assistance. The issue arises of whether an ethical duty can be shown under which governments, family-members, strangers, or others are ethically obliged to give the assistance that places disabled people on the same basis as the normally abled, and whether failure or refusal to give such assistance amounts to unethical discrimination. Ethical and legal systems that respect human rights require nondiscrimination on the basis of physical or mental disability.

Central to the quality of life, and perhaps at times to the very survival, of children and adolescents with spina bifida is their access to medical care. Distributive justice is concerned not with equal care, through which all members of a given society receive the same, but with equitable care. Equity requires that each person should be treated in accordance with his and her different needs. Disabled people have need of greater assistance than ordinarily able people if their lives are to be as satisfactory and fulfilling for them as the lives of able people are. Surgery, medication, physiotherapy, and similar health services and supplies may have to be made available to them, consistently with the means of their communities to maintain everyone's capacities to enjoy health, the ability to discharge usual social functions, and to avail themselves of social, educational, employment, recreational, and other opportunities. There is no right, of course, to forms of inappropriate, harmful, or futile care, even if disabled persons or their families demand it. Objective criteria may need to be set to establish what care is appropriate to meet standards of nondiscrimination, and what care is unreasonable to demand or provide.

Children and adolescents usually walk unaided, for instance, but many with spina bifida cannot do so. Because of the belief that such individuals should be able to live as normal a life as possible, however, many societies consider that an ethical and social duty exists to ensure that they have access to braces, crutches, and similar walking supports. That is, their spina bifida alone provides no basis for denying them means to walk when, with assistance, they can walk. However, some with the condition cannot walk even with assistance. If it is believed that they are nevertheless entitled equally with others to be mobile and not to be left bedridden, they may have to be afforded wheelchairs that they can propel themselves, provided that resources to supply and maintain wheelchairs are reasonably available. At the macroethical level of analysis, principles that support their allocation of resources in economically strong societies may not have the same force in poorer societies. If a patient's impairment is such that they cannot propel themselves, family members may bear ethical duties to move such children and adolescents so that, for instance, they can attend school and have a life of some variety and experience. Not every family can give time and energy to this purpose, and the wider community or society in general may bear ethical duties of aid. No general ethical duty can be shown to provide mechanical chairs to those able to operate controls, because such chairs are usually costly to provide and maintain. However, ethical duties are widely recognized to equip persons in wheelchairs to enjoy access to premises usually entered by steps by providing access for the disabled by ramps, and in countries where elevators are common, to supply them for those incapable of climbing stairs.

There are clearly limits to ethical duties to relieve a disabled person's disadvantages. Their access to schools and public buildings must usually be accommodated, and some societies believe that access to private premises the public is usually invited to enter, such as shops and commercial offices, should also be compelled, under principles and laws on nondiscrimination. However, there may be no ethical duty to equip physically disabled people to compete in such activities as track and field sports. This is not to say that no provision need be made for their recreation and sporting activities. Many sports are available to both usually mobile and less mobile competitors, such as gun and rifle shooting and archery. Further, athletic competitions may be undertaken among wheelchair-bound persons, and ethical duties may be shown to provide those able to propel their own chairs with opportunities for athletic competition. Even in resource-poor communities that do not give the priority to diversions and entertainments that richer societies can afford, due regard should be paid to a disabled person's play and entertainment.

Corrective or Compensatory Justice

Not all societies give the attention to private litigation that Western societies do, or believe that the private pursuit of compensatory awards through courts of law is suitable or adequate to remedy alleged wrongs. Nevertheless, particularly where health and social services are not available through publicly funded agencies, parents or other guardians of children born with spina bifida, and perhaps adolescents themselves approaching adulthood, may consider whether a court would award compensation, and whether a party with the means to pay could be shown to be legally at fault.

Parents' claims may be more successful than those of affected children and adolescents themselves. Parents' claims, usually described as "wrongful birth" actions, might be based on the failure of health care professionals to advise pregnant women to take tests that could indicate that their fetuses in utero were affected by neural tube defects, and the women's assertions that, had they learned of this, they would have exercised a legal option to terminate the pregnancy. Failure to inform women of the availability of alphafetoprotein screening and, for instance, fetal imaging services that would show an anomaly may be the basis for such claims. Where abortion is not lawful on the ground of fetal injury, of course, the failure of the opportunity for abortion is usually not compensatable. However, many legal systems, including those with restrictive abortion laws, allow performance of the procedure where a fetus is shown to be affected by a serious anomaly that would represent a serious handicap in a born child.

Awards of damages usually cover the costs of continued pregnancy and childbirth, but also include the costs of rearing a disabled child up to the end of the parents' legal responsibilities for their children's well-being, which in many Western countries occurs when the child is aged 16 or even 18. Accordingly, damages will be measured by the extent to which caring for all of the needs of a child or adolescent with spina bifida exceeds the costs of caring for an unaffected child. Damages will go beyond liability for medical care to include the costs of home nursing, special educational care, and provision of social, leisure, and recreational opportunities.

Since parents' awards may be limited to costs of care only until an affected child or adolescent is aged 18, 16, or a lower age at which parents' support responsibilities legally end, support thereafter may depend on the abilities of the affected children or adolescents to sue for compensation. Their claims may not need to be brought until they reach adult age. However, their actions are based on the claim that their mothers were given negligent medical care, and that the children that suffered a neural tube defect in utero should not have been born. These so-called "wrongful life" actions were initially disapproved of by the courts, not only because some approach human life as a divine gift that is a blessing and never "wrong," but also because damages may appear impossible to calculate. Courts often measure in money the difference between impaired and unimpaired life, but not all feel that they can measure the difference between impaired existence and what a New Jersey court in 1967 described as "the utter void of nonexistence." In time, however, more courts have come to recognize that the claim is really for the costs of the extraordinary care that handicapped people need to pursue a conventionally contented and fulfilled life, and make awards accordingly.

The basis of both wrongful birth and wrongful life claims depends on evidence of professional negligence. The birth of an affected child does not in itself show negligence, but if it can be established that tests were not advised that would have shown the unborn child's neural tube defect, or that tests were negligently conducted or test results negligently interpreted, children and adolescents may be able to recover compensation for the extraordinary expenses they will incur as adults living with spina bifida.

Beneficence

Since justice includes ethical duties of nondiscrimination, children and adolescents with spina bifida should be guaranteed the same entitlements to benefits enjoyed by unaffected children and adolescents in their families and communities. Accordingly, the ethical duty of doing good, beneficence, coincides with application of the ethical duty to act justly. Affected children and adolescents have no ethical claim to privileges, but have the same claim as others to fostering of their intellectual, artistic, musical, and other talents through access to schooling and higher educational opportunities. Similarly, they should have access to training for employment suitable to their intellectual and physical capacities, and the economic, industrial, and commercial environment their unaffected peers can be expected to enter. They should be afforded opportunities to participate in the culture of their social, age-related peers, for instance by being able to join youth groups. Such activities as dancing may be beyond their abilities, but they should be able to define the limits to their participation rather than have limits imposed on them by the attitudes, lower expectations, and reduced allocations of resources to their desires set by others.

Autonomy of Competent Persons

The autonomy of persons capable of making choices, and of bearing responsibility for them, is a central element of the ethical principle of respect for persons. Competence is specific to particular functions, so that persons who cannot make their own choices in more complex matters are often competent to exercise choices in the large majority of routine affairs. No individual is entirely autonomous, of course, since everyone is subject to constraints arising from circumstances beyond their reasonable control. The ethical duty regarding mentally competent children and adolescents with spina bifida, however, is to maximize their opportunities to exercise choices among the options available to them, and to avoid and prevent their subjection to patronizing and paternalistic attitudes that deny them choices they are capable of making. Children and younger adolescents are entitled to the advice and protective regard of parents, teachers, and comparable guardians that may be described as "paternalistic" or, in gender-neutral language, "parentalistic," but such advice and regard should be directed to the encouragement and growth of self-determination and responsibility in those who receive it. It should not be supposed that those with spina bifida are less capable of making decisions and choices than others, although the decisions and choices that have to be made in their circumstances may be different from those relevant to unaffected children and adolescents. Later childhood and adolescence are times of growing sexual awareness and awakening that adults often find inappropriate and difficult to channel. A physically impaired person's sexuality is often troublesome in institutional and family settings, but, as in other areas of their lives, the sexual interests of affected children and adolescents should be respected.

Protection of the Vulnerable

Where individuals are vulnerable and incapable of making or enforcing responsible choices, they are ethically entitled to protection. Vulnerability to discrimination based on any physical or mental disability is of special concern to children and adolescents with spina bifida, but vulnerability goes beyond their liability to be denied opportunities available to unaffected peers. There may be vulnerability to many forms of abuse, such as physical, sexual, emotional, and economic abuse, and to exploitation of their need for care. Institutions offering care may neglect their needs or divert resources given for their care to other purposes, including gaining unconscionable profits and treating dependent persons whose care staff members find it more satisfying to provide. Giving care to disabled, vulnerable children and adolescents often appears as a form of charity that brings credit to providers, and protects them from moral scrutiny and criticism. Where care is given without pay or other material reward, it may indeed conform to the highest level of moral dedication to others. A potential exists in many areas, however, to exploit vulnerable persons behind a screen of morality, and no person or agency, whether charitable, religious, or therapeutic in its commitment, is above ethical questioning and answerability. Persons and agencies providing for the needs of vulnerable children and adolescents with spina bifida should accept their liability to give an account of their practices, attitudes, and influence on those who depend on them. In an increasing number of countries, institutions create independent ethical review committees to monitor their conduct and provide advice on current and anticipated areas of ethical concern. Similarly, such committees may be established by governmental and other providers of resources to affected persons living in families in their communities to identify and resolve any abuse or exploitation of their dependency to which they may be subject.

Observance of Human Rights

Many ethical duties owed to persons vulnerable to discrimination and abuse on grounds of their physical or mental disability, age, or other characteristics outside their own control are now expressed not only in international human rights conventions, but also in historic and modern national constitutions. Citizens of all countries should review the constitutional and other laws of their own countries to see how effect is given to the ethical principles expressed in the United Nations' 1948 Universal Declaration of Human Rights. Many, if not all, countries have made a public ethical and legal commitment to individuals' achievement of the highest standard of health that each can attain, and to prohibit discrimination against disabled persons. Such recently endorsed international treaties as the Convention on the Rights of the Child embody principles already present in the laws of many countries. Such treaties allow endorsing countries to make an international declaration of their commitment to human rights principles present in their domestic systems of law and government. Accordingly, the human rights entitlements of children and adolescents with spina bifida to ethical care, treatment, and management are based on, and reinforced by, legal commitments that many countries have made at both international and domestic levels.

Developmental Factors, Health, and Psychosocial Adjustment of Children and Youths with Spina Bifida

Rune J. Simeonsson, Gail S. Huntington, Janey Sturtz McMillen, Deborah Halperin, and Darla Swann

Summary. For many children and youths with spina bifida, the gap resulting from functional limitations and the demands of the environment are likely to contribute to secondary conditions and a lower quality of life. This study describes the development of an initial information base, focusing on developmental factors in the manifestation of secondary conditions in children and youths. The subjects in this study were a subset from the larger study drawn for two age groups: 40 children (10–14 years) and 22 youths (15–18 years). In this prospective study, data were obtained on a range of physical, social, and psychological variables. Documentation of the prevalence of secondary conditions on the basis of self-report was made using the taxonomical dimensions of the Impairment, Disability, and Handicap codes of the ICIDH. This study was an initial effort to document secondary conditions associated with spina bifida, and to examine developmental differences in children and youths. These preliminary findings indicate that children and adolescents with spina bifida report relatively frequent impairments in the physical domain of latex allergy, balance, and weight. In the psychological domain, frequent disabilities are difficulties with problem solving, endurance, and lack of social skills. In the social domain, problems with isolation, exclusion, mobility, and family stress are generally reported more frequently for youths than children. These results extend earlier findings concerning children with spina bifida which reported increased emotional problems, and difficulties with visuomoter and mathematical tasks [14]. When children and youths do report difficulty living with spina bifida, these findings underscore the importance of documenting life experiences and adaptation from the child's as well as the family's perspective. In general, children and youths report a favorable quality of life.

The promotion of increased folic acid intake during pregnancy represents a significant medical advance in the prevention of spina bifida. Improved surgical techniques also represent advances in the management of the medical dimensions of spina bifida. At the same time, it is recognized that there are sequelae and complications secondary to medical aspects which result in poor adjustment and reduced quality of life for children and youths with spina bifida. Increasingly, it is clear that interdisciplinary initiatives should encompass not only

FPG Child Development Center, University of North Carolina, CB No. 8185, Chapel Hill, NC 27599-8185, USA intervention and rehabilitation, but also the prevention of secondary conditions [6] and improvement of well-being and quality of life [2]. In order to achieve the aim of the prevention of secondary conditions, a knowledge base of their natural history and epidemiology must be established. This study describes the development of such a knowledge base for the specific congenital condition of spina bifida, focusing on developmental factors in the manifestation of secondary conditions in children and youths.

What are secondary conditions of disability? As a relatively recent term [7], secondary conditions have not been clearly defined, nor consistently described. While the term may be relatively new, the underlying concept is certainly well established to define sequelae and complications of an underlying congenital or acquired condition [6]. To provide a coherent frame for developing public health initiatives to reduce or prevent secondary conditions, it is essential that criteria defining secondary conditions be operationalized. First, secondary conditions are the direct or indirect consequences of an underlying primary condition. The primary condition constitutes a necessary but not sufficient cause, in that not all primary conditions result in sequelae or complications. A second criterion is that secondary conditions reflect, to a significant degree, the interaction of the person with the environment. Viewed within a biopsychosocial model [1], development is constantly modified by the opportunities which the environment affords and the person's engagement with that environment, setting the stage for subsequent transactions. The nature of these interactions with the environment is likely to account for different expressions of secondary conditions in persons with the same primary impairment. Third, the nature and extent of expressed secondary conditions will vary as a function of age or developmental stage, so that some are more frequent in childhood (e.g., incontinence) and adolescence (e.g., isolation), whereas others are more frequent in adults (e.g., pressure sores). Fourth, secondary conditions are also mediated by individual differences in the form of personal traits and characteristics, such as motivation and behavioral style. These individual differences account for the fact that persons with the same impairment adapt differently to environmental demands, with a resultant variability in secondary conditions. Viewed individually and collectively, the above criteria are consistent with the premise that secondary conditions are preventable.

Secondary conditions may be physical, social, or psychological in nature. They may be unique to a given condition, or they may cut across various primary disabilities. Viewed in the context of the conceptual framework of the International Classification of Impairments, Disabilities, and Handicaps—ICIDH [15], secondary conditions are consistent with "handicaps as disadvantage in life roles." Secondary conditions may also be viewed as complications manifested as impairments and disabilities, as shown in Fig. 1. A number of secondary conditions of a physical nature [11], such as pressure sores [3] or contractures [16], may be manifested in several primary conditions involving impairment of movement. They may be reflective of risk factors such as inadequate or inappropriate care, lack of stimulation, or limited opportunities. Secondary conditions may be manifested in social aspects such as lack of peer interaction, isolation, and stigma associated with disability. They may also be expressed in psychological forms, such as lowered self-esteem, problems in adjustment to disability, and a heightened sense of dependence on families [5] or primary caregivers. Thus, while secondary conditions may vary in their form, they can be seen as reflecting a common basis, namely a gap between a person's ability characteristics and environmental demands.

For many children and youths with spina bifida, the gap resulting from functional limitations and the demands of the environment are likely to contribute to secondary conditions and a lower quality of life. Comprehensive models for interdisciplinary assessment and intervention efforts [9, 13] and public health prevention initiatives require data on the distribu-

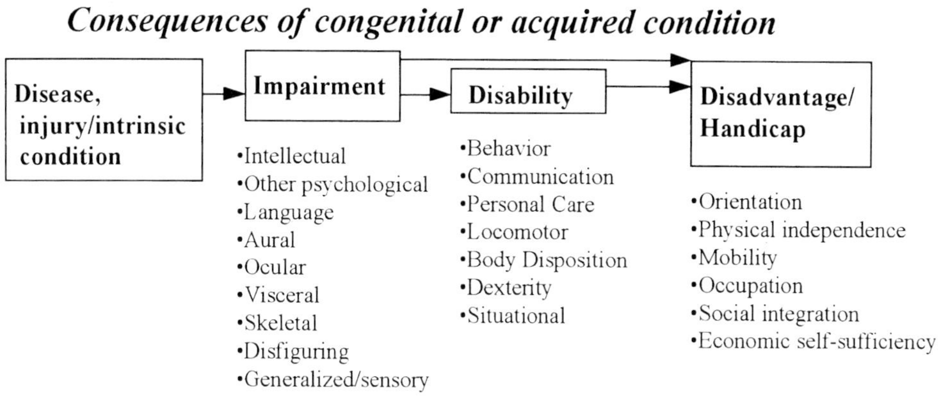

FIG. 1. International classification of impairments, disabilities, and handicaps [15]

tion of secondary conditions. Furthermore, an analysis of possible developmental differences in children and youths is important is this regard in order to identify potential risk and resilience factors, and to differentiate prevention initiatives. To this end, three research questions were examined in this study.

1. What is the distribution of selected secondary conditions in children and youths with spina bifida?
2. To what extent is there congruence between children and youths with spina bifida and their parents on perceived quality of life?
3. What is the relationship of secondary conditions to perceived quality of life in children and youths with spina bifida?

In answering these questions, the study builds on the conceptual and taxonomic framework of the ICIDH [15] to promote a consistent and comprehensive approach to documentation of disablement. By drawing on caregiver perceptions of secondary conditions and quality of life, the study will provide data that can contribute to an information base for planning future intervention and prevention initiatives.

Methods

Subjects

The Spina Bifida Project is an ongoing longitudinal study of 160 families who have a family member with spina bifida. Subjects for the study were recruited primarily through the University of North Carolina Hospitals' Physical Medicine and Rehabilitation Clinic and the Lenox Baker Children's Hospital Myelomeningocele Clinic. Other subjects were recruited through the North Carolina Spina Bifida Association. In addition to the longitudinal nature of the study, subjects were recruited into four age groups: early childhood (birth to 5 years), school age (6–11 years), adolescence (12–17 years), and young adult (18 years and above). The subjects in this study were a subset from the larger study drawn for two age groups: 40 children (10–14 years) and 22 youths (15–18 years). Summary demographic information is presented in Table 1. The current status of bowel and bladder continence as reported by the family are presented in Tables 2 and 3, respectively. As shown in the tables, there is a clear

TABLE 1. Subject characteristics

	Children	Youths
Subjects	40	22
Males	18	10
Females	22	12
Lesion level		
Thoracic	17%	14%
Lumbar	47%	68%
Sacral	35%	18%
Reporting shunt symptoms	12.2% (33)[a]	105 (20)[a]
Reporting orthopedic symptoms	53% (32)[a]	42% (20)[a]
Reporting bladder symptoms	62% (34)[a]	60% (19)[a]

[a] Number available for analysis.

TABLE 2. Family report of bowel continence difficulty

Description	Children ($n = 34$) (%)	Youths ($n = 20$) (%)
Incontinent	5.9	5
Frequent soiling	5.9	5
Mostly continent	11.8	40
Occasional soiling	55.9	0
Continent	20.6	50

TABLE 3. Family report of bladder continence difficulty

Description	Children ($n = 33$) (%)	Youths ($n = 20$) (%)
Incontinent	6.1	0
Frequent wetting	24.2	10
Occasionally wet	24.2	25
Mostly dry	30.3	45
Continent	15.2	20

developmental shift toward continence from childhood to adolescence, particularly for bowel contineence.

Measures

In this prospective study, data were obtained on a range of physical, social, and psychological variables. A battery of measures was administered to children and young adults with spina bifida, with alternate forms contingent upon the age of the subject and their ability to comprehend the instructions for a given task. Complementary measures were completed by a family member, typically the mother. Selected measures were also sent to community service providers of the subjects in order to assess their perception of the subject's functioning in schools or other settings outside the home. To address the questions in this study, data from a selected number of the measures will be used. The measures described below are the Secondary Conditions Questionnaire, the Demographic Medical History Questionnaire, and the Quality of Life Questionnaire.

Secondary Conditions Questionnaire

The Secondary Conditions Questionnaire was designed to assess the presence of secondary conditions of the physical, psychological, social, and academic domains among individuals. A Likert rating scale ranging from 0 (never a problem) to 5 (always a problem) was used for the respondent to indicate the degree to which any of the listed secondary conditions were a problem. Open-ended questions further enabled individuals to suggest ways of preventing the existence of these secondary conditions, and describe expectations for the future. Subjects at least 10 years of age, who were able to comprehend the instructions of the task, and their families completed this form. The family member version includes a section related to family concerns around raising a child with a disability. Internal consistency based on available data for the Secondary Conditions Questionnaire was estimated at 0.86 [8]. The correlation between parent and child ratings was estimated at 0.46. This measure yielded the following variables for analyses, coded by ICIDH domains: seven physical conditions coded as impairments, five psychological conditions coded as disabilities, and four social conditions coded as handicaps.

Demographic Medical History Questionnaire

The Demographic Medical History Questionnaire was used to document the individual's birth and medical history, including the areas of neurosurgery, orthopedics, urology, and other health issues. The final page of the questionnaire provides yearly updated information regarding current functional status, method of bladder/bowel control, current medications and symptoms, ambulation and educational/vocational status, and illness/hospitalization history over the previous 12-month period. This measure yielded the following variables for analyses: lesion level; shunt, bladder, and orthopedic symptoms; bowel and bladder continence status.

Quality of Life Questionnaire

Perceived quality of life was assessed quantitatively by asking the respondent to rate their quality of life on a 1–5 scale, with 1 representing poor and 5 representing excellent. Following the rating, the respondent was asked to describe the basis for their rating, which yielded information for qualitative analysis.

Procedures

All clinic patients received a letter describing the study in their preclinic packet. Those families who expressed an interest in participating were asked to sign a letter of consent. Research staff introduced the study measures to subjects and their families, and parents/caregivers were given the option of completing measures on their own or with a staff member. Parents were asked to complete measures regarding subject characteristics, subject and family functioning, and aspects of the environment. Subjects who were at least 10 years of age participated in an interview examining their perspectives of the effect of spina bifida on their lives, and completed other measures of subject functioning.

If a family was unable to complete all of the measures in the clinic setting, measures which the family could complete on their own were sent home with a self-addressed, stamped envelope. Other measures were completed over the telephone, with the family's permission. Medical file reviews were completed at the clinic's corresponding hospital.

Results

Documentation of the prevalence of secondary conditions was made on the basis of self-report using the taxonomical dimensions of the impairment, disability, and handicap codes of the ICIDH. For the dimension of impairment (Table 4), the most prevalent secondary conditions were latex allergy, balance problems, weight problems, and pain. While there was variability noted for several secondary conditions by age, of interest is the fact that three (skin breakdown, scoliosis, and pain) increase with age from children to youths, whereas reports of problems with latex allergy, weight, balance, and strength decreased with age.

For the dimension of disability (Table 5), measuring the reduced ability to perform activities, the most prevalent secondary conditions reported were problem solving, endurance, and lack of social skills. These were followed in descending order of prevalence by problems of learning/attention and poor body image. Of interest here is the fact that the self-reports showed an increasing developmental trend from child to youth for all disabilities.

Documentation of secondary conditions as a disadvantage through the handicap code (Table 6) revealed that the prevalence of secondary conditions was higher for youths than for children. A quarter of children and youths reported family stress as a problem. In regard to perceived quality of life (Table 7), the majority of children (19/32%) and youths (9/17%)

TABLE 4. Impairments reported by children and youths in the physical domain

Secondary condition	WHO ICIDH I-CODE	Children (n = 36) (%)	Youths (n = 20) (%)
Pain	48	22	25
Weight	70	33	25
Scoliosis	70	17	20
Balance	48	30	25
Latex allergy	87	36	30
Skin breakdown	92	5	20
Strength	94	19	10

TABLE 5. Disabilities reported by children and youths in the psychological domain

Secondary condition	WHO ICIDH D-CODE	Children (n = 36) (%)	Youths (n = 20) (%)
Endurance	71	28	40
Poor body image	10	11	25
Problem solving	14	33	60
Learning/attention	16	17	30
Lack of social skills	19	5	40

TABLE 6. Handicaps reported by children and youths in the social domain

Secondary conditions	WHO ICIDH H-CODE	Children ($n = 36$) (%)	Youths ($n = 20$) (%)
Mobility	3	11	30
Isolation	5	22	45
Exclusion	5	39	45
Family stress	7	25	25

WHO-ICIDH, World Health Organization-International Classification of Impairments, Disabilities, and Handicaps. H, handicap.

TABLE 7. Self-report on quality of life by children and youths

Age group	Poor	Fair	Good	Very good/Excellent
Children ($n = 32$)	–	5	19	8
Youth ($n = 17$)	–	3	9	5

reported a rating of good. The proportion who perceived their quality of life as fair or poor was relatively small: (5/32) for children and (3/17) for youths. The congruence between ratings by parents and their children was 37%, with 43% parental overestimation and 20% parental underestimation.

Discussion

This study was an initial effort to document secondary conditions associated with spina bifida and to examine developmental differences in children and youths. These preliminary findings indicate that children and adolescents with spina bifida report relatively frequent impairments in the physical domains of latex allergy, balance, and weight. In the psychological domain, frequent disabilities are difficulties with problem solving, endurance, and learning and attention of social skills. In the social domain, problems with isolation, exclusion, and mobility. Learning and attention are generally reported more frequently for youths than for children. These results extend earlier findings concerning children with spina bifida which reported increased emotional problems, and difficulties with visuomotor and mathematical tasks [14]. While children and youths do report difficulties in living with spina bifida, these findings underscore the importance of documenting life experiences and adaptation from the child's as well as the family's perspective. In general, children and youths report a favorable quality of life. The limited congruence in ratings of quality of life between parent and children supports the value of documenting the uniqueness of perspectives, which is consistent with recent findings by Young et al. [17].

An important factor contributing to variability in the expression of secondary conditions is the mediating role of environmental factors. The same underlying primary condition in two children may be modified or exacerbated by the presence of risk or protective factors. In addition to elements of the child's environment, these factors include individual differences specific to that child. At the level of the natural environment, a primary dimension may be limitations imposed by terrain or climate. In the constructed environment, risk factors are exemplified by dangerous, inaccessible, inefficient, or inconvenient settings in the form of stairs, doors, and difficult spatial arrangements. Physical risk factors include the lack of adaptive devices and technology to facilitate the achievement of basic activities of mobility and communication. Social and psychological risk factors may take the form of limited social contacts and psychological support. These social and psychological factors are clearly confounded or exacerbated by functional limitations of movement or communication. The interactive and dynamic nature of these risk factors is consistent with the biopsychosocial model [1] in which the effects are not simply additive but synergistic. A central factor that may mediate risk or resilience in these contexts is the nature and form of environmental supports in home and school. Personal factors in the form of behavioral style and personality characteristics often influence the manner of adaptation to the environment [4]. Such factors serve a protective function when a person is characterized by persistence, motivation, and self-esteem. Alternatively, limited motivation and persistence, as well as a sense of lack of control, may serve to place the individual at greater risk of secondary conditions. A long-term goal of this effort is to identify risk and resilience factors for the identification and development of programs to promote health and prevent secondary conditions in persons with developmental disabilities [10, 12]. To this end, priority needs to be placed on modifying physical aspects of the environment, increasing opportunities for social experiences in the school and community, and establishing policies which will promote access and participation for all children and youths.

Acknowledgment. Research supported by contract No. 731, Office on Disability and Health, Centers for Disease Control and Prevention.

References

1. Engel GL (1983) The biopsychosocial model and family medicine. J Fam Pract 16:409–413
2. Fuhrer MJ (1994) Subjective well-being: implications for medical rehabilitation outcomes and models of disablement. Am J Phys Med Rehabil 73:358–364
3. Harris MB, Banta JV (1990) Cost of skin care in the myelomeningocele population. J Pediatric Orthopedics 10:355–361
4. King GA, Shultz IZ, Steel K, Gilpin M, Cathers T (1993) Am J Occup Ther 47:132–140
5. Kokkonen J (1995) The social effects in adult life of chronic physical illness since childhood. Eur J Pediatr 154:676–681
6. Lollar DJ (1994) Preventing secondary conditions associated with spina bifida or cerebral palsy: proceedings and recommendations of a symposium. Spina Bifida Association of America, Washington
7. Marge M (1988) Health Promot for persons with disabilities moving beyond rehabilitation. Am J Health Promot 2:29–35
8. McMillen JS (1997) Child and family characteristics as predictors of child's quality of life. Diss Abstr Int 58 (8-A):3087 (University Microfilms No. AAM9803636)
9. Redaelli T, Cassinis A, Cosignani F, Conti B, Onofri MP, Dall'Acqua A (1992) Interdisciplinary treatment of spina bifida children. Paraplegia 30:683–689
10. Rosenbaum PL (1988) Prevention of psychosocial problems in children with chronic illness. Can Med Assoc J 139:293–295
11. Shurtleff DB (1986) Decubitus formation and skin breakdown. In: Shurtleff DB (ed) Myelodysplasia and exostrophies: Significance, prevention, and treatment. Grune and Stratton, New York, pp 299–311
12. Simeonsson RJ (1991) Primary, secondary, and tertiary prevention in early intervention. J Early Intervention 15:124–134
13. Watson D (1991) Occupational therapy intervention guidelines for children and adolescents with spina bifida. Child Care Health Dev 17:367–380
14. Wills K (1993) Neuropsychological characteristics of children with spina bifida/hydrocephalus. J Clin Child Psychol 22:247–265

15. World Health Organization (1980) International classification of impairments, disabilities, and handicaps. World Health Organization, Geneva
16. Wright JG, Menelaus MB, Broughton NS, Shurtleff D (1991) Natural history of knee contractures in myelomeningocele. J Pediatric Orthopaedics 11:725–730
17. Young NL, Yoshida KK, Williams I, Bombardier C, Wright JG (1995) The role of children in reporting their physical disability. Arch Phys Med Rehabil 76:913–918

Abstract

Social Welfare for Children with Spina Bifida

AKIIE H. NINOMIYA

Children with spina bifida have the same human rights as non-disabled children. Since the basic practice of human rights is to have QOL with the family, community, and school environments, the education of children with spina bifida ought to be in regular school circumstances. At the present time, the medical profession tends to control the life activities of children with spina bifida and discourage attending regular schools, which has a profound impact on their personality development. Ordinarily, the family, friends, and school community would play an important role. An integrated educational system is essential for personality development in a normal environment. The stage of self-identity is especially crucial for young adults with spina bifida, since the special school system separates them from regular school life, often creating personalities known as persons with disabilities. Peer groups have their own ideology, faith culture, etc., which provides an identity. However, persons with spina bifida might identify themselves as "disabled persons" and have difficulty participating in mainstream life.

The medical model could create dependency, and discourage autonomy and an independent way of life. However, the behavior model encourages patients to think and act as full citizens who have responsibility and rights in society, the medical profession's role being supportive with a service-oriented approach. This model promotes autonomy and a sense of independent living necessary to join mainstreaming.

The environmental model provides complete accessibility for patients with spina bifida, in terms of family, community, and societal life. A combination of the behavior and environmental models is very effective for the civil movement and mainstreaming. Independent living provides much more human rights as well as consumer rights than institutionalization, with medical and social welfare also being much less costly than in the medical model.

School of Policy Studies, Kwansei Gakuin University, Kobe, Japan

Contributors Index